Pathophysiology

Pathophysiology

Ivan Damjanov, MD, PhD

Professor, Department of Pathology and Laboratory Medicine
The University of Kansas School of Medicine
Kansas City, Kansas

With illustrations by Matt Chansky

SAUNDERS

ELSEVIER

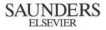

1600 John F. Kennedy Blvd.
Ste 1800
Philadelphia, PA 19103-2899

PATHOPHYSIOLOGY   ISBN-13: 978-1-4160-0229-1

Notice

Knowledge and best practice in this field are constantly changing. As new research and experience broaden our knowledge, changes in practice, treatment and drug therapy may become necessary or appropriate. Readers are advised to check the most current information provided (i) on procedures featured or (ii) by the manufacturer of each product to be administered, to verify the recommended dose or formula, the method and duration of administration, and contraindications. It is the responsibility of the practitioner, relying on their own experience and knowledge of the patient, to make diagnoses, to determine dosages and the best treatment for each individual patient, and to take all appropriate safety precautions. To the fullest extent of the law, neither the Publisher nor the Author assumes any liability for any injury and/or damage to persons or property arising out of or related to any use of the material contained in this book.

Library of Congress Cataloging-in-Publication Data

Damjanov, Ivan.
  Pathophysiology / Ivan Damjanov.—1st ed.
    p. ; cm.
  Includes bibliographical references.
  ISBN 978-1-4160-0229-1
  1. Physiology, Pathological. I. Title.
    [DNLM: 1. Pathology, Clinical—methods. QY 4 D161p 2009]
  RB113.D335 2009
  616.07—dc22   2007034333

Acquisitions Editor: William Schmidt
Managing Editor: Rebecca Gruliow
Design Direction: Steven Stave

Printed in China.

Last digit is the print number: 9 8 7 6 5 4 3 2 1

Preface

Pathology (from the Greek words *pathos,* meaning disease, and *logos,* meaning science) is the traditional name for the branch of basic medical sciences dealing with the study of diseases. In clinical medicine pathology comprises two main subdivisions, known as anatomic and clinical pathology. Anatomic pathology is also taught to medical students in the preclinical years of their curriculum. In some medical schools clinical pathology is taught as a special subject, but in most U.S. medical schools laboratory clinical pathology, simplified for didactic purposes, is taught as part of the clinical courses. In this context it is called Introduction to Clinical Medicine, Medical Propedeutics, Basic Clinical Skills, and many other similarly imaginative names. Despite a panoply of names, the common aim of all these courses is to introduce medical students to clinical medicine and to provide a bridge between basic sciences and clinical medicine. Most notably, these courses show medical students that their studies of biochemistry, anatomy, physiology, microbiology, or pathology were not in vain and that all these basic sciences are highly relevant for the understanding of disease processes.

The best way to teach medical students how to apply their knowledge of basic medical science to the study of disease in clinical settings is to concentrate on the pathologic basis of disease and illustrate pathologic changes in terms of changes in the body functions—that is, normal physiology. This hybrid science, based on the application of principles of pathology and physiology to clinical medicine, is called **pathophysiology.** The principles of pathophysiology are the basis of clinical medicine and are essential for the diagnosis of diseases, modern therapeutics, and the formulation of prognosis and restoration of health. This book was written to show medical students how to make this jump from basic sciences to the clinics and to encourage them to base their future clinical practice on principles of basic science.

Medicine is an applied science, and to practice in modern times one must have a good grip on all basic medical sciences, most notably physiology and pathology. I have spent most of my life teaching pathology to medical students, and I have always tried to base my teaching not on dissected cadavers but on clinical examples and in the context of the dynamic changes in the human body that are the principles of human physiology. Hence this book, which could also be called *dynamic pathology* or *physiology applied to clinical medicine* or just simply *clinical or laboratory pathology.*

The book is divided into 12 chapters. The first two chapters deal with generalities and show the student how to use the laboratory and to interpret the essential laboratory findings. For the sake of simplicity, I have concentrated only on basic chemical laboratory tests, which are used as salient examples of how to study patients' problems by applying laboratory techniques to the study of body fluids and tissue samples. In the third chapter I discuss the prototypical diseases, each one of which belongs to a major pathogenetic category, such as genetic diseases, circulatory diseases, metabolic diseases, diseases related to nutritional abuse or intoxication, infectious diseases, autoimmune diseases, neoplastic diseases, and diseases of unknown etiology. The remaining nine chapters deal with major organ systems; each illustrates the principal pathologic conditions affecting them.

Each chapter begins with a list of basic terms and definitions. These terms are subdivided into several categories, such as normal anatomy and physiology, symptoms or clinical entities. In all organ-based chapters, enough space is devoted to a review of normal anatomy and physiology as needed for the understanding of pathophysiology. Thereafter, I discuss the principal symptoms and laboratory findings. These principles are applied to the main diseases, which have been selected to show how the particular organ systems malfunction during various diseases. Each chapter concludes with several clinical cases and then questions and suggestions for discussion in the classroom.

Clinical medicine can be mastered only by observing patients, talking to them, examining them, treating them, and caring for them. Although I am sure most medical students cannot wait to enter the clinics and do just that, I hope this introductory text will allow them to consolidate their knowledge of basic medical sciences and prepare as well as possible for encounters with their patients—and for a life-long journey through practical medicine. I wish them luck on their journey, for as Cervantes put it so poetically, "Viajar es mejor que la posada." The trip may be more fun than reaching the imaginary goal. In the meantime, I urge students and professors alike to send me e-mails (idamjano@kumc.edu) with comments, suggestions, or criticism. May the force be with you!

Ivan Damjanov
Kansas City, Kansas

Contents

Chapter 1

LABORATORY MEDICINE

Introduction

Laboratory medicine is the branch of clinical medicine dealing with changes in the human body that can be detected only by analyzing the body's chemical components in the laboratory. Essential for the assessment of health status and various clinical problems, the services of laboratory medicine can be used for many purposes, but the most important applications are as follows:

- **Diagnostic disease-oriented laboratory testing.** Such testing is usually ordered by the attending physician and is part of the initial work-up on almost all patients. These tests are routinely performed in all hospitals and ambulatory medical facilities.
- **Pretreatment assessment of the patient's condition.** Laboratory tests are routinely performed for all persons entering a hospital for medical, surgical, or emergency treatment.
- **Follow-up after treatment.** Patients treated in hospitals or ambulatory clinics are regularly tested to determine the effects of treatment. For example, diabetics treated with insulin must regularly monitor their blood sugar levels to determine if their dosage of insulin or other medications is correct.
- **Screening for diseases.** Screening tests are performed for populations at risk for a certain condition, such blood lipid profiles in patients with a history of familial hyperlipidemia, or after a person reaches a certain age, such as prostate specific antigen test in men older than 55 years.
- **Periodic monitoring of the state of health.** Laboratory tests are typically part of the yearly medical examination recommended to monitor well-being. Additionally, they are almost invariably performed in special circumstances, such as pregnancy, infancy, and childhood. Many jobs require a pre-employment

medical examination and school districts mandate preadmittance examinations that include routine laboratory testing. Together with physical examination, laboratory testing represents the most important part of the yearly medical examination performed by numerous health care providers.
- **Research.** Laboratory tests are usually included in monitoring patients or normal persons being treated with new drugs (clinical trials) or those enrolled in research studies aimed at elucidating the pathophysiology of various diseases.

Laboratory Tests

Laboratory tests are performed on body fluids or tissue samples.

Laboratory tests can be classified as follows:

- Routine tests performed in most hospital laboratories
- Specialized tests performed only in specialized reference laboratories or under specific conditions and during complex medical procedures
- Emergency tests performed on short notice and reported immediately to the ordering physician

Routine laboratory tests are most often performed on blood and urine, but on occasion the same tests can be performed on other body fluids such as the cerebrospinal fluid; joint fluid; or effusions in the abdominal, thoracic, or other cavity.

Blood tests are performed usually in batteries, or panels, known as sequential multiple analysis (SMA-6, SMA-7, or SMA-12) (Table 1-1).

Blood may be submitted in tubes that either contain or do not contain anticoagulants. The tops of these tubes are color-coded to avoid confusion. Blood collected into a tube

KEY WORDS

Accuracy of a test   Statistical term reflecting the capacity of the test to measure the true value of an analyte.

Acute-phase proteins   Proteins that appear in increased concentration in blood in response to inflammation are called positive acute-phase proteins. This group includes C-reactive protein, transferrin, ceruloplasmin, fibrinogen, α_1-antitrypsin, and several others. Proteins, like albumin, whose concentrations are is decreased in response to inflammation, are called negative acute-phase proteins.

Alkaline phosphatase   Enzyme that hydrolyzes orthophosphoric esters, present in many cells of the body and in serum. Serum alkaline phosphatase is elevated in biliary obstruction, but it may also be derived from growing bones, bone undergoing remodeling (as in Paget's disease), osteoblastic metastases, and bone-forming tumors.

Aminotransferase   Also known as transaminase. A group of enzymes transferring amino groups from one amino acid to another. Alanine aminotransferase (ALT) and aspartate aminotransferase (AST) have clinical significance in liver function tests. ALT and AST are found in many other organs, and their serum concentration is elevated in other pathologic conditions as well (e.g., myocardial and lung infarctions).

Blood urea nitrogen (BUN)   Blood nitrogen present in the form of urea. This test does not measure nitrogen included in proteins, accounting for approximately 18% of total blood nitrogen. BUN is elevated in renal failure. Since urea is a highly diffusible molecule its blood concentration falls rapidly after renal dialysis. BUN can be increased due to heart failure, shock, dehydration, and many other conditions and is a less specific marker of renal failure than elevated levels of creatinine.

Calcium   A bivalent chemical element (Ca^{2+}) present predominantly in the extracellular compartment in ionized form or in the form of salts. It is essential for many cellular functions. Hypercalcemia may be caused by hyperparathyroidism or several nonparathyroid-related conditions such a malignant tumors with metastases to bone. Hypocalcemia is less common and may be caused by reduced absorption or increased loss of calcium. Increased and decreased serum concentrations of calcium are associated with distinct pathophysiologic consequences.

Carbon dioxide (CO_2)   Gas produced in the body during oxidative respiration of cells and exhaled through the lungs into the atmosphere. Carbon dioxide along with bicarbonate (HCO_3^-) forms the most powerful of the body's buffer systems in the blood. Hypercapnia (excessive CO_2) and hypocapnia (decreased CO_2) are mostly caused by respiratory and renal disturbances and are related to acid–base imbalance.

Chloride   A monovalent chemical element (Cl^-) mostly found in the extracellular fluid. In the serum it is a part of the anionic pool, but it can be also measured in urine and sweat.

Creatinine   The end product of creatine degradation, which is excreted in urine. Serum creatinine is elevated in renal failure (azotemia).

Glucose   Monosaccharide, formed from the degradation of glycogen, cellulose, and other complex carbohydrates. Blood glucose is elevated in diabetes mellitus and lowered in various conditions that cause hypoglycemia.

Lactate dehydrogenase (LDH)   Ubiquitous enzyme involved in the removal of hydrogen from lactate. The concentration of LDH in blood is elevated in conditions marked by widespread cell destruction.

Lipoprotein   A complex between proteins and lipids, found in the cell membranes and in the blood. By ultracentrifugation, blood lipoproteins can be separated into four categories: chylomicrons, very low density lipoproteins (VLDLs), low-density lipoproteins (LDLs), and high-density lipoproteins (HDLs). These lipoproteins carry other lipids, such as cholesterol, phospholipids, and triglycerides, throughout the body. Hyperlipidemia, which may be congenital or acquired, is associated with an increased risk for coronary atherosclerosis.

Phosphorus   A monovalent chemical element (P), which is present predominantly in the extracellular space (in the form of monophosphates [PO_4^-] and diphosphates [PO_4^{2-}]) or linked with calcium in complex salts that form the matrix of bones. Its metabolism is intimately linked with the metabolism of calcium. Inside the cells phosphorus is often attached to major macromolecules and energy-rich compounds such as adenosine triphosphate (ATP).

Plasma   Liquid portion of the blood, containing water, minerals, proteins, lipoproteins, and monosaccharides. Serum is plasma minus the clotting factors.

Potassium   A monovalent chemical element (K^+) predominantly found inside the cells, but also in the extracellular compartment. For example the ratio of K^+ inside the red blood cells and in plasma is 20:1. Hyperkalemia or hypokalemia are caused by several diseases and are associated with distinct pathophysiologic consequences, mostly pertaining to the contraction of cardiac and skeletal muscle.

Precision of a test   Statistical term for the consistency with which the same result can be obtained when applying the same test repeatedly to the same sample.

Predictive value of a test   Statistical term estimating the probability that a positive test result will identify a person with a disease ("true positives and false positives").

Protein   Group of macromolecules composed of amino acids. Proteins are essential for the maintenance of life, acting as structural elements, enzymes, membrane channels, and other vital cell components. They are also found in body fluids. Serum proteins can be divided by electrophoresis into two major groups: albumin and globulins. Hypoproteinemia may be caused by several diseases (most notably malnutrition, malabsorption of nutrients, and liver and kidney disease) and is associated with distinct pathophysiologic events.

Sensitivity of a test   Statistical term for the capacity of a test to correctly identify individuals who have the disease ("true positives and false negatives").

Specificity of a test   Statistical term for the capacity of a test to correctly identify individuals who do not have the disease ("true negatives and false positives").

Table 1-1 Common Laboratory Panels

SMA-6
Sodium
Potassium
Chloride
Carbon dioxide
Blood urea nitrogen
Glucose

SMA-12
Albumin
Alkaline phosphatase
Aspartate aminotransferase
Bilirubin
Calcium
Cholesterol
Creatinine
Glucose
Lactate dehydrogenase
Phosphorus
Protein (total)
Uric acid

aminetetraacetic acid (EDTA) or green-top tubes with lithium heparin, the red cells, leukocytes, and platelets remain in suspension inside the tube; the blood cells can be separated from the plasma by centrifugation. **Plasma** contains fibrinogen and all other coagulation factors and is used for specialized tests, such as measurement of the concentration of coagulation factors, lipids and lipoproteins, or folic acid. For the measurement of lactic acid or the optimal measurement of glucose, the blood is collected in gray-top tubes containing fluoride oxalate (an inhibitor of glycolysis), which does not interfere with the measurement of these analytes.

> **Pearl**
>
> > Serum is best defined as *defibrinated plasma*, which means it does not clot and cannot be used for the study of coagulation factors and substances entrapped in the fibrin meshwork of the clot.

Specialized tests are not performed in all hospital laboratories but are sent to highly specialized reference laboratories. Specialized tests often require that the specimens be collected in a specified manner or under highly controlled circumstances. Most of these tests are performed in specialized reference laboratories or manually by specially trained technicians. This category of tests includes the testing of rare oligominerals such as copper or selenium, certain hormones such as vasoactive intestinal polypeptide (VIP) or parathyroid hormone-related protein (PTHrP), certain drugs and toxins, and DNA analysis. Many tests that were considered specialized in the past have become routine. One example is the troponin test, which is today routinely performed on the serum of patients thought to have suffered a myocardial infarction. Testing for human immunodeficiency virus (HIV) or hepatitis C virus was initially performed only in specialized laboratories but is routine in most hospitals today.

that does not contain an anticoagulant (red tubes) will clot, and the red blood cells, leukocytes, and platelets will separate from the **serum** (Fig. 1-1). The separation of blood cells from serum can be accelerated by collecting the blood in tubes that are not coated with anticoagulant. Such tubes contain a gel at the bottom that activates clotting and promotes the separation of the clot from the serum ("red/green," also known as "tiger-top tubes" or "light green-mint tubes"). These tubes are used in the laboratories that perform automated testing. Serum contains all the normal minerals, enzymes, immunoglobulins, and proteins besides the coagulation factors, and is thus used for most routine laboratory tests.

If the blood is collected into a tube that contains anticoagulants, such as lavender-top tubes containing ethylenedi-

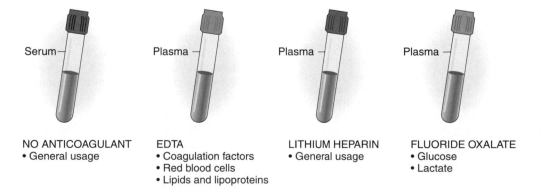

| NO ANTICOAGULANT | EDTA | LITHIUM HEPARIN | FLUORIDE OXALATE |
| Serum | Plasma | Plasma | Plasma |

NO ANTICOAGULANT
• General usage

EDTA
• Coagulation factors
• Red blood cells
• Lipids and lipoproteins

LITHIUM HEPARIN
• General usage

FLUORIDE OXALATE
• Glucose
• Lactate

Figure 1-1 Test tubes with color-coded tops. Red, no anticoagulant; lavender, ethylenediaminetetraacetic acid (EDTA); green, lithium heparin; gray, fluoride oxalate.

The samples for specialized tests are often collected in a unique manner. For example diurnal variation of hormones can be measured on several specimens collected at predetermined times. The sweat test for cystic fibrosis requires stimulation of sweat production with pilocarpine. Enzyme deficiency, which is the hallmark of some inborn errors of metabolism, requires tissue samples containing cells. DNA analysis requires samples containing nucleated cells from a buccal smear or white blood cells.

Emergency tests are performed on samples obtained during surgery or as part of the work-up on critically ill patients. Intraoperative testing for parathyroid hormone (PTH) may help the surgeon determine whether a PTH-secreting adenoma was removed. Analysis for drugs such as salicylic acid, acetaminophen, or digitalis may be important in diagnosing possible drug toxicity. Blood gasses and electrolytes are measured on an emergency basis in patients with acid–base disorders.

Good laboratory tests must be precise (reliable) and accurate and have high sensitivity and specificity.

In the United States the results for most analytes are expressed as **concentrations** in grams (g), milligrams (mg), micrograms (µg), or nanograms (ng) or as moles (mol) or millimoles (mmol) per liter (L), deciliter (dL), or milliliter (mL) of fluid. The activity of enzymes is expressed in **activity units** per liter (U/L). In other countries, laboratory data are reported according to the **Système International (SI),** using metric units. In many major U.S. hospitals, both systems are used in parallel.

Modern laboratories are highly automated, and the performance of tests is controlled at several levels to ensure high precision and accuracy.

The **precision,** or **reliability,** of a test can be determined by repeating the same test on the same sample. Ideally the same result should always be obtained, but in practice this does not always occur. So the standard deviation (SD) from the mean must be calculated for lab results. A highly precise test has a low SD, meaning that the results occur within a narrow range. In most instances the reference range is determined by adding 2 SD to the mean, which means that 95% of the results fall in that range, and only 1:20 (5%) fall outside it.

The **accuracy** of a test reflects how close the measured value is to the true value. An ideal test should have high precision and high accuracy. Like the target-shooting analogy shown in Figure 1-2, the outcome of each measurement should be as close as possible to the bull's eye ("true value") and the results should be as close together as possible (low scatter). These results can be graphically presented and typically have a bell-shaped (Gaussian) distribution with a low standard deviation from the mean. A test is unacceptable if it has high precision but does not reflect the true value (i.e., low accuracy). A test could have low precision but, if repeated several times, could have a statistically acceptable accuracy. Such tests have a wide

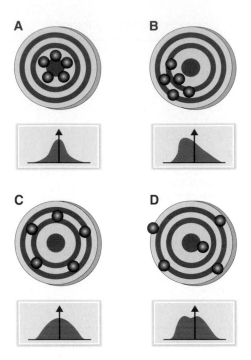

Figure 1-2 Precision and accuracy of tests. **A,** Ideal test has high precision and high accuracy. **B,** This test has high precision but low accuracy. **C,** This test has high low accuracy but overall it has high precision. **D,** This test has low precision and low accuracy.

standard deviation. Tests that have low precision and low accuracy are not used in clinical laboratories. Such tests may have a Gaussian distribution with a very high standard deviation or do not form a bell-shaped curve.

Good laboratory tests must have high sensitivity and specificity.

The diagnostic value of each laboratory test is expressed in terms of its specificity, sensitivity, predictive value, and efficiency as follows:

Specificity measures the incidence of "true negative" (TN) results; that is, normal values occur in all tested persons who do not have a disease—those who presented as "true negatives" or "false positives" (FP) (Fig. 1-3). Specificity is calculated according to the following formula:

$$\text{Specificity (\%)} = [\text{TN}/(\text{TN} + \text{FP})] \times 100$$

Sensitivity measures the incidence of "true positive" (TP) results among all persons who have the disease irrespective of whether they tested positively or negatively, thus representing a sum of "true positives" plus "false negatives" (FN). Sensitivity is calculated according to the following formula:

$$\text{Sensitivity (\%)} = [\text{TP}/(\text{TP} + \text{FN})] \times 100$$

A

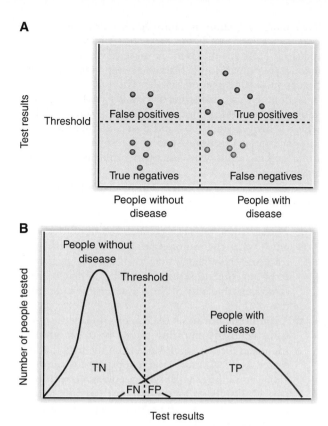

B

Figure 1-3 **A,** Sensitivity and specificity of laboratory tests. An average laboratory test will detect most persons who have a disease ("true positives"—TP), but some persons with the disease will not be detected ("false negatives"—FN). Some healthy persons will be also positive ("false positives"—FP), whereas most of those who are healthy will be negative ("true negatives"—TN). **B,** Raising the cut-off point increases specificity ("negativity in health"). Lowering the cut-off point increases the sensitivity of the test ("positivity in disease").

Pearl

> Specificity is thought of as *negativity in health.* Sensitivity is thought of as *positivity in disease.* High sensitivity is a hallmark of an ideal screening test. Tests of high specificity should be used for final diagnosis, especially if the treatment is risky or could have adverse consequences.

The specificity and the sensitivity of a test can be adjusted by raising or lowering the cut-off point for a positive result (see Fig. 1-3). A test with high specificity will be always negative in health; that is, it will be negative for both FP and TN. Tests with a high sensitivity will be

positive for all those who have a disease and will include all TP and FN.

Predictive value. The positive predictive value of a test predicts how many persons with a disease will have a positive result, whereas a negative predictive test predicts how many persons who do not have a disease will have a negative result. These predictive values are calculated according to the following formulas:

$$\text{Predictive value of a positive test (\%)} = [\text{TP}/(\text{TP} + \text{FP})] \times 100$$
$$\text{Predictive value of a negative test (\%)} = [\text{TN}/(\text{TN} + \text{FN})] \times 100$$

For example, if a test has a positive predictive value of 90%, it will be positive in 90% of persons with the disease, whereas 10% will have false negative results and will not be detected with this test. In a test with a 90% negative predictive value, 90% of all persons who do *not* have the disease will have a negative result, but 10% will have a false positive result.

Pearl

> The predictive value of a test depends on the prevalence of the disease in the tested population. The predictive value decreases as prevalence decreases.

Efficiency relates to the number of all correct results and is calculated according to the following formula:

$$\text{Efficiency (\%)} = [(\text{TP} + \text{TN})/(\text{TP} + \text{TN} + \text{FP} + \text{FN})] \times 100$$

Water and Sodium

Water, which accounts for approximately 60% of total body weight, is divided into two categories:

- **Intracellular volume** (ICV), containing 70% of the total water
- **Extracellular volume** (ECV) comprising the remaining 30% of total water, divided as **interstitial compartment** (22%) and **plasma** (8%)

Body water contains solutes that are unequally distributed in the ICV and ECV. Among these solutes are organic compounds, such as proteins, glucose, or lipids, and inorganics in the form of electrolytes and gases. Sodium (Na^+) is the most important electrolyte in the ECV, and potassium (K^+) is the most important electrolyte in the ICV (Fig. 1-4). Active maintenance of Na^+ and K^+ gradients across the cell membranes by energy-dependent pumps regulates the distribution of water in the body.

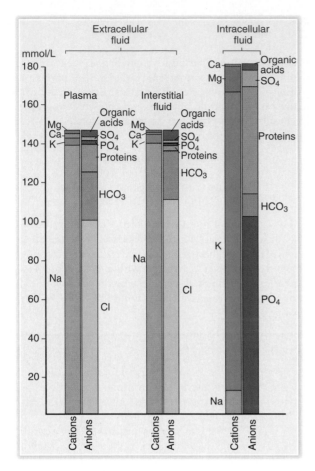

Figure 1-4 Concentration of electrolytes in plasma, interstitial fluid, and intracellular fluid. (Redrawn from Edwards, CRW, Bouchier AD, Haslett C, Chivers ER [eds]: Davidson's Principles and Practice of Medicine, 17th ed, Churchill Livingstone, Edinburgh, 1995, p 590.)

Sodium is the principal electrolyte in the extracellular volume.

The body of an adult man weighing 70 kg contains approximately 4200 mmol of Na^+. Approximately 50% of this is in the extracellular fluid, 40% is in the bone, and 10% is inside the cells. All the Na^+ in the extracellular and intracellular fluid and approximately 50% in bone form the so-called exchangeable sodium, which is in constant intercompartmental flux. Serum concentration of Na^+ is in the range of 135 to 145 mmol/L.

The concentration of sodium in the body depends on the amount of water and is controlled by kidneys and several hormones.

A regular diet contains more Na^+ than the body needs, and the intestines can absorb unlimited amounts of this mineral.

Thus intake of sodium is almost never a problem, and the body can adjust even if the exogenous salt is dramatically reduced. Most of the Na^+ is excreted in urine. Small amounts of Na^+ are lost in feces and sweat. Hence the excretion and loss equal the total intake (Fig. 1-5).

Sodium is in balance with body water content. A 70-kg adult male requires approximately 2.5 L of water, 2.1 L of which is derived from food and drinks and 400 mL from intermediate metabolism. Most of the water is excreted in urine, and the rest in feces and by insensible loss in exhaled air or perspiration.

Sodium balance is under the control of several physiologic mechanisms:

- **Thirst.** If one ingests too much sodium or loses too much water the osmoreceptors in the hypothalamus react to increase the osmolality of the plasma, thereby activating the thirst center. Intake of water brings down the osmolality of the plasma, ending the sensation of thirst.
- **Antidiuretic hormone (ADH, or arginine vasopressin).** Increased osmolality caused by a loss of water stimulates the release of ADH from the hypothalamic center. ADH stimulates the resorption of water in the kidney until the osmolality of the plasma is reduced to normal. Depletion of the intravascular volume may stimulate thirst and ADH release independently of the changes in osmolality.
- **Aldosterone.** Loss of ECV affects the glomerular filtration rate (GFR), causing a release of renin from the juxtaglomerular apparatus. Renin acts on angiotensinogen, which leads to an increased production of aldosterone from the zona glomerulosa of the adrenal cortex. Aldosterone promotes the exchange of Na^+ for K^+ or hydrogen (H^+) in the distal renal tubules, causing retention of Na^+ and expansion of the ECV.
- **Atrial natriuretic peptide (ANP).** ANP stimulates the kidneys to increase the excretion of Na^+ in urine.

Sodium plays a role in forming the electric charges across the cell membrane and in acid–base regulation and is the most important electrolyte regulating the osmolality of the extracellular fluid.

Even though Na^+ represents the most abundant ECV cation, its functions are not fully understood. It is known that Na^+ participates in several physiologic processes, the most important of which are as follows:

- **Acid–base balance.** Sodium is an important cation that binds to several anions such as chloride, phosphates, and bicarbonates. Thus, it plays an important role in the maintenance of the acid–base balance.

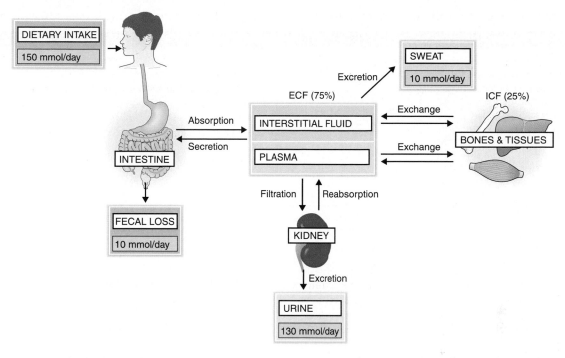

Figure 1-5 Sodium intake and excretion. ECF, extracellular fluid; ICF, intracellular fluid.

■ **Cell membrane polarity.** Sodium is distributed differentially inside and outside the cell; it contributes to the formation of the electric charges across the cell membranes. The maintenance of the Na^+ gradient across the cell membrane requires expenditure of energy, which is needed for the fueling of the Na^+/K^+ ATPase, the cell membrane pump, moving Na^+ and K^+ in or out of the cell.

■ **Osmolality of body fluids.** As the most abundant cation, Na^+ is essential for the maintenance of the osmolality of body fluids in the normal range from 285 to 295 mOsm/kg. Thus, Na^+ is essential for the maintenance of the volume of extracellular fluid (ECF), and indirectly also the volume of intracellular fluid. Even a small increase of osmolality of ECF stimulates osmoreceptors, which initiate thirst, ADH release, and water reabsorption in the kidneys. Reduced osmolality owing to overhydration reduces water intake and inhibits ADH secretion, allowing the excretion of water in urine.

Sodium concentration is the primary determinant of serum osmolality.

Osmolality of the serum depends mostly on the concentration of Na^+, and to a lesser degree of glucose and urea (expressed as BUN, blood urea nitrogen). The contribution of anions is less than 10% of the total value of serum osmolality, and thus a formula for calculating serum osmolality takes into account only Na^+, glucose, and BUN as follows:

$$\text{Serum osmolality} = 2 \times Na^+ \ (mmol/L) + \frac{\text{glucose (mg/dL)}}{18} + \frac{\text{BUN (mg/dL)}}{2.8}$$

Serum osmolality is measured to determine the water content of ECF and exclude the possibility of overhydration or dehydration. In such cases the measured osmolality corresponds to the calculated osmolality, and the difference is usually less than 10 mOsm/kg. When an osmolal gap (>10 mOsm/kg) occurs, the discrepancy between the measured and calculated osmolality is usually caused by the presence of a low-molecular-weight substance (e.g., alcohol, ethylene glycol) in the blood. The study of the osmolal gap is especially useful in patients who are comatose or suspected of intoxication. The most common causes of increased serum osmolality are listed in Table 1-2.

Hyponatremia may be classified as dilutional or depletional.

Hyponatremia is a common condition defined as a serum concentration of Na^+ below 136 mmol/L. Mild hyponatremia is found in 2 to 3% of all hospitalized patients. In most instances it is just a sign of illness, reflecting the inability of

Table 1-2 Causes of Altered Serum Osmolality

INCREASED OSMOLALITY	DECREASED OSMOLALITY
Increased content of normal components	Overhydration
Sodium (hypernatremia)	SIADH
Glucose (hyperglycemia)	Loss of sodium in excess to water
BUN (renal failure)	
Toxic substances in blood	
Alcohols (ethanol, methanol)	
Ethylene glycol (antifreeze)	
Acetone	
Loss of water in excess to sodium	
Dehydration	
Diabetes insipidus	

BUN, blood urea nitrogen; SIADH, syndrome of inappropriate antidiuretic hormone secretion.
Based on data from Bakerman S, Strausbauch P: Bakerman's ABC's of Interpretative Laboratory Data, 3rd ed, Interpretative Laboratory Data, Myrtle Beach, SC, 1998.

cells to maintain the normal gradient and flux of electrolytes across the cell membranes *("sick cell syndrome")*. Severe hyponatremia is usually a consequence of water intoxication.

Pathogenetically, hyponatremia may be classified as dilutional or depletional (Fig. 1-6).

Dilutional hyponatremia occurs under the following conditions:

- **Increased water intake.** This may occur due to obsessive water drinking (neurotic polydipsia), or in some lung cancer patients who have the paraneoplastic syndrome of inappropriate ADH secretion (SIADH).
- **Infusion of water.** Most often it is a consequence of inappropriate intravenous infusion of fluids, but occasionally it my be also related to massive use of enemas.

- **Decreased excretion of water.** This may be a consequence of heart failure or renal failure. In both conditions water is retained in the extracellular spaces.
- **Hypoproteinemia.** Inadequate production of serum proteins in end-stage liver disease (cirrhosis) or a loss of proteins in nephrotic syndrome or chronic protein-losing gastroenteropathy results in hypoalbuminemia. Since albumin concentration is partly responsible for the oncotic pressure that keeps fluids inside the blood vessels, hypoalbuminemia leads to a shift of water from the vessels into the interstitial spaces and consequent hypovolemia. This loss of fluid triggers the ADH and the renin–angiotensin–aldosterone response, resulting in a net retention of water and dilutional hyponatremia.

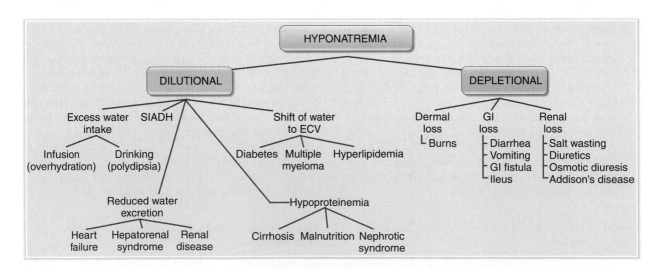

Figure 1-6 Pathogenesis of hyponatremia. It can be classified as *dilutional*, due to water excess, or *depletional*, due to a net loss of sodium. ECV, extracellular volume; GI, gastrointestinal; SIADH, syndrome of inappropriate antidiuretic hormone secretion.

■ **Shift of water from cells into the ECV.** This occurs in hyperglycemia of diabetes mellitus, paraproteinemia of multiple myeloma, or hyperlipidemia. In all these conditions, osmotically active substances in the blood and extracellular fluids cause a shift of fluids from the intracellular to the extracellular compartment. The total amount of Na^+ remains the same but it is diluted by the influx of water into the ECV.

■ **Syndrome of inappropriate antidiuretic hormone secretion (SIADH).** ADH may be secreted by some tumors. Such a paraneoplastic syndrome may cause "water poisoning" due to excessive retention of water in the kidneys under the influence of ADH.

Depletional hyponatremia occurs whenever a net loss of Na^+ occurs. Sodium may be lost through the gastrointestinal (GI) system or the kidneys, most often under the following conditions:

■ **Gastrointestinal loss**
   ■ Vomiting
   ■ Diarrhea
   ■ Sequestration of fluid in the intestine (e.g., paralytic ileus)
   ■ Gastrointestinal fistulas
■ **Renal loss**
   ■ Glycosuria of diabetes mellitus
   ■ Hypercalcemia associated with polyuria
   ■ Salt-wasting kidney diseases. This may occur in any chronic renal disease resulting in a loss of nephron function. The remaining nephrons become overloaded with urea, causing an osmotic diuresis and consequent depletion of Na^+ from ECV.
   ■ Diuretics, especially osmotic, or any form of diuretic overdose

■ Addison's disease, characterized by aldosterone deficiency. A lack of cortisol, which is necessary to excrete the water load, leads also to water retention. Thus, the hyponatremia in these patients is in part dilutional.
■ **Dermal loss**
   ■ Burns

<table>
<tr><td>Pearl</td></tr>
<tr><td>> The most common cause of hyponatremia is a combined loss of Na^+ and water, in which the lost Na^+ is not adequately replaced.</td></tr>
</table>

Symptoms of hyponatremia depend on the concentration of sodium and the way it has developed.

Hyponatremia is usually mild and, thus, asymptomatic. Slowly evolving hyponatremia, especially if dilutional, is well tolerated, and even if the Na^+ concentration drops to 100 mmol/L it may cause few if any symptoms. On the other hand rapidly developing hyponatremia of 120 or even 125 mmol/L may cause significant neurologic symptoms.

Symptoms are mostly related to depressed transmission of neural or neuromuscular signals and include muscle weakness, somnolence, and, in severe cases, coma.

Death, if it occurs, is usually related to the underlying disease rather than hyponatremia itself.

Hyponatremia may be associated with increased total body water levels, relative increase in extracellular water, loss of Na^+ in excess relative to body water or increase in total body water in excess to increased Na^+ (Table 1-3).

Table 1-3 Causes of Hyponatremia

PATHOGENESIS	MECHANISM	CLINICAL CONDITION	ECV
Increased total body H_2O	H_2O excretion ↓	SIADH Addison's disease Hypothyroidism	↑; no edema
	H_2O intake ↑	Psychogenic polydipsia	
Relative increase of H_2O in ECV	Shift of H_2O cells → ECV	Diabetes mellitus Hyperlipidemia Paraproteinemia	N
Reduced total body salt and water ($Na^+ > H_2O$)	Loss of Na^+ without proper replacement	Fever Burns Drugs (e.g., diuretics)	↓↓ (many conditions)
Increased total body water and salt ($H_2O > Na^+$)	Retention of Na^+ with H_2O excretion ↓↓	Cardiac failure, liver failure, renal failure	↑↑, +edema

↑, increase; ↓, decrease; ↑↑, marked increase; ↓↓, marked decrease; ECV, extracellular volume; SIADH, syndrome of inappropriate antidiuretic hormone secretion.
Based on data from Edwards CRW, Bouchier AD, Haslett C, Chivers ER (eds): Davidson's Principles and Practice of Medicine, 17th ed, Churchill Livingstone, Edinburgh, 1995.

When the plasma volume is reduced by 5% in chronic hyponatremia, ADH is released in spite of the osmoreceptor-generated inhibitory effects on its secretion. Due to the effects of ADH in chronic hyponatremia the volume of urine is reduced and it will be concentrated.

Treatment of hyponatremia should be directed at its causes and the correction of sodium–water balance. Water restriction will suffice in mild cases of dilutional hyponatremia. Severe hyponatremia may cause brain injury, but likewise, too rapid correction of hyponatremia with infusion of salts can cause central pontine myelinolysis.

Hypernatremia is clinically almost always a consequence of dehydration.

Hypernatremia is defined as serum concentration of Na^+ over 150 mmol/L. It is much less common than hyponatremia, but if it occurs, it has more severe clinical repercussions. Most affected patients are either very young or very old, critically ill, or neurologically impaired (e.g., patients in coma).

Theoretically, hypernatremia may result from a loss of water or a gain of Na^+. These changes lead to hyperosmolality, to which the body responds by either increasing water intake or conserving water excretion through the kidneys. The second compensatory mechanism includes the release of ADH, thereby reducing urinary excretion of water.

Drinking of water corrects hypernatremia in most instances. Clinically significant hypernatremia develops only in persons who have no access to water or are unconscious and cannot drink (e.g., comatose patients, persons in deep anesthesia, very old immobile persons, or infants). Hypothalamic injury may affect adversely the thirst center and thus cause hypernatremia. It also may lead to diabetes insipidus and excessive loss of water in urine due to ADH deficiency.

Water loss can occur through the kidneys, GI tract, or the skin:

- **Renal loss of water.** Hypernatremia is a symptom of **diabetes insipidus,** which may be central or nephrogenic in origin. **Central diabetes insipidus** may be primary (i.e., related to the injury of the hypothalamus or the posterior lobe of the pituitary) or secondary to drug treatment (e.g., lithium). **Nephrogenic diabetes insipidus** is a consequence of end-stage renal disease. In the postsurgical period, the patient may develop **renal tubular necrosis** and lose excessive amounts of water relative to Na^+, especially during the polyuric phase of tubular necrosis. Other iatrogenic causes of hypernatremia include the use of loop and osmotic **diuretics.**
- **Gastrointestinal loss of water.** Water may be lost during **diarrhea** or prolonged **vomiting,** but also because of prolonged suction through a **nasogastric tube. Osmotic cathartic agents** like lactulose may cause water loss.

- **Dermal loss of water.** Dermal loss occurs in extreme heat that evokes profuse **sweating,** but it is also encountered after extensive **burns.**

Excessive sodium intake or retention. Sodium retention occurs under the following conditions:

- **Adrenal cortical lesions.** Most commonly adrenal cortical abnormalities are responsible for hypercortisolism, causing Na^+ retention. Such hypercortisolism may be due to benign or malignant adrenal cortical tumors.
- **Corticosteroids.** Long-term use of corticosteroids in the treatment of rheumatoid arthritis, systemic autoimmune diseases, or nephrotic syndrome may also cause sodium retention.
- **Infusion of sodium-rich solutions.** This may occur while infusing sodium bicarbonate ($NaHCO_3$) during resuscitation, hypertonic saline feeding, administration of NaCl-rich emetics or enemas, or intrauterine injection of hypertonic saline.

Clinical findings depend on the nature of hypernatremia.

Clinically, hypernatremia must be always evaluated in the context of hydration of the body. If hypovolemia is present, urinary or intestinal water loss must be suspected. In euvolemic patients central or nephrogenic diabetes insipidus, dermal or respiratory loss of water, or inadequate intake of water (hypodipsia) must be considered. In hypervolemic patients an excess of mineralocorticoids, such as occurs in primary hyperaldosteronism, is a possibility (Fig. 1-7).

Symptoms depend on the degree of hypernatremia and usually appear when the Na^+ concentration reaches 155 to 160 mmol/L. The rate and the time over which hypernatremia develops are also important. Typically the affected person is thirsty, but many are either unconscious or too young to say so. There is oliguria. Neurologic symptoms, such as irritability, restlessness, confusion, and agitation, predominate. In some cases generalized muscle weakness is present. Low-grade fever from dehydration is present, and the skin appears flushed and dry. The plasma volume depletion in hypovolemic hypernatremia may adversely affect the function of the heart and the kidneys. It presents with hypotension, tachycardia, and renal failure due to hypoperfusion. Ultimately the patient becomes lethargic and comatose.

Treatment should include water replacement. Water should be first given by mouth, and if it must be given intravenously it should be administered as a 5% dextrose solution.

Pearl

> Hypernatremia is usually related to dehydration, which may be first suspected when noticing a high hematocrit. Spurious hyperalbuminemia is also a sign of dehydration.

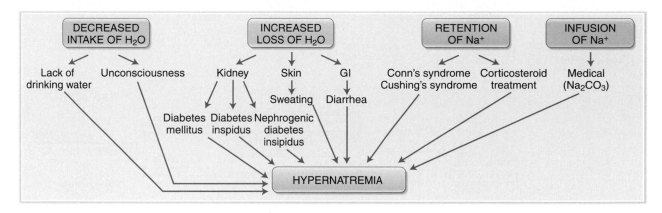

Figure 1-7 Pathogenesis of hypernatremia.

Chloride

Chloride is the major extracellular anion and it is tightly linked to intake, excretion and metabolism of sodium.

Chloride (Cl^-) is the major anion of plasma and interstitial fluids, accounting with bicarbonate (HCO_3^-) for most of the anionic charge of plasma. As such its functions include maintenance of hydration, osmotic pressure, and electrolyte balance. The reference range for chloride is 98 to 106 mmol/L.

Chloride is mostly bound to Na^+, forming the common salt (NaCl). Accordingly, its metabolism follows that of Na^+. The only exceptions occur in certain forms of metabolic acidosis and alkalosis.

- **Hyperchloremic metabolic acidosis.** Depletion of HCO_3^- in metabolic acidosis is usually accompanied by formation of organic anions, which will replace the lost HCO_3^-. If this does not occur, the gap is filled with Cl^-. Hyperchloremia in this condition is not accompanied by hypernatremia.
- **Hypochloremic metabolic alkalosis.** Metabolic alkalosis caused by a loss of Cl^- in the GI tract is associated with an anion gap that is filled with HCO_3^-. The concentration of Na^+ is in the normal range, and the condition can be treated with Cl^- infusion.

Pearl

> NaCl is excreted in sweat, but Cl^- is the preferred analyte measured in the sweat of children thought to have cystic fibrosis. Chloride concentration over 60 mmol/L in the sweat is diagnostic of cystic fibrosis. This is typically measured after pilocarpine stimulation.

Potassium

Potassium (K^+) is the principal intracellular cation.

The body contains somewhat less K^+ than Na^+ (3500 mmol), of which approximately 98% is inside the cells and only 2% is in the extracellular fluid. Ninety percent of the intracellular K^+ is in the exchangeable intracellular pool, whereas 8% is structurally bound to the bone, brain cells, and red blood cells. The extracellular K^+ may be exchanged with the rapidly exchangeable pool, and the shifts between these two pools occur quite often.

The plasma contains only 0.4% of the total body K^+. The normal reference interval in the serum is 3.5 to 5.0 mmol/L. It is slightly higher in serum than in plasma, because some K^+ is released from platelets during coagulation of blood.

Potassium balance is maintained primarily by the kidneys.

The normal diet contains enough K^+ and thus on average 100 mmol of K^+ is absorbed daily, 90 mmol is excreted by the kidneys, and the remaining 10 mmol is lost in feces and sweat (Fig. 1-8).

The kidneys can regulate the excretion of K^+, although approximately 30 mmol/day is excreted as obligatory renal loss. Potassium is filtered through the glomeruli but is almost completely absorbed in the proximal tubules (Fig. 1-9). The concentration of K^+ in the blood and the glomerular filtration rate (GFR) regulate K^+ excretion, because these two factors determine the amount of K^+ available in the interstitial fluid of the kidneys for the exchange that occurs in the distal tubule and the collecting duct.

Potassium reenters from the interstitial fluid into the cells of the distal tubules and collecting duct. A small part of it is actively secreted into the lumen, but mostly K^+ enters passively through diffusion. This diffusion occurs in response to the active reabsorption of Na^+ from

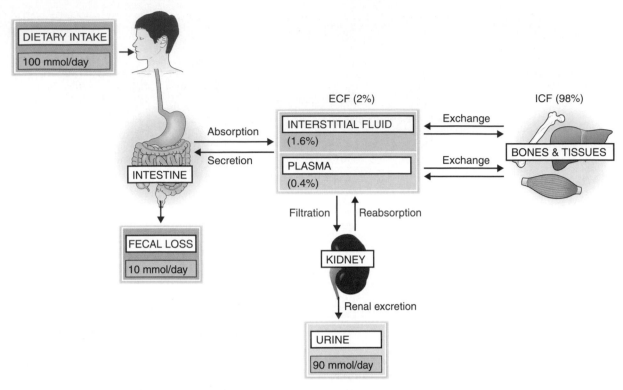

Figure 1-8 Potassium intake and excretion. Intake in the food is balanced by excretion in the urine and, to a smaller extent, in the feces and sweat (not shown here). Most of the K$^+$ is stored in the intracellular volume (ICV), and only 2% is found in the extracellular fluid volume (ECF). Only 0.4% of total K$^+$ is in the plasma. Most of the intracellular fluid (ICF) contains exchangeable K$^+$, but 8% is tightly bound in tissues. The balance of K$^+$ critically depends on the function of the kidneys. The modulators of K$^+$ excretion in the kidneys are the Na$^+$ and K$^+$ concentration in the plasma and inside the kidney compartments, aldosterone, acid–base balance, and the glomerular filtration rate (GFR).

the lumen of tubular and ductal cells. Active Na$^+$ reabsorption generates an electric membrane gradient, and K$^+$ and **hydrogen ions (H$^+$)** cross the membranes to neutralize these electric charges. Aldosterone promotes secretion of K$^+$ in the distal tubule but also promotes, reabsorption of Na$^+$, thus stimulating the sodium–potassium exchange (i.e., the excretion of K$^+$ in urine). Remember that aldosterone secretion is stimulated by the renin–angiotensin system, but can also be increased directly by a high intake of K$^+$.

The excretion of K$^+$ in urine depends also on the amount of Na$^+$ absorbed in the distal nephron. If Na$^+$ reabsorption is stimulated by diuretics, more K$^+$ will be needed to replace the reabsorbed Na$^+$.

Potassium and hydrogen ions are in a balance, and the excretion of K$^+$ in urine depends on the availability of H$^+$. In acidosis, the excess of H$^+$ favors the exchange of Na$^+$ for H$^+$. The urinary excretion of K$^+$ is reduced, and renal acidosis is therefore associated with hyperkalemia. The reverse happens in alkalosis, when less H$^+$ is available for exchange; higher excretion of K$^+$ results in hypokalemia, which is typical of renal alkalosis. The reverse is also true: Since

hypokalemia of any origin makes less K$^+$ available for the exchange with Na$^+$ in the distal nephron, hypokalemia tends to produce alkalosis.

Intercellular potassium concentration depends on the transmembrane exchange between the extracellular and intracellular pool of potassium.

The concentration of K$^+$ inside the cells is an order of magnitude (approximately 25 times) higher than in the interstitial fluid. Such a huge gradient can be maintained only by the constant work of the sodium–potassium adenosine triphosphatase (**Na$^+$/K$^+$ ATPase),** which requires a huge expenditure of energy. Cell injury caused by ischemia or toxins may reduce the energy supply or impair the function of ATPase, resulting in a net increase of the efflux of K$^+$ from the cells (Fig. 1-10).

Potassium is in an equilibrium with H$^+$, and the concentration of H$^+$ influences the flux of K$^+$ across the cell membrane. In acidosis, the high concentration of H$^+$ in the interstitial fluid favors its influx into the cell cytoplasm, where it displaces K$^+$. Acidosis is thus associated

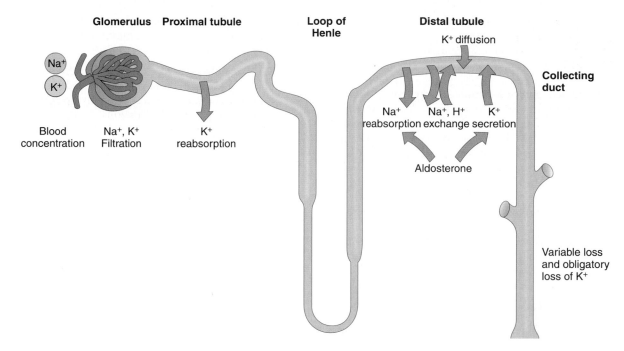

Figure 1-9 Potassium excretion in the kidney.

with hyperkalemia. Alkalosis favors the flux of H^+ and K^+ in the opposite direction and is thus associated with hypokalemia.

Potassium flux across the cell membrane may be promoted by **insulin.** Conversely a lack of insulin in diabetes favors efflux of K^+ from cells.

Hypokalemia is usually caused by increased loss or by redistribution of potassium in the body compartments.

Hypokalemia is most often related to an **increased loss** of K^+ in the urine, GI tract, or skin, but it may also be a consequence of the **redistribution** of K^+ from the ECF to the

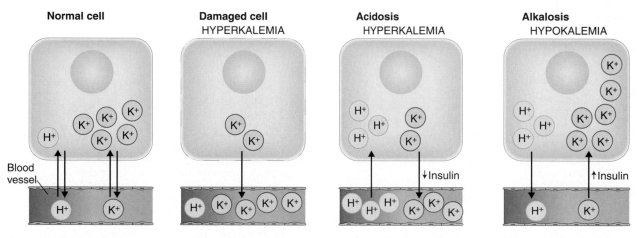

Figure 1-10 Potassium flux across the cell membrane. **A,** In the normal cell the intracellular potassium (K^+) concentration is several times higher than in the interstitial fluid. The gradient is maintained by the Na/K-ATPase in the cell membrane. **B,** Cell injury leads to a leakage of K^+ from the cytoplasm into the interstitial fluid. **C,** In acidosis the hydrogen ions (H^+) enter the cells from the interstitial fluid, displacing K^+, which is translocated into the interstitial fluid (hyperkalemia). Lack of insulin in diabetes mellitus favors efflux of K^+ from cells. **D,** In alkalosis the intracellular H^+ enters the interstitial fluid and the K^+ enters the cells, causing hypokalemia. Insulin also favors the entry of K^+ into the cells.

ICF compartment (Fig. 1-11). **Reduced intake** is rarely a problem, but may be encountered during starvation, in patients with anorexia nervosa, or in alcoholics on an unbalanced diet.

- **Increased gastrointestinal loss of potassium.** It can occur in several conditions. All GI secretions contain K^+. In patients who are vomiting or have diarrhea, K^+ is lost together with the water and Na^+. Prolonged use of laxatives may have the same effect. Prolonged loss of Na^+ may cause secondary hyperaldosteronism and an increased loss of K^+ in urine. Mucus, produced in excess by the inflamed mucosa or villous adenomas, also may deplete K^+ from the body.
- **Increased renal loss of potassium.** It occurs most often in patients treated with diuretics or those who have osmotic polyuria, as in diabetes. Mineralocorticoid excess as seen in primary hyperaldosteronism caused by adrenal cortical tumors is a rare cause of hypokalemia. Secondary hyperaldosteronism that occurs in end-stage kidney disease or in cirrhosis may also produce hypokalemia.
- **Redistribution of potassium.** It occurs during alkalosis, which favors the entry of K^+ into the cells, where it replaces H^+ that has entered into the ICF. Insulin administration promotes the entry of K^+ into the cells. Familial periodic muscle paralysis is a rare condition in which hypokalemia develops because of the entry of K^+ into the muscle cells.

Hypokalemia impairs transmission of neuromuscular impulses and weakens the contraction of muscles.

Hypokalemia may be asymptomatic, but if symptoms develop they most often pertain to organs, such as skeletal and cardiac muscle, smooth muscle, and nerves, whose function depends critically on the polarization and depolarization of cell membranes. The most common signs and symptoms of hypokalemia are as follows:

- **Cardiac.** Hypokalemia may cause arrhythmias and abnormal cardiac contractions associated with characteristic electrocardiographic (ECG) changes. These ECG changes include flattening or inversion of T waves, ST segment depression, and the appearance of U waves. Digitalis toxicity is increased.
- **Neuromuscular.** Generalized muscle weakness and hypotonia are present. Lethargy, depression, and confusion are occasionally encountered.
- **Gastrointestinal.** Slow peristalsis may cause constipation or ileus.
- **Metabolic/renal.** Alkalosis and polyuria due to decreased concentrating capacity of the kidneys may develop in some patients.

Hyperkalemia is caused most often by renal failure, metabolic disturbances, or tissue damage.

Hyperkalemia may develop due to **reduced excretion of K^+**, **massive release** from injured cells or in massive cell lysis, or the **redistribution of K^+** from ICV to ECV (Fig. 1-12). Even though hyperkalemia may develop due to **increased intake,** this rarely occurs.

- **Reduced excretion.** Most often hyperkalemia is a consequence of reduced excretion in end-stage kidney disease. Hyperkalemia usually appears after more than 80% of the nephrons are lost or damaged. Metabolic disturbances causing ketoacidosis also may reduce renal K^+ excretion. In Addison's disease hypoaldosteronism occurs, which also may reduce excretion of K^+ in the urine. Many drugs may affect the excretion of K^+ in urine, especially nonsteroidal anti-inflammatory drugs (NSAIDs), diuretics, and antihypertensive drugs.

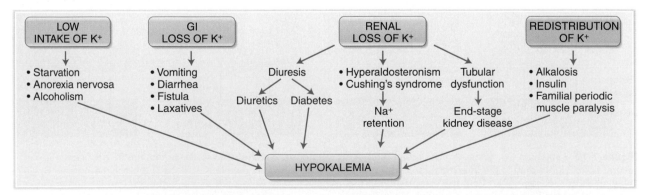

Figure 1-11 Causes of hypokalemia. Hypokalemia may develop owing to reduced intake of potassium (K^+), loss in the gastrointestinal (GI) system or kidneys, and redistribution of K^+ between the intracellular and extracellular fluid.

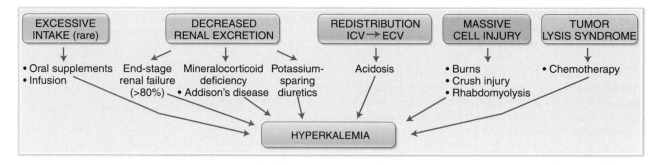

Figure 1-12 Causes of hyperkalemia. Hyperkalemia may be caused by reduced excretion in the kidneys, release of potassium from damaged or lyzed cells (e.g., tumor lysis syndrome), owing to the redistribution of potassium between the intracellular and extracellular fluid compartment, and rarely due to an increased intake of potassium. ECV, extracellular volume; ICV, intracellular volume.

■ **Massive tissue injury or cell lysis.** Hyperkalemia results from the release of K^+ from the intracellular space into the ECV. For example, burns, crush injuries, or rhabdomyolysis are usually accompanied by hyperkalemia. Massive tumor cell lysis following chemotherapy may cause severe hyperkalemia. This is most often encountered in the therapy for lymphomas and other tumors that respond to cytotoxic drugs.

■ **Redistribution of potassium from the ICV to the ECV.** Such an internal redistribution occurs most often in ketoacidosis of diabetes. Lack of insulin and severe hyperglycemia also may cause hyperkalemia. Hyperkalemic periodic paralysis is a rare muscle disease characterized by hyperkalemia and mytonia.

Pearls

> Hyperkalemia is a potentially lethal condition. If detected in the laboratory the pathologist must call in the finding by telephone to the clinician who submitted the blood sample.

> Spurious hyperkalemia results from a release of K^+ from hemolyzed red blood cells. Hemolysis and delayed separation of blood cells from serum are the most common causes of hyperkalemia in hospital laboratories.

Hyperkalemia causes cardiac arrhythmias that may be lethal.

Hyperkalemia accelerates the transmission of electric current in the heart, leading to arrhythmia. The characteristic ECG changes include initially peaked T waves. If the concentration of K^+ exceeds 6 mmol/L, the P waves disappear and the QRS complexes become widened. Ventricular arrhythmia ensues, progressing to fibrillation, which may have a lethal outcome.

Treatment of hyperkalemia requires immediate infusion of calcium gluconate to counteract the cardiotoxic effects of hyperkalemia. It should be followed by infusion of hypertonic glucose, which causes a release of insulin and thus promotes the entry of K^+ into the cells. Sodium bicarbonate infusion increases the pH of the ECF, and this alkalosis also promotes a K^+ shift into the cells.

Acid–Base Balance

Hydrogen ion concentration in body fluids is expressed as nanomoles per liter (nmol/L) or, as is more common in the United States, on a pH scale. The pH of a solution is the logarithm (base 10) of H^+ activity. Thus a solution containing hydrogen in a concentration of 100 nmol/L has a pH of 7.0. Values below pH 7 are considered to be in the acidic range, and those above pH 7 are alkaline. Thus a solution with an H^+ concentration of 50 nmol/L has a pH of 7.30, and a solution with a concentration of 125 nmol/L has a pH of 6.90.

Normal blood has an H^+ concentration of 40 nmol/L, or a pH of 7.40.

The pH of the blood varies in a narrow range from 7.35 to 7.45, primarily because the blood is well buffered. Hemoglobin—which buffers the changes in CO_2—and bicarbonate (HCO_3^-)—which buffers the fixed acids, such as lactate or sulfate—account for most of blood's buffering capacity. These two systems are also interconnected with each other and account for most of the buffering capacity of the blood. Phosphates and plasma proteins also may act as buffers, but they play a minor role.

Hydrogen ions produced in the intermediary metabolism are buffered or eliminated from the body to prevent acidification of the internal milieu.

Hydrogen ions are formed inside the cells during each of the major metabolic processes, including tissue respiration, glycolysis, lipolysis, or ureagenesis. From the ICV H^+ enters the interstitial fluids, where is it buffered primarily with

HCO_3^- to form a carbonic acid (H_2CO_3), which tends to dissociate into carbon dioxide (CO_2) and water (H_2O):

$$H^+ + HCO_3^- \rightleftharpoons H_2CO_3 \rightleftharpoons H_2O + CO_2$$

The binding of H^+ to HCO_3^- occurs fast, but the breakdown of H_2CO_3 takes longer. This process may be facilitated by carbonic anhydrase, an enzyme present in red blood cells and the kidney tubules. The CO_2 is exhaled in the lungs, and H^+ and H_2O are excreted in the kidneys.

The kidneys play a crucial role in eliminating the acids and forming the alkali of the bicarbonate buffering system.

Carbonic acid is cleaved in the kidney cells into H^+ and HCO_3^- (Fig. 1-13). Hydrogen ions are excreted in urine, and the recovered HCO_3^- is returned into the circulation. Hydrogen ions entering the urine are linked to phosphate and ammonia, which serve as the primary urinary buffers.

In addition to the recovery of bicarbonate, kidney cells have also a capacity to regenerate HCO_3^- from CO_2 and H_2O. Hence the kidneys play a major role in the maintenance of the acid–base balance: By removing H^+ from blood or adding HCO_3^- the kidneys make the blood pH rise into the alkaline range, and by reducing the excretion of H^+ in urine they lower the pH into the acidic range.

Acid–base disorders are classified as acidosis or alkalosis.

The pH of the blood is normally slightly alkaline. If the pH drops below the normal reference point the condition is clinically called acidosis, and if it rises above the upper limit it is called alkalosis. Acidosis and alkalosis are called metabolic if the main problem is related to the maintenance of the bicarbonate (HCO_3^-) concentration. A disturbance in the acid–base balance that is related to the maintenance of the P_{CO_2} concentration of blood is called respiratory acidosis or respiratory alkalosis. In some instances the underlying problems are complex and the condition is called mixed respiratory–metabolic acidosis or alkalosis.

In brief one can summarize the changes as follows:

- **Metabolic acidosis** is related to an accumulation of H^+ (acids) and a decrease of HCO_3^-. The loss of HCO_3^- may cause an anion gap that is filled in with fixed acids. The lungs compensate fast by exhaling CO_2, and thus in compensated metabolic acidosis P_{CO_2} is reduced.
- **Metabolic alkalosis** results from a loss of H^+ or a retention of HCO_3^-. Compensation occurs fast by reduced CO_2 expiration, which leads to an increased P_{CO_2}.
- **Respiratory acidosis** results from excessive retention of CO_2 in the lungs. The kidneys compensate over time by retaining HCO_3^-, which leads to a rise of blood HCO_3^-.

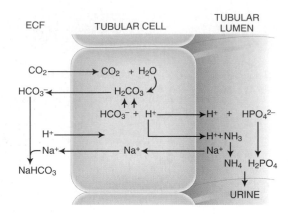

Figure 1-13 Buffering functions of the kidney. Kidneys excrete hydrogen ions (H^+) and return the recovered or regenerated bicarbonate (HCO_3^-) into the blood. Hydrogen in urine is buffered to phosphate or ammonia. The kidneys regenerate HCO_3^-, releasing it into the extracellular fluid, and also take up H^+, thus lowering the pH of the blood. ECF, extracellular fluid.

- **Respiratory alkalosis** results from excessive loss of CO_2 through the lungs. The kidneys compensate over time by increasing excretion of HCO_3^-, thus lowering the concentration of HCO_3^- in blood.

The primary disturbances leading to respiratory or metabolic acidosis and alkalosis are illustrated in Figure 1-14. Note that the values for acute respiratory acidosis and alkalosis vary from those in chronic respiratory acidosis and alkalosis, because it takes time for the kidneys to compensate for the abnormality. In contrast, there is no difference between acute and chronic metabolic acidosis or alkalosis because in metabolic disturbances of acid–base balance the respiratory compensation occurs immediately and does not change when the acute disorder progresses into a chronic state. The changes in simple and compensated acid–base disorders are summarized in Table 1-4.

The clinical diagnosis of simple acid–base disorders can be established by measuring the pH of an arterial blood sample in conjunction with the concentration of HCO_3^- and the P_{CO_2} (Fig. 1-15).

Metabolic acidosis results from a loss of bicarbonates and increased concentration of hydrogen ion in the extracellular fluid.

Metabolic acidosis is characterized by a rise of H^+ concentration; that is, lowering of the pH due to a reduced blood HCO_3^-: P_{CO_2} ratio below the normal 20:1 as shown in the following marked up Henderson-Hasselbalch formula:

$$\downarrow pH = pK + \log \frac{\downarrow [HCO_3^-]}{P_{CO_2}}$$

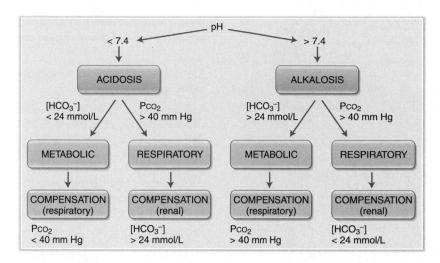

Figure 1-14 Clinical diagnosis of acid–base disorders. The arterial blood sample is analyzed by measuring its pH, concentration of bicarbonate (HCO_3^-), and carbon dioxide pressure (PCO_2). On the basis of these findings, the condition can be classified as acidosis or alkalosis, and further subclassified as respiratory or metabolic or respiratory, simple or compensated. (Modified from Guyton AC, Hall JE: Medical Physiology, 11th ed, WB Saunders, Philadelphia, 2000, p 399.)

Compensation occurs when the decreased pH of arterial blood stimulates the central chemoreceptors, provoking hyperventilation and an increased elimination of CO_2 through the lungs.

$$pH = pK + \log \frac{[HCO_3^-]}{\downarrow PCO_2}$$

In general terms respiratory compensation occurs fast after the onset of metabolic acidosis. One can calculate that the loss of each millimole per liter of HCO_3^- is compensated by 1.3 mm Hg of PCO_2. If the kidney is relatively healthy it will contribute over time to this compensatory effort by excreting

H^+ in form of NH_4^+, but if the patient is in end-stage kidney disease, renal compensation cannot take place.

Metabolic acidosis could have several causes, which could be arranged into the following four groups:

- **Loss of bicarbonate.** Bicarbonate is most often lost through the GI tract in diarrhea. It may be related to intestinal, pancreatic, or biliary drainage, and some forms of renal tubular acidosis.
- **Inability to excrete hydrogen ion through the kidneys.** Most often this occurs in end-stage kidney failure because the kidneys cannot form ammonia and excrete H^+ in the form of NH_4^+. It also can occur in hypoaldosteronism, when hyperkalemia in the kidneys inhibits

Table 1-4 Summary of Changes in Acid–Base Disorders

DISORDER	PRIMARY ABNORMALITY	BLOOD CHEMISTRY		
		pH	PCO₂	[HCO₃⁻]
Metabolic acidosis	HCO_3^- low	↓	→	↓
Compensated (respiratory CO_2)		—	↓	—
Metabolic alkalosis	HCO_3^- high	↑	→	↑
Compensated (respiratory retention CO_2)		—	↑	—
Respiratory acidosis	CO_2^- high	↓	↑	→
Compensated (renal retention HCO_3^-)		—		↑
Respiratory alkalosis	CO_2^- low	↑	↓	→
Compensated (renal excretion HCO_3^-)		—		↓

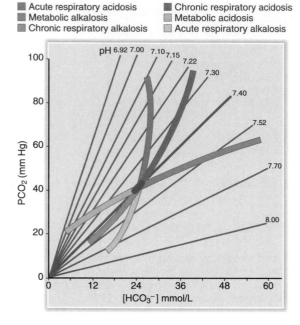

■ Acute respiratory acidosis   ■ Chronic respiratory acidosis
■ Metabolic alkalosis   ■ Metabolic acidosis
■ Chronic respiratory alkalosis ■ Acute respiratory alkalosis

Figure 1-15 Diagram of changes of blood pH, P_{CO_2}, and plasma concentration of HCO_3^- in compensated acidosis and alkalosis. (Modified from Constanzo LS: Physiology, WB Saunders, Philadelphia, 1998, p 280.)

the synthesis of NH_3. Hydrogen ions cannot be excreted in some forms of renal tubular acidosis.

■ **Excessive production of endogenous acids.** Most often this occurs in uncontrolled diabetes mellitus when the patients develop ketoacidosis or in tissue hypoxia when lactic acidosis develops. Since lactates are metabolized mostly in the liver, liver failure is also accompanied by lactic acidosis.

■ **Ingestion of fixed acids.** Ingestion of acids during poisoning with salicylates, methanol, or ethylene glycol can cause acidosis. These chemicals are transformed into acids (salicylic acid, formic acid, or glycolic acid/ oxalic acid, respectively), leading to the acidification of the interstitial fluids. Alternatively, these acids and their metabolites damage the liver cells, the primary site of lactic acid degradation, thus causing lactic acidosis.

Pearl

> Normal lactic acid concentration in the blood is 0.6 to 1.2. mmol/L, but it can rise 10 times higher during vigorous exercise. This rise is temporary, but if it persists it can give rise to lactic acidosis.

Lactic acidosis can be classified as type A or B. Type A is more common and is caused by hypoxic cell injury (as occurs in heart failure or shock) or severe exercise. Type B lactic aci-

dosis is found in severe liver disease and chronic alcohol abuse and may be related to ingestion of certain drugs and poisons.

Metabolic acidosis may be accompanied by a high anion gap.

Sodium and K^+ are the most abundant cations, and CO_2 and Cl^- the most abundant anions in blood. Using the concentration (expressed in millimoles per liter) for these analytes and inserting the measured values into the formula $(Na^+ + K^+) - (CO_2 + Cl^-)$, the normal anion gap can be approximated. It normally varies from 10 to 20 mmol/L. For example, in the following formula the concentrations are $Na^+ = 138$, $K^+ = 3.5$, $CO_2 = 25$, and $Cl^- = 100$. The anion gap is 16.5 mmol/L:

$$(138 + 3.5) - (25 + 100) = 16.5$$

In metabolic acidosis the anion gap may remain in the normal range, or it may be increased. The loss of HCO_3^2 in diarrhea, hypoaldosteronism, or certain forms of proximal or distal renal tubular acidosis and obstructive uropathy are associated with a normal anion gap. The loss of HCO_3^2 is compensated in such instances with reactive hyperchloremia. Increased acid in metabolic acidosis caused by ketoacidosis, lactic acidosis, end-stage renal disease, or ingestion of extraneous acids is not taken into account in the preceding formula, thus causing a widening of the anion gap. The most common conditions producing metabolic acidosis are listed in Table 1-5.

Metabolic acidosis may cause reduced cardiac output, especially if the pH drops below 7.2. Resistance to catecholamines may cause hypotension. Deep and rhythmic breathing *(Kussmaul breathing)* may develop, especially in ketoacidosis.

Table 1-5 Causes of Metabolic Acidosis

Acidosis with Normal Anion Gap
Gastrointestinal loss of bicarbonates
    Diarrhea
    Gastrointestinal, biliary or pancreatic fistulae
Renal diseases
    Obstructive uropathy
    Renal tubular acidosis
    Chronic pyelonephritis
Hypoaldosteronism
Hyperalimentation

Acidosis with High Anion Gap
Ketoacidosis
    Diabetes
    Alcohol abuse
Lactic acidosis
    Tissue damage and ischemia
    Liver insufficiency
End-stage kidney disease
Poisoning
    Salicylates
    Ethylene glycol
    Methanol

Pearl

> A mnemonic for the most common causes of metabolic acidosis with an anion gap is DEKALS. It is easy to remember it if you know that DK (diabetic ketoacidosis) is the most important form of this disease. The mnemonic stands for:
  Diabetic acidosis
  Ethylene glycol (antifreeze)
  Kidney failure
  Alcohols (ethanol and methanol)
  Lactic acidosis (low perfusion of tissues, e.g., shock, sepsis)
  Salicylate poisoning

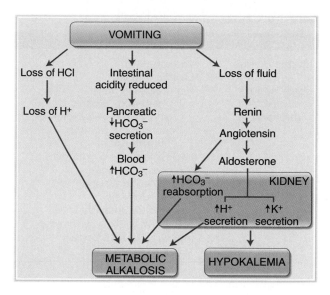

Figure 1-16 Metabolic alkalosis due to vomiting. (Modified from Constanzo LS: Physiology, WB Saunders, Philadelphia, 1998.)

Metabolic alkalosis results from excessive loss of hydrogen ions or excessive retention of bicarbonate.

Metabolic alkalosis may result from an excessive loss of H^+ through the GI tract or the kidneys, or a net gain of HCO_3^- due to excessive ingestion or renal retention. In either case the concentration of HCO_3^- increases, as shown in the marked-up Henderson-Hasselbalch equation:

$$\uparrow pH = pK + \log \frac{\uparrow[HCO_3^-]}{P_{CO_2}}$$

Compensatory changes take place fast through hypoventilation, resulting in reduced expiration of CO_2 and increased P_{CO_2} of blood:

$$pH = pK + \log \frac{[HCO_3^-]}{\uparrow P_{CO_2}}$$

Metabolic alkalosis is most often caused by vomiting of gastric contents (Fig. 1-16). Note that the gastric parietal cells form hydrochloric acid (HCl), which is secreted into the lumen. Each H^+ excreted into the lumen as HCl is compensated by a release of HCO_3^- into the interstitial fluids and blood. Normally, this HCO_3^- is utilized in the pancreas to neutralize the HCl of gastric acid that has reached the duodenum. If the gastric contents are vomited, no HCl reaches the duodenum and thus the stimulus for the pancreatic release is missing. Excess HCO_3^- in the blood forces H^+ to enter the cells, thus diminishing H^+ concentration in blood and consequently causing alkalosis of the blood.

Metabolic alkalosis is usually short-lived, and if it persists it is related to abnormal handling of bicarbonate and hydrogen in the kidneys.

In normal persons it is very difficult to induce a sustained alkalosis even if one were to infuse HCO_3^- into the circulation. If the kidney functions properly excess HCO_3^- is filtered in the glomerulus and is available for renal excretion. Persistence

of metabolic alkalosis implies inappropriate reabsorption of filtered HCO_3^-. Persistence of alkalosis occurs under three conditions:

- **Extracellular volume contraction.** A decreased ECV leads to a reduced glomerular filtration, with increased Na^+ reabsorption in the kidney. In the presence of Cl^- depletion Na^+ retention is followed by obligatory HCO_3^- reabsorption. Infusion of normal saline NaCl expands the ECV and provides enough Cl^-, thus correcting the alkalosis.
- **Potassium deficiency.** A K^+ deficiency may also enhance HCO_3^- reabsorption in the kidneys while increasing H^+ secretion into the tubular fluid. Potassium deficiency also forces H^+ from the extracellular fluid to enter the cells, further contributing to the alkalosis.
- **Mineralocorticoid excess.** Aldosterone promotes distal tubular reabsorption of Na^+ and reciprocal excretion of K^+ and H^+. Note that increased mineralocorticoid secretion can be primarily due to adrenal disturbances, such as Conn's or Cushing's syndromes, but it is also a reaction to volume contraction.

The latter form of hyperaldosteronism responds favorably to volume expansion with normal saline infusion; Conn's and Cushing's syndromes do not respond to infusion of normal saline. The most important causes of metabolic alkalosis are listed in Table 1-6.

Metabolic alkalosis is usually clinically dominated by symptoms of the underlying disease. Tetany may develop in some cases.

Table 1-6 Causes of Metabolic Alkalosis

PATHOGENESIS	CLINICAL CONDITION
Gastric H$^+$ loss	Vomiting
	Gastric drainage
Renal H$^+$ loss and HCO$_3^-$ retention	Hyperaldosteronism
	Primary (e.g., Conn's and Cushing's syndromes)
	Secondary (e.g., renal hypertension)
	Hypokalemia (e.g., diuretics, chronic diarrhea)
	Volume contraction (e.g., cirrhosis)
Net gain of HCO$_3^-$	Absorbable antacids (e.g., milk alkali syndrome)
	Ingestion of bicarbonate (e.g., baking soda)

Table 1-7 Causes of Respiratory Acidosis

PATHOGENESIS	DISORDERS AND DISEASES
Central nervous system depression	Trauma
	Intracranial hemorrhage
	Tumors
	Infections
	Severe hypoxia
	Drugs (e.g., opiates, barbiturates), anesthesia
Neuromuscular diseases involving respiratory muscles	Myasthenia gravis
	Muscular dystrophy
	Amyotrophic lateral sclerosis
	Guillain-Barré syndrome
	Cervical spinal cord injury
Chest wall/pleural disorders	Thoracic deformities (e.g., kyphoscoliosis)
	Pleural effusion
	Pneumothorax
Airway obstruction	Foreign body aspiration
	Drowning or strangulation
	Asthma
	Chronic bronchitis or bronchiolitis
Alveolar capillary block	Chronic interstitial pneumonitis
	Pulmonary edema
	Emphysema
Impaired perfusion of lungs	Massive pulmonary embolism
	Cardiac arrest

Respiratory acidosis is characterized by retention of carbon dioxide due to hypoventilation.

The primary disorder in respiratory acidosis is retention of CO$_2$ as shown in the Henderson-Hasselbalch formula:

$$pH = pK + \log \frac{[HCO_3^-]}{\uparrow P_{CO_2}}$$

The retention of CO$_2$ can result from the inhibition of respiration at several levels, such as due to injuries of the central respiratory center, paralysis of respiratory muscles, or lung diseases. The most important causes of respiratory acidosis are listed in Table 1-7.

Respiratory acidosis is invariably associated with hypoxia, the treatment of which requires correction of both hypoxia and hypercapnia. The CO$_2$ excess is buffered to a great extent inside the red blood cells, where the following reaction takes place:

$$CO_2 + H_2O \rightarrow H^+ + HCO_3^-$$

Excess H$^+$ is bound to hemoglobin and phosphates, which act as buffers. Additional compensation occurs in the kidneys where H$^+$ is excreted in the form of NH$_4^+$ and exchanged for HCO$_3^-$, correcting the acidity of the extracellular fluid as shown in the Henderson-Hasselbalch formula:

$$pH = pK + \log \frac{[HCO_3^-]}{P_{CO_2}}$$

In acute respiratory acidosis the pH of the blood is quite low, since the compensatory production of HCO$_3^-$ is inadequate (for each mm Hg of P$_{CO_2}$ only a 0.1 mmol/L of HCO$_3^-$ is produced). With time the kidneys compensate, producing sufficient amounts of HCO$_3^-$ (for each mm Hg

of P$_{CO_2}$ 0.4 mmol/L of HCO$_3^-$), and thus in chronic respiratory acidosis the pH returns closer to the normal range of values.

Symptoms are most often related to increased blood flow into the brain through the dilated blood vessels and secondary intracranial pressure elevation. Cardiovascular symptoms include reduced cardiac output and pulmonary hypertension.

Respiratory alkalosis is caused by hyperventilation, leading to an increasesd loss of carbon dioxide.

Loss of CO$_2$ is related to hyperventilation, which can be voluntary, drug-induced, related to several systemic or neurologic diseases, or related to hypoxemia. The most important causes of respiratory alkalosis are listed in Table 1-8.

In respiratory alkalosis the symptoms of the underlying disorder predominate. Acute hypocapnia can induce cerebral vasoconstriction with a feeling of lightheadedness, mental confusion, and syncope. Perioral and peripheral paresthesia may develop due to a drop **in ionized calcium (Ca^{2+})** concentration.

Table 1-8 Causes of Respiratory Alkalosis

PATHOGENESIS	DISORDERS AND DISEASES
Respiratory center stimulation	Voluntary hyperventilation
	Anxiety
	Reflex hyperventilation (e.g., pulmonary embolism)
	Fever and sepsis
	Drugs (e.g., salicylate poisoning)
	Brain diseases (e.g., tumor, stroke, meningitis)
	Liver disease (e.g., hepatic failure)
	Pregnancy
Hypoxemia	High altitude
	Pneumonia
	Right-to-left shunt heart failure
	Carbon monoxide poisoning
	Anemia
Mechanical ventilation	—

the exchangeable Ca^{2+} pool, including the plasma, extracellular fluid, and intracellular Ca^{2+}. The ratio of intracellular to extracellular Ca^{2+} is 1:10,000. This ratio is tightly controlled through energy-dependent calcium channels on the cell membrane.

The concentration of Ca^{2+} in plasma and interstitial fluid is tightly regulated and depends on the intake, the rate of absorption in the intestine, excretion through the kidneys, and the balance with the fixed calcium stores in the bones (Fig. 1-17). These metabolic processes are under the control mainly of parathyroid hormone, calcitonin, and vitamin D. Several other hormones, most notably thyroxin, cortisol, and growth hormone, also contribute to the metabolism of Ca^{2+}. The concentration of Ca^{2+} in plasma depends also on the pH of the blood and the concentration of albumin, which binds Ca^{2+}.

Pearl

> Acute respiratory alkalosis may rapidly reduce the concentration of unbound Ca^{2+} in blood and cause titanic contractions of the skeletal muscles.

Calcium

Calcium (Ca^{2+}) is the fifth most common element in the body. It is mostly found in the bones, which contain 99% of the total body Ca^{2+}. The remaining 1% of Ca^{2+} forms

Under physiological condition the concentration of Ca^{2+} in blood is in the range of 8.4 to 10.2 mg/dL (2.2–2.6 mmol/L). Approximately 45 to 50% of calcium is in an ionized form ("free calcium"), 40 to 45% is bound to serum

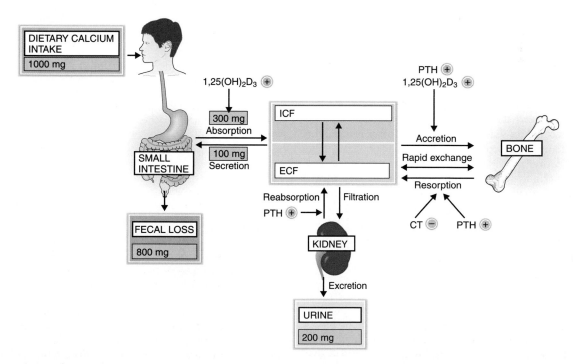

Figure 1-17 Calcium turnover under normal conditions. ECF, extracellular fluid; ICF, intracellular fluid; 1,25(OH)$_2$D$_3$, 1,25-dihydroxyvitamin D$_3$; PTH, parathyroid hormone; CT, calcitonin.

proteins, and 10 to 15% is bound to anions such as bicarbonate, phosphate, lactate, or citrate. Most of the protein-bound calcium is bound to albumin, accounting for 80% of this fraction. The remaining 20% of protein-bound calcium is bound to globulins. Binding of calcium to serum proteins occurs in a pH-dependent manner: more calcium is bound to albumin in alkalosis and less in acidosis. The most important clinical condition associated with an increased concentration of protein-bound calcium is **dehydration,** which can, however, be readily corrected by rehydration. **Paraproteinemia** of multiple myeloma is also characterized by an increased concentration of protein-bound calcium.

The concentration of Ca^{2+} acts as a trigger for the release of parathyroid hormone and is thus the critical physiological value essential for clinically evaluating calcium homeostasis. Unfortunately, current analytical methods measure only the total calcium concentration of calcium in the blood. To calculate the concentration of unbound Ca^{2+}, the concentration of albumin must be known. Thus in persons with **hypoalbuminemia,** total serum Ca^{2+} is low, yet there is no clinical evidence of hypocalcemia. The concentration of unbound Ca^{2+} in the serum of these persons is within normal limits, and accordingly the secretion of parathyroid hormone (regulated by the concentration of unbound Ca^{2+}) is also normal (Fig. 1-18).

The adjusted unbound Ca^{2+} concentration can be calculated according to the following formula:

$$\text{Adjusted serum } Ca^{2+} \text{ (mg/dL)} = \text{total Ca (mg/dL)} + 0.8[4.0 - \text{albumin (g/dL)}]$$

Using SI units for reporting the laboratory values in mmol/L, the adjusted unbound Ca^{2+} concentration is calculated according to the following formula:

$$\text{Adjusted serum } Ca^{2+} \text{ (mmol/L)} = \text{total Ca (mmol/L)} + 0.02[47 - \text{albumin (mmol/L)}]$$

These formulas provide only a rough estimate of Ca^{2+} concentration, and the true value can be measured only by complex techniques that are not readily available in routine hospital laboratory procedures. Estimates made by using these empirical formulas may give misleading results for Ca^{2+} in clinical conditions such as chronic renal failure, especially if patients are on maintenance hemodialysis or are experiencing hyperparathyroidism or chronic liver disease.

True hypocalcemia is most often related to disturbances of parathyroid hormone or vitamin D metabolism.

Hypocalcemia detected in the laboratory is most often "**spurious,**" meaning that it is related to low serum albumin concentration, alkalosis, or some artifact of blood collection (Fig. 1-19). Many diseases cause **hypoalbuminemia,** and consequently **pseudohypocalcemia** of this type is very common. In **alkalosis** the blood contains fewer free H^+ available for binding to albumin and thus

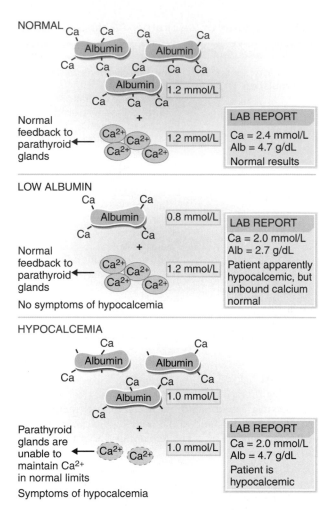

Figure 1-18 The binding of calcium to albumin. It should be noted that the laboratory measurements include both free calcium and calcium bound to albumin. (Modified from Gaw A, Cowan RA, O'Reilly DST, et al: An Illustrated Colour Text: Clinical Biochemistry, Churchill and Livingstone, Edinburgh, 1995.)

more Ca^{2+} binds to albumin, resulting in a decreased concentration of Ca^{2+}.

Pearl

> Prolonged application of the tourniquet during venipuncture may cause false hypercalcemia. Blood mistakenly drawn into tubes that contain EDTA or oxalate has an artificially low Ca^{2+} concentration because these anticoagulants bind Ca^{2+}.

Once these causes of spurious hypocalcemia have been excluded, it must be decided whether hypocalcemia is related to hypoparathyroidism or nonparathyroid disorders.

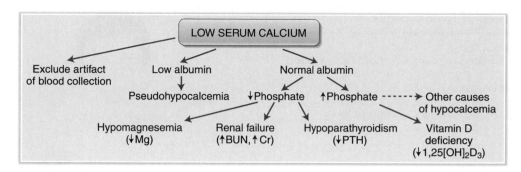

Figure 1-19 Causes of hypocalcemia. BUN, blood urea nitrogen; Cr, creatinine; Mg, magnesium; 1,25(OH)$_2$D$_3$, 1,25-dihydroxyvitamin D$_3$; PTH, parathyroid hormone.

Since the metabolism of calcium is closely related to that of phosphorus, serum concentration of Ca^{2+} and phosphorus will provide the initial clues about the possible causes of hypocalcemia. Additional studies may be needed by measuring serum levels of Mg^{2+}, 1,25-dihydroxyvitamin D$_3$ (1,25[OH]$_2$D$_3$), or PTH.

Hypocalcemia associated with hyperphosphatemia may be due to hypoparathyroidism or chronic renal failure, and less often to hypomagnesemia.

- **Hypoparathyroidism** may be congenital, as in Di-George syndrome, or acquired after inadvertent removal of the parathyroids during neck surgery.
- **Chronic renal failure** causes hypocalcemia primarily through hyperphosphatemia due to phosphate retention and inadequate hydroxylation of vitamin D into 1,25(OH)$_2$D$_3$. These conditions can be diagnosed by measuring serum PTH or by evaluating renal function and measuring serum BUN and creatinine, or 1,25(OH)$_2$D$_3$.
- **Hypomagnesemia** is also a possible cause of hypoparathyroidism. Magnesium ions are essential for the formation of the active form of PTH, and without Mg^{2+} hypocalcemia develops. It is characterized by low levels of PTH in serum due to a reduced PTH release. Since the PTH is not in an active form, a peripheral unresponsiveness to PTH results. Hypocalcemia can be promptly corrected by adding magnesium to the diet.

Hypocalcemia associated with hypophosphatemia is most likely related to disturbances of **vitamin D** intake and/or its metabolism. Vitamin D deficiency may have several causes, as follows:

- **Inadequate intake of vitamin D.** This is uncommon in the United States but could be encountered in the malnourished elderly and persons on special diets.
- **Rickets.** Vitamin D deficiency in childhood is uncommon in the United States. In other parts of the world it is usually related to inadequate exposure to sunlight.

- **Intestinal malabsorption.** Since vitamin D is a fat-soluble vitamin, malabsorption of fats due to intestinal, pancreatic, or biliary disorders may also cause vitamin D deficiency.
- **Renal or liver disease.** Since vitamin D is activated by hydroxylation in the kidneys and the liver, renal or hepatic insufficiency may cause signs of functional hypovitaminosis D. Inborn errors of metabolism affecting the hydroxylation of vitamin D (e.g., 1α-hydroxylase deficiency) may produce so-called **vitamin D–resistant rickets.**
- **Drug-related.** Certain drugs, such as anticonvulsants, may alter the metabolism of vitamin D in the liver and also cause hypocalcemia.

Hypocalcemia caused by vitamin D disturbances or deficiency may cause **secondary parathyroid hyperplasia,** which in turn will lead to a release of calcium and phosphorus from bones and subsequent osteomalacia. PTH is phosphaturic, but it also stimulates retention of calcium, contributing to the normalization of the Ca^{2+} levels in serum. All these aspects of calcium metabolism must be taken into an account when interpreting the laboratory data.

Hypocalcemia of acute onset may occur during acute necrosis of the pancreas due to the binding of calcium to fatty acids and deposition of these calcium soaps. Massive transfusion of citrated blood also may cause hypocalcemia.

Neonatal hypocalcemia may be idiopathic but may be caused by various rare **inborn errors of metabolism,** such as hyperphosphatemia, pseudohyperparathyroidism (peripheral PTH resistance), and vitamin D 1α-hydroxylase deficiency. The most important causes of hypocalcemia are listed in Table 1-9.

Hypocalcemia leads to functional disturbances of nerve cells and muscle cells.

Calcium is essential for the conductance of the neural impulses and generally for the function of nerve cells. It also plays an important role in the contraction of smooth, striated,

Table 1-9 Causes of Hypocalcemia

Spurious hypocalcemia
    Artifactual, related to technical errors during blood
    collection
    Hypoalbuminemia
    Alkalemia
Vitamin D deficiency or hydroxylation defects
    Dietary (e.g., rickets)
    Malabsorption
    1α-Hydroxylase deficiency
    Renal and liver diseases
    Drug-related
Hypoparathyroidism
    Absence of parathyroids (primary or secondary)
    Peripheral resistance to PTH
    Magnesium deficiency
Renal failure
    Acute renal failure
    Chronic renal failure
    Tumor lysis syndrome
Drugs (e.g., bisphosphonates, cisplatinum,
    anticonvulsants)
Transfusion of citrated blood
Acute pancreatitis
Neonatal hypocalcemia
Inborn errors of metabolism

PTH, parathyroid hormone.

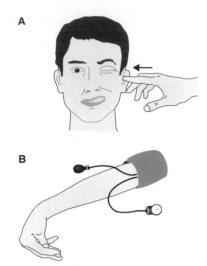

Figure 1-20 Signs of hypocalcemia. **A,** Facial spasm can be induced in hypocalcemia by pressure on the facial nerve *(Chvostek's sign).* **B,** Carpal spasm may be induced in persons with hypocalcemia induced by blood pressure-cuff tightening for at least 2 minutes *(Trousseau's sign).*

and cardiac muscle cells. Accordingly the symptoms of hypocalcemia include the following:

- **Neuromuscular symptoms.** Typically there is numbness and paresthesia, or muscle spasm and cramps. Spasm of the facial muscle *(Chvostek's sign)* or carpal spasm *(Trousseau's sign)* can be induced during physical examination (Fig. 1-20).
- **Cardiac signs.** These appear as abnormalities of cardiac rhythm and prolongation of QT interval in the ECG.
- **Behavioral changes.** Most of the mental symptoms are nonspecific, such as lack of alertness. Convulsions and loss of consciousness are rare manifestations of hypocalcemia, but may occur if the condition is not recognized and treated.

- **Laryngeal stridor.** This is usually related to laryngospasm.

Hypercalcemia is most often caused by primary hyperparathyroidism and malignant tumors.

Hypercalcemia is a common laboratory abnormality found in approximately 2 to 3 per 1000 persons whose blood was analyzed with a routine multichannel analyzer. Most of these patients have either no symptoms or the symptoms are so nonspecific that they are not easily linked to hypercalcemia. Most often hypercalcemia is caused by primary hyperparathyroidism or malignant tumors. Other causes of hypercalcemia are less common (Table 1-10).

Hyperparathyroidism is classified as primary, secondary, or tertiary.

- **Primary hyperparathyroidism** is most often caused by parathyroid adenoma and less often by primary parathyroid hyperplasia.

Table 1-10 Causes of Hypercalcemia

MOST COMMON CAUSES	LESS COMMON CAUSES	UNCOMMON CAUSES
Primary hyperparathyroidism	Granuloma (e.g., sarcoidosis)	Paget's disease
Malignant tumors	Hypervitaminosis D	Adrenal failure
Metastases to bone	Hyperthyroidism	Milk-alkali syndrome
Paraneoplastic syndromes	Drugs (thiazide)	Lithium therapy
Multiple myeloma, lymphoma		Hypermagnesemia
		Immobilization

- **Secondary parathyroid hyperplasia** may develop in patients with chronic renal disease.
- **Tertiary hyperparathyroidism** typically develops in the context of secondary hyperparathyroidism. In some of these patients the secretion of PTH becomes independent of Ca^{2+} levels in blood and cannot be medically regulated.

Excess PTH mobilizes calcium and PO_4^- from bones. In the kidneys it blocks the excretion of Ca^{2+} by promoting its reabsorption. PTH also stimulates the excretion of phosphorus and the hydroxylation of vitamin D in the kidney. Activated vitamin D increases the absorption of Ca^{2+} in the gut, promotes reabsorption of Ca^{2+} from primary filtrate in the kidneys, and promotes the PTH-mediated resorption of bone (Fig. 1-21).

Malignant tumors are a common cause of hypercalcemia, which may be a consequence of direct bone destruction by metastases or the action of osteolytic hormones and cytokines in osteolytic paraneoplastic syndromes.

Hypercalcemia is common in breast carcinoma patients who have **bone metastases.** Osteolytic metastases are readily seen on radiographs and are often associated with pathologic fractures. In patients with solid tumors who do not have metastases, hypercalcemia is most often caused by **parathyroid hormone-related polypeptide (PTHrP).** This hormone is most often produced by squamous cell carcinoma of the lungs, but it may be detected in the serum of other cancer patients as well. It acts on bone and kidneys like PTH. Hypercalcemia is associated with hypophosphatemia and increased PO_4^- excretion in urine. In contrast to primary hyperparathyroidism, excretion of Ca^{2+} in urine is increased and serum PTH is suppressed and undetectable.

Multiple myeloma and lymphomas secrete cytokines, such as interleukin-1 and tumor necrosis factor, which activate osteoclasts and thus cause lysis of bone trabeculae. In contrast to bone lysis in primary hyperparathyroidism, which also stimulates the osteoblasts, osteoclastic lesions are not coupled with new bone formation.

Vitamin D-related hypercalcemia may be found in **vitamin D intoxication.** Several granulomatous diseases, such as **sarcoidosis, tuberculosis,** or **fungal infections,** are characterized by hypercalcemia, which develops due to excessive formation of $1,25(OH)_2D_3$. Hypercalcemia of sarcoidosis can be suppressed by corticosteroid treatment.

Hyperthyroidism is quite often accompanied by hypercalciuria and hypercalcemia, which result from increased turnover of the bone. Prolonged **immobilization** may cause hypercalcemia in children, because the bone resorption exceeds new bone formation. In adults immobilization is a rare cause of hypercalcemia.

For treatment purposes hypercalcemia is subdivided into two groups: that associated with excess PTH, and unrelated to PTH.

Parathyroid hormone concentration in blood is easily measured and thus it is common to perform this test on most patients who have hypercalcemia. On the basis of these laboratory data hypercalcemia can be classified as PTH-mediated or non-PTH–mediated (Fig. 1-22). The most common conditions that manifest with increased or normal to decreased PTH concentration in blood are listed in Table 1-11.

Hypercalcemia is usually asymptomatic or it may present with symptoms related to several organ systems.

Hypercalcemia is usually asymptomatic, and the diagnosis is made by laboratory methods during routine testing or a work-up when some other disease is suggested. Once diagnosed hypercalcemia should be further investigated in the context of parathyroid activity and classified as either PTH-related or unrelated to PTH (see Fig. 1-22). PTH is elevated in hyperparathyroidism, but it is not detectable in the serum of patients with malignancy-associated hypercalcemia. As mentioned earlier hypercalcemia may be associated with hyperphosphatemia or hypophosphatemia. Urine usually contains increased amounts of Ca^{2+}. Measurements of PTHrP and $1,25(OH)_2D_3$ or serum Mg^{2+} are needed in some cases to prove the nature of malignancy-associated,

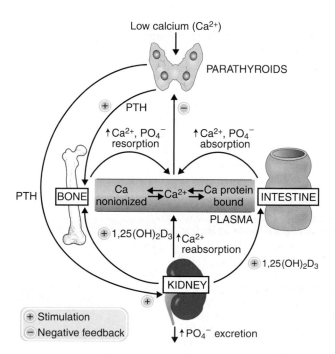

Figure 1-21 Pathogenesis of hypercalcemia in hyperparathyroidism. $1,25(OH)_2D_3$, 1,25-dihydroxyvitamin D_3; PTH, parathyroid hormone.

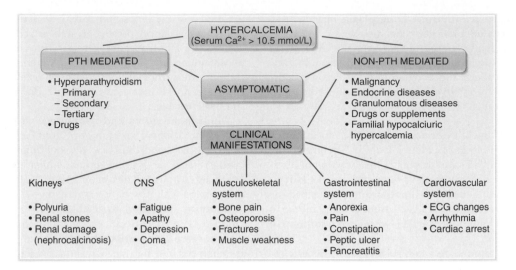

Figure 1-22 Causes and consequences of hypercalcemia. CNS, central nervous system; ECG, electrocardiographic; PTH, parathyroid hormone.

vitamin D-associated, or magnesium toxicity-related hypercalcemia.

Most patients have vague symptoms, such as fatigue, malaise, weakness, or depression. Various clinical signs and symptoms linked to hypercalcemia can be grouped by organ systems (only in retrospect) as follows:

- **Renal symptoms**—polyuria and polydipsia, renal calculi, nephrocalcinosis
- **Musculoskeletal symptoms**—bone pain, fractures, or demineralization and osteoporosis; muscle weakness and hypotonia; gout, pseudogout, and periarticular calcifications
- **Neurologic symptoms**—weakness, fatigue, apathy, or depression
- **Gastrointestinal symptoms**—abdominal pain, anorexia, constipation, peptic ulcer disease, pancre-atitis
- **Cardiovascular symptoms**—arrhythmia and ECG changes and, in extreme cases, even cardiac arrest

Phosphorus

The body contains approximately 600 g of phosphorus, which is equally distributed in the intracellular and the extracellular fluid. The bulk of the phosphorus (85%) is located in the bones and teeth (Fig. 1-23). Approximately 14% of phosphorus is inside the cells or bound to the organic extracellular matrix of soft tissue, and less than 1% is present in the extracellular fluid. Inside the cells it is present in the form of inorganic free anions or as part of various organophosphates, such as phosphoproteins, phospholipids, or nuclei acids and energy-rich compounds (ADP, ATP, cAMP, etc.).

In the extracellular fluid the blood phosphorus is present mostly as a mixture of monohydrogen and dihydrogen phosphates, known as alkaline (HPO_4^{-2}) and acid phosphate ($H_2PO_4^{-}$). Approximately 10% of serum phosphorus is bound to proteins, but in contrast to calcium this component is not important for estimating the total serum

Table 1-11 Causes of Hypercalcemia Related to Serum Parathyroid Hormone Levels

ELEVATED PTH	NORMAL/DECREASED PTH LEVELS
Primary hyperparathyroidism	Malignant tumors (measure PTHrP)
Secondary hyperparathyroidism	Endocrine disorders
Chronic renal failure	Hyperthyroidism
Vitamin D deficiency	Addison's disease
Tertiary hyperparathyroidism	Growth hormone excess
Drugs (e.g., lithium, theophylline)	Granulomatous diseases
Familial hypocalciuric hypercalcemia	Hypervitaminosis A and D
	Drugs (e.g., thiazides, tamoxifen)
	Immobilization of children and adolescents

PTH, parathyroid hormone; PTHrP, parathyroid hormone-related protein.
Based on data from Bourke E, Delaney V: Assessment of hypocalcemia and hypercalcemia. Clin Lab Med 1993;13:157–181.

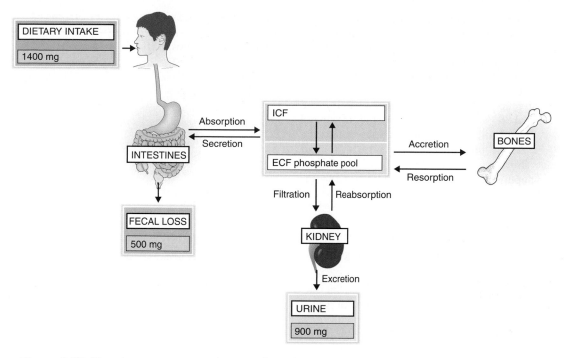

Figure 1-23 Phosphorus turnover under normal conditions. ECF, extracellular fluid; ICF, intracellular fluid.

concentration of phosphorus. The concentration of phosphorus in serum is expressed as milligrams or millimoles of elemental phosphorus, and it is normally 3 to 4.5 mg/dL (0.7–1.4 mmol/L).

The kidney plays the crucial role in the homeostasis of phosphorus. Alkaline and acid phosphates are filtered through the glomeruli in a ratio of 4:1, and the alkaline is converted into the acid as a result of H^+ secretion in the proximal tubules. Ninety-five percent of the filtered phosphate is then reabsorbed in the proximal tubule. PTH inhibits reabsorption of phosphate in the proximal tubule, promoting phosphaturia. Since the serum phosphorus and calcium are in a reciprocal relationship, hypophosphatemia resulting from excessive loss of phosphate in urine is associated with hypercalcemia.

Hypophosphatemia may result from inadequate absorption or increased loss of phosphorus or be due to a shift from the extracellular to the intracellular compartment.

Severe hypophosphatemia is rare, but modest reduction of serum phosphorus concentration may occur quite often, even though only temporarily. It reflects either reduced absorption or increased loss of phosphorus or its redistribution within the body. The causes of hypophosphatemia are listed in Table 1-12.

The normal American diet contains enough phosphorus, and a nutritional deficiency occurs only in severe malnutri-

tion. Nutritional recovery in such persons is also associated with hypophosphatemia, mostly due to the redistribution of phosphate into the cells due to increased carbohydrate

Table 1-12 Causes of Hypophosphatemia

Reduced Absorption and Intake
Chronic malnutrition
Chronic alcoholism
Abuse of phosphate-binding antacids (aluminum
  hydroxide)

Increased Loss/Removal
Hyperparathyroidism
Vitamin D deficiency
Hemodialysis
Peritoneal dialysis

**Shift of Phosphates from Extracellular
to Intracellular Space**
Insulin and carbohydrate metabolism
  Infusion of glucose or insulin
  Treatment of diabetic acidosis
  Nutritional recovery after starvation
  Hyperalimentation
  Severe burns
Alkalosis
  Respiratory alkalosis
  Bicarbonate infusion
Extracellular fluid volume expansion

metabolism. Abuse of phosphate-binding antacids, such as aluminum hydroxide, may prevent normal absorption.

Hyperparathyroidism leads to hyperphosphaturia and may cause hypophosphatemia. Likewise, vitamin D deficiency or disturbances in activation of vitamin D may cause hypophosphatemia.

Infusion of glucose or insulin, especially during the treatment of diabetic acidosis, leads to a shift of glucose into cells. Potassium, like phosphate, also moves into the cells from the extracellular space. A shift from acidosis to alkalosis may also contribute to this shift. Alkalosis itself may cause hypophosphatemia, especially if induced by bicarbonate infusion.

Hypophosphatemia may affect the function of muscles and the nervous system as well as oxygen delivery.

The symptoms of hypophosphatemia are nonspecific. Severe hypophosphatemia is characterized by muscle weakness, which may involve the respiratory muscles and cause respiratory insufficiency. Cardiac arrhythmia is also found. Neurologic symptoms include confusion, but in severe cases it may progress to coma with convulsions.

Hypophosphatemia results in a reduction of 2,3-diphosphoglycerate (2,3-DPG) in red blood cells, which adversely affects their ability to transport oxygen. Generalized hypoxia may result, and the vital organs may be imperiled. Hemolysis and hypercalciuria with excessive excretion of magnesium in urine are found during laboratory studies.

Phosphate may be given orally or intravenously, but when using the latter method, levels of serum calcium, phosphates, potassium, sodium, and chloride should be carefully monitored. Milk is a good source of phosphorus.

Hyperphosphatemia is most often caused by renal failure or extensive cell lysis.

The most common causes of hyperphosphatemia are listed in Table 1-13.

Chronic renal failure is the most significant cause of hyperphosphatemia. Renal injury prevents excretion of phosphorus. Hyperphosphatemia impairs further the already reduced synthesis of activated vitamin D ($1,25[OH]_2D_3$), which contributes to reducing the concentration of serum Ca^{2+} and secondary parathyroid hyperplasia.

Massive cell lysis under various conditions causes a release of intracellular phosphorus into the extracellular space. This occurs in the so-called tumor lysis syndrome during chemotherapy, rhabdomyolysis of skeletal muscles during strenuous effort or trauma (especially crush injury), and heat stroke. Massive liver necrosis or hemolytic reactions also cause hyperphosphatemia.

Table 1-13 Causes of Hyperphosphatemia

Pseudohyperphosphatemia
Hemolysis of blood
Multiple myeloma

Increased Intake
Rectal phosphate enema
Intravenous phosphate

Cell Lysis
Tumor lysis syndrome
Rhabdomyolysis/crush injury
Heat stroke
Hepatic necrosis
Severe hemolytic anemia/transfusion reaction

Diminished Excretion
Renal failure

Pearl

> Hemolyzed blood is a major source of spurious hyperphosphatemia.

Hyperphosphatemia leads to hypocalcemia and metastatic calcification.

Hyperphosphatemia of acute onset is associated with **hypocalcemia,** which may manifest with tetany and spastic contraction of skeletal muscles. Seizures and disturbances of cardiac rhythm ensue, and, in severe cases, the patient may die.

Hyperphosphatemia may cause **metastatic calcifications** in many systems. This occurs when the serum calcium × phosphorus product exceeds a critical value, and the calcium phosphate becomes insoluble. Most dangerous are deposits in the kidneys that may impair the ability of the kidney to excrete minerals and waste product and cause renal insufficiency. **Calciphylaxis** is a severe form of such calcification of skin, soft tissues, and vessels associated with dermal ulcerations.

Trace elements are found in very small amounts in the body, but most of them are essential for the maintenance of health.

The human body contains some 40 chemical elements. The nine major ones (hydrogen, oxygen, nitrogen, sodium, potassium, calcium, chloride, phosphorus, and sulfate) constitute 99% of the total body weight of chemical elements, whereas the remaining 1% are classified as oligominerals or trace elements. Many of these trace elements are essential for certain physiological processes, but it is also worth remembering that they may be toxic if present in high concentrations. These trace elements can be measured in body fluids and tissues, in which they are often bound to specific carrier proteins. The most important trace elements and their functions are listed in Table 1-14.

Table 1-14 Trace Elements

ELEMENT	PROTEIN CARRIER	FUNCTION	DISORDERS
Iron	Hemoglobin	Oxygen transport	Anemia
	Transferrin, ferritin	Transport, storage	—
	Cytochrome enzymes	Cell respiration	—
Copper	Ceruloplasmin	Transport, storage	Wilson's disease
		Coenzyme	—
Magnesium	—	Like calcium	—
Iodine	Thyroxin	Hormone function	Hypothyroidism
Selenium	Glutathione peroxidase	Antioxidant	Cardiomyopathy
Cobalt	B_{12} vitamin	—	Cardiomyopathy

Proteins

Proteins are essential components of all cells and are found in all extracellular fluids of the body. All living cells can synthesize proteins for internal purposes, but some, such as liver or plasma cells, also secrete proteins into the extracellular fluid. Proteins have numerous biologic functions and serve as structural elements of the cell membranes and organelles, as enzymes, carrier molecules, buffers, oncotic molecules, and so on.

With a few notable exceptions, such as immunoglobulins, most plasma proteins are produced by the liver. Inside the circulation plasma proteins perform complex functions, such as during the coagulation sequence, during which they may be consumed. Proteins are taken up by endothelial cells, macrophages, and specialized parenchymal cells such as hepatocytes or endocrine cells. Plasma proteins are filtered through the glomeruli and may be lost in urine, but are also secreted into various ECF compartments (e.g., pleural fluid) or into the gastrointestinal juices. Hence the study of plasma proteins may give some information about the functioning of many organ systems and numerous diseases such as:

- Infections
- Autoimmune diseases
- Hematologic diseases
- Liver diseases
- Gastrointestinal diseases
- Cardiovascular diseases

Proteins can be analyzed using several analytic methods, which can be chosen depending on desired degree of specificity.

Proteins can be measured not only in plasma and serum but also in various other body fluids, such as urine, pleural effusion, cerebrospinal fluid, and amniotic fluid. In most instances the first step involves quantification with laboratory instruments. In some instances, as in protein analysis of urine, a semiquantitative approach with a "dipstick" can be used.

The qualitative analysis of serum proteins may be limited to a crude measurement of the two major components, **albumin** and **globulin (A:G),** or it may involve more detailed separation of the protein fraction of serum. Under normal circumstances the A:G ratio is 3:1. Many inflammatory conditions change the A:G ratio by suppressing the hepatic production of albumin or by stimulating the production of immunoglobulins. In autoimmune hepatitis the A:G ratio may actually be reversed, and the serum may contain more globulin than albumin.

In some instances it may be necessary to target the study to a **specific protein,** such as ceruloplasmin in Wilson's disease or transferrin in hemochromatosis. Proteins that serve as enzymes may be quantitated by measuring their enzymatic activity, which is typically expressed as international units of enzymatic activity per fluid volume (e.g., IU/dL).

Electrophoresis is a relatively simple method used in the laboratory for analyzing serum proteins. In a solution exposed to electric current, serum proteins separate into five fractions labeled **albumin** and α_1, α_2, β, and γ **globulins** (Fig. 1-24). Each of the globulin fractions contains numerous proteins, only some of which are listed here. In some persons and in fetal blood and infants there is a sixth fraction called **prealbumin,** which contains transthyretin, a thyroid hormone and retinol-binding protein.

Albumin is the most abundant plasma protein, exceeding the globulins at a rate of 2:1.

Under normal circumstances the concentration of proteins in plasma is in the range of 6 to 8 g/dL. Albumin accounts for two thirds, and globulins for the remaining one third. Hence the A:G ratio is normally 2:1. The most important plasma proteins are briefly discussed here.

Albumin. Under physiologic conditions—that is, in slightly alkaline pH (7.35) albumin is negatively charged and

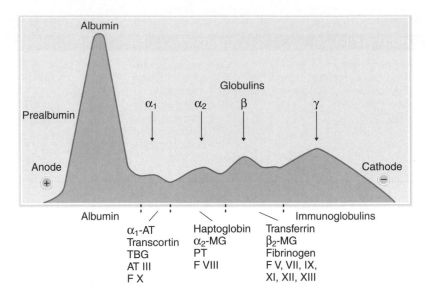

Figure 1-24 Serum protein electrophoresis. The proteins are separated into five major fractions, including albumin and four globulin fractions labeled α_1, α_2, β, and γ.

migrates fast toward the anode. Albumin has numerous physiological functions acting in the blood as

- Principal oncotic protein in the blood, accounting for 80% of oncotic activity of the plasma
- Buffer
- Source of amino acids for the synthesis of other proteins
- Transport protein for calcium, free fatty acids, bilirubin, hormones, drugs, and so on
- Antioxidant
- Regulator of capillary permeability

Plasma contains 3.5 to 5.2 g/dL albumin. Albumin is synthesized by the liver and lost in small amounts in urine (30 mg/24 hours) and feces. Increased concentration of albumin typically results in dehydration. Hypoalbuminemia may result from decreased synthesis of albumin in the liver or increased loss though the kidneys, intestines, or external body surface. Albumin synthesis is depressed in many diseases, most likely through the action of cytokines such as interleukin-6 (IL-6) (Table 1-15).

Pearl

> Spurious hypoalbuminemia is commonly seen in pregnancy. It is related to increased plasma volume.

- **α_1-globulin.** This fraction contains a_1-antitrypsin, a_1-fetoprotein, a_1-acid glycoprotein, and a_1-lipoprotein.
  - **α_1-antitrypsin,** a serine protease inhibitor, accounts for 90% of this fraction. In α_1-antitrypsin deficiency

Table 1-15 Causes of Hypoalbuminemia

Decreased Intake or Synthesis
Malnutrition
Chronic liver disease
Malabsorption syndrome
Cachexia of chronic disease

Increased Loss
Nephrotic syndrome
Protein losing enteropathy
Burns
Bleeding

the α_1-globulin fraction of serum is visibly decreased.

- **α_1-fetoprotein** (AFP) is a major fetal protein and is prominent in the serum of fetuses and infants. It is also increased in patients who have liver cell carcinoma and gonadal and extragonadal germ cell tumors. AFP is also increased in the serum of women who carry fetuses with Down syndrome or neural tube anomalies and atresia of the gastrointestinal tract.
- **α_2-globulin.** This fraction contains α_2-macroglobulin, haptoglobin, and ceruloplasmin.
  - **α_2-macroglobulin** is a protease inhibitor that has a molecular weight of 750 kD and is thus one of the largest proteins in the blood. In nephrotic syndrome, its concentration is increased in part because it is not lost in urine and in part because its synthesis is increased to compensate for the loss of albumin and provide oncotic strength to plasma.

- **Haptoglobin** binds free hemoglobin during intravascular hemolysis and serves to clear hemoglobin from the circulation.
- **Ceruloplasmin,** a copper-containing protein with ferroxidase activity, is important for transport of iron and copper. It is decreased in Wilson's disease, a disorder of copper metabolism. Ceruloplasmin is an **acute-phase protein,** and its concentration in plasma is increased in various diseases as well in pregnancy.
- **β-globulin.** This fraction contains transferrin, C3 and C4 complement, β₂-microglobulin, fibrinogen, and C-reactive protein.
  - **Transferrin** is the major iron-transporting protein, and its concentration correlates with the total iron-binding capacity (TIBC) of the serum. Transferrin concentration is reduced in chronic anemia.
  - **Complement factors C3 and C4** are involved in many inflammatory and immune reactions. C3 and C4 concentration in blood is reduced in active autoimmune disorders, such as systemic lupus erythematosus.
  - **β₂-microglobulin** is the light-chain portion of the class I human leukocyte antigen expressed on nucleated blood cells and cells forming many tissues. β₂-microglobulin is filtered in the glomeruli, but almost all of it is reabsorbed and a decreased concentration of this protein in plasma is found only in the presence of tubular malabsorption. Its concentration in blood is increased in patients who have B-cell lymphoma and leukemia or multiple myeloma.
  - **Fibrinogen** is a high-molecular-weight protein involved in coagulation. The coagulation cascade leads to the polymerization of fibrinogen into fibrin, which forms the meshwork of the clot.
- **γ-globulin.** This fraction contains predominantly immunoglobulins and C-reactive protein.
  - **Immunoglobulins.** There are five classes of immunoglobulins, called so because they participate in the immune reactions. IgG accounts for 80% of total immunoglobulins, whereas IgA and IgM account for 15%. IgE and IgD are found in small amounts. **Hypogammaglobulinemia** is a feature of primary (congenital) or secondary immunodeficiencies. **Hypergammaglobulinemia** may be polyclonal, as in infections or chronic autoimmune diseases, or monoclonal, as in multiple myeloma (Fig. 1-25).
  - **C-reactive protein (CRP)** is an important component of the γ-globulin fraction that participates in many inflammatory processes. Under normal circumstances it is present in barely detectable amounts (<10 mg/dL), but in infection or any form of physiologic stress and in many chronic diseases its serum concentration may increase a thousand times (Fig. 1-26). At this point it may become visible even in routine electrophoresis. C-reactive protein can be used for monitoring infectious diseases, chronic conditions such as rheumatoid arthritis, and rejection of transplanted organs. In patients with chronic coronary heart disease or angina pectoris CRP is also predictive of future coronary occlusions. C-reactive protein is the principal acute-phase reactant, and as such its serum concentration correlates well with erythrocyte sedimentation rate (ESR). Other acute-phase proteins are listed in Table 1-16.

The catalytic activity of certain serum enzymes may be measured in the clinical laboratory for diagnostic purposes.

Enzymes are proteins that catalyze certain chemical reactions. The activity of an enzyme can be determined by measuring the rate of the chemical reaction catalyzed by the enzyme. Enzymes are classified as oxidoreductases, transferases, hydrolases, lyases, isomerases, and ligases. Among the thousands of enzymes in the body only a few are important from the diagnostic point of view. Some of these enzymes appear in the

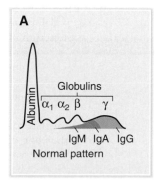
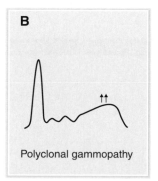
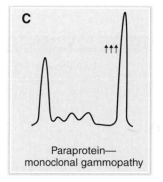
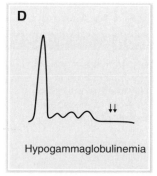

Figure 1-25 Serum electrophoresis patterns. **A,** Normal serum, **B,** Polyclonal gammopathy, **C,** Monoclonal gammopathy, **D,** Hypogammaglobulinemia.

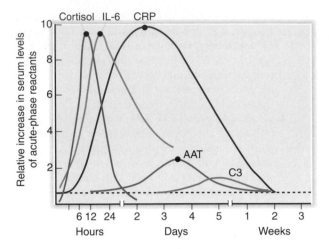

Figure 1-26 Response to acute disease. It includes a release of cortisol, interleukin, and acute-phase proteins. AAT, α_1-antichymotrypsin; C3, complement; CRP, C-reactive protein; IL-6, interleukin-6.

blood, and their activity can be measured in serum. Examples of serum enzymes with diagnostic significance follow:

■ **Aminotransferases.** These enzymes catalyze the transfer of amines from one amino acid to another. **Aspartate aminotransferase (AST)** and **alanine aminotransferase (ALT)** are two enzymes typically included in the laboratory panel known under the name of liver function tests (see Chapter 9). AST is found mostly in the mitochondria of liver cells, but 20% is found in the cytosol. ALT is located only in the cytosol. Both enzymes leak out of the damaged liver cells and appear in blood. AST and ALT are elevated in the serum of patients who have acute viral hepatitis or toxin- or drug-induced liver cell necrosis. Both AST and ALT are found in other organs besides the liver, but in proper context they are very sensitive markers of liver cell injury.

■ **Alkaline phosphatase.** This enzyme manifests in blood in several isoforms. In a healthy person the

blood contains predominantly the isozyme derived from the bone. It may be increased in growing children and persons who have osteoblastic lesions—osteoblastic tumors. Increased activity of alkaline phosphatase is encountered in biliary obstruction, which stimulates the synthesis of alkaline phosphates in hepatocytes. Combined with bilirubin, alkaline phosphatase is a good marker of biliary obstruction.

■ **Lactate dehydrogenase (LDH).** This ubiquitous enzyme appears in the serum in five isoenzymes. Increased activity of LDH in serum is found in **neoplastic states;** when LDH is released from tumor cells; or in conditions marked by **cell lysis** or **tissue injury,** such as massive hemolysis, myocardial infarction, renal infarction, shock, and many others. The analysis of LDH isozymes was previously used in the diagnosis of myocardial infarction, characterized by a ratio between isozyme LD_1 and LD_2, and a reversal of the $LD_1:LD_2$ ratio over the value of 1, colloquially known as "$LD_1:LD_2$ flip."

■ **Creatine kinase (CK).** This enzyme is found in skeletal and striated muscle; in blood it appears in the form of three isoforms known as CK-MM, CK-MB, and CK-BB. Creatine kinase is a sensitive marker of muscle injury, but the use of CK-MB as a marker of myocardial infarction has been diminished due to the widespread use of troponins.

Protein degradation products are excreted in urine, and their elevated concentration in serum may be a sign of renal failure.

Urea and creatinine are the two most important protein degradation products normally found in blood. Urea is produced in the liver from ammonia—the main end product of protein degradation. Creatinine is derived from the skeletal muscle creatine and phosphocreatine.

Blood urea nitrogen (BUN) concentration in normal healthy persons is in the range of 10 to 15 mg/dL (3.6 and 5.4 mmol/L, respectively). Since urea is excreted in urine,

Table 1-16 Acute-phase Proteins

PROTEIN	PRINCIPAL FUNCTION	DEGREE OF ELEVATION IN DISEASE
C-reactive protein	Proinflammatory	+++
Serum amyloid A	Proinflammatory	+++
α_1-Antichymotrypsin	Protease inhibitor	++
α_1-Acid glycoprotein	Tissue repair	++
Ceruloplasmin	Copper transport	++
Transferrin	Iron transport	++
Fibrinogen	Coagulation	++
Haptoglobin	Free hemoglobin binding	+
Hemopexin	Free hemoglobin binding	+
C3 complement	Proinflammatory	+

Based on data from Marshall WJ, Bangert SK: Clinical Biochemistry: Metabolic and Clinical Aspects, Churchill Livingstone, New York, 1995.

Table 1-17 Major Lipoprotein Classes

PROPERTY	CHYLOMICRONS	VLDL	LDL	HDL
Origin	Intestine	Liver	VLDL	Intestine, liver, other LP
Protein content	1%	10%	20%	50%
Major lipid	TG (90%)	TG (90%)	Cholesterol (50%)	PL (25%) Cholesterol (20%)
Transport function	TG from GI tract to liver	TG out of liver	Cholesterol relay	Cholesterol transport to the liver

GI, gastrointestinal; HDL, high-density lipoprotein; LDL, low-density lipoproteins; LP, lipoprotein; PL, phospholipids; TG, triglyceride; VLDL, very low density lipoprotein.

BUN is elevated in persons with renal failure, prerenal failure due to renal hypoperfusion, shock, or volume depletion. Other causes of elevated BUN are GI bleeding, stress, drugs (e.g., aminoglycosides), and corticosteroids. Decreased BUN is found in starving patients or those with liver failure, overhydration, or polyuria and nephritic syndrome. Infancy and pregnancy also may cause elevated BUN. Severe elevation of BUN over 150 mg/dL is almost invariably a sign of renal failure. However, since the concentration of BUN depends on so many factors, it is less reliable for estimating early stages of renal failure than creatinine.

Creatinine concentration in blood is in the range from 0.6 to 1.0 mg/dL (53–88 μmol/L). Creatinine production is relatively constant, approximately 20 mg/kg/day. It is removed almost exclusively by the kidney. Since 85% of filtered creatinine is removed in urine, its rise in the blood is a sensitive indicator of reduced GFR.

Lipids and Lipoproteins

The lipids occur in plasma in two major forms: cholesterol and triglycerides. Both of these lipids are insoluble in water and must be complexed with apoproteins to form one of the four lipoproteins: chylomicrons, very low density lipoproteins (VLDLs), low-density lipoproteins (LDLs), and high-density lipoproteins (HDLs). The main features of these four classes of lipoproteins are listed in Table 1-17.

Lipoproteins can be separated one from another by centrifugation or by electrophoresis, which is done in detailed studies of lipoprotein disorders. In a routine laboratory work-up it is customary to determine only the concentration of total triglycerides, total cholesterol, LDL cholesterol, and HDL cholesterol.

The desirable levels of serum lipids are as follows:

- Triglycerides, males 40 to 160 mg/dL; females 35 to 135 mg/dL
- Total cholesterol below 200 mg/dL
- LDL cholesterol below 100 mg/dL
- HDL cholesterol over 60 mg/dL

Hyperlipidemias are classified as primary (genetic) hyperlipoproteinemias or secondary dislipoproteinemias.

Familial hypercholesterolemia, the most common single-gene defect related hyperlipidemia affecting 1:500 Americans, is associated with an elevation of both cholesterol and triglycerides. Familial combined hyperlipidemia, a polygenic disorder representing the most common form of primary hyperlipidemia, is characterized by a highly variable pattern of lipid disorders. Numerous conditions are associated with secondary dislipoproteinemia. The changes in the blood lipids in the most common forms of secondary hyperlipidemia are listed in Table 1-18.

Table 1-18 Causes of Secondary Hyperlipidemiaw

CONDITION	CHANGES IN SERUM LIPIDS		
	TRIGLYCERIDES	CHOLESTEROL	HDL CHOLESTEROL
Diabetes mellitus	+	+/−	−
Obesity	+	+/−	−
Alcoholism	+/−	+	+
Hypothyroidism	+/−	+	+/−
Nephrotic syndrome	+/−	+	+/−
Biliary obstruction	+/−	+	+/−
Antihypertensive drugs	+	+/−	−

+, elevated; −, lowered; +/−, unchanged or only slightly increased.

Carbohydrates

Carbohydrates are absorbed from the food and processed in the liver, which serves also as their main storage site. Carbohydrates are stored in the liver as glycogen and are released into the blood mostly as glucose. Glucose is an important source of energy for many organs. Skeletal muscles preferentially utilize glucose during the initial stages of exercise. The brain critically depends on the constant supply of glucose, which is the only fuel this organ can use. Even though the blood contains relatively small amounts of the total body glucose it can be readily measured. The glucose concentration of blood is tightly controlled hormonally and is kept within a close range from 70 to 105 mg/dL (3.9–5.8 mmol/L). Hyperglycemia is most often caused by diabetes mellitus. Hypoglycemia is most likely caused by overzealous treatment of diabetes. The most important causes of hypoglycemia are listed in Table 1-19.

Table 1-19 Most Important Causes of Hypoglycemia

Drugs
Insulin and other antidiabetic drugs
β-Adrenergic antagonists
Sulfonamides

Major Organ Failure
Liver, kidney, heart failure
Shock and sepsis

Malnutrition
Anorexia nervosa

Hormone Deficiencies
Adrenal failure
Hypopituitarism

Tumors
Insulin producing tumors (e.g., insulinoma of pancreas)
IGF producing tumors (e.g., leiomyosarcoma)
Glucose-storing and -consuming tumors (e.g., hepatocellular carcinoma)

IGF, insulin growth factor.

CASE STUDIES

Case 1 PROLONGED VOMITING DUE TO PYLORIC STENOSIS

Clinical history A 5-week-old infant boy was hospitalized because of prolonged projectile vomiting that occurred after each feeding over the period of several days.[1]

Physical findings The boy appeared to be in great distress. He was dehydrated, lethargic, and his breathing was shallow. The radiographic study of the upper GI tract revealed pyloric stenosis.[2]

Laboratory findings Sodium 140 mmol/L, potassium 3.1 mmol/L, chloride 95 mmol/L, pH 7.54, P_{CO_2} 45 mm Hg, bicarbonate 40 mmol/L.[3]

Outcome The child was rehydrated and the electrolyte and acid–base imbalance was corrected to prepare the child for surgery. Following pylorotomy the child recovered completely and did not have any more problems.

Questions and topics for discussion
1. What is lost during prolonged vomiting? What are the consequences?
2. What is pyloric stenosis? What is the cause and underlying pathology of this disease in infants?
3. Interpret these laboratory findings and explain their pathogenesis and significance.

Case 2 LOSS OF CONSCIOUSNESS FOLLOWING A DRUG OVERDOSE

Clinical history A 20-year-old man was found comatose in a public bathroom, with a rubber band around his arm and a syringe next to him. He was transferred to the emergency department.

Physical findings The patient was unconscious and his breathing was shallow. Auscultation revealed prominent crackles over both lungs, and the chest radiograph showed signs suggestive of pulmonary edema.

Laboratory findings The blood was drawn for blood gas analysis, and the following data were obtained: pH 7.30, P_{CO_2} 56 mm Hg, bicarbonate 24 mmol/L, P_{O_2} 70 mm Hg.[1]

Outcome The patient was treated and recovered completely.[2]

Questions and topics for discussion
1. Which acid–base disturbance has developed?
2. What is the treatment of this condition?

Case 3 FREQUENT URINATION, THIRST, AND CONSTANT COUGH IN A CHRONIC SMOKER

Clinical history   A 60-year-old man, known to smoke two packs of cigarettes per day for 40 years, complained that he has a constant urge to urinate.[1] He was also constantly thirsty and drank at least 4 to 5 L of fluid per day.[2] He also complained that he coughed a lot and produced abundant sputum.

Physical findings   Chest auscultation findings were consistent with chronic bronchitis. Chest radiograph revealed a mass in the hilum of the right lung.[3] Radiographic examination of the skeleton disclosed no abnormalities. No other abnormalities were found.

Laboratory findings   Serum calcium 12.0 mg/dL, serum phosphorus 2.4 mg/dL. Serum parathyroid hormone (PTH) was not detectable.[4]

Lung biopsy revealed that the mass was a malignant tumor.[5]

An additional blood sample was drawn, and the serum was sent to a reference laboratory to measure parathyroid hormone-related polypeptide (PTHrP).[6]

Outcome   PTHrP test was positive. The lung tumor was resected and the patient's condition, including the urinary problems, improved.[7]

Questions and topics for discussion
1. What are possible causes for frequent urination in a 60-year-old man? What additional information would you need to decide about further work-up?
2. What is the medical term for increased thirst and drinking of large amounts of fluid? What could cause such symptoms?
3. What is the lung mass? What work-up would you recommend for such a patient to determine the nature of the lung lesion?
4. Why was the test for PTH ordered?
5. How could a lung tumor cause frequent urination and increased thirst? Which histologic type of lung cancer would you expect to find under these conditions?
6. What is PTHrP? Why would you measure this hormone in this patient?
7. Why did the urinary problems improve? List all the diseases you would mention in the epicrisis on discharging this patient from the hospital.

Case 4 POISONING WITH ANTIFREEZE

Clinical history   A homeless person was found lying unconscious next to a gas station, and an empty bottle of antifreeze was found next to him.[1] He was transferred to the hospital. He was placed into the intensive care unit, and a venous blood sample was sent to the lab.

Laboratory findings   Na 135 mmol/ L, K 4.0 mmol/L, Cl 92 mmol/L, glucose 100 mg/dL, BUN 40 mg/dL, creatinine 3.0 mg/dL, pH 7.28, bicarbonate 18 mmol/L.[2–4]

Outcome   Following intensive therapy[5] the patient recovered.

Questions and topics for discussion
1. What is the toxic substance in antifreeze? What are the signs of antifreeze poisoning?
2. Does this patient have acidosis or alkalosis, and is it respiratory or metabolic?
3. Is there an anion gap in the blood? Please explain what is happening.
4. Is there an osmolal gap?
5. What is the treatment of this form of poisoning?

Chapter 2

SIGNS AND SYMPTOMS

Introduction

The clinical diagnosis of disease is based on the recognition and proper interpretation of its manifestation, commonly known as signs and symptoms. The term **symptom** is used for features that are recognized subjectively by the affected person, whereas **signs** are more objectively noticeable and can be recognized by the nurse or doctor during physical examination, by ancillary methods and tests, by another person associated with the patient, or by the patient himself or herself.

Most symptoms and many signs are usually described during the medical history interview when the patient presents to the physician. Other signs are discovered during the **physical examination** and clinical work-up. The most important findings detected by physical examination are listed in Table 2-1.

The ultimate significance of all signs and symptoms discovered during the initial work-up is not always obvious, and the physician must often use inductive and deductive reasoning in interpreting them. Often it is necessary to formulate one or more working hypotheses and develop a list of various similar conditions to be included in the **differential diagnosis.** Many of these conditions must be excluded by additional testing until the tentative diagnosis is reached (Fig. 2-1). This tentative diagnosis functions as a working hypothesis until confirmed by other means, which often include definitive or pathognomonic pathologic findings. Prior to instituting any therapy, it is desirable to make the **definitive diagnosis** formulated in terms of precise etiology, **pathogenesis, pathophysiology,** and **underlying pathology.**

The signs and symptoms of various diseases may be classified as **systemic** or centered on a **specific organ system.** The important and common systemic signs and symptoms are described here, but most of the organ system-centered signs and symptoms will be discussed in subsequent chapters. Table 2-2 contains a list of the most common systemic and organ-centered signs and symptoms encountered in general medical practice.

Table 2-1 Clinical Findings That Can Be Noted During Physical Examination

Overall Assessment
Extent of distress and severity of disease
Mental status
Mobility and the degree of incapacity
Vital signs (temperature, pulse rate, respiratory rate, blood pressure)

Review of Systems
Ear, nose, and throat inspection (including otoscopy)
Eye inspection (assessment of movement and reactions, fundoscopy)
Neck inspection and palpation
Cardiovascular system (auscultation of heart sounds or murmurs, signs of cyanosis or edema)
Respiratory system (ease of respiration, percussion, and auscultation for respiratory sounds, extraneous sounds)
Abdominal organs (palpation and percussion to determine the size of the liver and spleen, fluid or intra-abdominal masses, auscultation of bowel sounds)
Extremities (including joints, muscles, and neural reflexes)
Skin and hairy scalp (inspection and palpation)

Fatigue

Fatigue, or tiredness, is the normal physiologic response to demanding exercise or any other prolonged physical or mental activity. Physiologically, it can be most easily

Anorexia Lack of appetite sometimes associated with aversion to food.

Cachexia Generalized weakness, wasting, and weight loss caused by cancer or other debilitating chronic diseases.

Coma State of deep unconsciousness accompanied by a loss of responsiveness to external stimuli. The depth of coma can be graded; in the most severe form it is irreversible.

Edema Localized or generalized excessive accumulation of fluid in the interstitial spaces of various tissues or body cavities. When generalized it is called anasarca.

Fatigue Feeling of tiredness and inability to perform optimally. It occurs physiologically at the end of prolonged effort or as a sign of disease.

Fever (pyrexia) Increased body temperature over the upper limits of normal. It may be a physiologic response to endogenous or exogenous influences that accelerate the metabolism or raise the body temperature. Most often it is a consequence of diseases that produce endogenous pyrogens acting on the hypothalamic thermoregulatory center.

Headache (cephalalgia) Pain in the head caused by a variety of mechanisms affecting the intracranial or extracranial structures of the head.

Hemorrhage (bleeding) Escape of blood from the vessels into the tissues, hollow organs, or external environment.

Pain Unpleasant or distressing feeling based on a psychological reaction to sensory stimuli generated in specialized nerve endings in the skin, muscles, and many internal organs.

Sign Manifestation of a disease that can be recognized objectively by medical examination.

Symptom Manifestation of a disease recognized subjectively by the affected patient.

Syncope (faint, swoon) Temporary loss of consciousness related to a sudden onset of generalized cerebral ischemia.

Weight loss Voluntary or involuntary loss of body mass, empirically defined as exceeding 5% of the body weight over a 6-month period.

---

measured in the **muscles,** which, when fatigued, cannot maintain a contraction or respond progressively slowly to stimuli, until finally no reaction can be elicited from them. In such cases the muscles are simply depleted of fuel in form of nutrients (e.g., glycogen) and energy-rich compounds like creatine phosphate or adenosine triphosphate (ATP) (Fig. 2-2). The accumulation of lactic acid and the acidification of the internal milieu inhibit actin–myosin interaction and muscle cell contraction. Increased concentration of phosphorus in the cytosol affects the release of calcium from internal stores (e.g., sarcoplasmic reticulum), preventing its catalytic action on the contractile fibers.

Psychological fatigue can ensue after prolonged mental effort, excitement, stress, and even lack of sleep. The underlying pathogenesis of psychological fatigue is less well known. Both muscle fatigue and psychological fatigue are relieved by rest.

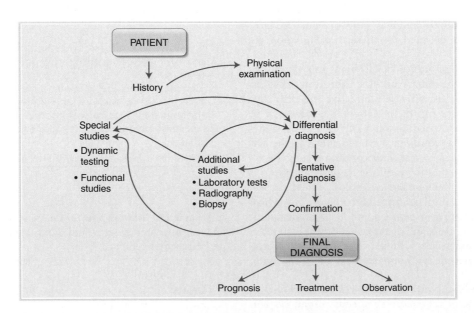

Figure 2-1 Diagnostic work-up. The complexity of the work-up varies from patient to patient, but in most instances it begins with the taking of history and physical examination. Simple or complex ancillary methods are used to arrive at a tentative (provisional) diagnosis, which, if confirmed, is used to formulate the prognosis and the treatment plan.

Table 2-2 Most Common Signs and Symptoms Encountered in General Medical Practice

PHYSICAL		PSYCHOLOGICAL/NEUROLOGIC/SENSORY
SYSTEMIC	**LOCALIZED**	
Fatigue	Pain	Anxiety
Fever	Headache	Depression
Weakness	Back pain and joint pain	Insomnia
Anorexia	Chest and abdominal pain	Irritability
Weight loss	Cough	Loss of mental prowess
Weight gain	Nasal discharge	Loss of consciousness
Swelling*	GI symptoms	Dizziness and vertigo
Itching and rash*	Shortness of breath	Gait and movement disorders
Bleeding*	Palpable ``lumps and bumps´´	Hearing loss
		Visual problems

*May be both systemic and localized. Note also that this classification includes certain entities that could belong to more than one rubric and that some physical signs and symptoms are actually manifestations of psychological/neurologic disturbances.

Fatigue is a common sign of disease.

Fatigue is a common complaint, especially in chronic diseases and after surgery or trauma. Sometimes it is even the leading symptom prompting the patient to see the doctor. Patients use the term *fatigue* rather loosely, and thus it is important to determine whether they mean exhaustion, lack of energy, weakness, or even boredom. In 50% to 60% of cases the feeling of fatigue is **psychogenic,** in 30% to 50% of cases it has an **organic** cause, and in the remaining 20% it is of **undetermined cause.** If the patient is older than 40 years of age, organic disease is found to be the underlying cause of fatigue in over 80% of cases.

Psychogenic fatigue (also known as central fatigue) is characterized by an aversion to doing anything. It is usually present before the patient gets out of bed. It fluctuates during the week and is usually less pronounced over the weekend or on holidays. It is not relieved by rest. **Anxiety states, depression,** and **sleep disorders** also may cause fatigue, which is most likely multifactorial.

Pharmacologic causes of fatigue include sleeping pills, tranquilizers, and some antihypertensive drugs. Cytostatics used in the treatment of cancer have complex effects on the intermediary metabolism and can also cause fatigue by inhibiting the normal energy-generating processes or by causing the formation of toxic byproducts. Recreational **drug abuse** is frequently associated with fatigue.

Fatigue related to systemic disease is usually mild or nonexistent in the morning but worsens during the day. It may be caused by hypothyroidism, adrenal insufficiency, chronic heart disease, lung diseases, hematologic diseases such as anemia, myelodysplastic syndrome or multiple myeloma, cirrhosis, uremia, cancer, chronic infections, and autoimmune disorders, to mention the most important ones. **Neuromuscular disorders,** such as muscular dystrophy, myasthenia gravis, multiple sclerosis, and Parkinson's disease cause fatigue with muscle weakness. The most common organic causes of fatigue are listed in Table 2-3.

Chronic fatigue syndrome is a clinical entity characterized by long-standing tiredness with no obvious physical or psychological basis. The cause of this syndrome is unknown, but it seems to be linked to psychological reactions to minor stresses in daily life. Many other explanations have been proposed and explored, but no definitive conclusion has yet been reached. The hypothesis that it is related to viral infection is not proven, even though many patients complain of upper respiratory and pharyngeal swelling and some even have enlarged lymph nodes.

The clinical diagnosis of chronic fatigue syndrome is made only if the symptoms last more than 6 months.

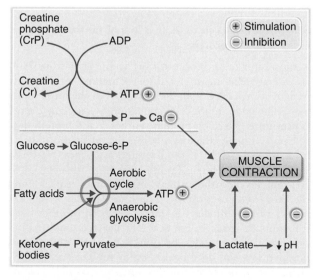

Figure 2-2 Muscle fatigue. ADP, adenine diphosphate; ATP, adenine triphosphate.

Table 2-3 Organic Causes of Fatigue

CATEGORIES OF DISEASES	CLINICAL EXAMPLES
Cardiovascular	Congestive heart failure, MI
Respiratory	Chronic obstructive pulmonary disease, asthma
Hematologic	Anemia, MDS, multiple myeloma
Endocrine	Hypothyroidism, hyperthyroidism, adrenal insufficiency
Hepatic	Cirrhosis, chronic hepatitis
Renal	Chronic renal failure
Neurologic/muscular	Myopathies, neuropathies, myasthenia gravis, multiple sclerosis
Cancer	Any form of cancer can cause fatigue
Autoimmune	Rheumatoid arthritis, SLE
Other	Obesity, malnutrition, alcohol abuse, effects of medication, radiation therapy

MDS, myelodysplastic syndrome; MI, myocardial infarction; SLE, systemic lupus erythematosus.

Muscle and joint pain are common, and headache is a prominent complaint. The extent of fatigue worsens during the day and after exertion. Other symptoms include fever that comes and wanes, abdominal pain, muscle pain, and difficulty in concentrating or sleeping. Organic symptoms such as sore throat and enlargement of lymph nodes may suggest chronic infection or neoplasia, but detailed clinical studies usually cannot prove any structural abnormalities. The laboratory studies are usually noncontributory. The treatment should include supportive measures and should be planned for each person individually, but no treatment regimen devised to date has proved successful.

Weight Loss

Weight loss results when the intake of calories is insufficient to meet the energy requirements of the body. Weight loss may be **voluntary,** as occurs in persons who are dieting, or **involuntary,** as when a caloric deficit occurs due to exogenous or endogenous factors beyond voluntary control. Medically significant involuntary weight loss is empirically defined as loss of 5% of body weight documented over a 6-month period.

Weight loss due to a loss of fluid is called **dehydration.**

Overall, weight loss can result under the following conditions:

- **Insufficient intake of food.** The causes vary over a broad range from famine related to poverty, to voluntary reduction of food intake, or that resulting from psychiatric diseases such as anorexia nervosa and bulimia.
- **Malabsorption of nutrients.** This can occur, for example, in chronic pancreatitis, intestinal malabsorption syndromes, intestinal lymphoma, amyloidosis, scleroderma, and chronic liver disease.
- **Loss of metabolites and nutrients.** Nutrients can be lost due to prolonged vomiting, diarrhea, or drainage through fistula tracts. In diabetes mellitus glucosuria and diarrhea may also cause a loss of metabolites, such as glucose loss in urine and protein loss in the stool.
- **Increased demand for nutrients and calories.** An increased demand for nutrients and calories occurs physiologically during infancy and childhood, as well as during pregnancy. Pathologically increased demand may occur in the course of chronic infections, after burns, and in patients who have malignant tumors. Metabolic disorders such as hyperthyroidism cause hypermetabolism requiring more calories.

The initial work-up for a patient who complains of weight loss must first determine if the weight loss is voluntary or involuntary. In cases of involuntary weight loss, document not only the extent but also the duration of the loss and investigate the possible causes. Determine whether the food intake is normal or decreased (Fig. 2-3). If food intake is adequate the weight loss might be related to inadequate absorption or to excessive loss or utilization of calories caused by various metabolic diseases. On the other hand, if food intake is decreased, determine whether the patient has normal or decreased appetite and then ascertain the causes of these conditions.

Starvation results initially in a loss of fat followed later on by a loss of protein.

Reduced intake of calories during voluntary fasting, famine, or anorexia nervosa results in marked loss of body weight in the range from 20% to 50% of the initial body mass. The body responds to starvation by reducing energy expenditure, reducing protein synthesis, and protein degradation. Initially, the loss involves the fat tissue, followed by a reduced weight of the liver and intestines. However, if energy intake remains low, the weight of the heart, skeletal muscles, and the kidneys also becomes reduced, and the skin becomes atrophic. The brain, however, remains intact, and the intellect is not affected. Most other body functions are reduced. For example, heartbeat and respiration slow, the muscles become weak, and the gonads produce less sex hormones. Severe protein-energy deficiency results in **marasmus,** a severe form of body wasting most commonly encountered in famine-ridden parts of Africa.

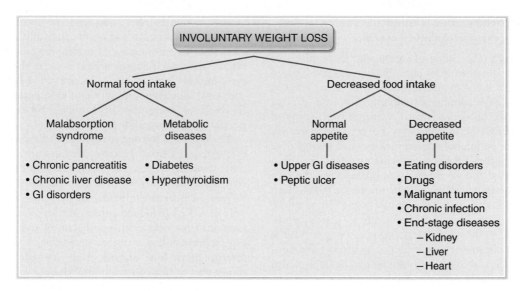

Figure 2-3 Algorithm for diagnosis of involuntary weight loss. GI, gastrointestinal.

Cachexia is characterized by involuntary weight loss caused by the complex effects of cancer or chronic diseases on the body.

Cachexia is a syndrome characterized by weakness and weight loss encountered in patients who have cancer or certain chronic infectious diseases, such as tuberculosis or AIDS. The weight loss is typically accompanied by muscle wasting, and thus the patient feels tired, weak, and unable to work. The overall basal metabolic rate is increased, with changes involving the metabolism of proteins, carbohydrates, and fats. Increased degradation of **proteins** is accompanied by increased BUN and creatinine, anemia, and hypoalbuminemia. Reduced utilization of **glucose** and increased gluconeogenesis result in hyperglycemia, increased concentration of plasma lactate, and insulin resistance. Free **fatty acids** in the blood are increased due to unsuppressed free fatty acid mobilization from peripheral fat stores.

The pathogenesis of **cachexia in cancer patients** is complex and not fully understood. Several factors play a potential role, such as:

- **Obstruction of the gastrointestinal tract.** Carcinoma of the stomach and esophagus may interfere with the ingestion of food. Carcinoma of the head of the pancreas may obstruct the common bile duct and prevent the influx of bile or pancreatic juices.
- **Anorexia.** Patients lose appetite, which in part could be due to a loss of taste for sweet, sour, and salty foods. Some patients, like those who have gastric or liver cancer, develop aversion to meat, whereas others develop a dislike for coffee or chocolate.

- **Early satiety.** Increased blood glucose due to poor utilization or low levels of insulin may suppress appetite. Increased plasma concentration of proteins and amino acids mobilized from the muscle may act on the satiety center and suppress appetite.
- **Increased energy expenditure.** The tumor acts as a parasite and may consume more energy than normal tissues. In addition, the competition for nutrients between the tumor and the host leads to metabolic disturbances in the host, including hypermetabolism, which, in turn, leads to an increased energetic inefficiency.
- **Cytokines released in response to tumor growth.** Tumor necrosis factor (also known as *cachectin*), interleukin 6 (IL-6), and many other cytokines could be responsible for anorexia, hypermetabolism, and many other metabolic abnormalities, such as muscle proteolysis and apoptosis.
- **Therapy.** Weight loss is in many cases due to chemotherapy, known to cause nausea, vomiting, diarrhea, altered taste, and pain. Surgery could also cause increased weight loss by increasing energy expenditure or by affecting food intake.

Fever

Fever is an abnormal elevation of the body temperature above the upper limit of normal daily variation (i.e., >37.8°C [100°F] orally or 38.2°C [100.8°F] rectally). Remember that body temperature is lower in the morning (37.2°C) and reaches it upper limit of normal (37.7°C) in the evening. Overall, the temperature is lower in older people, hence the clinical dictum "the older the colder."

Normal body temperature is under the control of the hypothalamic thermoregulatory center.

Heat generated in the course of various metabolic processes and normal action of muscles and other organs is dissipated mostly through the skin and some internal organs such as lungs and the upper aerodigestive system. The entire process of thermoregulation depends on the proper functioning of the hypothalamic thermoregulatory center, which receives input from the peripheral sensors for cold and warm in the skin and central thermal receptors in the hypothalamus. Skin receptors respond to external temperature, whereas the central receptors respond to the temperature of the blood. Both signals are integrated and compared with the setting of the hypothalamic thermostat. If the temperature exceeds the upper limit set by the thermostat, signals are sent to the periphery to dissipate the heat. This occurs through the vasodilatation of dermal blood vessels, which fill with warm blood, allowing the blood to transmit the excess heat to the exterior of the body by radiation or convection. Central signals also activate sweat glands, stimulating heat loss by evaporation. Shivering of skeletal muscles may increase peripheral heat production (Fig. 2-4).

Fever results from action of endogenous pyrogens on the hypothalamic thermostat.

Under normal conditions the hypothalamic thermoregulatory center adjusts the peripheral loss of heat to match heat production, thus keeping the body temperature in a range roughly between 37°C and 38°C. In many inflammatory diseases the set point of the hypothalamic thermostat occurs at a higher temperature, which reduces the dissipation of heat in the periphery and leads to hyperthermia. This resetting of the thermostat results from the action of cytokines released from activated macrophages and, to a lesser extent, activated T lymphocytes. Because they cause fever, these mediators of inflammation are called B lymphocytes. The most important among them are interleukins (IL-1α, IL-1β, IL-6), tumor necrosis factors (TNF-α, TNF-β), and interferons (IFN-α, IFN-β, IFN-γ).

Endogenous pyrogens do not act directly on the thermoregulatory center. Instead, they act on the endothelial cells of a highly vascular part of the wall of the third ventricle, called *organum vasculosum laminae terminalis* (OVLT). Under the influence of pyrogens the endothelial cells of OVLT produce prostaglandin PGE$_2$, which diffuses into the adjacent hypothalamus and, by acting on the thermoregulatory center, raises the set point for thermoregulation. The signals from the thermoregulatory center lead to vasoconstriction of dermal vessels, cessation of sweating, and shivering of muscles, thereby reducing the dissipation of heat (Fig. 2-5).

Fever can result from infections or noninfectious disease.

Fever is a common sign of infections, but it can occur in the course of many other diseases (Table 2-4). Thus it is customary to classify fever as infectious or noninfectious. If the cause cannot be identified, it is classified as fever of unknown origin (FUO).

Fever of infectious origin. Almost any acute or chronic infectious disease may cause fever. As a rule, infection should be the first diagnosis considered in all febrile

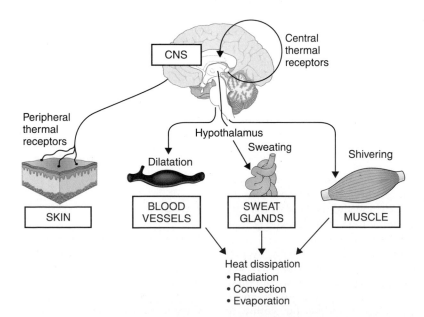

Figure 2-4 Regulation of temperature. CNS, central nervous system.

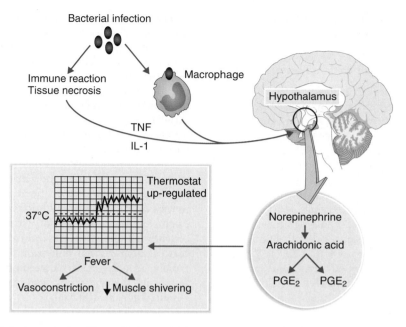

Figure 2-5 Pathogenesis of fever. IL-1, interleukin-1; PGE, prostaglandin; TNF, tumor necrosis factor.

patients, especially if the fever is of sudden onset, associated with other signs of inflammation, and localizing symptoms point to a site of infection. Only after infection has been excluded as a possible cause is it advisable to consider other causes of fever.

Pearl

> Afebrile infections most often occur in very old or very young persons, but can also be seen in middle-aged adults who have congestive heart failure or chronic renal insufficiency.

Fever related to noninfectious diseases. Endogenous pyrogens can be released by inflammatory cells infiltrating various organs affected by autoimmune diseases, following tissue necrosis after infarction, in crystalline arthropathy (e.g., gout), and as part of a drug reaction. Pyrogens may be released from many other cells, especially endothelial cells in the blood vessels, fixed macrophages such as hepatic Kupffer cells, glial cells, and dermal Langerhans cells. Parenchymal tissue cells—such as keratinocytes of the skin, nasal and bronchial, or intestinal epithelial cells—also can produce cytokines that act as pyrogens. Tumor cells are a well-known source of pyrogens. Fever is especially common in patients who have lymphoma, renal cell carcinoma, and primary or secondary tumors of the liver.

Fever of unknown origin. For clinical purposes FUO is defined as temperature over 38.3°C (101°F) lasting at least 3 weeks, for which the cause could not be found after 1 week of intensive investigation. Most diseases that evade early diagnosis turn out to be either infectious or neoplastic. Even under the best of all possible conditions, the cause

Table 2-4 Common Causes of Fever

Infectious diseases
    Acute infection (e.g., influenza)
    Chronic infection (e.g., tuberculosis, AIDS)
Autoimmune diseases
    Rheumatoid arthritis
    Systemic lupus erythematosus
Thrombosis, hemorrhage, and infarction
    Myocardial infarction
    Cerebrovascular incident
    Retroperitoneal hematoma
    Thrombophlebitis of leg veins
Crystalline arthropathy
    Gout
Metabolic disorders
    Hyperthyroidism
    Alcoholic hepatitis
Drug reaction
Neoplastic diseases
    Lymphoma
    Renal cell carcinoma
    Liver tumors (primary and secondary)

of fever cannot be determined in about 10% to 15% of patients.

Acute fever may have adverse effect on several organs.

It is generally believed that mild elevation of body temperature helps the body combat infection by accelerating the metabolism and all defense mechanisms. Roughly speaking, for each degree (centigrade) rise in temperature, the basal metabolic rate increases by approximately 10%, and otherwise healthy individuals can readily tolerate body temperature up to 40.5°C (105°F). As temperature rises, the heart and respiratory rates are increased. The body's own attempts to reduce the temperature include sweating and chills. Fever also affects the central nervous system, typically causing headache. High temperatures may cause convulsions, especially in children.

Extreme hyperthermia beyond 42.1°C (108°F) may damage the endothelium of blood vessels and cause disseminated intravascular coagulation (DIC). Microvascular thrombosis leads to ischemic tissue injury, especially in the brain and the heart. Hypotensive shock and neurologic signs of cerebral ischemia develop, and the patient may fall into coma and die.

Heat stroke results from prolonged exposure to high environmental temperatures. The affected person has high fever, but does not sweat, indicating a failure of central thermoregulation. Most often it is seen during summer heat waves, typically affecting the elderly and those who have been incapacitated by alcohol or drugs. These patients usually lapse into coma and often die.

Pearl

> Very high fever over 41.5°C (106.7°F) is usually not of infectious origin. Most often it is a consequence of stroke or other intracranial lesions. The only infections that should be considered in the differential diagnosis are encephalitis and meningitis.

Pain

Pain is an unpleasant feeling; that is, a psychological reaction to sensations that begin with the stimulation of peripheral sensors. Pathogenetically it includes four sequential components:

- Stimulation of the sensory nerve endings or nociceptors
- Transmission of the afferent sensory nerve impulse
- Modulation of the impulse in the sensory centers
- Cognitive and emotional interpretation of the sensory input

The pain pathway has two parts: the peripheral part, involving the nociceptors and sensory nerves, and a central part, involving the cortical centers (Fig. 2-6).

Nociceptors. As the term implies (*nociceptor* is derived from the Latin words *nocere*, meaning hurting, *receptor*, meaning receiver), the main function of receptors for pain is to recognize mechanical, thermal, or chemical impulses that could damage the body and consequently elicit a reaction that will minimize that damage. Nociceptors are free nerve endings widely distributed in the skin, soft tissues, skeletal muscles, and joints. Internal organs are sparsely supplied, but almost all major organs, except the brain, have nociceptors.

Nociceptors can be classified as thermal, mechanical, chemical, or polymodal nociceptors. They include fast myelinated mechanical Aδ fibers and slow unmyelinated polymodal C fibers. In addition to nociceptors pain can originate from other sensory stimuli. For example, the distention of the intestines stimulates local **mechanoreceptors,** causing visceral dull pain. Pacinian corpuscles, the rapidly adapting mechanoreceptors of the skin, are also found in the mesentery and the pancreas, and their stimulation generates pain.

The nociceptors respond to external stimuli by transmitting afferent nerve signals and also by secreting mediators of inflammation such as substance P. The nerve impulses also travel efferently through interconnecting axons **(axonal reflex),** provoking a vascular response. The release of these mediators acts on endothelial cells of the local blood vessels, inducing increased permeability and also stimulating them to secrete cytokines. Hence the entire area becomes inflamed **(neurogenic inflammation).** The mediators of inflammation, such as bradykinin or cytokines, act on nociceptors, increasing their responsiveness **(peripheral sensitization).** Peripheral sensitization is associated with **hyperalgesia,** an increased feeling of pain and a reduced threshold to pain. Conversely, stimulating other sensory endings, such as low-threshold mechanoreceptors Aα and Aβ, may reduce the sensation of pain.

Central nervous system response. From the early stages of pain transmission, as soon as the impulses reach the sensory centers in the brain, pain has also a psychological **component.** It evokes emotions and can be modulated by cognitive mechanisms. For example it is well known that in the heat of the battle or during sporting events an injured person can withstand pain that would otherwise be perceived as intolerable. The intensity of the pain can be reduced by reducing the level of consciousness (e.g., by anesthesia), distracting the person's attention, and by a variety of palliative effects that produce a placebo effect. Fear and expectations also may modify the perception of pain.

The reaction to pain can be modified in the brain by cortical impulses and by the activation of other subcortical centers. At the cellular level a major role is played by small-molecular-weight polypeptides called **endorphins.** These polypeptides bind to opioid receptors on sensory neurons, modifying the perception of the pain. Opioid drugs and other analgesics also have similar effects.

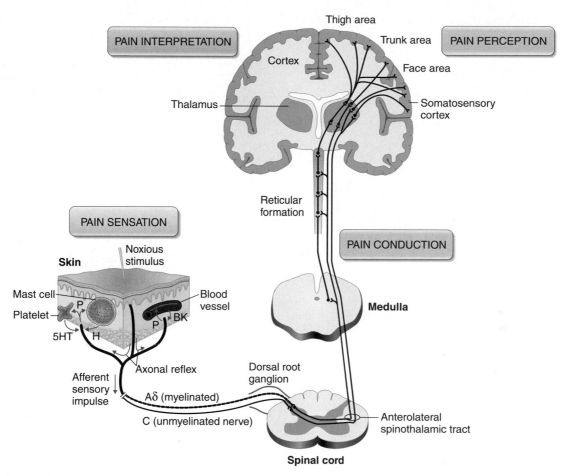

Figure 2-6 Pathogenesis of pain. BK, bradykinin; H, hydrogen; 5HT, 5 hydroxytryptamine (serotonin); P, phosphate.

Pain can be classified as organic or psychogenic.

Because pain has both sensory and psychological components, it is best to classify it as predominantly organic or predominantly psychogenic (Fig. 2-7). **Organic pain** can be explained in terms of underlying pathology, whereas **psychogenic pain** eludes such explanation and its cause may be quite puzzling.

Organic pain resulting from excessive or prolonged stimulation of peripheral nerve endings is called nociceptive pain (Fig. 2-8). **Nociceptive pain,** which originates in the skin and subcutaneous tissues, typically corresponds to innervation of anatomic dermatomes and is called somatic pain. **Somatic pain** is typically sharp, severe, and pricking. Pain originating from the parietal peritoneum or pleura is known as parietal pain but in essence is identical to somatic pain. **Parietal pain** can be localized or diffuse. **Localized pain,** such as pain in the right lower abdominal quadrant in appendicitis, can pinpoint the nature of the disease that precipitates it. However, pain can also be **referred** to a site quite distant from the site of original pathology. Diffuse parietal

pain is typically seen in peritonitis when the entire surface of the abdominal cavity is inflamed. Typically the patient tries not to move, and any movement, such as coughing or vomiting, exacerbates the pain. Pain originating from the nerve endings in internal organs is called **visceral pain.** Visceral pain is usually poorly localized and is most intensively felt in the midline of the abdomen or thorax. Pain is often dull, but it may also be colicky and cause a feeling described by the patients as gnawing or burning.

Neuropathic pain results from an injury to the peripheral sensory nerves or nerves in the spinal cord and brain. Typical examples of neuropathic pain are back pain due to the compression of spinal nerves by a degenerated intervertebral disk, herpes simplex neuropathy involving the facial nerve, or pain due to spinal cord injury.

Psychogenic pain cannot be readily explained, but that does not preclude its resulting from some underlying pathology. Typical examples are chronic headache and back pain, which can be quite crippling and represent some of the most common problems encountered in daily medical practice.

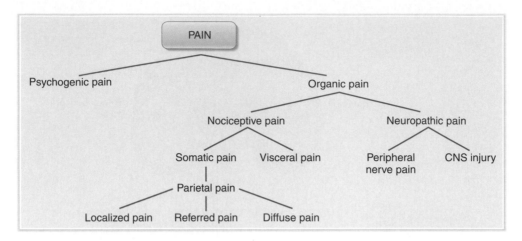

Figure 2-7 Classification of pain. CNS, central nervous system.

Headache can be caused by organic diseases or functional disturbances involving the intracranial and extracranial structures.

Headache is a very common complaint, and although it may be crippling it is rarely life-threatening. Approximately 75% of all people experience headache from time to time, 50% have at least one headache a month, and 5% have headaches daily. Women are affected twice as often as men. Family history is found in two thirds of all headache patients.

Headache can be classified as acute or chronic. Chronic headaches are often recurrent. Pathogenetically, the headaches can be classified as primary or secondary, and as related to intracranial or extracranial causes (Fig. 2-9).

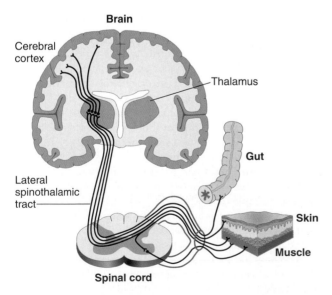

Figure 2-8 Transmission of nociceptive and visceral impulses.

Primary headache. Diagnosis is made by excluding potential organic causes of headache, such as sinusitis or brain tumors, and by observing symptom presentation and the localization and distribution of pain (Fig. 2-10).

■ **Migraine headache.** This very common type of headache affects approximately 10% of all women. The attack is thought to result from initial vasospasm followed by a dilatation of intracranial and extracranial arteries. The distribution of pain is variable. Three clinical forms are recognized. **Migraine with aura** is associated with a premonitory aura or prodrome of neurologic symptoms. Most common is scintillating scotoma, a bright spot in the center of the visual field that flickers and changes color. The patient may feel "pins and needles in the fingers" and tingling in the area of the nose, mouth, and lips *(digitolingual paresthesia)* (Fig. 2-11). Occasionally hemiparesis may ensue, but in most cases the neurologic symptoms resolve spontaneously. **Migraine without an aura** is characterized by throbbing pain. **Complicated migraine** is characterized by the persistence of neurologic symptoms even after the headache has ceased. Migraine pain can be precipitated by various agents, such as alcohol, monosodium glutamate (used for preparing some Asian-style food), estrogens, and many others. It occurs more often under certain circumstances, such as in the premenstrual period, after exposure to bright light, or during changes in weather.

■ **Tension headache.** Headache caused by tension is the most common form. Although the pathogenesis is not understood, it most likely is multifactorial in etiology and could have several pathogenetic mechanisms. Tension headache has a strong psychological component and is often precipitated by stress or emotional conflict. Of all the forms of headaches, tension headaches vary the most with regard to type of onset,

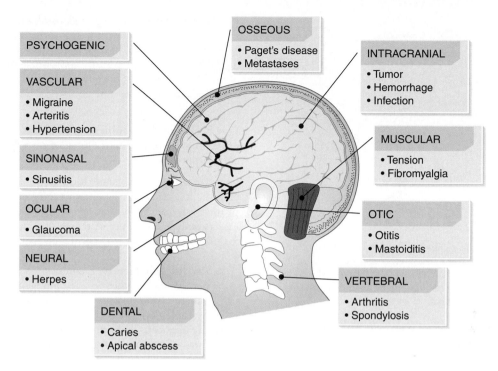

Figure 2-9 Headache.

character, location, severity, and duration. Most often the pain is bilateral and associated with tightness and "muscle tension," usually in the neck. The so-called headband distribution, or pain across the brow and top of the head, is often mentioned. Subjective tenderness over the temporalis muscle and the "trigger points" felt within the area of the trapezius muscle have been noted in many cases.

■ **Cluster headaches.** This form of recurrent headache presents with severe unilateral periorbital or temporal lancinating pain that may last from 15 minutes to

3 hours. The name *cluster headaches* is actually derived from their occurring closely together in both time and location. The pain recurs regularly and typically occurs almost always in the same location. In contrast to the migraine headache, which is relieved by sleep, cluster headaches occur more often on awakening. Periorbital pain may be associated with eye symptoms, such as tearing, or stuffy nose. Cluster headaches are much more common in men than women and are refractory to standard treatment with analgesics.

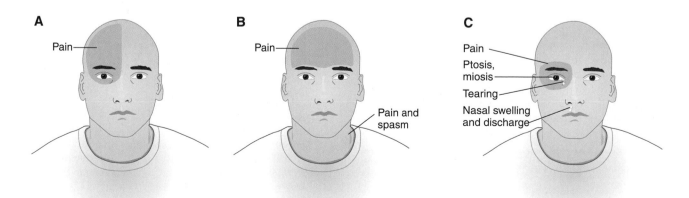

Figure 2-10 Distribution of pain in primary headache syndromes. **A,** Migraine. **B,** Tension headache. **C,** Cluster headaches.

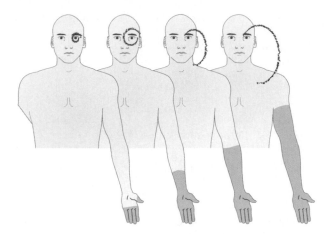

Figure 2-11 Migraine. The prodrome includes scotoma and paresthesias of the fingers, extending to the arm and the face, especially around the nasolabial area. (Redrawn from Branch WT, Jr: Office Practice of Medicine, 3rd ed, WB Saunders, Philadelphia, 1994.)

Secondary headaches. Such headaches are related to organic lesions in the intracranial and extracranial structures or accompany chronic diseases of unknown etiology, systemic infections, or drugs. These headaches are related to pathologic changes in extracranial and intracranial structures.

- **Extracranial structures.** Nociceptors are found in essentially all extracranial structures, including the skin, muscles, specialized organs, and parts of the respiratory and digestive system. The calvarium is insensitive, but the periosteum is richly innervated. Thus, pain can result from the stimulation of nociceptors in any of these anatomic sites. It can be secondary to muscle spasm, contraction of arteries, temporal arteritis, inflammation of the mucosa of the nasal sinuses, or increased intraocular pressure, as well as many other causes.
- **Intracranial structures.** The brain itself dose not contain sensory receptors. Likewise the pia and arachnoid and most of the dura are insensitive to pain. Intracranial pain originates from the traction, displacement, compression, or inflammation of pain-sensitive intracranial structures. These include the dura at the base of the brain, arteries, venous sinuses and the major veins, and cranial nerves V, VII, IX, and X. Irritation of the upper cervical nerves also gives rise to headache.

Pearl

> Brain tumors account for less than 1% of severe headaches, but the patients usually describe them as the "worst headache of my life."

The clinical diagnosis of pain depends on detailed history and physical examination, as well as special tests if indicated. The adage that careful history taking may help in diagnosing 80% of disease is especially appropriate in the diagnosis of headaches. The most important causes of secondary headaches are listed in Table 2-5.

Low back pain is a multifactorial disease with a strong psychological component affecting over 50% of all elderly persons.

Low back pain in an acute form may occur at any age. Chronic low back pain is one of the most common complaints in persons older than age 60 years. Its causes are not understood, but in most instances it is multifactorial and includes the following pathogenic mechanisms:

- **Psychogenic factors.** Depression, stress, and anxiety play important roles in the pathogenesis of low back pain, and any treatment must take into account these psychological aspects of the disease.
- **Ligamentous sprain.** Pain is related to deep structures of the back, and the patient typically tries to limit movement to reduce pain.
- **Fibromuscular pain.** Fibromyalgia that is lessened by stretching or movement suggests that the pain is of fibromuscular origin. Muscular pain may be associated with tenderness to palpation.
- **Sciatica.** Back pain associated with sciatica (pain radiating along the sciatic nerve) may be caused by herniation of intervertebral disks, causing the compression of the nerve roots of the sciatic nerve (Fig. 2-12). Such pain is

Table 2-5 Causes of Secondary Headaches

Systemic causes
  Viral infection (e.g., influenza)
  Hypertension
  Anemia
  Alcohol
  Drugs
Head and neck infection
  Acute upper respiratory infection
  Chronic sinusitis
  Otitis media
Chronic diseases of unknown origin
  Giant cell (temporal) arteritis
  Glaucoma
  Temporomandibular joint disorders
  Cervical spine disorders
Intracranial diseases
  Tumors of the brain
  Intracranial bleeding
  Intracranial infection (brain abscess, encephalitis, meningitis)

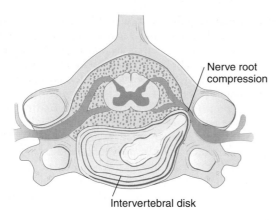

Figure 2-12 Radicular pain due to the compression of the spinal nerve roots by the herniated intervertebral disk.

increased by straining during the Valsalva maneuver, coughing or sneezing, or by lifting an extended leg. Spinal stenosis is a rare cause of the same symptoms.

Chest pain may be caused by a variety of conditions, including diseases of the heart, esophagus, lungs, and thoracic cage.

Chest pain may be related to the skin, subcutaneous tissue, muscle, ribs, and vertebrae making up the thoracic cage, or it may be visceral and originate in the internal organs (Fig. 2-13). With a few exceptions chest pain results from the stimulation of nociceptors. Several distinct forms of pain are recognized as follows:

- **Dermal pain.** Skin lesions irritate the sensory nerves and are usually well localized and readily visible during physical examination. Herpes zoster causes neuritic pain along the sensory spinal nerves and is typically limited to anatomic dermatomes.
- **Myalgia.** Muscle pain may occur in a variety of conditions, such as trauma, hematoma, myositis, strain, and relative ischemia due to excessive effort of untrained muscles. Muscle pain may have a considerable psychologic component, and in anxious persons it may be mistaken for cardiac pain.
- **Ostalgia.** The periosteum of the ribs and vertebrae is well-innervated, and any mechanical injury due to compression or inflammation extending to the bones from adjacent tissues may cause intense pain. Metastases to the thoracic vertebrae may cause back pain limited to specific dermatomes.
- **Posterior root pain.** This neuropathic pain is usually caused by compression of nerves as a result of deformities of the thorax, or by narrowing of the intervertebral spaces due to degeneration of an intervertebral disk. Dorsal root pain is usually sharp and accentuated by motion, such as occurs during bending of the arms or torsion of the trunk.
- **Pleural pain.** The parietal pleura is densely innervated, whereas the visceral pleura is insensitive. Irritation of parietal pleura produces sharp pain, which is perceived as if originating in the overlying skin. It is described as sharp, knifelike, and accentuated by respiratory movements.
- **Esophageal pain.** Distention of the esophagus or disturbances of peristalsis cause pain that is most

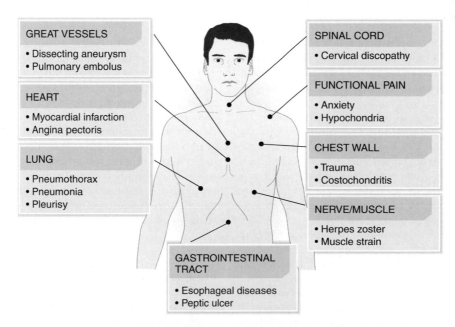

GREAT VESSELS
- Dissecting aneurysm
- Pulmonary embolus

HEART
- Myocardial infarction
- Angina pectoris

LUNG
- Pneumothorax
- Pneumonia
- Pleurisy

SPINAL CORD
- Cervical discopathy

FUNCTIONAL PAIN
- Anxiety
- Hypochondria

CHEST WALL
- Trauma
- Costochondritis

NERVE/MUSCLE
- Herpes zoster
- Muscle strain

GASTROINTESTINAL TRACT
- Esophageal diseases
- Peptic ulcer

Figure 2-13 Most important causes of chest pain.

often substernal. Esophageal pain may be projected around the chest or resemble pain originating from other thoracic viscera. Heartburn is a form of substernal pain that occurs due to regurgitation of gastric contents after a meal. However, even this pain may extend over the precardial area and be confused with heart pain.

- **Cardiac pain.** This pain occurs typically in ischemic heart disease. It is discussed in greater detail in Chapter 4.
- **Pericardial pain.** The visceral pericardium (epicardium) does not have sensory receptors, and the parietal pericardium is weakly innervated by pain fibers. Nevertheless, pericarditis may cause pain, which is most often substernal or to the left of the sternum. Such pain most likely results from the reaction of adjacent structures in the mediastinum or the parietal pleura.

Abdominal pain may originate from most intra-abdominal organs and may be classified as visceral or somatic (parietal).

Abdominal pain may originate from any of the abdominal organs but most often it is related to problems in the digestive system. Pain originating from the internal organs is called visceral, whereas pain arising from the dermatomes or parietal peritoneum is called parietal or somatic. Abdominal pain coming from outside the abdominal area is called referred pain. Abdominal pain may have metabolic, toxic, neurogenic, and psychogenic causes.

- **Visceral pain.** Visceral pain is typically vague and poorly localized. Most often gastrointestinal pain is perceived as centered on the midline, with the upper gastrointestinal tract projecting to the epigastrium, midgut projecting to the periumbilical area, and the terminal colorectal pain referring to the suprapubic area. Pain may be crampy, especially when resulting from spastic contraction, distention, or twisting of intestines.
- **Parietal.** Pain originating from skin, subcutaneous tissue, muscle, and the parietal peritoneum is typically steadier and more localized. Visceral pain can become parietal once the parietal peritoneum becomes involved. For example, in acute appendicitis, which begins as a midline periumbilical pain, the sensation shifts to the right lower quadrant once the inflammation extends to the overlying parietal peritoneum.
- **Referred pain.** Pain stemming from thorax, spine, or lower extremities may project onto the abdomen. It is usually perceived as superficial and localized to a specific dermatome.
- **Metabolic or toxic pain.** Pain may be a prominent feature of some metabolic diseases such as porphyria or diabetic acidosis. Lead poisoning may manifest as abdominal colic.

- **Neurogenic pain.** Radicular pain due to the compression of sensory spinal nerves may manifest as abdominal pain. Tabes dorsalis, a feature of secondary syphilis, may also manifest as abdominal pain. This pain is a form of radicular pain related to chronic meningitis, which constricts the sensory nerves branching from the paraspinal ganglia and entering into the posterior columns of the spinal cord.
- **Psychogenic pain.** In some instances the cause of abdominal pain cannot be determined and so should be assumed to be psychogenic. Persistent pain of undefined origin can be quite incapacitating and may profoundly affect the patient or lead to numerous medical examinations or unnecessary medical and surgical procedures. The cause of pain usually remains unknown.

Abdominal pain must be systematically evaluated to assess its mode of onset, duration, nature (severity, constancy), and factors that aggravate it or relieve it (e.g., association with meals, position of the body, menstrual cycle). The location of pain can provide valuable diagnostic information because various pathologic processes manifest with pain in different locations (Fig. 2-14).

Joint pain is usually caused by multifactorial disorders involving the synovium and the periarticular connective tissue.

Pain involving the joints is a very common complaint. It may be acute or chronic and involve a single joint (**monoarticular pain**) or many (**polyarticular pain**). Acute pain is often related to the causative events, such as trauma, or specific disease, such as rheumatoid arthritis, gout, or bacterial infection of the joint (Fig. 2-15). The causes of chronic pain are usually less obvious and are often ascribed to poorly defined or multifactorial diseases, such as degenerative joint disease (DJD), fibromyalgia, or chronic bursitis.

Pain may be associated with characteristic clinical findings, such as accumulation of an exudate or transudate in the articular cavity. In patients who have hemophilia pain is usually associated with accumulation of blood (hemarthrosis). In rheumatoid arthritis chronic pain of the hands is accompanied by ulnar deviation and deformities (Fig. 2-16). DJD involving the hand may produce fusiform swelling of distal interphalangeal joints (Heberden's nodes) and less often swelling of the proximal interphalangeal nodules (Bouchard's nodes), whereas the phalangeal-metacarpal joints are not affected. The most common causes of joint pain are listed in the Table 2-6.

Weakness

Weakness is a loss of muscle strength. The affected person is unable to initiate a muscle action, so weakness should therefore not be confused with easy fatigability (i.e., inability to

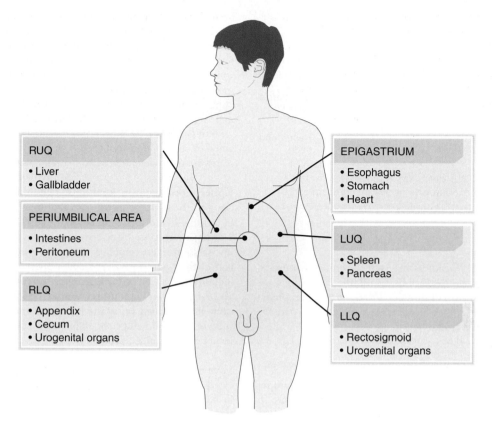

Figure 2-14 Abdominal pain. The point of greatest tenderness may have several locations. LLQ, left lower quadrant; LUQ, left upper quadrant; RLQ, right lower quadrant; RUQ, right upper quadrant.

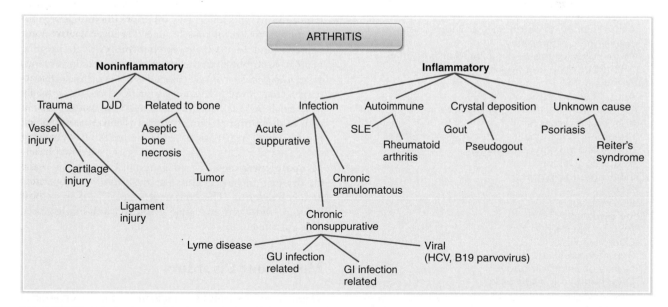

Figure 2-15 Joint pain is related to pathologic changes involving the cartilage, bone, synovium, bursae, or tendons. DJD, degenerative joint disease; GI, gastrointestinal; GU, gastrourinary; HCV, hepatitis C virus; SLE, systemic lupus erythematosus.

A   **B**

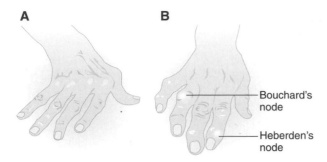

Bouchard's
node

Heberden's
node

Figure 2-16 A, Ulnar deviation in rheumatoid arthritis
B, Bouchard's and Heberden's nodes manifesting as fusiform swelling of interphalangeal nodes in degenerative
joint disease.

sustain an action). Weakness may affect groups of muscles,
such as proximal or distal muscles of the extremities, or
involve an entire region of muscles. **Paralysis** and **paraplegia**
are terms used for severe regional muscle weakness in patients
who have suffered a stroke.

Muscle weakness results from neuromuscular diseases.

Voluntary actions of the muscles depend on proper
innervation of the alpha motoneurons, which originate in
the anterior horn of the spinal cord (Fig. 2-17). This **lower
motor neuron** is in synaptic connection with the upper
motor neuron emanating from the cerebral cortex and the

Table 2-6 Common Causes of Joint Pain

Trauma
   Acute injury with tearing of cartilage or ligaments
   Neurogenic arthropathy
   Postsurgical or prosthesis-related arthropathy
   Hemarthrosis in hemophilia
Infections
   Acute viral or septic bacterial
   Chronic nonspecific or granulomatous
Autoimmune diseases
   Rheumatoid arthritis
   Systemic lupus erythematosus
   Systemic sclerosis
Crystalline arthropathies
   Gout
   Pseudogout
Bone diseases
   Aseptic necrosis
   Osteoporosis
   Bone tumors
Diseases of unknown origin
   Degenerative joint disease
   Fibromyalgia
   Chronic bursitis
   Chondromalacia

brainstem. The **upper motor neuron** includes **pyramidal**
corticospinal and corticobulbar tracts, as well as **extrapyramidal** tracts, including the following: rubrospinal, pontine
reticulospinal, medullary reticulospinal, lateral vestibulo-
spinal, and tectospinal. The **cerebellum** regulates both
movement and posture and is important for the maintenance of the synergy of muscle actions. Pathologic changes
in any of these structures affect muscle function and cause
weakness. Hence, weakness may be classified as neuropathic
when related to lesions of the upper or lower motor neuron,
or myopathic when related to primary muscle disease.

Upper motor neuron weakness. The injury is typically located in the brain or spinal cord and may be a consequence
of trauma, hemorrhage, or a space-occupying lesion, such as
a tumor or abscess. Muscle weakness may be profound and
involves entire anatomic regions (e.g., *hemiplegia,* in which
half of the body is paralyzed). It is often associated with an
inability to talk or properly enunciate sounds (*dysarthria* or
dysphonia) or an inability to swallow (*dysphagia*). It is typically accompanied by spasticity. If the movements recover
they may remain sluggish. Rapid movements are more affected than sustained action.

Lower motor neuron weakness. The injury is typically located in the anterior horn of the spinal cord, but it can also
be found in the brainstem or at the level of axons as they
leave the spinal cord and enter the skeletal muscle. Typically
it occurs in amyotrophic lateral sclerosis (Lou Gehrig's disease), a disease of unknown origin affecting the anterior horn
motor neurons or the upper motor neurons.

   The loss of alpha motoneurons weakens muscle action
because the normal recruitment of motor units takes place
during normal muscle contraction. The loss of gamma
motoneurons, which normally innervate the muscle spindle,
contributes to loss of muscle tone. Damaged lower motor
neurons tend to discharge spontaneously in an irregular
manner, contributing to the fine muscle contractions known
as *fasciculation.* Even if fasciculation is not evident electromyography may reveal *fibrillation potentials,* related to discharges
from single muscle fibers. Muscle weakness is more prominent in distal than proximal muscles of the extremities, and
it is associated with a loss of tendon reflexes.

Myopathic weakness. Weakness results from primary muscle diseases, including muscular dystrophies, myopathies,
and polymyositis. The contractile capacity of muscles is
reduced, and electromyography usually shows a decreased
unit potential.

Movement Disorders

Voluntary movements are modified by the impulses from
extrapyramidal motor centers in the basal ganglia. Diseases
affecting the striatum, globus pallidus, subthalamic nucleus,

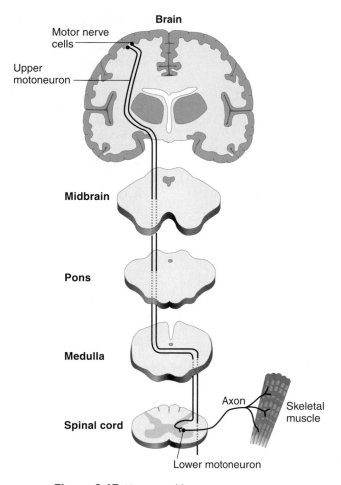

Figure 2-17 Upper and lower motoneurons.

and the substantia nigra cause movement disorders also known as dyskinesia. They may be classified as hyperkinetic, characterized by excessive motor activity, or hypokinetic, in which the motor activity is reduced.

Hyperkinetic movements result from a loss of inhibition of impulses from upper motor centers.

Hyperkinetic movements result from a loss of inhibitory control mechanisms that normally regulate the impulses emanating from the upper motor centers. The most important abnormal hyperkinetic movements are as follows:

Tics. These rapid involuntary movements, such as eye blinking or facial spasm, are repetitive but not rhythmic. Tics may be simple or complex and are occasionally associated with pain *(tic douloureux)*. Tics are common in children but tend to disappear on their own. Tics are a feature of **Tourette's syndrome,** an autosomal dominant disease that predominantly affects males. These patients usually have *complex motor tics* on the face (e.g., blinking, frowning,

sniffing) and *phonic tics* (e.g., throat-clearing, grunting, barking). In about 50% of cases the patient experiences a compulsive urge to curse *(coprolalia)*.

Tremor. This is a form of rhythmic repetitive muscle contraction alternating with relaxation. Tremor may occur physiologically due to cold or fatigue, hyperthyroidism, or some drugs (e.g., caffeine).

Tremor due to neurologic disorders is classified as either resting (if present while the person is at rest) or intentional (if the person is moving). **Resting tremor** is a feature of Parkinson's disease. **Intentional tremor** is related to cerebellar lesions and is often seen in multiple sclerosis. Postural tremor is observed when a patient tries to hold a position, such as holding the arms stretched out. Flapping of the hands that occurs in such a position is known as **asterixis** and is a common sign of end-stage liver disease (Fig. 2-18).

Chorea. Chorea is characterized by rapid involuntary jerky movements of hands, feet, and face, merging with the normal voluntary movements. It may be combined with **athetosis,**

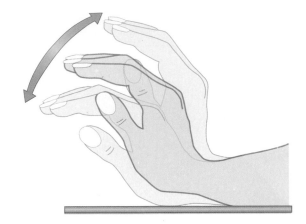

Figure 2-18 Asterixis. The extended hand shows characteristic flipping movement.

slow writing movements involving the muscles of the entire extremity. It is a feature of Huntington's disease and rheumatic fever *(Sydenham's chorea)* but may be also induced by certain drugs, and may even occur without obvious reasons during pregnancy.

Myoclonus. Characterized by a sudden contraction of muscles, myoclonic contractions may occur in normal healthy persons while they are falling asleep. Myoclonus may be a feature of myoclonic epilepsy, Alzheimer's disease, and Creutzfeldt-Jakob disease, and is also seen in some metabolic diseases such as end-stage renal disease. It may also follow traumatic brain injury or ischemic stroke. It is called **action myoclonus** because it may be precipitated by voluntary movement.

Pearl

> Hiccup is a form of myoclonus due to the contraction of the diaphragm.

Parkinson's disease is a prototypical hypokinetic movement disorder.

Parkinson's disease is a progressive neurodegenerative disorder affecting the substantia nigra, locus ceruleus, and related dopaminergic basal ganglia. In primary Parkinson's disease, which accounts for 90% of all cases, the cause is unknown. Secondary Parkinson's disease could be caused by drugs interfering with the action of dopamine in the basal ganglia, toxins such as carbon monoxide, intracerebral bleeding due to repetitive trauma, encephalitis, or tumors. The movement disorders include:

- **Hypokinesia and loss of involuntary movements.** Overall the patient is less mobile. The face appears rigid and expressionless. The blinking is reduced. The speech is monotonous.
- **Tremor.** It is most prominent at rest and occurs at a rate of 4 to 6 cycles per second. Initially it is confined to one anatomic site, such as one hand, but with time it tends to become generalized. It is more pronounced under emotional stress and it is less prominent during voluntary movements.
- **Bradykinesia.** Voluntary movements are slow; however, no muscle weakness is present.
- **Rigidity.** Limbs resist passive movement. Rigidity accounts for the typical flexed posture.
- **Gait abnormalities.** The patient needs time to get up from a sitting position. The gait is shuffling and unsteady, and the normal movement of arms that occurs during walking is reduced. Sudden stopping or accelerating is a problem.

The most common clinical features of Parkinson's disease are presented in Figure 2-19.

Gait Disorders

Walking is an extremely complex activity involving the cortex, subcortical centers, cerebellum, spinal cord, and the skeletal muscles. Coordinated locomotion also requires maintenance of balance through the input from the sensory impulses in the inner ear and the sensory endings in the muscle spindle. Gait disorders can develop for many reasons and are best classified as neurologic and nonneurologic. Presented in a systematic manner, the gait disturbances are listed as follows:

- **Disorders of motor control.** These include major catastrophic cerebral insults such as intracranial hemorrhage and head trauma, both of which may cause complete or partial paralysis. Many neurologic diseases affect the gait, including Parkinson's and Huntington's diseases and multiple sclerosis. Alcohol and many psychotropic drugs also interfere with the normal gait.
- **Sensory disorders.** Tabes dorsalis caused by syphilis or the degeneration of posterior columns due to vitamin B_{12} deficiency cause sensory disruption and loss of proprioception, adversely affecting gait.
- **Muscle diseases.** Primary muscular dystrophies are characterized by gait disorders, and in Duchenne's muscular dystrophy most patients are confined to a wheelchair by the time they start going to elementary school.
- **Orthopedic disorders.** Skeletal deformities, trauma, or degenerative joint disease adversely affect gait.

The most common cause of gait disturbance is pain, followed by deformities caused by trauma and orthopedic disorders.

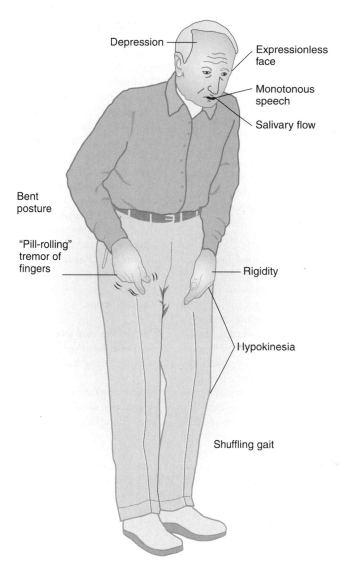

Depression

Expressionless face

Monotonous speech

Salivary flow

Bent posture

"Pill-rolling" tremor of fingers

Rigidity

Hypokinesia

Shuffling gait

Figure 2-19 Parkinson's disease. Clinical features include shuffling gait, tremor, rigidity, and lack of facial expression.

Syncope

Syncope (fainting, passing out) is a transient sudden loss of consciousness with a loss of postural tone and prompt spontaneous recovery. It is caused by cerebral ischemia, related to either cardiovascular or noncardiovascular factors. Several forms of syncope are recognized, but in all of them a disproportion occurs between the cardiac ejection volume and the arterial vascular space that must be filled with blood. The most important causes of syncope are as follows:

- **Pump failure.** Syncope occurs in many cardiac diseases but is most often related to conduction disturbances.
- **Obstruction of blood flow.** Valvular disease may impede outflow of the blood from the left ventricle,

and pulmonary embolism may obstruct the outflow from the right ventricle.

- **Reduced venous return to the right heart.** Increased pooling of blood in the venous system reduces the cardiac output and also results in low blood pressure.
- **Hypovolemia.** Any loss of blood, especially if copious and sudden, reduces cardiac output.
- **Systemic or localized vasodilatation.** Dilatation of arteries supplying blood to the major organs may change the hemodynamics and, by redirecting the blood into some parts of the body, reduce the flow to the brain.
- **Cerebral arterial vasoconstriction.** Selective vasoconstriction occurs in hypocapnia.

Clinically it is important to determine whether syncope is of **cardiac origin** or **noncardiogenic,** and if so, to which specific pathogenic mechanism it is related (Fig. 2-20).

Cardiac syncope. Pump failure of sudden onset is most often caused by *bradyarrhythmia* or *tachycardia.* Congenital or acquired valvular disorders may cause a sudden drop in the outflow of blood from the heart. Most often it is caused by aortic stenosis. Hypertrophic cardiomyopathy may cause syncope due to subvalvular obstruction of the aortic orifice. Malfunctioning cardiac prostheses are yet another important cause of fainting. Thromboemboli also may obstruct blood flow. Fainting is a common symptom in persons who have cardiac myxoma temporarily obstructing the flow of blood from the left atrium into the left ventricle.

Vasomotor syncope. Most often occurring in young women, vasomotor syncope is related to increased vagal tone and inadequate sympathetic regulation of the peripheral circulation. Typical episodes are precipitated by stress, pain, or a frightful event and are associated with premonitory symptoms such as nausea, sweating, blurring of vision, or tachycardia. The affected person regains consciousness when laid down. Syncope during **swallowing** is also related to a vasovagal reflex. A large bolus of food entering the esophagus stimulates the vagus nerve, thus causing peripheral vasodilatation and bradycardia, reducing the blood pressure, and causing cerebral ischemia. **Carotid sinus syncope** that occurs on compression or massage of the carotid sinus is also caused by peripheral vasodilatation. **Micturition syncope** typically occurs in elderly men who go to the bathroom during the night and faint while emptying the bladder. It is probably of vasovagal origin, but the exact mechanism of fainting is not understood.

Orthostatic (postural) hypotension. This vasomotor syncope occurs on standing up from a supine position. It is related to inadequate reflex vasoconstriction that normally occurs when rising from a lying to an upright position. Normally, when we stand up the blood return to the heart is temporarily reduced with consequently diminished cardiac output. To prevent a disproportion between the cardiac output and the arterial space, reflex vasoconstriction ensues to reduce the arterial space. If this reflex vasoconstriction does not take place, incomplete filling of brain vasculature causes ischemia and fainting occurs. On lying down the syncope is reversed. Orthostatic hypotension occurs without obvious reasons in elderly men (**idiopathic orthostatic hypotension),** but is even more common in those who have autonomic system dysfunction such as is often seen in **diabetes mellitus.** Persons treated with **adrenergic blockers** or those who have lost blood due to **massive bleeding** are especially susceptible to fainting. Hypotension due to **anaphylactic drug reaction** may cause syncope.

Posttussive and postdefecation syncope. Syncope develops due to reduced venous return into the right heart, caused by increased intrathoracic pressure (Valsalva maneuver).

Hyperventilation syncope. It results from hypocapnia and respiratory alkalosis, which cause cerebral vasoconstriction and dilatation of other blood vessels, leading to cerebral ischemia.

Cerebral syncope. Syncope can occur in the prodrome of epileptic fits or during transient ischemic attacks. The brain is dependent on a normal supply of glucose, and thus hypoglycemia induced by high insulin levels may result in loss of consciousness.

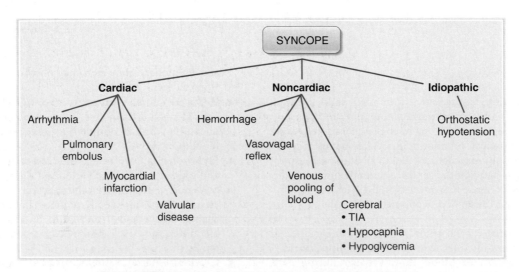

Figure 2-20 Causes of syncope. TIA, transient ischemic attack.

Coma

Coma is a sleeplike state in which the affected person has closed eyes and cannot be aroused by verbal or mechanical stimuli. Such stimuli can evoke reflex responses and other stereotypic and noncognate reactions, but the consciousness cannot be regained to enable the patient to become aware of his or her surroundings. Patients who have been in coma for a long time may open up their eyes, but are still unconscious and unresponsive to external stimuli. Such a condition is called a **vegetative state.** In these patients the reflexes and automatic movements are nevertheless preserved and the sleep–wake cycle is intact.

A lesser degree of unconsciousness from which the patient can be awakened by vigorous stimulation is called **stupor.** A mild degree of unconsciousness from which the patient can be awakened with words or shaking is called **drowsiness.** It is usually associated with **confusion,** a state in which the patient shows incoherence and cannot reason properly.

The causes of coma include structural brain lesions, metabolic disturbances, drugs, and toxins.

Coma results from injuries to the cortex and the thalamic and brainstem nuclei forming the *reticular-activating system (RAS).* RAS involves several nuclei, such as serotonin-containing raphe nuclei and the norepinephrine-containing nucleus ceruleus. RAS is connected in several ways with the cortex and is instrumental in arousal and awakening the forebrain. RAS regulates sleep and through its links with the cortex is essential for maintenance of consciousness. The cortex and RAS can be injured by many structural and metabolic brain lesions (Fig. 2-21).

Structural lesions. Coma develops only if both hemispheres of the brain are affected. If the lesion is localized to one hemisphere, the circulatory changes and edema typically af-

Table 2-7 Structural Causes of Coma

Traumatic brain injury
Hemorrhage
  Cerebral
  Subarachnoid
  Subdural
Infarcts
  Embolic occlusion
  Thrombotic occlusion
  Hypotensive
Infection
  Abscess
  Encephalitis
  Meningitis
Tumors

fect the contralateral hemisphere and cause compression of the vital centers on the opposite side as well. The most important structural causes of coma are listed in Table 2-7.

Metabolic and toxic causes. Coma is encountered in the course of end-stage renal or hepatic failure, metabolic diseases such as diabetes, disturbances of mineral maintenance, and acid–base imbalance. Drugs and toxins are important causes of coma. The most important metabolic and toxic causes of coma are listed in Table 2-8.

The depth of coma can be assessed by monitoring the respiratory pattern, eye reactions, and muscles of the extremities.

Supratentorial lesions usually progress in an orderly and predictable manner, affecting first the cortex and then the deeper brain structures and finally inhibiting the vital

Table 2-8 Metabolic and Toxic Causes of Coma

Hepatic failure
Renal failure
Diabetes mellitus
Hyperglycemia
Lactic ketoacidosis
Hypoglycemia
Hyponatremia
Hypercalcemia
Adrenal insufficiency
Hypothyroidism
Sepsis
Epilepsy
Drugs and toxins
  Alcohol
  Opiates
  Barbiturates
  Benzodiazepines
  Anticonvulsants

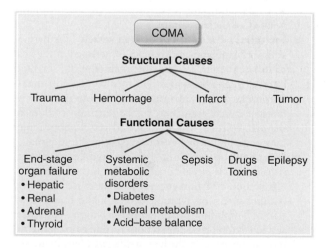

Figure 2-21 Causes of coma.

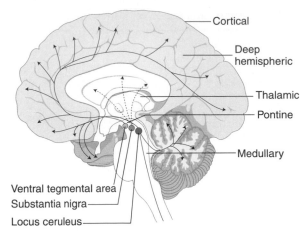

Figure 2-22 Depth of coma. Coma related to supratentorial causes first manifests with cortical inhibition and deepens by involving deeper subcortical structures, finally ending in the inhibition of the vital centers in the pons and the medulla oblongata.

centers in the pons and medulla oblongata (Fig. 2-22). The disease level may be assessed by observing respiratory movements, pupillary reaction, oculomotor reflexes, and motor responses of the extremities as follows:

- **Diffuse cerebral cortical depression.** Respiration is normal, but sometimes hyperventilation occurs. The pupils are in midposition and normally reactive, and the extraocular reflexes are intact. The extremities are hypotonic or hypertonic.
- **Diffuse deep-hemispheric depression.** Sustained hyperventilation and alkalosis are present, or inspirations assume a waxing–waning pattern typical of Cheyne-Stokes respiration. The pupils are in midposition and normally reactive, and the extraocular reflexes are intact. The extremities are diffusely hypertonic and show decorticate response to strong stimulation.
- **Thalamic impairment.** Cheyne-Stokes periodic breathing and possible periods of sustained hyperventilation are present. The pupils are small but reactive to light. Third-nerve paresis is evident, and the medial and superior rectus muscles show weakness, thus allowing eyes to be in an abducted position. The muscles of the extremities show a decerebrate response to noxious stimuli.
- **Pontine impairment.** Breathing is irregular with periods of apnea. The pupils are unreactive and either in midposition or very narrow. Sixth-nerve paresis is evident, affecting the lateral rectus muscle; or complete ophthalmoplegia is present. Extremities show flaccid quadriplegia and no decerebrate or decortication responses.
- **Medullary impairment.** Breathing is of irregular depth and pattern (*ataxic breathing*) with prominent

apneic periods. Pupils are dilated and unreactive. Ophthalmoplegia is complete. Flaccid quadriplegia is the rule, and no decerebrate or decorticate responses can be evoked by strong stimuli.

Edema

Edema is an excessive accumulation of fluid in the interstitial spaces of various tissues or in body cavities. It may be localized or generalized, in which case it is called **anasarca.** The accumulation of fluid in the abdominal cavity is called **ascites,** or **hydroperitoneum. Hydrothorax** refers to pleural effusion, **hydropericardium** to accumulation of fluid in the pericardial sac. Clinically, edema may be **visible** on inspection, or it may be **palpable** like the pitting edema of lower extremities that occurs in heart failure.

Edema develops due to disturbances of blood or lymph flow, lowering of the osmotic pressure of the plasma, or increased permeability of the wall of small blood vessels.

Edema results under conditions that favor efflux of fluids out of the blood vessels. Four principal causes of edema can be identified (Fig. 2-23) as follows:

- **Increased venous and capillary pressure.** Obstruction of the venous blood outflow by thrombi or increased venous pressure due to heart failure is transmitted into the capillaries, where it causes increased efflux of fluid into the interstitial spaces. This typically occurs in the lungs during left heart failure or in the lower extremities and peritoneal cavity in right heart failure.
- **Reduced oncotic plasma pressure.** Hypoalbuminemia is the most common cause of reduced oncotic pressure of the plasma. It occurs in chronic liver disease when the synthesis of albumin is reduced or in nephrotic syndrome and protein-losing enteropathy when albumin and other proteins are lost from the body at an increased rate.
- **Increased permeability of blood vessels.** The permeability of capillaries and venules is increased in the area of inflammation, leading to increased efflux of fluid into the interstitial spaces. The mediators of inflammation released from inflammatory cells into the interstitial spaces may contribute to the retention of fluid in the extravascular spaces. Increased vessel permeability may occur in burned skin or the brain after trauma.
- **Lymphatic obstruction.** Since the fluid from the interstitial spaces is in part drained through the lymphatics, obstruction of lymphatic vessels may cause edema by backpressure. This typically occurs due to the obstruction of lymph flow by tumors in the lymph nodes, after surgical lymph node dissection, or due to parasitic infections obstructing the lymphatics (e.g., "elephantiasis" of lower extremities in filariasis).

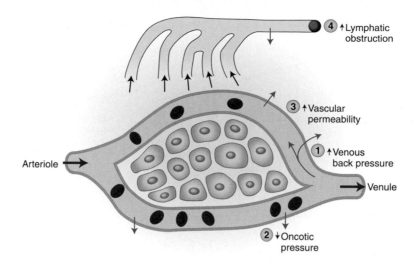

Figure 2-23 Principal causes of edema. Numbers in this figure correlate to those in Figure 2-24.

From the clinical point of view, edema can be classified pathogenetically or by its location (Fig. 2-24). In many clinical conditions edema is multifactorial in origin. Thus, in chronic heart failure edema is in part due to increased venous pressure and in part related to the expansion of the extracellular fluid content due to the retention of sodium. The accumulation of ascites fluid in liver disease is in part related to increased portal hypertension due to the abnormal structure of the liver and in part due to hypoalbuminemia. Obstruction of the hepatic lymph flow and the renal retention of sodium also contribute to the formation of ascites. The most important clinical forms of edema are presented in Figure 2-25.

Bleeding

Bleeding (hemorrhage) is a process during which the blood escapes from the blood vessels or the heart. Depending on the source, bleeding can be classified as cardiac, aortic,

arterial, capillary, or venous. The most common forms of hemorrhage are illustrated in Figure 2-26, but most of these disorders are discussed in greater detail in subsequent chapters. The pathogenesis of bleeding is discussed in Chapter 6.

Skin Changes

Skin lesions may take many forms and be either localized or widespread. They may be caused by primary skin diseases or may evolve in response to systemic diseases. These systemic diseases may be infectious, immune-mediated, metabolic, circulatory, or neoplastic.

Skin lesions are classified as primary or secondary. Secondary skin lesions develop from the primary lesions as they enlarge or become infected, or may simply be due to scratching and mechanical irritation.

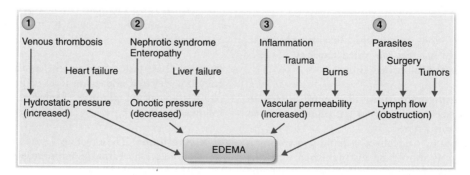

Figure 2-24 Pathogenesis of edema. 1, Hydrostatic edema occurs due to increased venous pressure, forcing the efflux of fluid from the vessels into the interstitial spaces. 2, Oncotic edema results from reduced oncotic pressure of the plasma that cannot retain the fluid inside the vessels. 3, Inflammatory edema develops due to increased permeability of the vessel wall. 4, Lymphatic edema develops due to an obstruction of lymphatic flow.

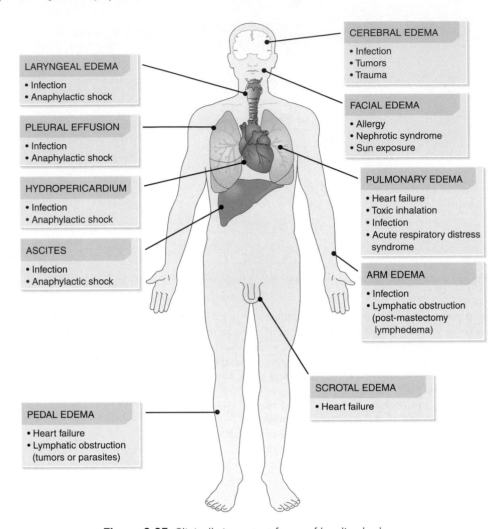

Figure 2-25 Clinically important forms of localized edema.

Primary skin lesions develop due to several mechanisms.

Primary skin lesions are shown in Figure 2-27. The most important causes of these lesions are briefly discussed here.

Macule. These flat lesions manifest as a localized change in the skin color. Large macules are called **patches.** Macules and patches include the following lesions:

- **Brown hyperpigmentation.** This may be seen in the form of freckles or café au lait pigmentation in neurofibromatosis type I.
- **Depigmentation.** Localized depigmentation is called *vitiligo.* It should be distinguished from the generalized lack of pigment occurring in congenital albinism.
- **Skin hemorrhages.** Small pinpoint hemorrhages are called *petechiae,* larger spots are called purpura, and those larger than 5 mm are called *ecchymoses.* Fresh

hemorrhages are red, but with time they become greenish or yellow due to the degradation of hemoglobin into biliverdin and bilirubin.
- **Drug exanthemas.** Drug reactions may cause inflammatory changes in the dermis and dilatation of blood vessels, which manifests as localized erythema.

Papule. These lesions are small (less than 1 cm in diameter) but elevated above the level of normal skin. Larger papules are called **plaques.** Examples of papules are as follows:

- **Xanthoma.** These yellow lesions result from an accumulation of lipid-filled macrophages in the dermis in hyperlipidemia.
- **Lichen planus.** The papules of this immune-mediated disease are flat-topped and silvery white.
- **Warts.** These lesions are caused by human papillomavirus.

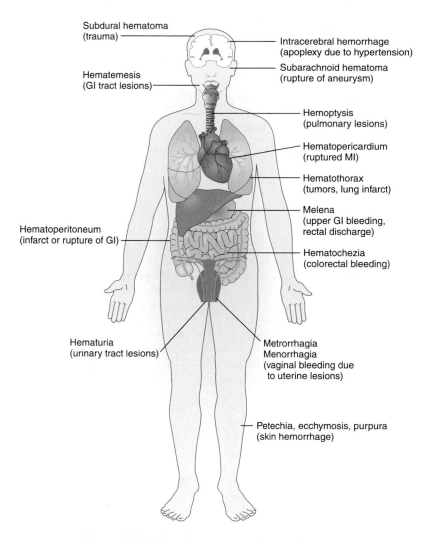

Figure 2-26 Clinically important forms of bleeding.

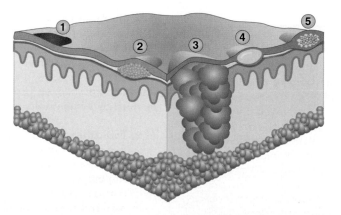

Figure 2-27 Primary skin lesions. 1, Macule. 2, Papule. 3, Nodule. 4, Vesicle. 5, Pustule.

- **Molluscum contagiosum.** These papules result from poxvirus infection. Typically the papules have a centrally depressed area ("umbilication").
- **Condyloma latum.** This lesion is typical of secondary syphilis. It appears in crops most often on the palms and intertriginous areas, which are described as "copper-colored."
- **Nevus.** This brown lesion results from the accumulation of pigment-bearing nevus cells. Nevi can be congenital or acquired.
- **Seborrheic keratosis.** This benign epithelial tumor is usually small and brown.

Certain childhood exanthemas, such as measles, manifest as red macular and papular eruptions.

Plaque. These lesions resemble papules but are much larger. They may arise from confluent papules or from papules that have enlarged. Examples of plaques are:

- **Psoriasis.** This primary skin disease, which may begin with formation of papules, is characterized by multiple erythematous plaques covered by silvery scales.
- **Atopic dermatitis.** These immune-mediated lesions of children begin as *spongiotic papules* showing edema of the epidermis over a mildly inflamed dermis. With time the epidermis undergoes hyperplasia, becomes thicker, but still retains its markings *(lichenification)*. These lesions cause itching and usually enlarge due to scratching and secondary infections. The spectrum of changes includes dry and wet oozing lesions of variable duration and is called **eczematous rash.**
- **Dermal infections.** Various fungal infections, tuberculosis of the skin, or leprosy may present in the form of plaques.
- **Disease of unknown origin.** Sarcoidosis, a granulomatous disease of unknown origin, may manifest with plaques or nodules. Granuloma annulare and erythema multiforme are also diseases of unknown cause that tend to form plaques. Some of these diseases are simply called *chronic nonspecific dermatitis.*

Pearl

> *Eczema,* a term derived from the Greek word meaning "boiling over," is often used as a synonym for atopic dermatitis. However, it is also used for many other skin lesions that have the same morphology. It is imperative to diagnose the causes of eczemas that can be treated, such as those related to atopy or other forms of allergy, environmental factors (e.g., chemicals or dust particles), or drugs. When all these potential causes are excluded, a group of diseases remain that do not respond to treatment and carry the label of chronic nonspecific dermatitis.

Nodule. This is a solid mass measuring more than 0.5 cm in diameter. The following are examples of dermal nodules:

- **Benign tumors.** Many dermal tumors are included in this group, such as lipoma and schwannoma.
- **Primary or metastatic carcinoma.** These nodules are often ulcerated or necrotic on their surface.
- **Rheumatoid nodule.** These lesions are granulomas that develop in the course of rheumatoid arthritis.
- **Erythema nodosum.** This disease of unknown origin is characterized by granulomatous inflammation of the dermis and subcutis.

Vesicle. This raised lesion resembles a papule but is filled with fluid. Larger vesicles are called **bullae.** Vesicles or bullae are found in the following diseases:

- **Herpes simplex.** This viral disease most often manifests with grouped vesicles on the lips, usually during or after a viral infection ("cold blisters"). Herpes genitalis affects the external genitalia.
- **Herpes zoster.** The vesicles are located along the peripheral nerves corresponding to anatomic dermatomes. The lesions typically result from the activation of the dormant varicella zoster herpesvirus, which has remained in the spinal ganglia after a childhood infection.
- **Contact dermatitis.** Poison ivy reaction is the prototypical example of this type IV hypersensitivity reaction. In sensitized persons linear streaks of papules and vesicles develop within 24 to 48 hours after contact with the oil (urushiol) from the leaves of poison ivy (*Rhus* sp.).
- **Pemphigus vulgaris.** This type II autoimmune disease is mediated by antibodies to desmosomal proteins and is characterized by formation of intraepidermal vesicles. Bullae are found on the skin and mucosae, most often involving the mouth.
- **Bullous pemphigoid.** This type II autoimmune hypersensitivity disease is characterized by the formation of subepidermal bullae due to the action of antibodies to basement membrane components. Groin, axillae, and flexural areas are most often involved.
- **Burns.** Grade I and II burns damage the epidermis and cause transudation of fluid in between the damaged epidermal cells into the space that separates the epidermis from the dermis.

Pustule. A pustule is a papule that contains pus. Diseases manifesting with pustules include:

- **Folliculitis.** This is a bacterial infection of hair follicles. Pus can be expressed by lateral pressure, but it may spread and involve adjacent follicles as well.
- **Impetigo.** This superficial infection is most often caused by *Staphylococcus aureus.* The pustules are superficial and typically found on the face of children. They rupture easily and heal without scarring.

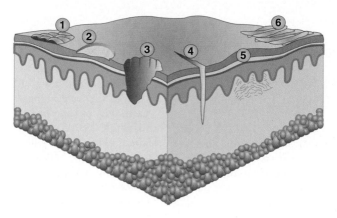

Figure 2-28 Secondary skin lesions. 1, Crust. 2, Erosion. 3, Ulcer. 4, Fissure. 5, Scar. 6, Scale.

■ **Acne.** This is a chronic infection caused by *Propione-bacterium acnes* involving the hair follicles and adjacent sebaceous glands.

Secondary skin lesions develop from primary lesions.

Secondary skin lesions develop from primary lesions that have been irritated, traumatized, exposed to humidity, or treated (Fig. 2-28). The most important secondary skin lesions are listed here:

■ **Crust.** Also known as a scab, a crust is composed of clotted blood or plasma and cell debris. Typically it develops at the site of previous vesicles and bullae or pustules. Crusts derived from plasma are yellow, those derived from blood are red, and those derived from pus are yellow or greenish.
■ **Erosion.** This superficial, partial loss of epidermis heals without scarring. Linear erosions caused by scratching are called **excoriations.**
■ **Ulcer.** An ulcer is a full-thickness loss of epidermis extending into the dermis. It heals with scarring.
■ **Fissure.** This is a crack in the skin extending vertically into the dermis.
■ **Scar.** A scar is a residue of the healing of wounds and other deep skin lesions. It is characterized by an accumulation of connective tissue. Hypertrophic scars are called **keloids.**
■ **Scale.** This thickening of the skin results from hyperproliferation of epidermis and inadequate desquamation of keratinocytes.

Generalized Eruptions

Skin lesions may be localized or widespread. Generalized (widespread) rashes or eruptions either are caused by primary skin diseases or are dermal manifestations of a systemic disease. The diagnosis is made in context, by taking a detailed history, performing a physical examination, and employing ancillary methods whenever needed. Generalized eruptions are classified on the basis of the morphology of the skin lesions and their distribution.

The most important generalized eruptions are listed under the heading of the most common clinical patterns (Table 2-9).

Table 2-9 Clinically Important Generalized Skin Eruptions

Eczematous eruptions
  Atopic dermatitis of children
  Allergic contact dermatitis
Papullosquamous eruptions
  Psoriasis
  Lichen planus
  Lupus erythematosus
  Fungal infections (e.g., tinea corporis, tinea versicolor)
Vesicobullous eruptions
  Erythema multiforme
  Staphylococcal scalded skin syndrome
  Viral infections (e.g., varicella)
  Autoimmune bullous diseases (e.g., pemphigus vulgaris, bullous pemphigoid)
Pustular eruptions
  Acne
  Staphylococcal and streptococcal skin infections
Purpuric eruptions
  Thrombotic thrombocytopenic purpura
  Idiopathic thrombocytopenic purpura
  Vasculitis
  Bleeding disorders

CASE STUDIES

Case 1 WEIGHT LOSS AND NIGHT SWEATS IN A 50-YEAR-OLD MAN

Clinical history   A 50-year-old white civil engineer, who was until recently in excellent health, complained of a 10-kg weight loss and feeling weakness the whole day.[1] He also noticed that he wakes up in the middle of the night drenched in sweat.[2] He eats normally and has a normal appetite.[3] Lately he has noticed that he gets nauseated when eating meat and drinking alcohol.[4]

Physical findings   He is in good physical condition but appears tired and apprehensive. He has mild fever of 38.2°C. His pulse rate is 92 beats per minute, and his blood pressure is 120/80 mm Hg. He has enlarged lymph nodes in the right supraclavicular area of the neck.[5]

Laboratory and clinical findings   A lymph node biopsy revealed adenocarcinoma.[6] Additional radiographic studies and upper gastrointestinal endoscopy with biopsies of the stomach were ordered.

Outcome   The patient was treated with chemotherapy but he died 18 months after the first visit to the doctor.[7]

Questions and topics for discussion
1. How do you define involuntary weight loss? What is the definition of weakness? What could cause weight loss and weakness?
2. What could cause night sweats? What is the pathogenesis of night sweats?
3. What is appetite and how is it regulated? Does this man have anorexia?
4. What is nausea? What is the significance of the aversion to certain foods and drink?
5. What are the possible causes of localized enlargement of the lymph nodes in the neck? What additional procedures or testing are necessary to make the diagnosis?
6. What is the significance of a pathologist's report stating that the neck lymph node contains adenocarcinoma? Is this a primary tumor or a metastasis? If it is a metastasis, where could the primary tumor most likely be?
7. Why did this patient die?

Case 2 HEADACHES IN A 20-YEAR-OLD WOMAN

Clinical history   A 20-year-old black college student complained of headaches that did not respond to her usual over-the-counter analgesic medication.[1] Her family history was interesting in that her mother and grandmother also had periodic severe headaches.[2] Lately she has had bouts of headaches at least once a week that typically have begun early in the morning while she was getting up from bed.[3] The pain would be throbbing, usually on the left side of her face, and was worse when she was moving than when lying down.[4] The pain would last 4 to 5 hours and would subside spontaneously. The pain was preceded by a feeling of anxiety and restlessness, and before it would begin she would notice flashing lights and partial loss of vision. She would feel tingling in her fingers and around the mouth and would become tongue-tied.[5]

Physical findings   Noncontributory.

Laboratory findings   Noncontributory.

Outcome   She was given medication and instructed to take some of these pills prophylactically before the headache begins and some for the relief of symptoms. She responded well to the treatment.[6]

Questions and topics for discussion
1. Define headache, and discuss the differences between acute and chronic headache.
2. Is the family history important for the diagnosis of headaches?
3. Is the fact that the headaches recur and occur in the morning important for diagnosis?
4. Are the location, quality, and intensity of the pain important for the diagnosis? Describe these clinical aspects of the disease as they typically define the most common forms of headache.
5. Does this patient have neurologic symptoms? Define *premonitory aura, paresthesia,* and *scotoma.* Do you think that the patient might have these symptoms?
6. What kind of medication would you prescribe?

Case 3 UNCONSCIOUS 50-YEAR-OLD MAN BROUGHT IN TO THE EMERGENCY DEPARTMENT

Clinical history   A 50-year-old man was found lying unconscious in front of the house where he lived. His wife called the ambulance service and accompanied him to the emergency department.

At the time of admission he was still unconscious but was smelling of alcohol.[1] The wife told the physicians that he was drinking quite often but did not have any serious diseases. She reported that he did not have diabetes, epilepsy, or hypertension and that he was not using street drugs.[2]

Physical findings   The head showed contusion and hematoma over the frontotemporal area on the left side. The eyes were reactive to light, and the eyeballs showed no deviation. He was breathing slowly and laboriously. The pulse was 50 beats per minute. Glasgow Coma Scale gave a score of 7.[3]

Laboratory findings   Blood alcohol levels were 200 mg/dL.[4]

Clinical and radiology findings   A computer tomography scan revealed a subdural hematoma.[5]

Outcome   A craniotomy was performed and the subdural hematoma surgically removed.[6]

The patient recovered.

Questions and topics for discussion
1. Is this patient in coma? How do you define coma? You assume the obvious, that the patient was so drunk that he passed out. Could there be some other causes for him being unconscious? Discuss some possibilities.
2. Why is it important to ask about all of the diseases and social habits of a comatose person?
3. What is the Glasgow Coma Scale? Is somebody with a score of 7 on that scale in coma?
4. Is the concentration of alcohol in the blood high enough to cause coma?
5. What is the pathogenesis of subdural hematoma?
6. How is subdural hematoma removed, and what are the consequences of this surgical intervention?

Case 4 SHORTNESS OF BREATH AND SWELLING OF LEGS IN A 70-YEAR-OLD MAN

Clinical history   A 70-year-old man complained that he is short of breath while going up the stairs to his bedroom. He has also noticed that his legs are swollen.[1] In addition he also complains of a dull pain in the upper abdomen on both the right and the left side.[2] From time to time he has pain on the left side of the chest, especially while walking or playing tennis.[3]

Clinical findings   Pleural effusion was noticed on the right side. The liver and the spleen are enlarged, and a small amount of fluid is present in the abdominal cavity.[4] Coronary angiography disclosed narrowing of both major coronary arteries.[5]

Outcome   Coronary angioplasty with stenting was performed.[6]

Questions and topics for discussion
1. What is the significance of these symptoms, and what could cause them?
2. What is the possible cause of upper abdominal pain?
3. What is the differential diagnosis of left-sided thoracic pain?
4. Explain the pathogenesis of hydrothorax, hepatomegaly, splenomegaly, and ascites in this patient.
5. What is the final diagnosis?
6. How are coronary angioplasty and insertion of stents performed?

Chapter 3

SYSTEMIC DISEASES

Introduction

The foundations of modern medicine may be traced to the nineteenth century when the principles of exact sciences were first applied to the study of the human body and its diseases. The teachings of cellular pathology, founded by Rudolf Virchow in the 1860s, have dominated our view of health and disease ever since. The original concepts have been modified since then by new discoveries and expanded by the contributions of other basic sciences, especially biochemistry, biophysics, and molecular biology.

Contemporary clinical medicine is based on scientific principles and the application of basic sciences to the study of health and diseases. Clinical medicine is also an empirical discipline and as such must be pragmatic and practical. Thus, the clinician must study diseases not only to better understand them but also to cure, prevent, or eradicate them. For each disease the clinician must determine its:

- **Etiology**—what caused it.
- **Pathogenesis**—how did it develop.
- **Pathology**—what anatomic changes it produced.
- **Pathophysiology**—what functional consequences it has.
- **Clinical features**—what signs and symptoms it produced.
- **Treatment** and **outcome**—how to cure it and how to predict the final prognosis.

For practical purposes diseases can be classified as **organ-centered** or **systemic.** For example, Alzheimer's disease involves the brain and is thus classified as an organ-centered disease. Gout is a metabolic disorder that affects many organs and is therefore classified as a systemic metabolic disease. Acute appendicitis is an example of an organ-based infection, but if untreated, appendicitis may give rise to bacteremia and become a systemic disease. The line separating organ-based and systemic diseases is fuzzy

and often arbitrary. Furthermore, even a strictly organ-based disease such as cirrhosis due to hepatitis C usually produces systemic disturbances, and many systemic diseases, such as systemic lupus erythematosus, first manifest with symptoms of skin or kidney disease. Thus, in this book we use the terms *organ-centered* and *systemic* with the understanding that many organ-centered diseases have systemic effects, and, conversely, many systemic diseases may be organ-centered.

Systemic diseases are classified according to their pathogenesis as follows:

- Genetic
- Metabolic
- Toxic
- Circulatory
- Infectious
- Immune
- Neoplastic

In this chapter we discuss several diseases that could be used as prototypes for all other diseases in each of these eight categories. We use **hereditary hemochromatosis** as an example of a genetic disease because it illustrates how a mutation of a gene encoding a single protein (HFE—involved in regulating the intestinal absorption of iron) can affect multiple organ systems. We discuss **gout** as an example of a metabolic disease and show how the same metabolic abnormality (**hyperuricemia**) has several causes and still produces the same set of clinical signs and symptoms. As an example of toxic diseases we discuss alcohol abuse. **Alcoholism** demonstrates how substance abuse can cause major health problems. The complexities of circulatory disturbances are discussed in the example of **shock** and closely related multiple organ failure. Acquired immunodeficiency syndrome (**AIDS**) is our example of a systemic infectious disease, illustrating the consequences of the primary viral infection and bacterial, viral, fungal, and parasitic

Acquired immunodeficiency syndrome (AIDS)   Immunodeficiency induced by human immunodeficiency virus (HIV) infection, characterized by a low count of helper T cells (CD4$^+$ cells) and opportunistic infections involving the skin, FI system, lungs, or the central nervous system.

Alcoholism   Pattern of alcohol intake resulting in psychophysical dependence on alcohol and dysfunction in one or more of five aspects of living: marital, social, legal, occupational, or physical.

Autoimmune diseases   Group of chronic diseases characterized by abnormal immune reactions to self antigens. Such diseases may be accompanied by overproduction of autoantibodies or abnormal T-cell reactions, and pathological or functional changes in various organs.

Carcinoma   Malignant neoplasm of epithelial origin.

Gout   Metabolic disease characterized by hyperuricemia and a deposition of monosodium urate crystals in joints and soft tissues.

Hereditary hemochromatosis   Common genetic disease associated with abnormal intestinal absorption of iron and iron overload that damages several vital organs, most notably the liver, islets of the pancreas and other endocrine organs, the heart, and the skin.

Hypersensitivity   Increased reactivity to exogenous or endogenous antigens, characterized by an overproduction of antibodies or abnormal cell-mediated reactions. Hypersensitivity to foreign antigens is also called allergy.

Hyperuricemia   Increased concentration of uric acid in blood in excess of the empirically determined upper limit of normal (>7 mg/dL for females, >8 mg/dL for males); it may be asymptomatic or it may be lead to a deposition of urate crystals in tissues, resulting in gout, urate nephropathy, or urolithiasis.

Sepsis   Presence of infectious pathogens or their derivatives in blood. Clinical consequences of sepsis are called septicemia and include fever, loss of vascular tone, and at least some signs of shock and multiple organ failure.

Shock   Set of systemic circulatory and metabolic disturbances involving numerous body functions caused by inadequate blood perfusion of vital organs.

Systemic lupus erythematosus (SLE)   Multisystem autoimmune disease of unknown origin characterized by the formation of circulating immune complexes and their deposition in numerous anatomic sites.

superinfections that complicate this disease complex. As an example of autoimmune disorders we examine **systemic lupus erythematosus (SLE),** an immune complex-mediated **hypersensitivity** reaction that can affect numerous organs. Finally, the systemic effects of a malignant tumor are illustrated by discussing **carcinoma of the lung,** not only because it is the number one cause of cancer-related death, but also because of its multiple systemic effects.

Hereditary Hemochromatosis

Hereditary hemochromatosis is a common autosomal recessive disorder marked by iron storage caused by abnormal absorption of iron in the intestines. In approximately 85% of cases hereditary hemochromatosis is caused by a mutation of the *HFE* gene, encoding a protein (HFE) that regulates the absorption of iron in the duodenum. The remaining 15% of cases are classified as non-*HFE*-related hereditary hemochromatosis.

The ***HFE* gene** is linked to the HLA-A locus on the short arm of chromosome 6 (6p). A mutation accounting for the cysteine-to-tyrosine substitution at amino acid 282 (called the C282Y mutation) inactivates the protein. Homozygotes are found at a rate of 1:220, and heterozygotes at a rate of approximately 1 in 10 persons. The signs of the disease occur only in 20% of homozygotes because the mutated gene has low penetrance. C282Y mutation is found in more than 85% of patients of northern European origin, but in only 60% of those of Mediterranean origin. Another mutation involving the substitution of histidine to aspartic acid at position 63 (H63D) is found in some persons, but it is not associated with iron overload unless combined by C282Y mutation on the other allele.

Unregulated absorption of iron in the duodenum leads to iron overload.

Under normal circumstances iron is absorbed in the duodenum mostly in form of ferrous (Fe^{2+}) iron (Fig. 3-1). The absorption of iron depends on the iron stored in the body, but normally enterocytes in the duodenum absorb only 10% of the total amount of iron entering the duodenum (i.e., 1–2 mg, from the 10–20 mg of iron ingested) daily in the typical American diet.

Low iron stores increase iron absorption in mature enterocytes on the surface of the intestinal villi. These cells absorb iron through the action of divalent metal transporter 1 *(DMT-1)*. Absorbed iron is in part stored in the enterocytes and in part transported into the interstitial fluid by a laterobasal protein called *ferroportin*. The activity of DMT-1 and ferroportin is normally suppressed by *hepcidin,* a regulatory protein circulating in the plasma. Hepcidin prevents abnormally high absorption of iron in the duodenum. It is synthesized by the liver in response to iron. Hepcidin also inhibits the release of iron from macrophages. Plasma hepcidin levels are low in persons with hereditary hemochromatosis.

The absorption of iron depends also on the transferrin iron sensors, which are expressed on the immature crypt cells. Note that these sensor cells do not participate in the absorption of iron in the intestine; instead they express receptors for transferrin and HFE gene product, which prime them to become absorptive enterocytes by activating the DMT-1/ferroportin system.

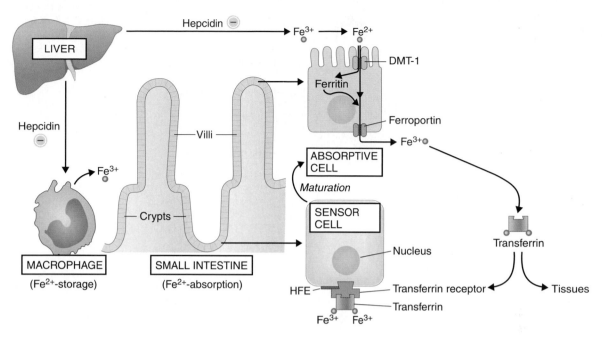

Figure 3-1 Iron absorption. The absorption of iron in the duodenum depends on the total iron stores of the body. Total iron body stores are reflected in the saturation of transferrin, the principal iron transport protein in the plasma. Transferrin binds to the immature precursors of normal enterocytes, which serve as iron sensors in the intestine. *HFE* gene product on these immature cells acts together with the transferrin receptor to differentiate into absorptively active enterocytes. Absorptively active enterocytes take up ferrous iron through the action of divalent metal transporter 1 (DMT-1). Absorbed iron is either stored in the cytoplasm as ferritin or transferred to the interstitial space by the basolateral protein called ferroportin. The action of DMT-1 and ferroportin in enterocytes and ferroportin in macrophages is regulated hepcidin, a liver-derived plasma protein. In hemochromatosis liver secretes less hepcidin than normal, and the *HFE* mutation affects its normal function.

In hereditary hemochromatosis the mutation of *HFE* leads to an uncontrolled absorption of iron in the duodenum. The total iron stores, which are normally around 2.5 g for women and 3.5 g for men can be increased 10 to 20 times and even more. The saturation of the iron transport protein transferrin is also increased, and the excess iron is also excreted into the urine.

Iron is deposited in the form of *ferritin,* which aggregates into *hemosiderin* granules. Hemosiderin may be detected in many organs, where it causes tissue injury and functional disturbances. Excess iron also results in the formation of free radicals, which have the following adverse effects:

- **Inactivation of enzymes.** Free radicals inhibit vital intracellular processes, such as oxidative respiration; protein synthesis; and transmembrane transport of fluids, minerals, and macromolecules.
- **Fibrosis.** Cell death caused by free radicals is accompanied by repair, during which the fibrous tissue replaces the parenchymal cells.
- **Carcinogenesis.** The interaction between iron-generated free radicals and nucleic acids may lead to DNA mutations, or activation of oncogenes and clonal proliferation, especially in the liver.

Iron overload causes pathologic changes in several vital organs.

Hemochromatosis may damage many organs, but most often the pathologic changes are seen in the liver (95%), skin (90%), pancreas (65%), joints (35%), and the heart (15%) (Fig. 3-2). Clinical symptoms usually manifest after age 40. Symptoms are 5 to 10 times less common in women, because normally women lose blood during menstruation and are thus less prone to accumulate iron. The symptoms occur later and are typically encountered several years after the onset of menopause.

Liver. Iron accumulates in Kupffer cells, hepatocytes, and even in bile duct cells (Fig. 3-3). Deposits of iron pigment lead to fibrosis, gradually progressing to frank cirrhosis. Clinically these changes are associated with hepatomegaly, portal hypertension with splenomegaly, and esophageal varices. Other signs and symptoms of liver failure are also present in advanced cases. Liver cell carcinoma develops in 20% to 30% of patients with cirrhosis.

Skin. Brown hyperpigmentation occurs in almost all patients who have cirrhosis. The hyperpigmentation, often described as "bronzing," is due to accumulation of hemosiderin in dermal macrophages and the increased amount of melanin in the epidermis.

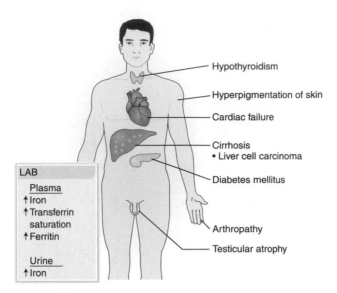

Figure 3-2 Hemochromatosis. Iron accumulates in major organs causing tissue injury.

Endocrine glands. Accumulation of hemosiderin in the pancreas is associated with diabetes and related to injury of the islets of Langerhans. Diabetes mellitus develops more readily in persons who have a genetic predisposition and a family history of diabetes. Other endocrine organs may be affected as well, most notably the thyroid and the gonads. Testicular atrophy and consequences of reduced testoster-

one production (e.g., loss of libido, erectile dysfunction, gynecomastia) are common.

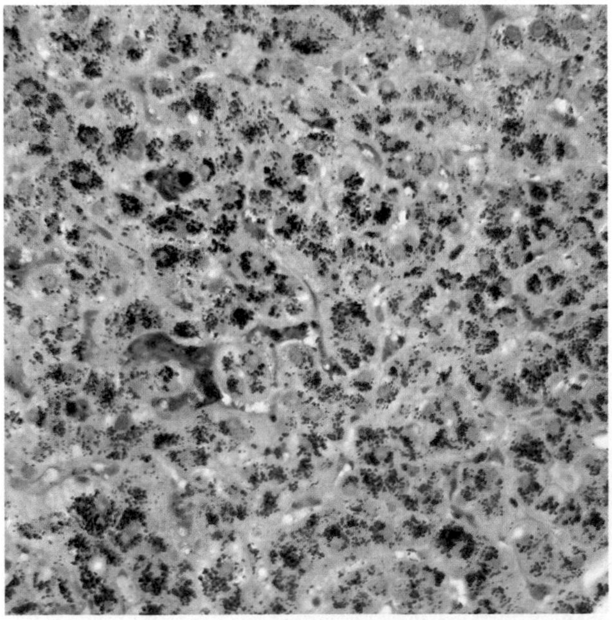

Joints. Deposits of hemosiderin cause joint injury typically associated with calcification of synovium and secondary changes in the adjacent bone. Many joints can be affected, but for unknown reasons the disease tends to begin with symptoms related to the second and third metacarpophalangeal joints.

Heart. Deposits of iron in the myocardium lead to cardiopathy with pump failure, dilatation of the heart, and conduction abnormalities.

Hemochromatosis is associated with diagnostic changes in iron metabolism.

Hemochromatosis is characterized by markedly increased body iron stores. The iron stores can be assessed with the use of several tests as follows:

- **Total plasma iron.** Normal plasma contains iron in a concentration of 50 to 170 μg/dL (9–30 μm/L). In hereditary hemochromatosis plasma iron concentration is usually increased to over 200 μg/dL.
- **Transferrin saturation.** Normally approximately 35% of serum transferrin is saturated with iron. In hereditary hemochromatosis the saturation of transferrin is over 50% and can be as high as 100%.
- **Serum ferritin.** Normal serum contains less than 200 μg/dL of ferritin. In hereditary hemochromatosis serum ferritin is over 1000 μg/L. An elevation of serum ferritin by 1 μg/L corresponds to approximately 65 mg of iron in the body stores.

Figure 3-3 Hemochromatosis. Hemosiderin, demonstrated in this slide of a liver biopsy specimen as bluish pigment resulting from the Prussian blue reaction, is seen in the form of granules in liver cells and Kupffer cells.

■ **Urinary iron excretion.** Normally the urine collected over 24 hours contains less than 2 mg of iron. In hereditary hemochromatosis urinary excretion is increased at least five times over the normal limit.

Pearl

> Serum transferrin saturation over 50% in a fasting person is highly suggestive of hemochromatosis.

These tests are usually performed as a battery to avoid false positive or negative results. For example, the serum ferritin level is markedly increased after extensive liver cell necrosis. Serum iron levels may be elevated in chronic alcoholics. Transferrin is a negative acute-phase protein, and its production is reduced in response to acute and many chronic diseases, as well as to malnutrition. Hence, its relatively high rate of saturation may be misleading sometimes.

Deposits of iron in the liver can be estimated subjectively in **liver biopsy** specimens stained with Prussian blue reacting with hemosiderin (see Fig. 3-3). Furthermore, the iron content of the liver biopsy specimen can be quantitated biochemically and expressed as iron in milligrams per gram of liver tissue. Liver containing increased amounts of iron appears *denser than normal on CT or MRI* examination. **Genetic testing** provides the final diagnosis. Genetic testing should also be offered to first-degree relatives. Treatment includes weekly phlebotomy to reduce the total iron content of the tissues.

Gout

Gout is a syndrome that includes hyperuricemia and periodic deposition of uric acid crystals in tissues, leading to formation of tophaceous nodules and recurrent crystal-mediated arthritis or renal injury. The reasons for the deposition of uric acid crystals are not fully understood, and the role of hyperuricemia in the pathogenesis of gouty arthritis has not been fully defined. To appreciate the complexity of gout and its relationship to hyperuricemia consider the following facts:

■ Only 2% to 3% of adults develop gout, even though 10% of the total adult population has hyperuricemia, defined empirically as an elevation of uric acid concentration in blood over 7 mg/dL (0.41 mmol/L). There is a sex-related difference in uric acid metabolism, and thus the actual upper limit of normal is 7 mg/dL for females and 8 mg/dL for males.

■ Over 90% of persons who have hyperuricemia never develop gout. This is most notable among cancer patients, 25% of whom have hyperuricemia, yet few of them ever develop gouty arthritis.

■ Gout is much more common in men than in women. The male to female ratio for this disease is 9:1. The serum concentration of uric acid is lower in women than in men, but this explains only in part the considerably lower incidence of gout in women.

Although hyperuricemia does not always cause gout, it is associated with an increased risk of gouty arthritis: in persons with normal uric acid the risk of gout is 1% and in those with concentrations 2 to 3 mg/dL above the upper limit of normal, the risk rises 20% to 30%. In general terms, the higher the concentration of uric acid the higher is the risk of gout.

Pearl

> During an attack of gouty arthritis uric acid is within normal limits in approximately 30% patients. Most likely this related to the periodic nature of hyperuricemia in these persons.

Uric acid concentration in blood depends on the balance between production and excretion of uric acid.

Uric acid is the end product of the degradation of adenine and guanine. The immediate metabolic precursor of uric acid is xanthine (Fig. 3-4). Xanthine may be produced directly from guanine or from hypoxanthine through the action of xanthine oxidoreductase. This enzyme has a dual function, acting as oxidase and dehydrogenase. It also transforms xanthine into uric acid. Although the breakdown of nucleic acids occurs in all tissues, uric acid is produced only in organs, such as the liver and the intestines, that contain xanthine oxidoreductase.

Overproduction of xanthine is prevented by hypoxanthine-guanine phosphoribosyl transferase (HGPRT), the primary enzyme involved in the so-called salvage pathway, which replenishes the inosinic and guanylic acid pools. Inosinic acid may be converted into adenylic acid and guanylic acid, both of which have a negative feedback effect on the formation of inosinic acid from phospho-α-D-ribosylpyrophosphate (PRPP).

The body contains approximately 1800 mg of uric acid, one third of which is turned over daily. Approximately two thirds of all uric acid is derived from the degradation of the purines, adenine and guanine (Fig. 3-5). The remaining third is derived from the diet. Two thirds of uric acid is eliminated from the blood in urine, and the remaining third through the intestines.

Ionized uric acid binds to sodium, and in blood it is predominantly found in the form of monosodium urate. Under physiologic conditions monosodium urate is saturated at a concentration of 6.8 mg/dL (415 μmol/L), and at higher concentrations one would expect it to precipitate and form crystals. This, however, does not occur, because

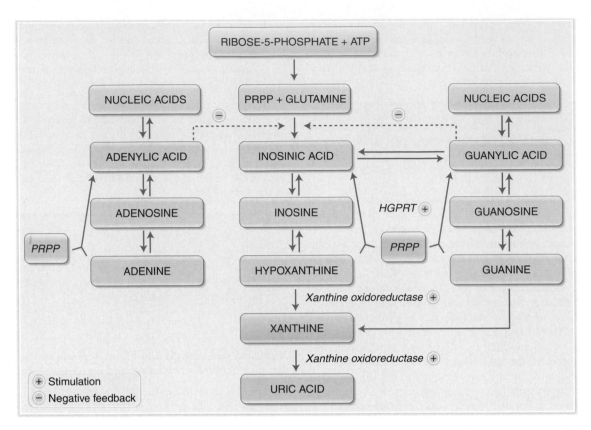

Figure 3-4 Formation of uric acid. Uric acid is formed from xanthine, and is the end product of the degradation of adenine and guanine. Note that inosinic acid forms from phospho-α-D-ribosylpyrophosphate (PRPP) under negative feedback control (dotted line), and that the overproduction of xanthine from hypoxanthine and guanine is regulated by hypoxanthine-guanine phosophoribosyltransferase (HGPRT) in the so-called salvage pathway.

the blood contains some stabilizing substances that prevent such crystallization. The solubility of monosodium urate decreases at low temperature, which accounts for the deposition of urate crystals in the joint tissue of the big toe during attacks of gouty arthritis.

Uric acid is filtered in the glomeruli, but almost all of it entering the proximal tubule is reabsorbed. Uric acid is then secreted back into the tubules and again reabsorbed to a large extent, so that only 10% of the uric acid is finally excreted into the urine. One third of the blood uric acid is excreted into the lumen of the intestine, where it undergoes uricolysis by the normal intestinal flora.

Hyperuricemia may develop due to overproduction or underexcretion of uric acid.

Hyperuricemia can result from overproduction or underexcretion of uric acid. Excessive dietary intake of purines can play a role under both conditions. Furthermore, in some patients both overproduction and underexcretion of uric acid occur. Alcohol, one of the most common triggers of gouty arthritis, can stimulate overproduction and prevent excretion.

Overproduction of uric acid is found in an isolated form in only 10% of all patients with gout. The defect can be **primary,** as in some inborn errors of metabolism, or **secondary,** when the excessive production of purines is related to increased cell lysis or turnover.

■ **Primary uric acid overproduction.** The prototype of this condition is **Lesch-Nyhan syndrome.** This inborn error of purine metabolism related to the deficiency of HGPRT is a rare X-linked cause of primary hyperuricemia. The deficiency of HGPRT results in a dysfunction of the salvage pathway and an overproduction of uric acid and gout of early onset. Several other genetic diseases also produce hyperuricemia, but fortunately these conditions are rare.

■ **Secondary hyperproduction of uric acid.** Uric acid overproduction typically occurs in tumor lysis syndrome after chemotherapy. Chemotherapy-induced killing of tumor cells results in a release of purine and pyrimidines from damaged nuclei; purines are then metabolized into uric acid. Leukemia, lymphoma, and chronic hemolytic

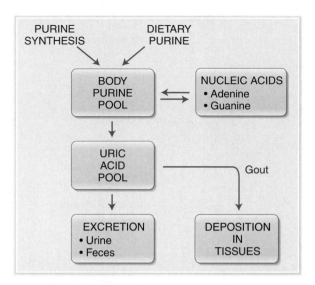

Figure 3-5 Metabolism of purines. Purines are derived from food, are newly synthesized, or formed from DNA. Purines are metabolized into uric acid, which is excreted in the kidneys or the intestines. Deposition of uric acid crystals in tissue leads to gout.

anemia also cause hyperuricemia. Chronic diseases characterized by epithelial proliferation—such as psoriasis or excessive bone formation, such as occurs in Paget's disease of bones—are also associated with overproduction of uric acid.

Overproducers of uric acid excrete uric acid in the urine in excess of 750 to 1000 mg/day, which may lead to the formation of uric acid stones in the urinary system. Overproduction of uric acid should be suspected if the attack of gout occurs at an early age, if there is a family history of early onset of gout, or if the uric acid renal stones are the first clinical sign of hyperuricemia.

Underexcretion of uric acid accounts for hyperuricemia in 90% of all patients with gout. These patients excrete less than 700 mg of uric acid per day. The causes include the following:

■ **Chronic renal disease.** Hyperuricemia occurs relatively late in the course of chronic renal failure, only after the disease has destroyed a significant number of nephrons. Patients who have polycystic kidney disease also cannot properly excrete uric acid in the urine.

■ **Drugs.** Hyperuricemia may be a side effect of treatment with diuretics, especially thiazides. Chronic ingestion of salicylates also may affect the tubular function and cause hyperuricemia. Levodopa and cyclosporine also cause hyperuricemia.

■ **Toxins.** The best know example is lead, which affects the excretion of uric acid in proximal tubules ("saturnine gout"). Alcohol can also reduce uric acid excretion in the kidneys.

■ **Metabolic disturbances.** Hyperuricemia is most often caused by lactic acidosis. Hyperparathyroidism and hypothyroidism may also affect renal tubular function and cause retention of uric acid.

Deposits of uric acid crystals in the joints cause inflammation.

Patients who have hyperuricemia tend to form deposits of monosodium phosphate in the connective tissue capsule of joints. These aggregates, called **microtophi,** may then spontaneously release monosodium urate into the synovial fluid, or a larger bolus of it is released due to mechanical trauma. Crystals in the synovial fluid have an irritating effect on the synovium and also have a chemotactic effect on neutrophils, which enter the joint cavity, thus contributing to the inflammation. The crystals also become coated with complement and immunoglobulin from exudated plasma. Complement and immunoglobulin act as opsonins, thus enabling the neutrophils to phagocytize the crystals. Activated neutrophils also produce oxygen radicals, arachidonic acid derivatives, and cytokines, which stimulate inflammation, cause vasodilation, and increase vascular permeability. These events account for the redness of the joint and its swelling. Crystals ingested into the phagocytic vacuoles of neutrophils tend to pierce the lysosomes, thus allowing a discharge of lytic enzyme into the extracellular space. Once initiated, the inflammation is autocatalytic and self-sustained, lasting for several days until it slowly abates (Fig. 3-6).

Chronic deposits of uric acid crystals lead to the formation of tophi.

Microscopic aggregates of monosodium urate crystals tend to enlarge with time until they transform into nodular masses visible by the naked eye or in radiographs in the periarticular bone. These nodules are called **tophi** (from the Latin word *tophus,* meaning porous stone). Most often they are found around the joints and the subchondral bone or subcutaneous tissue (Fig. 3-7). Typical locations are the metatarsophalangeal joint of the big toe, Achilles and infrapatellar tendons, the elbow and fingers, or the pinna of the ear. Tophi may form also in internal organs, such as the kidneys, but less commonly than in subcutaneous sites and around joints.

The formation of tophi is directly related to the duration of gout and the severity of hyperuricemia. They almost never occur in asymptomatic hyperuricemia.

Tophi act as space-occupying lesions and may cause pain, deformities of joints, and chronic inflammation. Bulging tophi may ulcerate the skin, and those inside the bone may erode the bone and cause large defects.

Hyperuricemia may damage kidneys and cause nephrolithiasis.

Prolonged hyperuricemia may affect the function of renal tubules (urate nephropathy). Deposits of monosodium phosphates are found in the medulla, where they may cause tissue

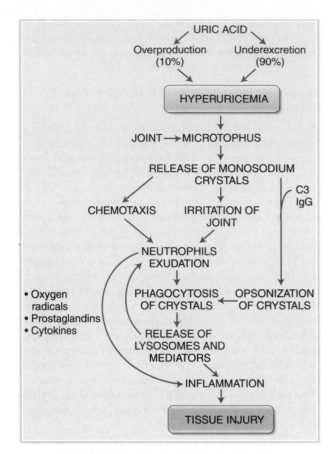

Figure 3-6 Acute arthritis in gout. Crystals of monosodium urate initiate the inflammation and act as chemoattractants for neutrophils. Crystals are covered with immunoglobulin and complement C3, which serve as opsonins, facilitating the phagocytosis of crystals. Lytic enzymes released from phagocytic vacuoles contribute to inflammation.

injury and predispose a person to secondary infection (pyelonephritis). Uric acid stones are formed in acid urine. The incidence of calcium phosphate stones is also increased.

Alcoholism

Ethyl alcohol (ethanol) is present in all alcoholic beverages such as beer, wine, or hard liquor. At least 70% of adults in the United States drink alcoholic beverages occasionally, but only about 10% of those drink excessive amounts that could adversely affect health. Still, alcohol abuse is widespread, and probably 10 to 12 million Americans are chronic alcoholics. Alcohol-related health problems account for a significant number of hospital admissions, traffic accidents, family violence, and chronic professional disability.

The following definitions are useful for considering the adverse effects of alcohol:

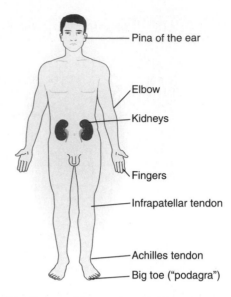

Figure 3-7 Gout and hyperuricemia. The most common sites of monosodium urate crystal deposition.

Acute intoxication (drunkenness). Psychological and somatic consequences of alcohol overdose. Like intoxication with other psychotropic substances alcohol intoxication is characterized by a depression of the central nervous system (CNS). Depending on the amount of alcohol consumed CNS depression may manifest as sedation and drowsiness, loss of motor coordination, delirium, or loss of consciousness that may progress to lethal coma.

Chronic alcoholism. A pattern of chronic alcohol consumption that is accompanied by psychological and physiologic signs of alcohol abuse and dependence.

Alcohol abuse. A repetitive pattern of drinking that continues even though it has adverse effects in one or more of the following five spheres of life: marital, social, legal, occupational, or physical. The consensus opinion of a scientific panel of the American Psychiatric Association is that a diagnosis of alcohol abuse should be used only if the patient has been drinking excessively for more than a month and he or she does not meet the criteria for alcohol dependence.

> **Pearl**
>
> > **Problem drinker** is a term used for persons who abuse alcohol, but if adverse consequences of drinking are pointed out to them, they can change their behaviors and stop drinking.

Alcohol dependence. This term is used to describe uncontrollable alcohol intake associated with tolerance to the effects of alcohol and symptomatic withdrawal when alcohol is not available. The diagnosis is made if at least three of the criteria listed in Table 3-1 are met.

Alcohol has direct effects on the brain.

Alcohol acts on brain cells as a toxin. It changes the fluidity of cell membranes, affecting the transmission of neural impulses, thus causing depression of neural activity. Alcohol has a sedative effect on most neural centers, but the suppression of some centers may lead to a loss of inhibition of others. This may induce a feeling of relaxation or good mood, as well as increased motor activity or uncontrolled emotions. The effects are dose-dependent and can be predicted roughly from the blood alcohol concentration (Fig. 3-8) as follows:

- 50 mg/dL (11 mmol/L)—sedation
- 50 to 150 mg/dL (11–33 mmol/L)—loss of motor coordination
- 150 to 200 mg/dL (33–43 mmol/L)—delirium
- 300 to 400 mg/dL (65–87 mmol/L)—unconsciousness and coma or respiratory arrest

Blood alcohol concentration can be reliably predicted from the breath test, which is routinely used by law enforcement to check for alcohol intoxication in drivers. Most of the states define legal intoxication with alcohol as a blood alcohol level of 100 mg/dL (22 mmol/L) in a person driving a motor vehicle.

Alcohol is metabolized in the liver.

Alcohol is absorbed in the stomach and small intestine, from which it is transported into the liver. In liver cells alcohol is metabolized through the action of alcohol dehydrogenase in the cytosol, P_{450} cytochrome (CYP2E) in the smooth endoplasmic reticulum of the microsomal fraction, and catalase in peroxisomes (Fig. 3-9).

Table 3-1 Criteria for the Diagnosis of Alcohol Dependence

1. The individual drinks more than he/she means to, *often.*
2. The individual is unsuccessful at cutting down.
3. Much time is spent thinking about getting a drink, or when the next drink will be taken.
4. There are frequent ill effects from drinking, such as absence from work, or being drunk or hung over at work.
5. The individual gives up important nondrinking activities.
6. The individual continues to drink even though it causes problems in family or with health.
7. A tolerance for alcohol has developed.
8. The individual has physical withdrawal symptoms.
9. The individual takes substances to relieve withdrawal symptoms.

Modified from Greene HL, Fincher RM, Johnson WP (eds): Clinical Medicine, 2nd ed. St. Louis, Mosby, p. 748, 1996.

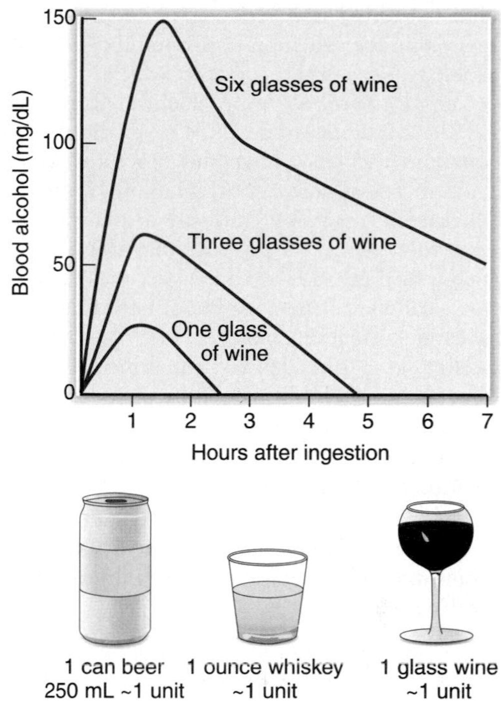

Figure 3-8 Acute alcohol intoxication. The blood concentration depends on the amount of alcohol ingested. The approximate blood alcohol levels for a 70-kg man are shown, using a 120-mL wine glass as a unit. The average alcohol content of wine is 11–13 mg/dL, beer 4–6 mg/dL, and whiskey or other hard liquors 40–45 mg/dL. The alcohol is cleared from the body at the same rate irrespective of the type of drink that was ingested.

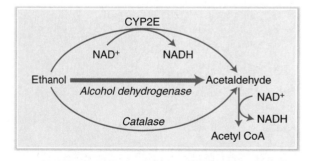

Figure 3-9 Three enzymes play a key function in the metabolism of alcohol in liver cells: alcohol dehydrogenase, CYP2E (cytochrome P_{450} enzyme in the smooth endoplasmic reticulum of the microsomal fraction), and catalase in peroxisomes. Alcohol dehydrogenase is the most important liver enzyme involved in oxidation of alcohol, transforming it into acetaldehyde, which is then oxidized to acetylcoenzyme A (CoA). Nicotine adenine dinucleotide (NAD^+) is reduced to NADH in this process, as well as during the action of CYP2E, a toxic metabolite, which is in turn oxidized to acetyl CoA by aldehyde dehydrogenase.

Alcohol dehydrogenase is the most important liver enzyme involved in the oxidation of alcohol. It oxidizes alcohol into acetaldehyde, a toxic metabolite, which is in turn oxidized to acetyl coenzyme A by aldehyde dehydrogenase. Nicotine adenine dinucleotide (NAD^+) is the cofactor for both oxidation reactions and in this process is reduced to NADH. An increased ratio of NADH to NAD^+ inhibits the NAD^+-dependent oxidation of lactate to pyruvate, leading to lactic acidosis. A lack of pyruvate may cause hypoglycemia, which is further exacerbated by poor intake of nutrients in chronic alcoholics. Beta oxidation of fatty acid is reduced and triglyceride formation enhanced, leading to fatty change in liver cells (Fig. 3-10). Hence, alcohol metabolism in the liver ultimately results in the formation of *toxic products* and *metabolic disturbances* affecting the function of liver cells. If these changes persist, fatty liver may progress into alcoholic steatohepatitis and finally into cirrhosis.

Chronic intake of alcohol and associated vitamin deficiencies may affect adversely the brain and peripheral nerves.

Chronic alcohol consumption is typically associated with **tolerance,** a condition in which the chronic alcoholic can drink much more than a novice and still show fewer signs of intoxication. On the other hand if an alcohol-dependent person is denied access to alcohol, he or she can present with signs of **alcohol withdrawal syndrome.** The severity of symptoms varies from mild tremulousness ("the shakes") to delirium tremens, seizures, and even death. Alcohol withdrawal occurs during the first 24 hours and is accompanied by physical signs and symptoms, such as facial flushing, tachycardia, and irritability.

Chronic alcoholics often have neurologic symptoms, but most of these seem to be related to a nutrient deficiency of vitamin B_1 (thiamine).

- **Wernicke's encephalopathy** is characterized by confusion, ophthalmoplegia, nystagmus, ataxia, and peripheral sensory-motor neuropathy.
- **Peripheral neuropathy** may be the only neurologic finding in some patients. It includes both motor and sensory symptoms, such as weakness; pain; paresthesia; and a loss of touch, position, vibration, and deep tendon reflexes.
- **Korsakoff's psychosis** is characterized by amnesia, an inability to learn, and a tendency for confabulation.

Chronic alcohol intake has adverse effects on the cardiac and skeletal muscles.

Alcohol interferes with the metabolism of muscle cells and is also toxic to both cardiac and skeletal muscle cells. Many chronic alcoholics have a deficiency of vitamin B_1 (thiamine), which may adversely affect the heart.

- **Skeletal muscle.** Alcoholic muscle injury may manifest clinically as progressive weakness and wasting. During bouts of heavy drinking rhabdomyolysis can ensue, producing a marked elevation of creatine kinase in the blood and renal tubular necrosis due to the obstruction of renal tubules with cytoplasmic detritus released from skeletal muscle cells that have undergone rhabdomyolysis.
- **Heart.** Chronic alcohol abuse may cause cardiomyopathy. In part it is due to the toxic effects of alcohol on cardiac myocytes and in part it is related to thiamine deficiency ("beri-beri heart"). Acute overindulgence with alcohol may cause arrhythmia or bouts of tachycardia ("holiday heart").

Alcohol abuse may induce numerous metabolic changes and affect any organ in the body.

Chronic alcohol abuse and related nutritional deficiencies may have adverse effects on the hematopoietic, endocrine, and gastrointestinal systems, but it is often impossible to determine whether such effects are due directly to alcohol toxicity or are a consequence of deficiencies of vitamins, iron, and other nutrients. For example anemia in chronic alcoholics is often macrocytic and it could be related to folic acid deficiency, poor nutrition, or toxic effects of alcohol on the bone marrow. Reduced resistance to infection is probably related to the adverse effects of alcohol on white blood cells, but the real causes for this abnormality are unknown. Increased incidence of gout in chronic alcoholics is related to the additional production and reduced excretion of uric acid. The most common consequences of chronic alcohol abuse are shown in Figure 3-11.

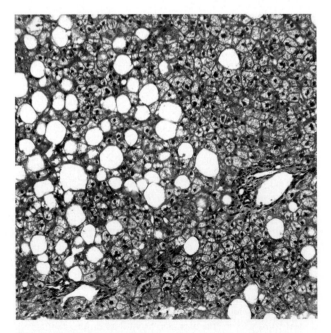

Figure 3-10 Biopsy specimen demonstrating fatty liver caused by alcohol abuse.

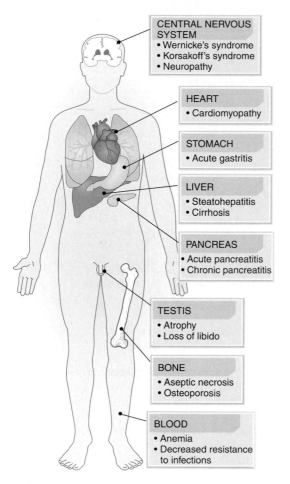

CENTRAL NERVOUS SYSTEM
• Wernicke's syndrome
• Korsakoff's syndrome
• Neuropathy

HEART
• Cardiomyopathy

STOMACH
• Acute gastritis

LIVER
• Steatohepatitis
• Cirrhosis

PANCREAS
• Acute pancreatitis
• Chronic pancreatitis

TESTIS
• Atrophy
• Loss of libido

BONE
• Aseptic necrosis
• Osteoporosis

BLOOD
• Anemia
• Decreased resistance to infections

Figure 3-11 The most common clinical consequences of chronic alcohol abuse.

Shock

Shock is a hemodynamic disturbance characterized by systemic hypoperfusion resulting in inadequate oxygen supply to vital organs. Shock can be pathogenetically classified as:

■ **Cardiogenic shock.** The prototype of this form of shock is cardiac pump failure that develops in myocardial infarction.
■ **Hypovolemic shock.** The circulatory disturbances result from inadequate intravascular volume, as typically seen after massive blood loss due to bleeding.
■ **Distributive shock.** Shock results from massive dilatation of blood vessels and a subsequent disproportion between the blood volume and the capacitance of the vasculature, as typically seen in septic shock.

In many instances shock may have more than one cause and is thus mediated by several pathogenetic mechanisms

(Fig. 3-12). Likewise, shock may begin in one form and evolve into another. For example hypovolemic shock due to blood loss may cause hypoxic injury of the heart. Hence, it becomes cardiogenic shock that continues even after the blood loss has been replaced.

Cardiogenic shock may be caused by several mechanisms that reduce the cardiac output.

Cardiac output depends on ventricular filling during diastole and on the strength of ventricular contraction during systole. Cardiogenic shock may result from various processes interfering with diastolic filling (**preload**), myocardial **pump failure**, or an obstruction of the outflow (**afterload**) as follows:

■ **Decreased preload.** Venous return of blood into the right atrium may be reduced due to hemorrhage, loss of plasma in severe burns, fluid loss in diarrhea, or influx of fluid into the peritoneal cavity in acute pancreatitis.
■ **Mechanical obstruction of venous return.** Thromboemboli of the pulmonary veins may obstruct pulmonary blood flow and thus completely stop the return of blood into the right ventricle. Tension pneumothorax may compress the pulmonary veins and produce the same effect.
■ **Impaired diastolic dilatation of the ventricles.** Pericardial tamponade due to hemopericardium or constrictive pericarditis may prevent normal dilatation of the ventricles during diastole and thus reduce the preload. Impaired ventricular filling is encountered in ventricular tachyarrhythmia, as well as in hypertrophic or constrictive cardiomyopathy.
■ **Contractile insufficiency.** Pump failure can occur in myocardial infarction, various forms of myocarditis, or dilated cardiomyopathy. Ventricular arrhythmias also weaken the contractile strength of the heart.
■ **Valvular obstruction.** Increased afterload due to structural changes of the aortic or pulmonary valves may reduce cardiac output.
■ **Valvular insufficiency.** Incomplete closure of valves allows backflow of the blood, reducing its forward propulsion. At the same time the reflux of blood increases the strain on the ventricular myocardium, incrementally diminishing its pumping capacity.

Hypovolemic shock results from a loss of fluid from the vascular space.

In hypovolemic shock the volume of circulating blood is reduced. Volume reduction can be a consequence of several pathologic processes as follows:

■ **Bleeding.** Massive bleeding with a loss in excess of 500 mL causes hypotension, reduces venous return, and lowers cardiac output. Bleeding in such volume occurs most often from arteries, but may develop

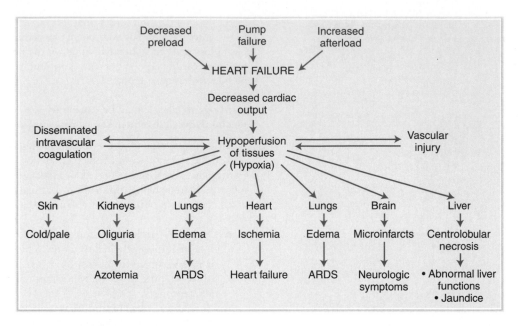

Figure 3-12 Cardiogenic shock. ARDS, acute respiratory distress syndrome.

from veins under pressure, as in esophageal varicose veins, in portal hypertension, or from the heart. The causes include trauma, spontaneous rupture of an aortic aneurysm, bleeding esophageal varices, bleeding peptic ulcer, ruptured ectopic pregnancy, or a pregnant uterus during or after the delivery.

■ **Fluid loss.** Loss of extracellular fluid may occur in persons who have suffered severe body burns. Vomiting, severe diarrhea, and polyuria also may cause excessive fluid loss.

■ **Pooling of fluid in the intestines.** Pooling can occur during paralytic ileus or be due to intestinal volvulus or obstruction by tumors.

■ **Pooling of fluid in body cavities.** Ascites and hydrothorax may reduce the volume of circulating blood.

■ **Anasarca.** Increased vascular permeability as seen in septic shock or anaphylactic shock is associated with generalized edema and with reduced volume of fluid in circulation.

Distributive shock results from vasodilation, increasing the capacitance of the vascular system.

Distributive shock is characterized by marked dilatation of blood vessels. Under such conditions a disproportion results between the volume of blood, which is normal, and the capacitance of the vascular space, which is increased. The possible causes of distributive shock include the following:

■ **Sepsis.** Severe bacterial infection may cause a massive release of bacterial endotoxins, which may stimulate several body reactions. The most important among

these is the **systemic inflammatory response system (SIRS),** a systemic response mediated by cytokines and mediators of inflammation produced by macrophages and white blood cells in the blood. The mediators of SIRS, such as tumor necrosis factor (TNF), interleukins, nitric oxide (NO), and others act on arterioles, capillaries, or venules, causing their dilatation and creating subsequent pooling of blood in the peripheral circulation. Reduced return of blood into the heart decreases the preload with a consequent drop in cardiac output, resulting in hypotension.

■ **Anaphylactic shock.** Vasodilation encountered in type I hypersensitivity reaction to foreign proteins (including *Hymenoptera* venom) or drugs is mediated by vasoactive substances released from mast cells coated with immunoglobulin E (IgE). Vasodilation, which is typically associated with increased vascular permeability, is mostly caused by histamine stored in mast cell granules.

■ **Neurogenic shock.** Brain trauma and intracranial hemorrhage are typically associated with widespread dilatation of blood vessels. This results from the increased intracranial pressure on the vasomotor centers, especially in the abdominal organs, and consequent splanchnic pooling of blood. Spinal cord injury also leads to vasodilation.

■ **Drugs.** Vasoactive drugs may cause massive dilatation. Overdose with narcotics acting on the medullary centers may cause coma with peripheral vasodilation. Anesthesia may also cause hypotension. Adverse drug reactions may manifest as anaphylactic shock.

Table 3-2 Circulatory Changes in Various Forms of Shock

TYPE OF SHOCK	PERIPHERAL VESSELS	CARDIAC OUTPUT	PULMONARY WEDGE PRESSURE/ CENTRAL VENOUS PRESSURE
Cardiogenic	Constricted	Low	High
Hypovolemic	Constricted	Low	Low
Distributive	Dilated	Normal or high	Normal or low

Initial stages of shock are followed by compensatory reactions aimed at reducing the subsequent adverse effects.

All forms of shock are initially characterized by hypotension and reactive tachycardia. In cardiogenic and hypovolemic shock the blood vessels of the skin are constricted and the extremities appears pale, cold, and clammy. In distributive shock the extremities appear warm and well perfused and there is low peripheral vascular resistance. In contrast to the low cardiac output associated with cardiogenic and hypovolemic shock, cardiac output in distributive shock is high. In cardiogenic shock the pulmonary wedge pressure is high, whereas in the hypovolemic type it is low. In distributive shock it may be low or normal (Table 3-2).

In hypovolemic shock caused by massive blood loss the first compensatory reaction is activation of the baroreceptor reflex (Fig. 3-13). The hypovolemia causes hypotension, which triggers an increase in sympathetic outflow and reactive tachycardia. Sympathetic stimulation also favors peripheral vasoconstriction, thus increasing peripheral resistance.

Hypoperfusion of the kidneys leads to low urinary output and also activates the renin–angiotensin system. Angiotensin II is a potent vasoconstrictor, which further promotes the constriction of arterioles, thus increasing total peripheral resistance (TPR). At the same time angiotensin II stimulates the release of aldosterone from the adrenal glands, which spurs renal reabsorption of sodium and fluid retention. Peripheral dilatation of capillaries reduces the capillary pressure, thus facilitating the entry of fluid from the interstitial spaces into the capillaries. All these mechanisms increase the volume of blood in the venous system and thus increase the preload. Improved contractility of the heart combined with increased preload leads to an increase in cardiac output.

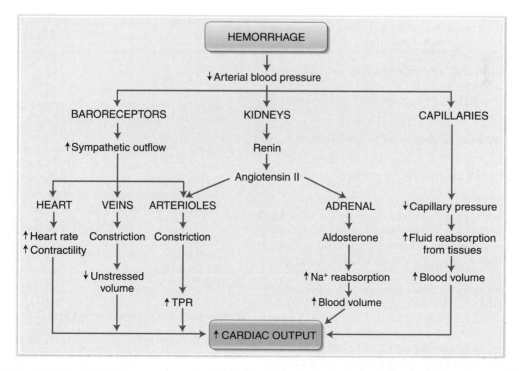

Figure 3-13 Hypotensive shock. Massive hemorrhage results in hypotension, which elicits a rapid baroreceptor response and activation of the sympathetic system, as well as renal release of renin. The aim of these reactions is to adjust the body to the blood loss and to compensate for it by increasing cardiac output. TPR, total peripheral resistance.

Shock leads to multiple organ failure.

Hypoperfusion of the tissues causes ischemia of endothelial cells in the terminal microvasculature. Injury to endothelial cells affects their capacity to react to physiologic stimuli and also leads to increased permeability and formation of edema. Ischemic injury to endothelial cells triggers disseminated intravascular coagulation (DIC), which, combined with hypotension, produces significant ischemia in the parenchymal organs. As a consequence, dysfunction of all major organs ensues, clinically manifesting as multiple organ failure. The following important manifestations of shock are seen in moribund patients:

- **Disseminated intravascular coagulation.** Microvascular thrombi are seen in major organs.
- **Diffuse alveolar damage of acute respiratory distress syndrome (ARDS).** The lungs are edematous and show widespread deposits of fibrin along the alveolar lining ("hyaline membranes"). These changes correlate with the respiratory problems seen in many shock patients (i.e., tachypnea and dyspnea), and are unresponsive to oxygen therapy.
- **Renal tubular necrosis.** It correlates with low urinary output (oliguria) progressing to anuria.
- **Centrolobular necrosis of the liver.** Necrosis of the liver accounts for the increased levels of serum aspartate aminotransferase (AST) and alanine aminotransferase (ALT) and prolongation of prothrombin time.
- **Ischemic necroses in the myocardium.** These focal changes correspond to hypoperfusion of the heart and contribute to pump failure.
- **Edema and focal ischemic changes in the brain.** These changes are seen only in terminally ill comatose patients who have the most advanced form of shock.

Clinically the severity of shock can be graded from mild to severe.

Shock can be mild and readily treatable or severe and refractory.

- **Mild shock.** The patient is in distress but conscious. The blood pressure is lower than normal and accompanied by tachycardia. Tachypnea and mild dyspnea are also present. Urinary output is reduced, but not severely.
- **Moderate shock.** As shock progresses, the patient becomes confused and restless, and hypotension and oliguria become more pronounced. Respiratory distress develops, and oxygen needs to be administered. Lactic acidosis is a sign of widespread hypoxic cell injury.
- **Advanced shock.** This stage of shock is dominated by multiple organ failure (Fig. 3-14). The patient is either agitated or apathetic and may lapse into coma. The blood pressure is very low and often unmeasureable.

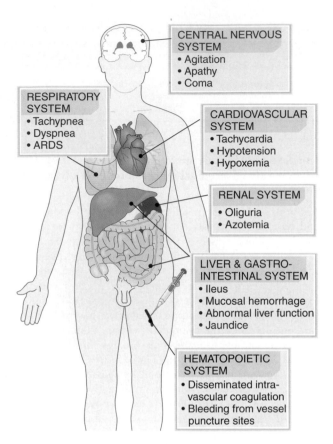

Figure 3-14 Multiple organ failure in shock. All major organs are involved. ARDS, acute respiratory distress syndrome.

Breathing is labored, and the patient requires assisted ventilation and develops signs of acute respiratory distress syndrome. The pulse is fast (tachycardia). The blood is poorly oxygenated, and the patient does not respond to the administration of oxygen. Urinary output is markedly reduced (oliguria progressing to anuria), and the laboratory tests show rising azotemia and metabolic acidosis. Coagulopathy indicative of DIC is common and typically associated with a bleeding tendency. Liver function tests are abnormal, and jaundice is often present. Mortality in this stage of shock is high.

Acquired Immunodeficiency Syndrome

AIDS is the final stage of infection with the human immunodeficiency virus (HIV).

HIV is a lentivirus from the family Retroviridae that has a predilection for infecting CD4 helper T cells and monocyte/macrophages. The virus is cytotoxic and capable of destroying parts of the immune system, engendering immunodeficiency in most infected persons. Within 10 years of the initial infection 50% of all untreated infected persons develop AIDS, 30% develop a milder form of immunodeficiency, and 20% remain asymptomatic.

HIV infection occurs most often through contact with infected blood or during sexual intercourse.

In addition to CD4 lymphocytes, HIV also infects monocytes and tissue macrophages, dendritic cells in the skin and lymph nodes, and microglial cells of the central nervous system. Virus can be isolated from the body fluids of infected persons, including blood, urine, saliva, tears, semen, milk, amniotic fluid, and spinal fluid.

The infection is most often transmitted by contact with the infected blood or body fluids. Modern testing of blood products has considerably reduced the risk of infection through transfusion, but has not completely eliminated it (the risk is very low, 1: 675,000). Hence, the groups most at risk are as follows (in decreasing order):

- **Infants of HIV infected mothers.** Over 90% of all infants born to HIV-infected mothers are also infected.
- **Sexual partners of infected persons.** Unprotected sex remains the highest risk factor for HIV infection among adults, especially in underdeveloped countries.
- **Intravenous drug abusers**
- **Recipients of multiple blood transfusions of pooled blood derivatives** (e.g., hemophiliacs)

- **Health care providers.** Needle pricks carry a slight risk of infection, estimated to be around 0.3%.

HIV infection can be divided into three phases: acute infection, latency phase, and AIDS.

The signs and symptoms of HIV infection are often nonspecific, and in many cases the infection is not even recognized until serologic evidence becomes available. In typical cases HIV infection can be divided into three phases (Fig. 3-15).

Acute retroviral syndrome. This term is used for a set of symptoms that develop in 40% to 70% of all acutely infected persons and includes fatigue. Antibodies to HIV-related antigen gp120 and other antigens are undetectable by enzyme-labeled immunoassay (ELISA) for 4 to 12 weeks ("window period"), but the presence of virus can be demonstrated by measuring the viral RNA or p24 antigen in the blood.

Symptoms appear 2 to 8 weeks after infection but vary from one person to another. These symptoms are nonspecific but most often include the following:

- Fatigue (95%)
- Fever (95%)
- Sore throat (75%)
- Lymphadenopathy (75%)
- Myalgia (60%)
- Rash on the trunk or face (50%)
- Headache (35%)

The pathogenesis of these symptoms has not been elucidated completely. Fatigue and fever are considered to be mediated by cytokine released from infected macrophages.

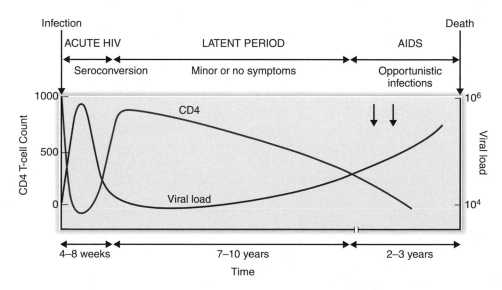

Figure 3-15 HIV infection. Typically the infection has three phases: Acute HIV syndrome, a latent period, and clinical AIDS. Viral load rises during the acute phase but drops down to very low levels during the latent period. It rises again during the AIDS phase. The CD4 count shows a progressive decline even during the latent phase, reaching a critical low level in the AIDS phase.

Sore throat and lymph node enlargement are related to the reaction of interdigitating cells and the hyperplasia of lymphoid follicles in the tonsils and other lymphoid organs. The skin rash is possibly related to immune complexes formed to viral antigens, but could also be related to proinflammatory cytokines. Headache occurs in approximately one half of all patients and is related to aseptic meningitis, characterized by an increased number of lymphocytes in the cerebrospinal fluid and slight hyperproteinemia.

Latency phase. This period lasts several years but in 80% of all infected persons immunodeficiency will develop over a period of 10 years. The rate of progression to immunodeficiency varies and is generally slower in younger than older persons. Many patients are asymptomatic or have only nonspecific symptoms. The symptoms and signs most often include the following:

- **Lymphadenopathy** (30–60%). Lymph node enlargement is typically persistent, lasting more than 3 months and involving at least two groups of lymph nodes outside the inguinal area.
- **Mucocutaneous infections** (5–10%). These include genital or oral herpesvirus infection, varicella-zoster infection, or hairy leukoplakia.

- **Skin diseases.** The incidence of seborrheic dermatitis is increased, and in patients who have psoriasis the symptoms may be more pronounced.
- **Bacterial pneumonia.** Infections with *Streptococcus pneumoniae* or other bacterial agents of pneumonia occur four times more often than in the general population.

The CD4 counts continue to decrease but typically remain over 200 cells/μL. Antibodies to HIV antigens are detectable by ELISA. However, these antibodies are inefficient in controlling the proliferation of the virus, which tends to mutate often, thus eluding the activated humoral and cellular immune responses.

Acquired immunodeficiency phase. Over a period of 4 to 10 years, the CD4 counts drop below 200 cells/mL, predisposing the affected person to opportunistic infections. Either one of these two criteria (i.e., CD count, 200 cells/mL or an AIDS-defining opportunistic infection) is sufficient for the diagnosis of AIDS. Essentially all organ systems can be affected (Fig. 3-16).

Acquired immunodeficiency syndrome is dominated by signs of opportunistic infections.

Central nervous system. HIV infects the brain by entering the central nervous system (CNS) in macrophages. The brain

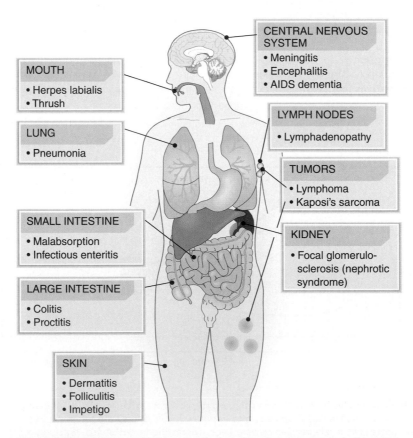

Figure 3-16 Pathologic changes and clinical findings associated with AIDS.

and the meninges can thus be affected by the virus itself or by an increased incidence of superinfections. The most important aspects of CNS involvements are as follows:

■ **HIV encephalopathy.** This term covers a broad spectrum of neurologic and behavioral symptoms. Over a period of time it may lead to **dementia.** Dilatation of the lateral ventricles of the brain is a sign of brain atrophy and is commonly found in patients with AIDS. Such a low-pressure **hydrocephalus** may occur in those who have dementia but also in those who have no major mental deficiencies.

■ **Aseptic meningitis.** It is most often present at the time of seroconversion, but may occur in later stages of the disease as well. Meningitis is considered to cause headache and probably contributes to the hydrocephalus. It must be distinguished from the more ominous forms of meningitis caused by the opportunistic infections.

■ **Opportunistic infections** are common in AIDS patients and may involve the brain or the meninges. Depending on the causative agent the brain infections may be localized, as in infection with *Toxoplasma gondii,* or widespread, as in cytomegalovirus (CMV) infection. Localized destructive infection may produce mass effects with severe headache, neurologic motor or sensory symptoms, or loss of consciousness. Meningitis may be caused by viruses, fungi (e.g., *Cryptococcus neoformans*), or bacteria (e.g., *Mycobacterium tuberculosis*).

■ **Peripheral neuropathy** is a common complication of HIV infection, but it may also be related to opportunistic infections (e.g., infections with CMV, herpes simplex virus, or herpes zoster). It may also be a consequence of the toxic side effects of drugs used to treat HIV.

Respiratory system. Pulmonary infections caused by bacteria occur at an increased rate in the latency phase of HIV infection but become even more pronounced in the later stages of the disease. Opportunistic infections with the fungus *Pneumocystis jiroveci* (formerly known as *Pneumocystis carinii*) are, however, one of the most common AIDS-defining infections that occur in heavily immunosuppressed persons. Other infectious pathogens include the bacterium *Mycobacterium tuberculosis* and the fungi *Candida albicans, Aspergillus flavus, Blastomyces dermatitidis, Histoplasma,* and other less common fungi.

Gastrointestinal system. The entire upper and lower gastrointestinal (GI) system may be involved. The most important clinical signs and symptoms suggesting GI involvement are as follows:

■ **Nausea and vomiting.** The causes of these symptoms are complex, but often they contribute to the **weight loss, anorexia,** and generalized **weakness** of the AIDS patient.

■ **Oral infections.** Most often such infections are caused by viruses and fungi. Herpes labialis is caused by herpes simplex virus, thrush is caused by *Candida albicans,* and hairy leukoplakia is related to Epstein-Barr virus infection.

■ **Esophagitis.** It is caused by fungi or viruses.

■ **Diarrhea.** This very common feature of AIDS may be related to HIV or opportunistic infections. In some cases it is related to medication. The opportunistic infections may be caused by *Mycobacterium avium intracellulare, Cryptosporidum* sp., *Giardia intestinalis, Campylobacter jejuni,* or *Clostridium difficile.*

■ **Liver disease.** AIDS often causes functional disturbances evidenced in abnormal liver function tests. In patients who are infected with hepatitis virus B or C HIV infection may cause a flare-up of the chronic liver infection.

Hematopoietic and lymphoid system. AIDS is associated with prominent changes in the lymph nodes, bone marrow, and the peripheral blood. The most prominent signs are:

■ Lymph node enlargement
■ Anemia
■ Leukopenia
■ Thrombocytopenia
■ Lymphoma. An increased incidence of lymphoma is a long-term risk even in treated patients. The incidence of extranodal lymphomas, such as CNS lymphoma, is increased.

Skin. Itching is a common symptom, and sometimes it is related to small papules or nodules ("itchy bumps"). In some instances it is related to a specific fungal infection, but in many others the cause remains undetermined.

AIDS can aggravate any preexisting skin diseases. Its effects on seborrheic dermatitis and psoriasis are well known, and occur even before the AIDS stage. AIDS also predisposes the patient to uncommon infections. For example infection with *Rochalimaea henselae,* the cause of cat-scratch disease, may manifest in the form of bluish red nodules. Some infections are more severe than in other people. For example herpes simplex virus may present with deep ulcerations that take a long time to heal. Chronic viral infections, such as human papillomavirus infection, may become exacerbated, leading to formation of numerous **warts. Kaposi's sarcoma** is related to infection with herpesvirus type 8. This vascular tumor most often affects the skin, but is often multifocal and involves internal organs as well.

Other organs. Opportunistic infections and the HIV infection itself may involve other organs as well and thus cause the following diseases:

■ Cardiomyopathy
■ HIV-related nephrotic syndrome
■ Myopathy
■ Arthropathy
■ Adrenal insufficiency

- Retinopathy
- Cervical dysplasia/neoplasia

Systemic Lupus Erythematosus

SLE is a multisystemic **autoimmune disease** of unknown origin characterized by the formation of circulating immune complexes and their deposition in numerous organs. SLE predominantly affects women of child-bearing age (20–40 years of age), and is nine times more common in women than men.

SLE is a multifactorial disease under the influence of genetic, hormonal, and environmental factors.

The etiology and pathogenesis of SLE are not fully understood. All the available data indicate that the symptoms and signs of the disease result from a dysregulation of the immune system and a loss of self tolerance. The immune system of the affected person reacts against a number of self antigens, causing pathologic changes in many organs (Fig. 3-17).

The disease is multifactorial and is under the influence of genetic, hormonal, and environmental factors.

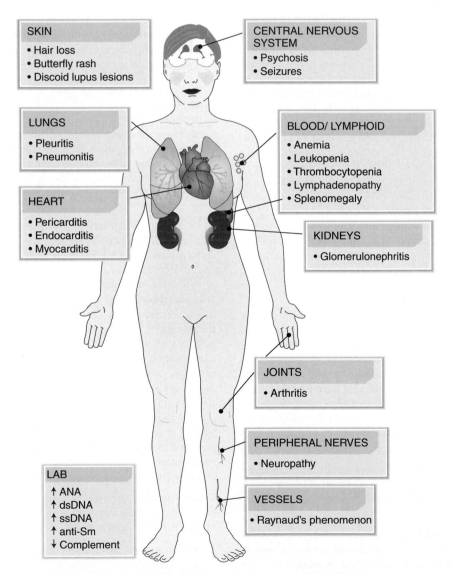

SKIN
- Hair loss
- Butterfly rash
- Discoid lupus lesions

CENTRAL NERVOUS SYSTEM
- Psychosis
- Seizures

LUNGS
- Pleuritis
- Pneumonitis

BLOOD/ LYMPHOID
- Anemia
- Leukopenia
- Thrombocytopenia
- Lymphadenopathy
- Splenomegaly

HEART
- Pericarditis
- Endocarditis
- Myocarditis

KIDNEYS
- Glomerulonephritis

JOINTS
- Arthritis

PERIPHERAL NERVES
- Neuropathy

LAB
- ↑ ANA
- ↑ dsDNA
- ↑ ssDNA
- ↑ anti-Sm
- ↓ Complement

VESSELS
- Raynaud's phenomenon

Figure 3-17 Pathologic changes and clinical findings owing to immune complex deposition in systemic lupus erythematosus. ANA, antinuclear antibody; dsDNA, double-stranded DNA; ssDNA, single-stranded DNA; anti-Sm, anti-Smith antibody.

Genetic predisposition. A familial predisposition to immune diseases may be found in a significant number of SLE patients. Genetic predisposition is suggested by the following findings:

- **Racial and ethnic differences.** The incidence of SLE varies from one population of women to another. Its incidence is three to four times higher in black women than in white women. The incidence of SLE is also high in Native American women, and the disease is very prevalent in China.
- **High concordance in monozygotic twins.** The concordance of the disease is close to 50% in monozygotic twins and is much higher than in heterozygotic twins.
- **Linkage to certain histocompatibility antigens.** HLA-DR2 and HLA-DR3 are associated with a three-time higher risk of SLE than other HLA haplotypes.
- **Genetic deficiencies of the complement system.** These deficiencies that affect the immune reactions are found in adult populations at a rate of 1:10,000 but may be found in 6% of all SLE patients.

Hormonal factors. SLE presents clinically most often during the second and third decade. During the reproductive years its incidence is nine times higher in women than in men. Even in prepubertal children SLE is more common in girls than in boys, but the female to male ratio is only 4:1 in children. After menopause the preponderance of women decreases as well.

Menarche, pregnancy, and even the use of oral contraceptives may precipitate the clinical onset of symptoms. In experimental animals that have a genetic form of SLE, ovariectomy may reduce the severity of the disease. All these data suggest that female sexual hormones play an important pathogenetic role, most likely facilitating the appearance of clinical symptoms.

Environmental factors. Several exogenous factors are known to precipitate the appearance of symptoms or adversely influence the course of the disease.

- **Ultraviolet light.** Exposure to sunlight plays an important role in the appearance of the skin rash. The rash is often seasonal and is typically most prominent on the face or the sun-exposed parts of the chest and the hands. The exact mechanism of this photosensitivity is not understood, but it seems that ultraviolet light has several effects. It stimulates keratinocytes to secrete cytokines, which promote local inflammation in the skin. It also may directly or indirectly alter the permeability of the dermal capillaries. Permeable capillaries allow circulating immune complexes to diffuse into the tissue and toward the epidermal–dermal basement membrane, where they are deposited, activating complement and producing skin injury.
- **Viruses.** Common viral infections aggravate symptoms of SLE. Many epidemiologic findings suggest a link between viral infections and SLE, but no definitive pathogenetic link between an infectious agent and the autoimmune disease has been found. A high incidence of autoantibodies among the family members of the affected patients and among the laboratory technicians dealing with the blood of such patients also suggests a possible infectious agent.
- **Drugs.** A number of drugs may produce an SLE-like syndrome, the most important among which are chlorpromazine, hydralazine, isoniazid, and methyldopa. In contrast to typical SLE, drug-induced lupus is equally common in men and women and it does not lead to complement consumption. Clinically, no renal or neurologic symptoms accompany drug-induced SLE, and the symptoms disappear after the drug has been discontinued.

SLE is characterized by an overproduction of antibodies that form immune complexes or are cytotoxic.

Patients with SLE produce antibodies directed at a variety of antigens, such as DNA, RNA, cell surface proteins, phospholipids, and other tissue components. The reasons for the overproduction of various antibodies are not fully understood. All the evidence indicates that the initial defect lies in helper or suppressor T cells, and that polyclonal B-lymphocyte activation is a secondary consequence of one or several T-cell defects.

The antibodies damage tissue in two ways: as immune complexes that are deposited in tissues or as cytotoxic antibodies that damage and kill cells. Activation of the complement cascade and the formation of biologically active complement fragments or complexes are essential for both of these effects.

Immune complexes. Antibodies to internal cell components cannot enter cells. Nevertheless these antibodies form immune complexes with the cell components that have leaked into the blood from damaged or dead cells. These circulating immune complexes, such as those directed against DNA or RNA, may be deposited in many organs. Typically this occurs in anatomic sites where the ultrafiltration of plasma leads to the formation of body fluids. The most common sites of immune complex deposition are the glomerular basement membranes, serosal surfaces of thoracic and abdominal organs, synovial membranes of the joints, choroid plexus of the lateral cerebral ventricles, or the choroids of the eye. Deposits are also seen in the skin along the epidermal–dermal junction. Activation of complement, which binds to the deposited immune complexes, leads to inflammation in these sites. The removal of complement containing immune complexes is defective, and thus the immune complexes remain in tissue longer than in otherwise healthy persons.

Cytotoxic antibodies. Antibodies directed to specific cell surface molecules react with cell surface antigens expressed on red blood cells, leukocytes, platelets, or endothelial cells. These antibodies also activate complement and kill cells either through complement-mediated mechanisms or by facilitating cell destruction by macrophages. Cytotoxic antibodies cause hemolytic anemia, leukopenia, or thrombocytopenia. They also mediate vasculitis at the site of endothelial cell injury.

Antibodies to nuclear antigens have diagnostic value.

Because antibodies to nuclear component cannot enter into cells, they are not cytotoxic. These antibodies can be readily detected in the blood of affected persons, but are often found in unaffected relatives and even other family members. These antibodies are of diagnostic significance and are useful for distinguishing SLE from closely related autoimmune disorders.

Antinuclear antibodies (ANAs). These antibodies are detected by testing the binding of patient's serum to nuclei of cells grown in tissue culture. The SLE patient's serum may contain antibodies to DNA, RNA, histones, and other nuclear proteins. After incubation, the patient's serum is washed and the antibodies bound to the nuclear components are detected by adding a fluoresceinated rabbit immunoglobulin reactive with human immunoglobulins. Four patterns could be detected by immunofluorescence microscopy as follows:

- **Diffuse pattern.** The entire nucleus stains because the antibodies react nonselectively with nucleic acid and protein components of the chromatin. This pattern is seen most often in SLE.
- **Speckled pattern.** This pattern is also commonly seen in SLE. It results from the binding of antibodies to nuclear proteins, such as histones and ribonucleoproteins.
- **Rim pattern.** In this pattern the staining is limited to the peripheral parts of the nucleus underlying the nuclear membrane. It results mostly from antibody binding to native double-stranded DNA. It is seen in up to 60% of SLE patients.
- **Nucleolar pattern.** Staining limited to the nucleolus is rarely seen in SLE and is typical of systemic sclerosis.

In clinical practice the ANA test is used for screening purposes, because it is positive in more than 95% of patients with SLE. However this test is also positive in most patients with systemic sclerosis, drug-induced lupus, and in Sjögren's syndrome and a significant number of persons with polymyositis or dermatomyositis. Confirming a diagnosis of SLE requires additional tests that are more specific (even though less sensitive) for SLE, such as antidouble-stranded DNA and Smith antigen (anti-Sm). These tests are listed in Table 3-3.

Procoagulant antibodies are found in approximately one half of all SLE patients.

Patients suffering from SLE produce not only antinuclear antibodies, but also antibodies to cell surface and cytoplasmic antigens. This accounts for the frequent presence of antibodies that cannot be fully explained and for the false positive syphilis test in which cardiolipin is used as the test antigen. This cross-reactivity with cardiolipin is found in only 50% of SLE patients—those who have so-called **antiphospholipid antibodies.** These antibodies react with phospholipids complexed plasma proteins and are also known as **lupus anticoagulant** because they interfere with the coagulation process in vitro. In vivo, these antibodies actually accelerate coagulation and are a cause of a **hypercoagulation syndrome.** It is called **secondary antiphospholipid antibody syndrome,** in contrast to the primary antiphospholipid antibody syndrome, which occurs in patients who do not have SLE. These

Table 3-3 Prevalence of Antinuclear Antibodies in Systemic Lupus Erythematosus

ANTIBODY	PREVALENCE IN SLE PATIENTS (%)	COMMENT
ANA	>95	Present in most autoimmune diseases
Antidouble-stranded DNA	40–60	Highly specific for SLE
Anti-Sm (protein core of small nuclear ribonucleoprotein)	20–30	Highly specific for SLE
U1RPN (nuclear ribonucleoprotein)	30–40	Highly specific for SLE
Antihistone	50–70	Positive in >95% drug-induced lupus
SS-A (Ro) (ribonucleoprotein)	30–50	Positive in >85% Sjögren's syndrome
SS-B (La) (ribonucleoprotein)	10–15	Positive in >70% Sjögren's syndrome

ANA, antinuclear antibody; SLE, systemic lupus erythematosus.

two syndromes are characterized by widespread thrombosis involving many organs.

Clinical features of SLE are protean, but some organ systems are involved more often than the others.

It is customary to say that the clinical features of SLE are protean, meaning that they are highly variable and unpredictable. The most common signs and symptoms are listed in Table 3-4.

The diagnosis of SLE is made if certain clinical and laboratory criteria are met.

In order to standardize the clinical diagnosis the American College of Rheumatology has defined diagnostic criteria, and by consensus it was agreed that the diagnosis should be made only if 4 or more of the 11 criteria are found (Table 3-5).

Pearl

> A mnemonic to remember the criteria for SLE has been devised by R. Leonard (Ann Rheum Dis 2001;60:638) as follows: **A RASH POINts MD.** It stands for **A**rthritis, **R**enal disease, **A**NA (positive antinuclear antibody), **S**erositis (pleurisy or pericarditis), **H**ematologic disorders, **P**hotosensitivity, **O**ral/nasopharyngeal ulcers, **I**mmunologic disorders, **N**eurologic disorders, **M**alar rash, **D**iscoid rash.

The clinical activity of SLE can be monitored by measuring the concentration of complement or by monitoring the function of the involved organs.

SLE is a chronic disease but its activities may wane and then again flare up spontaneously or due to treatment. Active disease leads to a consumption of complement, and thus the total concentration of complement is a useful indicator of disease activity. As soon as the disease is under control complement levels in the blood normalize. The most common finding on the day of the flare-up is reduction of antidouble-stranded DNA antibody titers. Serologic tests are not predictive of later flare-ups.

The activity of lupus nephritis may be monitored by periodic examination of urinary sediment and also by studying the renal functions with the standard tests such as BUN and creatinine. The flare-up of glomerulonephritis results in an "active sediment," which typically contains red blood cells, red blood cell casts, and white blood cell casts. Loss of glomeruli is accompanied by increased serum concentration of BUN and creatinine proportionate to the reduced glomerular filtration rate. Overall, renal involvement confers poor prognosis. A renal biopsy is usually performed to assess the

Table 3-4 Clinical Signs and Symptoms of Systemic Lupus Erythematosus

Constitutional symptoms
   Fatigue, malaise
   Fever
   Weight loss
Blood and lymphoid system related
   Anemia
   Leukopenia
   Thrombocytopenia
   Hypercoagulability
   Lymphadenopathy
   Splenomegaly
Skin related
   Photosensitivity
   Malar or discoid rash
Joint and muscle related
   Arthritis
   Myositis
Kidney related
   Microscopic hematuria and proteinuria
   Nephritic syndrome
   Nephrotic syndrome
Nervous and sensory system related
   Seizures
   Psychosis
   Peripheral neuropathy
   Visual problems
Respiratory system related
   Pleuritis
   Pneumonitis
Cardiovascular system related
   Pericarditis
   Endocarditis (Libman-Sacks)
   Raynaud's phenomenon
   Vasculitis
Gastrointestinal system related
   Chronic hepatitis

---

extent of the tissue injury and the activity of the renal disease. Mild mesangial proliferative glomerulonephritis has a relatively good prognosis, but diffuse and global proliferative glomerulonephritis that is unresponsive to treatment has a poor prognosis.

Lung Cancer

Lung cancer is the leading cause of cancer-related death in the United States and Europe. Even though it is more common in men than women, the incidence of lung cancer in women is on the rise. In both men and women it is related to tobacco smoking. Other risk factors such as exposure to radon, asbestos, and radioactive minerals are significantly less important than smoking.

Table 3-5 Criteria for the Diagnosis of Systemic Lupus Erythematosus as Defined by the American College of Rheumatology

CRITERION	DEFINITION
Malar rash	Fixed facial erythema over the malar area, sparing the nasolabial folds
Discoid rash	Erythematous patches with raised border covered with adherent keratotic scales and follicular plugging
Photosensitivity	Skin rash related to exposure to sunlight
Oral/nasopharyngeal ulcers	Ulceration is usually painless
Arthritis	Nonerosive arthritis involving two or more peripheral joints
Serositis	Inflammation with or without effusion involving pleura or pericardium
Renal disease	Persistent proteinuria greater than 3+ or presence of cellular casts
Neurologic disorder	Seizure or psychosis in the absence of other explanation
Hematologic disorder	Hemolytic anemia, neutropenia (<4000/mL), lymphocutopenia (<1,500/mL), or thrombocytopenia (<100,000/mL)
Immunologic disorder	Antibodies to native DNA or to Smith antigen, or phospholipids
Antinuclear antibody (ANA)	ANA in a high titer unrelated to drugs known to produce drug induced lupus syndrome

Modified from Hochberg MC: Updating the American College of Rheumatology revised criteria for the classification of systemic lupus erythematosus. Arthritis Rheum 1997;40:1725.

More than 90% of all lung cancers originate from the bronchial epithelium and are thus called bronchogenic. Accordingly most lung cancers are located in the central hilar area. Peripheral carcinomas, such as adenocarcinomas of bronchiolar origin and mesotheliomas originating from the pleura, are less common.

Common lung cancers are microscopically subclassified into two groups: small-cell carcinoma and nonsmall-cell carcinomas. The latter group comprises several microscopic variants, such as squamous cell carcinoma, adenocarcinoma, and large-cell carcinoma, which are often intermixed one with another (Table 3-6). Irrespective of their histologic type, lung cancers tend to metastasize the same way. Initial metastases are usually through the lymphatic system to the local lymph nodes. Hematogenous metastases lead to metastases in the brain, liver, bones, and, for some unknown reasons, quite often to the adrenal glands (Fig. 3-18).

Table 3-6 Histologic Forms of Common Lung Cancer

Non–small-cell carcinoma (80%)
   Squamous cell carcinoma (35%)
   Adenocarcinoma (35%)
   Large-cell carcinoma (10%)
Small-cell carcinoma (20%)

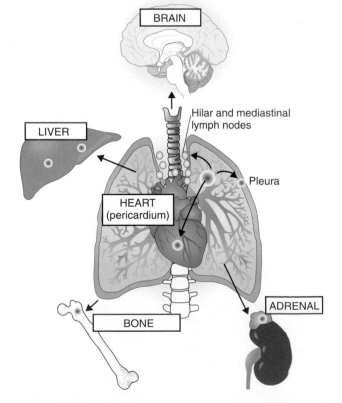

Figure 3-18 Lung cancer. Tumors tend to metastasize to local lymph nodes and distant sites such as brain, liver, bones, or adrenals.

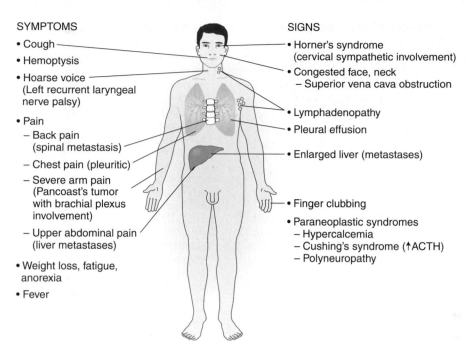

Figure 3-19 Clinical signs and symptoms of lung cancer. ACTH, adrenocorticotropic hormone.

Signs and symptoms of lung cancer depend on the location of the tumor.

For clinical purposes lung cancers are classified as either central (hilar) or peripheral (Fig. 3-19). Central tumors originate from major bronchi, whereas the peripheral tumors originate from bronchioli or bronchiolar epithelium trapped in scars, and from the mesothelium lining the pleura.

Central tumors tend to present with cough, dyspnea, hemoptysis, bronchial obstruction leading to bronchiectasis, or recurrent lung infection. Auscultation may reveal wheezing.

Peripheral tumors are more often asymptomatic and may be discovered during routine radiographic examination of the chest. Symptoms include pleuritic pain, pleural effusion, and dyspnea.

In addition to local symptoms many patients with lung cancer have systemic signs of neoplasia, such as weight loss, loss of appetite, malaise, and fatigue. The most common signs and symptoms are listed in the Table 3-7.

The pathogenesis of the signs and symptoms is briefly outlined as follows:

- **Cough.** It occurs in approximately 75% of all patients and is the most common finding in patients with lung cancer. Cough results from bronchial inflammation and direct irritation of nerve endings in the bronchi.
- **Dyspnea.** Shortness of breath results from the obstruction of major bronchi. It is usually associated with wheezing resulting from the passage of air through the narrowed bronchi. Changes that occur distal to the obstruction, such as atelectasis or bronchiectasis with mucous plugging and recurrent infections, reduce the respiratory capacity of the lungs.
- **Chest pain.** It results from the compression of nerve endings in the pleura or the major nerves. Superior sulcus tumors, known as **Pancoast's tumors,** cause pain that radiates into the upper inner arm due to the compression of the eighth cervical and first thoracic

Table 3-7 Clinical Signs and Symptoms of Lung Cancer

Very common
Cough
Dyspnea
Chest pain
Weight loss, fatigue, anorexia
Fever
Less common
Hemoptysis
Clubbing of fingers
Hoarseness
Superior vena cava syndrome
Hepatomegaly with pain
Bone pain
Neurologic symptoms
Paraneoplastic syndromes

nerves. **Horner's syndrome,** comprising ptosis, enophthalmus, miosis, and anhidrosis of one eye, results from compression of paravertebral and sympathetic nerves and ganglia.

- **Weight loss, fatigue, and anorexia.** These symptoms result from the systemic effects of the tumor and the cytokines secreted by the body defense systems in response to neoplasia.
- **Fever.** It results from the inflammation that occurs in the bronchi due to the irritation by the tumor. Obstruction of the bronchi predisposes the patient to chronic bronchitis, bronchiectasis, and pneumonia, which are often complicated by infection. Necrosis of larger tumor masses results in a release of endogenous pyrogens, which act on the hypothalamic thermoregulatory centers to cause fever.
- **Hemoptysis.** Bleeding is found in approximately one third of lung cancer patients. It is usually recognized as blood-stained sputum. Massive hemoptysis is uncommon.
- **Clubbing of fingers.** The pathogenesis of this sign is not fully understood. It is often a part of the **hypertrophic pulmonary osteoarthropathy,** characterized by proliferation of connective tissues around the joints and joint pain. It could be related also to hypoxia, since it is found in cyanotic patients suffering from other chronic lung and cardiac diseases.
- **Hoarseness.** It results from the compression of the left recurrent laryngeal nerve, which passes through the mediastinum as it reenters the larynx from below. Hoarseness results from the paralysis of the left vocal cord and is usually found in patients who have left upper lobe tumors.
- **Superior vena cava syndrome.** It manifests as upper thoracic and neck congestion resulting from the compression of the superior vena cava by mediastinal extension or mediastinal lymph node involvement by lung cancer.
- **Hepatomegaly, bone pain, and neurologic symptoms.** These symptoms result from distant metastases, which are very common in patients with lung cancer.

Paraneoplastic syndromes in patients with lung cancer depend on the microscopic type of cancer.

Lung cancer patients have metabolic disturbances that in many cases are related to the hormones that are paradoxically secreted by the tumors. Lung cancers affect other organs systems through immune or metabolic mechanisms, which are not fully understood. A list of paraneoplastic syndromes that could occur in lung cancer patients is given in Table 3-8.

Hormonal paraneoplastic syndromes are found in approximately 10% of lung cancer patients. Small-cell carcinoma, which originates from the neuroendocrine cells of the

Table 3-8 Paraneoplastic Syndromes in Lung Cancer Patients

Endocrine
   Hypercalcemia
   SIADH secretion
   Cushing's syndrome
Neuromuscular
   Lambert-Eaton syndrome
   Subacute cerebellar degeneration
   Dermatomyositis
Hematological
   Anemia
   Leukemoid reaction
   DIC
Dermatologic
   Acanthosis nigricans
   Hyperkeratosis
   Hyperpigmentation
Renal
   Nephrotic syndrome

DIC, disseminated intravascular coagulation; SIADH, syndrome of inappropriate antidiuretic hormone secretion.

bronchi, is much more often associated with such paraneoplastic syndromes than other forms of cancer. Carcinoid tumors, low-grade malignant tumors composed of well-differentiated neuroendocrine cells, also produce paraneoplastic syndrome quite often.

The most common endocrine paraneoplastic syndromes in patients with small-cell carcinoma are syndrome of inappropriate antidiuretic hormone secretion (SIADH), Cushing's syndrome, and Lambert-Eaton syndrome of periodic myasthenia-like muscular paralysis. Hypercalcemia resulting from the hypersecretion of parathyroid hormone-related polypeptide is encountered in patients who have squamous cell carcinoma.

The final diagnosis of lung cancer is based on radiologic and pathologic findings.

Radiologic examination is essential for the diagnosis of lung cancer as well as for its staging and follow-up after treatment. Lung cancer typically manifests as a radiologically visible mass. Mediastinal masses usually represent metastatic lesions in the lymph nodes. With the advent of modern radiologic imaging techniques it is possible to detect very small lesions, and theoretically an early lung cancer screening program could be launched. However, for the time being mass screening for lung cancer seems to be impractical. In patients who have radiologic abnormalities it is imperative to secure the diagnosis by biopsy and pathologic examination. The biopsy of central tumors can be performed bronchoscopically, whereas the peripheral tumors are best reached by transthoracic fine-needle aspiration biopsy.

CASE STUDIES

Case 1 BLEEDING FROM THE MOUTH AND DIABETES IN A 55-YEAR-OLD MAN

Clinical history A 55-year-old man was admitted because he noticed blood in his saliva several times, and an hour before admission he experienced massive bleeding from his mouth.[1] He also complained of heaviness under his left rib cage and noticed that he had an increased girth.[2] He denied alcohol consumption and smoking and said that he does not use any drugs. He never received any blood transfusions.[3]

Family and past history His father died of liver failure at the age of 60 years. Like his father he has diabetes, which is medically controlled.[4]

Clinical findings Mild ascites and enlargement of the liver and spleen were found during the physical examination. The skin was darkly pigmented, and spider angiomata were evident on the chest. Upper GI endoscopy revealed esophageal varices.[5] The bleeding site was identified and cauterized.

Laboratory findings Laboratory results included elevated blood sugar, low serum albumin, normal liver function tests, and normal prothrombin time.[6] Iron levels in blood were high, and the transferrin saturation was 65%. The urine contained more than 3 mg iron per 24 hours.[7]

Liver biopsy A transjugular liver biopsy revealed liver cell nodules surrounded by fibrous strands with massive deposition of iron in Kupffer cells, hepatocytes, and bile duct cells.[8]

Outcome The patient underwent treatment, which included weekly phlebotomies (450 mL of blood per week for 6 months). His condition did not improve and he underwent orthotopic liver transplantation.[9]

Questions and topics for discussion
1. What is the technical term for bleeding from the mouth? Can you be sure about the source of bleeding? What are the possible causes of such bleeding?
2. What do these symptoms suggest? What could cause a sensation of "heaviness" on the left side underneath the rib cage?
3. Why is it important to exclude alcohol and drug abuse in this patient?
4. Is the family history important in patients who have diabetes mellitus? Is this most likely type I or type II diabetes?
5. What diagnosis is suggested by all these clinical features?

6. Do these clinical laboratory findings support your clinical impression? Correlate and explain the clinical and the laboratory findings.
7. What is the diagnosis suggested by these laboratory findings?
8. What is the significance of the liver biopsy findings?
9. How common is the recurrence of the primary disease in the transplanted liver?

Case 2 SUDDEN ONSET OF PAIN IN THE RIGHT BIG TOE

Clinical history A 40-year-old man came back from a wedding and during that night he woke up because of severe pain in his right foot.[1,2] During the wedding he was dancing several hours, he ate a lot, and drank both wine and hard liquor. He also noticed that the joint between the big toe and the foot was swollen, red, and felt warm, and he could not step on that foot.[3] Since the pain did not subside he came to the emergency department.

Family and past history His father died of heart failure. The patient was obese and had mild hypertension. He has been treated for diabetes for 3 years, and the diseases seemed to be under control.[4]

Clinical findings The right first metatarsal joint was swollen, red, warm, and painful to palpation.

Laboratory findings Serum uric acid was elevated. Leukocytosis was present, and erythrocyte sedimentation rate (ESR) was increased.[5]

Arthrocentesis A few drops of turbid fluid were obtained from the affected first metatarsal joint. The analysis of joint fluid gave a count of 10,000 white blood cells/μL. Urine sediment examined under the polarizing microscope revealed needle-shaped negatively birefringent crystals.[6]

Outcome The patient was treated with nonsteroidal antiinflammatory drugs and improved. Three years later he came back complaining of blood in the urine and excruciating back pain. The diagnosis of urolithiasis was made.[7]

Questions and topics for discussion
1. What are the possible causes of foot pain? Could this be a bunion?
2. Is the time of onset of the pain important for diagnosis? Is the pain potentially related to the wedding that he attended the day before the onset of symptoms?

3. Is the diagnosis of arthritis justified in this case or should the disease be called podagra? Is it monoarticular or polyarticular? What could be the cause of this disease?

4. Does the history of diabetes and hypertension in this obese patient help in the diagnostic work-up? Explain.

5. What is the significance of hyperuricemia? Is he most likely an overproducer or underexcreter of uric acid? Do all persons who have hyperuricemia develop joint disease? What is the significance of leukocytosis and elevated ESR?

6. What is arthrocentesis? When should it be performed? Interpret these findings. What differential diagnosis should be considered in this case? Which crystal-related joint diseases do you know?

7. Explain the pathogenesis of urolithiasis in this case. What is the most likely composition of these urinary stones?

Case 3 FACIAL RASH AND SWELLING IN A PREGNANT 20-YEAR-OLD WOMAN

Clinical history   A 20-year-old woman, who is 6 months pregnant, came to her regular obstetric check-up complaining of a rash over her nose and cheeks. The rash worsens while she is outside in the garden.[1] She also reports swelling in her face, arms, and legs, and especially around the knee joints, which were painful. She attributed all these changes to her pregnancy, which was otherwise uneventful.[2]

History and physical examination   Her mother had severe rheumatoid arthritis for years.[3] The patient had been healthy until now. On physical examination the extremities showed prominent edema. Systolic and diastolic hypertension (150/100 mm Hg) were present.

Laboratory findings   There was mild anemia and hypoalbuminemia. Urine analysis revealed proteinuria and mild hematuria. The urinary sediment contained red blood cell casts and fragmented red blood cells.[4] She also had a positive ANA test (titer of 1:572) and antibodies to double- and single-stranded DNA and Smith antigen.[5] A kidney biopsy was performed and revealed focal mesangial proliferative glomerulonephritis, with deposits of IgG, IgM, IgA, and complement C3 in the mesangial areas and in the glomerular basement membranes.[6]

Outcome   The patient was treated with steroids and improved.

Questions and topics for discussion

1. List the conditions that could cause a facial rash. Does pregnancy predispose to facial rash? Is the worsening of the rash outdoors indicative of photosensitivity?

2. Is the swelling of the extremities and face to be expected during pregnancy? What could cause such swelling?

3. What is the significance of this family history?

4. Interpret these laboratory findings and find out whether this patient has preeclampsia or something else. Explain the pathogenesis of hypoalbuminemia and anemia.

5. Interpret these serologic findings and specify how they could help you distinguish SLE from dermatomyositis, Sjögren's syndrome, systemic sclerosis, or mixed connective tissue disease.

6. What is the prognosis of this renal disease? Is this considered to be a mild or severe form of glomerulonephritis?

Case 4 PROLONGED COUGHING AND WEIGHT LOSS IN A 60-YEAR-OLD MAN

Clinical history   A 60-year-old man asked medical assistance for prolonged coughing accompanied with abundant sputum that has been bothering him for the last 3 months.[1]

History and physical examination   The patient smokes two packs of cigarettes per day and has done so since he was 18 years old.[2] He was short of breath and often expectorates mucus or slightly blood-tinged viscous material. He has lost 15 pounds over the last 3 months and has no appetite.[3] He felt tired and depressed.

Radiologic findings   A 3-cm mass was found in the right hilum, and the mediastinum appeared widened.[4]

Laboratory findings   Mild anemia and mild leukocytosis were evident, and the ESR is elevated. He also had mild hypercalcemia, but all other mineral levels were within normal limits.[5]

Biopsy   A transbronchial biopsy was performed, and the pathology report indicated that the patient has a malignant tumor.[6]

Questions and topics for discussion

1. What are the possible causes of prolonged cough?

2. Can you calculate the cigarette-pack-per year history for this patient? What are the health risks related to smoking?

3. What are the possible causes of weight loss?

4. What is the significance of this radiologic finding? What step should be undertaken next?

5. Interpret these laboratory findings. Do they suggest a diagnosis of malignancy or an inflammatory lung disease? What is the possible pathogenesis of hypercalcemia?

6. Is this malignant tumor most likely a carcinoma, a sarcoma, or a mesothelioma?

Chapter 4

CARDIOVASCULAR DISEASES

Introduction

The cardiovascular system is one of the vital organ systems and its failure is one of the major causes of morbidity and the major cause of death in the Western world. The following epidemiologic facts show why the cardiovascular diseases are important for many human populations:

- More than 50% of all deaths in the United States and Western Europe are caused by cardiovascular diseases.
- Atherosclerosis is the most common chronic multifactorial degenerative disease and is especially prevalent among the elderly.
- Hypertension affects millions of Americans and is one of the most prevalent chronic diseases.
- Congenital heart diseases are found in 5 per 1000 newborns.

- Many cardiovascular diseases, such as atherosclerosis, are preventable or treatable if recognized early (e.g., arterial hypertension). It is thus encouraging to note that the incidence of cardiovascular disease has decreased in the United States over the last 40 years. Public health initiatives to reduce smoking, combat hyperlipidemia, and motivate people to exercise and follow a healthier life style have had noticeable effects on the incidence of cardiovascular diseases and their major complications. Major advances have been made also in the early diagnosis of cardiovascular disease, treatment based on interventional cardiology, and heart transplantation.

Cardiovascular diseases have many causes, but most of them are multifactorial. The relative clinical significance of various cardiovascular diseases is presented graphically in Figure 4-1.

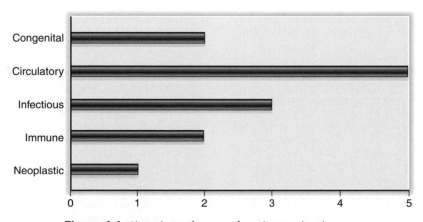

Figure 4-1 Clinical significance of cardiovascular diseases.

KEY WORDS

Anatomy and Physiology

Actin   Contractile protein that with myosin forms the filaments in sarcomeres.

Angiotensin   Vasoactive substance formed from angiotensinogen through the action of renin. It plays an important role in the pathogenesis of hypertension.

Aorta   Largest artery in the body, conveying arterial blood from the heart to the periphery.

Arteriole   Small muscular vessel serving as precapillary sphincter at the interface between the muscular arteries and capillaries.

Artery   Thick-walled muscular or elastic blood vessel conveying arterial blood from the heart to the arterioles.

Atrial natriuretic peptide   Family of vasoactive polypeptide hormones produced by the heart and vascular cells; important for the regulation of heart function and blood pressure.

Atrium   Chamber of the heart connected to systemic or pulmonary veins on one side and separated by a valve from the ventricle on the other. The heart has two atria: the right and the left atrium.

Conduction system of the heart   System of specialized cells capable of generating and conducting the electric currents essential for the automatic rhythmicity of the heart. It includes the sinoatrial node, atrioventricular node, the bundle of His and its main branches, and Purkinje fibers.

Coronary arteries   Arteries providing blood to the heart. Two major arteries originate in the aorta from the coronary sinuses. The left coronary artery has two main branches: the left anterior descending (LAD), providing the blood to the anterior side of the left ventricle and the anterior part of the ventricular septum; and the left circumflex (LCX), which provides blood to the lateral side of the left ventricle. The right coronary artery (RCA) usually gives rise to the posterior descending artery (PDA). The PDA originates from the RCA in 90% of the population designated as having right coronary dominance. In 10% of cases left coronary dominance occurs, and the PDA originates from the LCX.

Endocardium   Inner layer of the heart, forming the surface of the cardiac chambers. It is continuous with the endothelium of the great vessels.

Frank-Starling law   The power of ventricular contraction increases proportionately to the initial lengthening of its muscle fibers by end-diastolic filling.

Myocardium   Thickest layer of the atria and ventricles, composed of contractile cardiac myocytes.

Myoglobin   Oxygen-binding heme protein found in cardiac and skeletal muscle cells. It may spill out into the blood from necrotic muscle fibers and is thus a marker of myocardial cell necrosis occurring after myocardial infarction.

Myosin   Contractile protein forming the microfilaments in many human cells and most prominently the myofibrils in cardiac myocytes.

Pericardium   Outer layer of the heart, composed of a mesothelial layer and underlying connective tissue. It covers the subepicardial fat tissue, which contains the branches of the coronary arteries and veins.

Renin   Polypeptide hormone synthesized by juxtaglomerular (JG) cells in the kidney. It acts on angiotensinogen and is thus important for the aldosterone-mediated retention of sodium and water in the kidneys. It is synthesized in response to hypoperfusion of kidneys and is the primary mediator of renal hypertension.

Sarcomere   Functional contractile unit of each cardiac myocyte. It consists of thick filaments (myosin) and thin filaments (actin) and the regulatory proteins, troponins and tropomyosin.

Sarcoplasmic reticulum   Smooth endoplasmic reticulum in cardiac myocytes, composed of interconnected vesicles that serve as a calcium reservoir of these cells.

Septum   Part of the heart separating the left atrium from the right atrium, and the left ventricle from the right ventricle. It consists of fibrous tissue (fibrous septum) and muscle (muscular septum).

Troponin I and T   Sarcomeric proteins regulating the contraction of myofibrils. In myocardial infarction these proteins are released into the blood. The elevation of troponin I or T in blood is evidence of myocardial necrosis.

Valve   Mobile part of the cardiac orifice that separates atria from ventricles or the ventricles from the great vessels. Valves consist of a fibroelastic core covered with the endocardium. The mitral and tricuspid valves are attached to the papillary muscles with chordae tendineae. The aortic and pulmonary valves are semilunar and not attached to the muscles. At their base the valves are anchored to the annulus fibrosus, forming the connective tissue skeleton of the heart.

Ventricle   Cardiac chamber that has a thick muscular wall accounting for most of the contractile power of the heart. The heart has two ventricles, the right and the left ventricle, separated one from each other by a predominantly muscular septum.

Signs and Symptoms

Arrhythmia   Collective term used to describe several abnormalities of heartbeat, it includes, among others, tachycardia, bradycardia, premature ventricular beat, atrial or ventricular fibrillation, flutter, conduction defects, and heart block.

Bradycardia   Slow heartbeat, usually under 50 beats per minute.

Clubbing of fingers   Condition in which the amount of subcutaneous soft tissue of the terminal phalanges is increased, with curving of the nails, giving the fingers a drumstick appearance. It is commonly seen in cyanotic congenital heart diseases, such as tetralogy of Fallot. It is also encountered in chronic lung diseases with long-standing ventilatory problems.

Congestive hepatomegaly   Enlargement of the liver due to chronic passive accumulation of venous blood in the liver owing to right heart failure.

C-reactive polypeptide, or protein (CRP)   Acute-phase reactant secreted by the liver in response to cytokines released from inflammatory cells. Its concentration is elevated in blood in various inflammatory conditions, including the inflammation that occurs inside atherosclerotic blood vessels. As such it is an independent predictor of the risk for complications of atherosclerosis.

Creatine kinase (CK)   Enzyme released from damaged or necrotic cardiac and skeletal muscle. The cardiac isoenzyme (CK-MB) is elevated in the blood after myocardial infarction.

Cyanosis   Bluish or purplish tinge to the skin and mucosae that becomes visible once the unoxygenated hemoglobin concentration exceeds 5 g/100 mL of blood, or the overall oxygen saturation is less than 85%. It may be classified as central or peripheral.

Dyspnea   Shortness of breath that may be acute or chronic, episodic or continuous, exertional or resting. Usually it is a symptom of heart or lung disease. Exertional dyspnea or paroxysmal nocturnal dyspnea is usually a sign of heart disease.

Edema   Accumulation of fluid in tissues and body cavities. Cardiogenic edema involves either lungs and pleural cavity (in left heart failure) or peripheral tissues of the lower extremities and abdominal cavity (in right heart failure).

Hypertension   Elevated blood pressure in the arteries. It may be primary or idiopathic (90%), if the cause of hypertension is unknown, or secondary if the cause of hypertension is known. The most common causes of secondary hypertension are renal, endocrine, or vascular diseases.

Intermittent claudication   Sudden pain in the lower extremities, precipitated by walking; it is so severe that it will cause limping or might force the affected person to stop walking. It is typically a consequence of atherosclerotic narrowing of major leg arteries.

Ischemia   Localized circulatory disturbance resulting in the interruption of blood flow into an anatomic area. Most often caused by thrombotic or atheromatous occlusion of the arterial lumen.

Orthopnea   Shortness of breath that occurs when the patient lies down. It is usually a sign of lung disease because the vital capacity is normally reduced in supine position.

Paroxysmal nocturnal dyspnea   Form of dyspnea that occurs in patients with heart failure several hours after lying down. It is caused by increased venous return and the failure of the heart to propel the blood, leading to pulmonary congestion and edema and shortness of breath that wakes the patient.

Pulmonary edema   Accumulation of fluid in the alveoli and interstitial spaces of the lung. It may be a consequence of transudation of serum in left ventricular failure, during early stages of ARDS, or as an inflammatory exudate in early stages of pneumonia.

Pulmonary hypertension   Increased pressure inside the pulmonary artery and its branches. It may be a consequence of primary lung disease or chronic pulmonary congestion due to left heart failure or mitral valve disease. Pulmonary hypertension poses a strain on the right ventricle, causing its hypertrophy ("cor pulmonale").

Syncope   Loss of consciousness due to hypoperfusion of the brain by blood.

Tachycardia   Rapid heartbeat, in adults usually over 90 heartbeats per minute.

Cardiovascular Diseases and Pathologic Lesions

Amyloidosis of the heart   Deposition of fibrillar extracellular material that binds Congo red and is β-pleated when examined by electron diffraction analysis. It may be part of generalized amyloidosis or may present as an isolated cardiac amyloidosis. Deposits of amyloid in the cardiac interstitium cause restrictive cardiomyopathy.

Anastomosis   Connection between two vessels or two hollow organs. Vascular anastomoses may be between two arteries or two veins or they may be arteriovenous (A-V).

Aneurysm of aorta or arteries   Localized dilatation of an artery, caused most often by atherosclerosis, but also by syphilis or various forms of arteritis. Berry aneurysms of the circle of Willis are congenital.

Aneurysm of the ventricle   Dilatation of the ventricular lumen, most often as a late complication of myocardial infarction. The wall of the aneurysm is composed of fibrous scars and does not contract with the surrounding myocardium. Thrombi form within large ventricular aneurysms.

Angina pectoris   Chest pain caused by cardiac ischemia related to stenosis, partial occlusion, or spasm of the coronary arteries. Three main forms are recognized: (1) stable or classical angina; (2) unstable or crescendo angina or preinfarctional angina; and (3) Prinzmetal's angina, which is characterized by pain at rest, caused by functional narrowing of coronary arteries due to spasm.

Atheroma   Hallmark of atherosclerosis, presenting as a bulging of the wall of the aorta or a circumferential narrowing of smaller elastic arteries. It consists of a central core composed of lipids, cell debris, and foam cells, and a fibrous cap covering it on the luminal side. Complicated atheromas may be calcified, or ruptured and filled with coagulated blood.

Atherosclerosis   Common multifactorial disease of aorta and major elastic arteries, causing numerous diseases, such as coronary artery disease and cerebrovascular accidents (strokes).

Atrial fibrillation   Disturbance of normal atrial contraction, which is replaced by irregular twitching, best recognized by electrocardiogram (ECG). May predispose patient to formation of atrial mural thrombi.

Atrioventricular (AV) block   Disturbance of cardiac conduction characterized by an inability to transmit electric signals from the atrium to the ventricles.

Calcific aortic stenosis   Narrowing of the aortic orifice due to the calcification of the valves. It is most often caused by wear and tear of old age, but can be a complication of congenital bivalvular aortic orifice and rheumatic endocarditis.

Carcinoid heart disease   Cardiac disease caused by serotonin and other vasoactive substances released from gastrointestinal carcinoids that have metastasized to the liver. Cardiac changes include tricuspid and pulmonary valve stenosis and insufficiency and fibrosis of the atrial and ventricular lumen resulting from subendocardial fibrosis induced by vasoactive substances.

Cardiac tamponade   Compression of the heart by fluid, usually blood, that has entered into the pericardial sac. The pressure exerted by the fluid prevents the diastolic filling of the cardiac chambers and is usually fatal.

Cardiogenic shock   Systemic circulatory collapse caused by cardiac pump failure. It is characterized by hypotension and hypoperfusion of vital organs, causing ischemia of the brain, heart, kidneys, and other organs. Most often it is a complication of myocardial infarction.

Cardiomyopathy   Term used to describe primary myocardial diseases unrelated to coronary atherosclerosis, hypertension, or infectious or rheumatic carditis. Cardiomyopathy may occur in three forms: (1) dilated cardiomyopathy, (2) hypertrophic cardiomyopathy, and (3) restrictive cardiomyopathy.

Congestive heart failure   Clinical condition characterized by stagnation of blood retrograde to the failing heart. Left heart failure causes chronic passive congestion and edema of the lungs, whereas right heart failure results in congestive hepatomegaly, pitting edema of the lower extremities, ascites, and splenomegaly.

Constrictive pericarditis   Form of chronic pericarditis or pericardial fibrosis encasing the heart and preventing its expansion during diastole. The cause of constrictive pericarditis is most often unknown, and it is assumed to be a complication of a healed viral pericarditis. Radiation, tuberculosis, or tumors can cause the same changes.

Cor pulmonale   Clinical condition characterized by dilatation and strain of the right ventricle and possible right ventricular failure. Most often it is caused by left ventricular failure, but also by any other condition causing pulmonary hypertension.

Dilatation of the heart   Widening of the cardiac chambers, usually due to the stretching of cardiac myocytes. Dilatation of the ventricles is the first adaptation to an increased demand for cardiac output, and during this response the dilatation is beneficial and reversible.

Endocarditis, infectious   Inflammation caused by a bacterial infection of the valves or mural endocardium of the heart chambers. Bacteria destroy the valves, causing valvular defects and disturbing blood flow; emboli may occur and cause systemic symptoms.

Floppy valves   Congenital or acquired myxomatous degeneration of the valves accompanied by accumulation of sulfated glycosaminoglycans and a loss of collagen and elastic fibers. Mitral valve disease is found in 1% to 2% of adults; other valves are involved less often.

Hemopericardium   Accumulation of blood in the pericardial cavity. It may be caused by bleeding from the cardiac chambers or the root of the aorta.

Hypertensive heart disease   Complex heart disease caused by elevated arterial pressure. It is characterized by left ventricular hypertrophy and relative ischemia of the myocardium, which cannot get enough blood for its needs. Hypertension also predisposes to coronary atherosclerosis, which will contribute to myocardial ischemia.

Ischemic heart disease (IHD; also known as coronary heart disease)   Group of circulatory diseases caused by inadequate oxygen due to coronary insufficiency. Most often it is caused by atherosclerotic narrowing or occlusion of coronary arteries. The most important clinical forms of IHD are (1) angina pectoris, (2) myocardial infarct, (3) congestive heart disease, and (4) sudden cardiac death.

Left ventricular failure   Pump failure of the left ventricle manifesting with hypoperfusion of organs with arterial blood (forward failure) and stagnation of the blood in the lungs. It manifests with pulmonary congestion and edema.

Left ventricular hypertrophy   Thickening of the left ventricular myocardium. Most often it is caused by arterial hypertension, but it may also be caused by stenosis of the aortic orifice or insufficiency of the mitral valve. It is also found in cardiomyopathies.

Libman-Sacks endocarditis   Sterile endocarditis typically found in systemic lupus erythematosus. Most often it affects the mitral valve.

Mitral valve incompetence (also known as mitral insufficiency or mitral regurgitation)   Functional disturbance resulting from the inability of the mitral valves to close completely during systole.

Mitral valve prolapse   Synonym for floppy mitral valve (*see* Floppy valves)

Mitral valve stenosis   Functional disturbance resulting from the narrowing of the mitral orifice and valves, which cannot open completely during diastole. Most often (99%) it is a consequence of rheumatic endocarditis.

Myocardial infarct, subendocardial   Ischemic necrosis of the subendocardial zone of the myocardium, most often circumferential. Typically caused by hypoperfusion without complete anatomic occlusion of a coronary artery. It is most often found in shock or as a complication of myocardial infarction. In typical cases it presents without Q wave changes in the ECG ("non-Q wave infarction"), and is not accompanied by pericarditis.

Myocardial infarct, transmural   Localized area of ischemic necrosis of the myocardium caused by occlusion of a coronary artery. Most often it is a complication of thrombosis developing at the site of ruptured atheroma. Thromboemboli from the left ventricle are a less common cause.

Myocarditis   Inflammation of the myocardium accompanied by necrosis of cardiac myocytes. Etiologically classified as (1) infectious or (2) noninfectious.

Myxoma   Benign cardiac tumor most often found in the left atrium (75%), less often in the right atrium (24%), and very seldom in other cardiac chambers. Tumor protrudes into the lumen of the atria and may act as a "ball-valve." As such, it may temporarily occlude the mitral or tricuspid orifice and interrupt the blood flow. Also, parts of the tumor may detach and thus give rise to emboli.

Myxomatous degeneration of cardiac valves   Deformation of cardiac valves accompanied by accumulation of sulfate glycosaminoglycans and a loss of normal collagen and elastic fibers forming the central core of the valves. In most instances the cause is unknown. It may occur in inborn errors of metabolism such as the Marfan's syndrome and Ehlers-Danlos syndrome or various mucopolysaccharidoses. The mitral valve is most often involved, but all valves can be affected.

Pericarditis   Inflammation of epicardium and pericardium (i.e., the visceral and parietal layer of the pericardial sac). It can manifest in several pathologic forms: serous, fibrinous, fibrinohemorrhagic, purulent, fibrous, or calcific.

Rheumatic heart disease   Immune-mediated disease initiated by antigens on beta-hemolytic streptococci, usually after a streptococcal pharyngitis ("strep throat"). Clinically it is diagnosed by documenting the rheumatic fever (using the Jones criteria), establishing the link between the heart disease and the streptococcal infection (ASO titers high), and proving that the heart is damaged. Rheumatic carditis most often affects the cardiac valves of the left side of the heart.

Right ventricular hypertrophy   Thickening of the wall of the right ventricle, typically caused by pulmonary hypertension. The most common cause of right ventricular hypertrophy is left ventricular hypertrophy.

Rupture of the ventricle   Perforation of the wall of the left ventricle, usually caused by ischemic necrosis (transmutable infarct). Blood penetrates through the ventricular wall, filling the pericardial cavity and causing death due to pericardial tamponade.

Shunt   A passage that allows abnormal blood flow between two cardiac chambers on the opposite sides of the septum dividing the left from the right heart. Blood flows through the shunt from the higher pressurized chamber to the chamber that is under less pressure.

Stenosis   Narrowing of the lumen of a blood vessel or a cardiac orifice.

Tamponade (more correctly "cardiac tamponade")   Compression of the heart by the fluid accumulating in the pericardial sac. The most common cause of cardiac tamponade is hemopericardium.

Tricuspid valve insufficiency   Functional disturbance resulting from incomplete closure of the tricuspid valves. May be congenital or acquired. Acquired tricuspid valve insufficiency can be a consequence of endocarditis or carcinoid heart disease.

Truncus arteriosus   Congenital heart disease related to incomplete separation of the aorta from the fetal pulmonary artery. In this disease the aorta and the pulmonary artery form a single large blood vessel originating from the heart.

Valvular calcification   Dystrophic calcification affecting valves previously damaged by endocarditis, or resulting from the wear and tear of old age. Congenitally abnormal or lax valves are especially prone to calcification.

Valvular insufficiency   Circulatory disturbance caused by incomplete closure of a cardiac valve, resulting in regurgitation of blood from one chamber of the heart or a great vessel into another one of the heart chambers.

Valvular stenosis   Circulatory disturbance caused by narrowing of the orifice, usually caused by incomplete opening of the valves during systole or diastole.

Normal Structure and Function

ANATOMY AND HISTOLOGY

The cardiovascular system comprises the heart and blood vessels, which are classified as arteries, arterioles, capillaries, venules, and veins. The right heart pumps the blood into the lungs, where it is oxygenated and returned to the left heart for distribution through several parallel arterial pathways into the peripheral tissues (Fig. 4-2). This chapter focuses mostly on the heart, and the blood vessels are discussed only as they contribute to heart diseases and their peripheral manifestations.

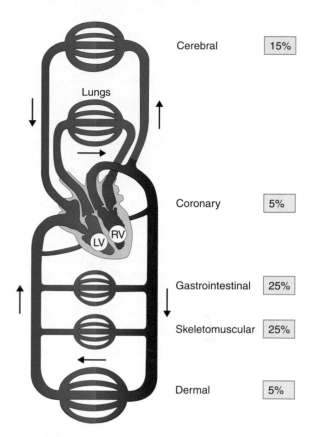

Figure 4-2 The circulatory system consists of two systems: the pulmonary and the systemic, both of which have an arterial, a venous, and a capillary part. LV, left ventricle; RV, right ventricle.

The heart is located in the mediastinum of the thoracic cavity.

The heart is located inside the pericardial sac, which is itself located in the lower (supradiaphragmatic) part of the mediastinum. The heart occupies the central portion of the mediastinum, extending slightly to the right from the midline and projecting with its apex toward the left lateral side (Fig. 4-3). The great vessels (i.e., the superior and inferior vena cava, the aorta, the pulmonary artery, and the pulmonary veins) are attached to the heart at its "base," which is located cranially and to the right of the apex. The contours of the heart are clearly visible in anteroposterior (AP) radiographic films.

Pearl

> Plain AP films may be used to assess the enlargement of the heart, dilatation of the aorta, or the accumulation of fluid inside the pericardial cavity.

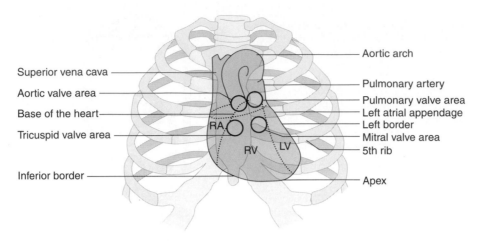

Figure 4-3 Anatomic location of the heart in the thorax. In a radiograph the right border is made of the contours of the right atrium (RA) and right ventricle (RV). The inferior border is made of right ventricle and on the left lateral side of the apex of the left ventricle (LV). The left border is made of the contours of left atrial appendage and left ventricle, and along the upper margin the aortic arch.

In adults the anterior mediastinum contains the remnants of the thymus, which does not affect the function of the heart unless enlarged due to thymoma or lymphoma. The posterior side of the heart is in anatomic contact with the esophagus and the thoracic aorta. Transesophageal echocardiography may be used to assess the left atrium lying on the esophagus, but it may also provide data on the entire heart.

The heart has four chambers and can be functionally divided into a right and a left part.

The heart has two atria and two ventricles (Fig. 4-4). The right atrium and ventricle contain unoxygenated ("venous") blood, which has an oxygen saturation between 72% and 80%. The contracting right heart pumps the blood into the lungs, where is it oxygenated. The left atrium and ventricle contain oxygenated ("arterial") blood with an oxygen saturation of 95% or more. The left ventricle propels the oxygenated blood into the periphery through the aorta and the arteries.

The atria and the ventricles and the great arteries are separated one from another by valves. These valves open and close during the cardiac contraction cycle, thus allowing the orderly flow of blood from one compartment to another. The closure and opening of the valves and the cardiac contractions account for the pressure gradients that develop differentially in each chamber.

The right atrium receives the venous blood from the upper and the lower venae cavae. The venous blood enters the right ventricle through the right atrioventricular (AV) orifice, which is tricuspid. The blood is pumped by the ventricle through a tricuspid pulmonary orifice into the pulmonary artery. The oxygenated blood returns to the heart through the pulmonary veins, which convey it to the left atrium. From the left atrium the blood passes through the left AV orifice, which is bicuspid and called mitral, and enters the left ventricle. The left ventricle pumps the blood into the aorta through the aortic valve.

The entire heart, except the endocardium, receives oxygenated blood through two coronary arteries.

Most human hearts have two coronary arteries, which originate from the coronary sinuses in the initial part of the thoracic aorta (Fig. 4-5).

The right coronary artery provides the blood for the entire right ventricle, the posterior side of the left ventricle, and the posterior side of the interventricular septum. In 90% of people it gives rise to the posterior descending coronary artery and is therefore by convention considered to be the **dominant artery.** It also provides the blood to the sinoatrial (SA) node in 60% and to the AV node in 90% of people.

The left coronary artery branches within 2.5 cm of its origin, giving rise to the left anterior descending (LAD) and left circumflex artery (LCX). The LAD provides blood to the anterior wall of the left ventricle, the apex of the heart, and the anterior part of the interventricular septum. The LCX provides the blood for the lateroposterior wall of the left ventricle.

Pearl

> The heart is positioned diagonally, and thus the posterior wall of the ventricles is clinically known as the heart's inferior surface. Accordingly, the pathologic term *posterior wall infarct* is clinically known as an inferior infarct.

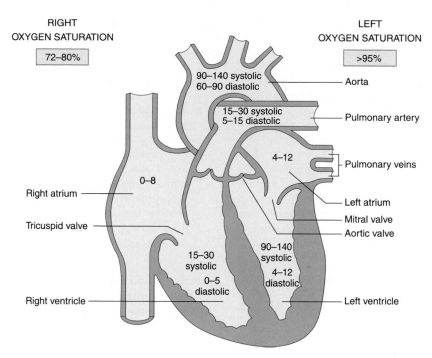

RIGHT
OXYGEN SATURATION

72–80%

LEFT
OXYGEN SATURATION

>95%

90–140 systolic
60–90 diastolic — Aorta

15–30 systolic
5–15 diastolic — Pulmonary artery

4–12 — Pulmonary veins

Right atrium — 0–8

Tricuspid valve

— Left atrium
— Mitral valve
— Aortic valve

15–30
systolic
0–5
diastolic

90–140
systolic
4–12
diastolic

Right ventricle — — Left ventricle

Figure 4-4 Cross section through the right and left heart and the great vessels. The range of systolic and diastolic pressures in each chamber is indicated. The oxygen saturation of blood in the right heart ranges from 72% to 80%, and is 95% or more in the left heart.

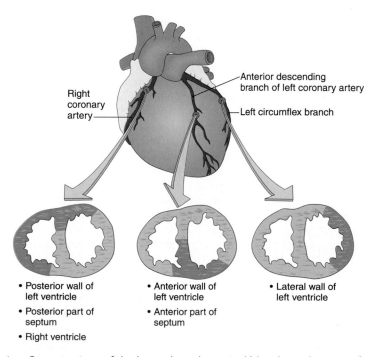

Right
coronary
artery

Anterior descending
branch of left coronary artery

Left circumflex branch

- Posterior wall of
  left ventricle
- Posterior part of
  septum
- Right ventricle

- Anterior wall of
  left ventricle
- Anterior part of
  septum

- Lateral wall of
  left ventricle

Figure 4-5 Coronary arteries. Cross sections of the heart show the typical blood supply areas of each of the three major coronary arteries.

The coronary arteries are located subepicardially on the external surface of the heart. The major veins follow the arteries. Because of their location these major vessels are not compressed by the contracting myocardium during the systole—a period of the cardiac cycle when the coronaries actually dilate to accommodate the influx of oxygenated blood. Coronary arteries have β_2-adrenergic receptors, which react to stimuli from sympathetic nerves, thereby causing coronary vasodilatation. Parasympathetic stimulation also causes mild coronary vasodilatation.

Due to their location in the epicardial fat tissue the coronary arteries are at a distance from the endocardium. The nourishment of the endocardium is, however, not affected by this distance because the endocardium receives oxygen and nutrients from the ventricular blood. The zone that is at risk for hypoxia, however, is the subendocardial myocardium, which is beyond the supply zone from the ventricles and is the last to receive the blood from the coronary arteries.

Pearl

> Subendocardial infarcts (also known as non-Q wave infarcts) are typically found in shock and other hypoperfusion states. These infarcts develop because the subendocardial myocardium is the last part of the ventricular muscle to receive oxygen from the coronaries, and if the blood pressure drops, it is the first to become ischemic.

The coronary arteries and their major branches are considered to be functionally terminal arteries. Although there are 40-μm or smaller caliber anastomoses between the major coronary arteries, these anastomoses are not sufficient to compensate for the occlusion of one coronary artery or its major branches. If a coronary artery become progressively stenotic these anastomoses can increase in size and become functional and provide blood to the relatively ischemic portion of the heart supplied normally by the other coronary.

Pearl

> So-called paradoxical infarcts, that is, infarcts that develop in the left coronary artery supply zone due to a thrombus in the right coronary, and vice versa, are a consequence of newly developed anastomoses due to the gradual narrowing of the coronary artery that normally provides the blood to the infarcted area.

The heart is composed of three layers: endocardium, myocardium, and pericardium.

The inside of the heart is covered with endocardium, which is a layer continuous with the endothelium of blood vessels. The endocardium also covers the surface of the valves. The myocar-

dium, or the muscle layer, is the primary contractile component of the heart. The pericardium forms the pericardial sac and also covers the external surface of the heart as epicardium.

The myocardium is composed of two types of cells called cardiac **myocytes:** conducting cells and contractile cells.

- The conducting cells form the SA and AV node, the intra-arterial atrial internodal tracts, the AV node, the bundle of His, and the Purkinje system.
- The contractile myocytes form the bulk of the heart wall. Cardiac myocytes are striated muscle cells with centrally placed nuclei and well-developed cytoplasm. These branching cells are interconnected one with another through gap junctions called intercalated discs allowing easy passage of electric current through the myocardium.

Contractile function of cardiac myocytes depends on the proper functioning of sarcomeres and supporting structures in the cytoplasm.

Contractile units in the cytoplasm of cardiac myocytes are called **sarcomeres** (Fig. 4-6). They are composed of thick myosin filaments interdigitating with thinner actin filaments and a number of contraction-regulating proteins, such as tropomyosin and troponins (C, I, and T). During contraction the myosin filaments slide along one another, whereas during relaxation they slide in the opposite direction.

The overlapping of actin and myosin filaments accounts for the striation of cardiac myocytes. Three regions are recognized by light microscopy: two lighter regions called I (isotropic), and a darker region called A (anisotropic). By electron microscopy the central part of the I region contains the Z line. Normal sarcomeres, measured from one Z line to another, vary in length from 1.5 μm in contracted muscle cells in systole to 2.2 μm in stretched muscle fibers in diastole.

The cell membrane of myocytes, also known as **sarcolemma,** invaginates into the cytoplasm, forming the so-called **transverse tubular system** (T tubules). The T system is an important regulator for the flux of calcium ions from outside into the cells and from one cellular compartment to another (Fig. 4-7). The T tubules are closely linked to the **sarcoplasmic reticulum,** a system of cisterns that serve as the main intracellular store of calcium. The sarcoplasmic reticulum and the T tubules form an integral system essential for the rapid transmission of electrical stimuli and the contraction–relaxation of myocytes.

PHYSIOLOGY

Cardiac contractions depend on the interaction of the external innervation and the endogenous conduction system of the heart.

The heart receives parasympathetic innervation from the vagus and sympathetic innervation from sympathetic ganglia. The cholinergic parasympathetic stimuli, which are

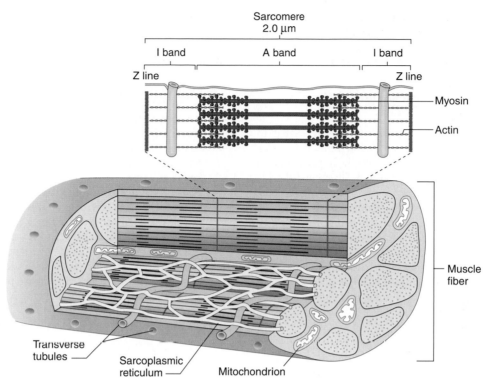

Figure 4-6 Sarcomeres. These basic contractile units consist of thick myosin and thin actin filaments that slide along each other in one direction in systole and the other in diastole. (Modified from Boon NA, Colledge NR, Walker BR [eds]: Davidson's Principles and Practice of Medicine, 20th ed. Churchill-Livingstone, Edinburgh, 2006.)

under normal circumstances predominant, stimulate the heart through the AV and SA node. Vagal stimulation has a negative chronotropic and inotropic effect; that is, it slows down the heartbeat and reduces the strength of the cardiac contraction. Sympathetic stimuli transmitted mostly through β₁-adrenergic receptors have a positive chronotropic and inotropic effect. Sensory nerves, important for the cardiac reflexes, exit the heart through the vagus nerve.

The automatic contractility of the heart is regulated through the SA and AV node and the conduction system of the myocardium. The SA node is the source of initial

impulses and accounts for the normal "sinus rhythm." The depolarization wave is transmitted from the SA node to the internodal and interatrial fibers, which causes depolarization of the right and left atrium. The electric impulses cannot freely pass into the ventricle because the annulus fibrosus blocks their propagation. The only way that the impulses can get into the ventricle is by reaching first the AV node located on the atrial side of the annulus fibrosus. From the SA node the electric impulses enter the bundle of His, which penetrates the annulus fibrosus and allows the stimuli to pass from the atrium to the ventricle. Then they reach the

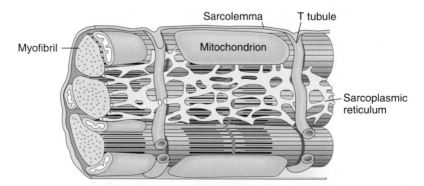

Figure 4-7 Transverse tubular system and sarcoplasmic reticulum. The T tubules represent invaginations of the sarcolemma.

Purkinje fibers and are transmitted to cardiac myocytes, causing their depolarization. These electrical events can be traced externally and if superimposed on one another can be recorded as an electrocardiographic tracing (Fig. 4-8).

Cardiac myocyte contraction begins with the depolarization of the sarcolemma.

The contraction of cardiac myocytes is closely related to changes in the plasma membrane. Sarcolemma, the plasma membrane of cardiac myocytes, is selectively permeable to ions. The differential distribution of ions inside and outside the myocytes accounts for the electric charge of the cells membrane, which in a resting cell is approximately -90 mV. If the cell is stimulated, the potential is reduced to a critical level, called *threshold potential*, whereupon the cell membrane undergoes depolarization, which is completed spontaneously according to the *all-or-none law*. The cell membrane is then repolarized by several mechanisms, and the cycle is repeated automatically.

The cardiac myocyte's **action potential,** or the change in the membrane potential that occurs after the cell has been adequately stimulated, can be divided into five phases (Fig. 4-9):

- **Phase 0 (fast upstroke)** characterized by an opening of fast Na^+ channels and an influx of sodium. Upstroke ends when the Na^+ channels are inactivated.
- **Phase 1 (partial repolarization)** resulting from inactivation of Na^+ channels and rapid opening and closure of K^+ channels. Efflux of K^+ accounts for partial repolarization.
- **Phase 2 (plateau)** resulting from the opening of the voltage-sensitive Ca^{2+} channels, which allows the influx of Ca^{2+} counterbalanced by a slow efflux of K^+.
- **Phase 3 (repolarization)** due to closure of Ca^{2+} channels and an efflux of K^+, leading to repolarization of the cell membrane. The excess of Na^+ inside the cell and a net loss of K^+ are corrected by active pumping of Na^+ and K^+ across the cell membrane by Na^+/K^+ ATPase.

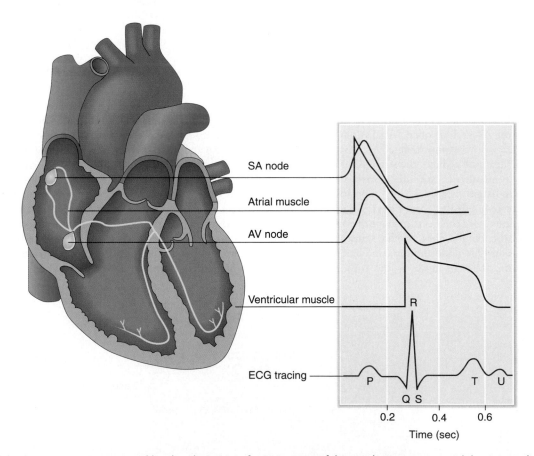

Figure 4-8 Electric currents generated by depolarization of various parts of the conduction system and the myocardium. Superimposed one over another these electric impulses can be registered as the normal electrocardiographic (ECG) tracing. AV, atrioventricular; SA, sinoatrial. (Modified from Boron WF, Boulpaep EL [eds]: Medical Physiology. Saunders, Philadelphia, 2003.)

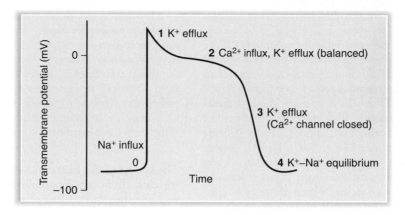

Figure 4-9 Action potential of cardiac myocytes. Each of the five phases is characterized by an influx or efflux of Na+, K+, and Ca²⁺.

■ **Phase 4 (forward current)** characterized by mild gradual depolarization of cell membrane due to Na⁺ influx accompanied by mild K⁺ efflux. During this phase the cell rests, and potential rises slowly to reach the initial threshold for the next depolarization.

Contraction of sarcomeres requires a marked increase of cystosolic calcium concentration so that it could start binding to troponin C.

During phase 2 of the myocyte action potential Ca²⁺ enters into the cytoplasm through the calcium channels and is transferred into the sarcoplasmic reticulum (Fig. 4-10). The entry of extracellular Ca²⁺ acts as a trigger for discharge of large amounts of Ca²⁺ stored inside the cisterns of the sarcoplasmic reticulum and to a lesser degree in mitochondria. Once the concentration of cytosolic calcium has risen 10-fold Ca²⁺ binds to troponin C, which inactivates troponin I, allowing it to induce conformational changes in tropomyosin, the principal regulator of actin–myosin interaction. Tropomyosin deblocks actin, allowing it to interact with myosin. This interaction is a multistep process that ultimately leads to contraction of the sarcomeres.

After the contraction occurs the calcium dissociates from tropomysin, which inhibits actin–myosin interaction, leading to relaxation of the sarcomeres. Free Ca²⁺ is pumped by Adenosine triphosphate (ATP)-dependent calcium pumps back into the sarcoplasmic reticulum and mitochondria, where it is stored. It is also exchanged for Na⁺ across the plasma membrane and extruded from the cell cytoplasm into the interstitial space. During the next action potential the entire cycle is repeated.

Pearl

> Digitalis and related cardiac glycosides increase the concentration of calcium in cardiac myocytes, thus stimulating the contraction of the heart.

Contraction of the myocytes results in systole and the expulsion of the blood from the ventricles, whereas during diastole the ventricles dilate and fill with blood.

The cardiac cycle has two phases: systole, during which the myocardium of the ventricles contracts, and diastole, during which the ventricles dilate. The force of cardiac contraction is influenced by several factors, the most important of

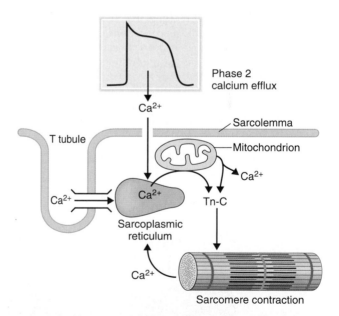

Figure 4-10 The role of calcium (Ca²⁺) in mediating the contraction of sarcomeres. The entry of Ca²⁺ from outside the cell triggers the release of Ca²⁺ from the sarcoplasmic reticulum and to a lesser extent from mitochondria. Free cytoplasmic Ca²⁺ binds to troponin C, which interacts with other troponins and tropomyosin enabling the contraction of sarcomeres. At the end of the contraction Ca²⁺ is released from the sarcomeres and returned to the sarcoplasmic reticulum. Tn-C, troponin C.

which are the preload, contractility of the myocytes, and the afterload (Fig. 4-11).

Preload refers to the end-diastolic volume (i.e., the amount of blood in the ventricles just before the contraction). The contraction of the ventricles increases in proportion to the increased preload (i.e., the venous return to the heart). This is in keeping with the **Frank-Starling law of the heart,** which states that "volume of blood ejected by the ventricle depends on the volume present in the ventricle at the end of diastole." Many years after Frank and Starling defined their law, it was shown that the increased end-diastolic pressure leads to lengthening of the sarcomeres, which thereupon contract more forcefully (Fig. 4-12). In other words the energy of contraction is proportional to the initial length of the cardiac muscles. The Frank-Starling law works only within limits: if the optimal lengthening of sarcomere is exceeded, the contractions become less powerful.

Increased contractility (positive inotropic effect) refers to faster contraction of myocytes or increased velocity of shortening at a constant preload. It can be achieved by sympathetic stimulation or with drugs that have, like digitalis, a positive inotropic effect. Sympathetic stimulation also has a **positive chronotropic effect;** that is, it increases the heart rate, which also contributes to increased cardiac output.

Decreased contractility (negative inotropic effect) is encountered under pathologic conditions, such as coronary heart disease, hypoxia, and acidosis. In such conditions the heart cannot increase cardiac output in response to increased end-diastolic pressure.

Afterload refers to the pressure and resistance against which the ventricles work. In the left ventricle, afterload may be caused by narrowing of the arteries or arterial hypertension, as well as by narrowing of the aortic valves by rheumatic disease or calcification. Afterload to the right ventricle results from various conditions causing pulmonary hypertension or left ventricular failure. Afterload must be overcome by increased cardiac work, but ultimately the heart fails.

The action of the heart occurs in repetitive cycles, which include coordination of myocardial contractility and opening and closing of valves.

The cardiac cycle can be monitored by recording the pressure in various chambers or in the aorta, by measuring the volume of blood in various chambers, by recording the electric potential in electrocardiographic (ECG) tracings, and by monitoring the opening and closing of valves using a cardiac phonograph (Fig. 4-13).

The cardiac cycle begins with the formation of an action potential inside the sinus node. This occurs during diastole when the muscle is relaxed and the ventricles dilated. Through the opening of the mitral and tricuspid valves the ventricles fill until the pressure inside the ventricles reaches the pressure in the atria. This part of the heart cycle is called **diastasis.** The impulses generated in the SA node are transmitted to the atrial musculature. Spreading of the depolarization through the atria is seen in ECG as the **P wave.** The impulses also reach the AV node from which they enter into the ventricles. The 0.10-second delay in the relay of the impulses to the

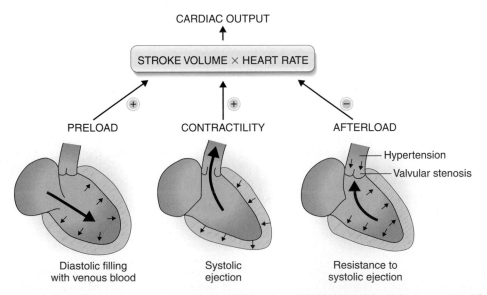

Figure 4-11 Cardiac output depends on the preload, the afterload, and the contractility of the heart. (Modified from Price AS, Wilson LM: Pathophysiology. Clinical Concepts of Disease Processes, 6th ed. Mosby, St. Louis, 2003.)

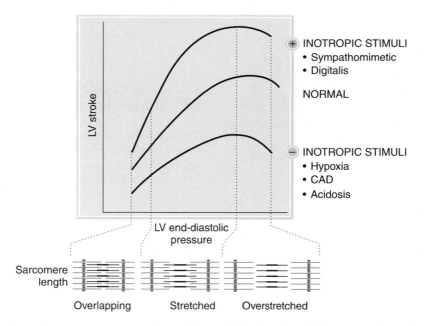

Figure 4-12 Ventricular performance curve according to the Frank-Starling law of the heart. The cardiac output. The left ventricular (LV) stroke increases proportionately to the end-diastolic pressure (i.e., the length to the sarcomere). If the maximum permissible length is exceeded, the LV stroke decreases. Positive inotropic stimuli increase the LV stroke. Negative inotropic stimuli decrease contractility and reduce the LV stroke. CAD, coronary artery disease.

atrial muscles and the entry of the electric current into the ventricles allows enough time for the **atrial contraction,** which typically precedes ventricular contraction before the arteriovenous (A-V) valves close.

The depolarization of the ventricles shows up in the ECG as the **QRS complex,** which leads to systolic contraction of the ventricles. At the beginning of systole the A-V valve closes to prevent the reflux of blood into the atrium once the ventricle begins contracting. The closure of the A-V valve is heard as the **first heart sound (S₁).** It is low in pitch and continues relatively long after the closure. Initially the ventricular *contraction is isovolumic,* but then the aortic valve opens and the blood **ejection phase** begins. During this phase the blood is ejected into the aorta from the left ventricle and into the lungs from the right ventricle. At the end the volume of the blood in the ventricles decreases dramatically.

At the end of systole the aortic valve closes and diastole begins with **isovolumic relaxation** of the ventricles. The closure of the aortic valve is heard as the **second heart sound (S₂).** At the end of the isovolumic relaxation the A-V valve opens and the **rapid filling (inflow) phase** of diastole begins; the cycle is then repeated. The **third cardiac sound (S₃)** can be heard during the period of rapid filling in young persons; in older persons S₃ is a sign of ventricular dysfunction. The **fourth cardiac sound (S₄)** is produced by atrial contraction. These phases of the systole

and diastole are presented in Figure 4-14. Heart sounds are shown in Figure 4-15.

The four phases of the ventricular systole and diastole can be best presented as a pressure–volume loop.

Changes in the ratio of left ventricular volume and intraventricular pressure during the four periods of the cardiac cycle are shown in Figure 4-16. This pressure–volume loop has four parts, as follows:

- **Diastolic filling.** At point A the mitral valve opens, allowing the influx of blood from the atrium. The volume in the ventricle increases, but the pressure rises only minimally.
- **Isovolumic contraction.** At point B the mitral valve closes and the ventricle begins contracting. The pressure in the ventricle rises.
- **Ejection.** At point C the aortic valve opens and the period of ejection of blood into the aorta begins. The intraventricular pressure continues rising but then declines slightly. The volume of blood in the left ventricle drops from 120 mL to less than 50 mL.
- **Isovolumic relaxation.** At point D the aortic valve closes and the ventricle begins relaxation. The intraventricular pressure and the volume of blood in it are low. Then the cycle repeats.

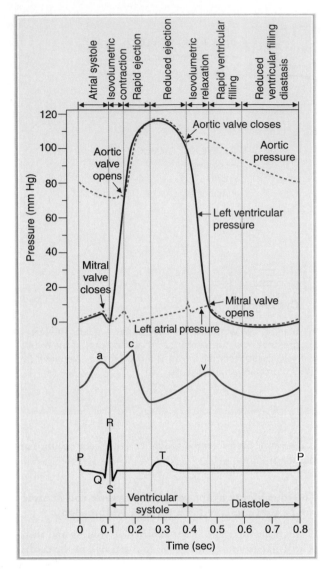

Figure 4-13 Electrical and mechanical events during the cardiac cycle. (Modified from Guyton AC, Hall JE, Textbook of Medical Physiology, 10th ed. Saunders, Philadelphia, 2000, p. 99.)

The ejection fraction is usually about 60% of the total blood volume in the ventricle.

At the end of diastole each ventricle contains approximately 110 to 120 mL of blood, known as **end-diastolic volume.** **Stroke volume** output during systole equals 70 mL, and the remaining 40 to 50 mL is called the **end-systolic volume.** The **ejection fraction** is calculated as the percentage of end-diastolic volume that is ejected from the ventricle. In normal healthy persons it is in the range of 60%. Stroke volume output can be increased during strong cardiac contractions, which reduce the

end-systolic volume to 10 to 20 mL, as well as by increasing the end-diastolic volumes of the ventricle (Fig. 4-17).

Clinical and Laboratory Evaluation of Cardiac Diseases

The evaluation of suspected cases of cardiovascular disease includes taking a complete history and performing a physical examination, standard laboratory tests, and specialized tests aimed at detecting specific diseases.

FAMILY AND PERSONAL HISTORY

Family and personal history may provide valuable clues about the nature of cardiovascular disease (Table 4-1). Many cardiovascular diseases are multifactorial and have a tendency to affect several members of a family. Some, such as congenital heart diseases, are typically found in children; others, such as cardiomyopathies, may be diagnosed at any age. Still others, such as atherosclerosis and congestive heart failure, are more prevalent in the elderly.

SIGNS AND SYMPTOMS OF HEART DISEASES

Symptoms and signs of cardiovascular disease vary from one patient to another. Bear in mind that the most prevalent cardiovascular disease, atherosclerosis, affects the arteries in many parts of the body and can manifest with cardiac, cerebral, or renal symptoms, just to mention a few. Here we concentrate predominantly on heart disease and discuss the most important signs and symptoms pointing to a specific heart disease. The most important signs and symptoms noticed by taking the patient's history and performing the physical examination are as follows:

- Chest discomfort and pain
- Palpitations
- Dyspnea
- Edema
- Cyanosis
- Syncope
- Cardiac murmurs
- Abnormal pulse
- Jugular venous pulse
- Hypertension

Chest discomfort and pain are common symptoms that may be of cardiac or noncardiac origin.

Chest discomfort and pain are closely related sensations that vary in intensity. Minor pain may be perceived as discomfort, and pain often begins as discomfort that gradually

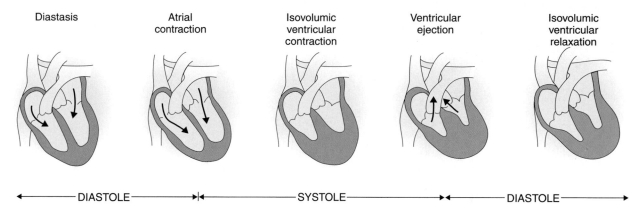

Figure 4-14 Phases of ventricular filling and contraction.

intensifies. Clinically it is customary to subdivide chest pain into two groups: cardiac and noncardiac. The most common causes of acute chest discomfort and pain are listed in Table 4-2.

Cardiac pain may be classified as ischemic or pericardial.

Cardiac pain is transmitted to the cerebral sensory cortex through the sympathetic and parasympathetic autonomic nerve fibers. The parasympathetic fibers are part of the

vagus nerve. The sympathetic sensory fibers enter the upper five to six thoracic and lower cervical ganglia and from there interconnect with afferent fibers leading the sensations into the sensory cortex. Because these sensory fibers communicate with other sensory nerves it is not always possible to determine the exact origin of pain. Accordingly it is important to remember that pain originating from many other organs may be perceived as cardiac, and conversely, pain of cardiac origin may be misinterpreted as stemming from other organs.

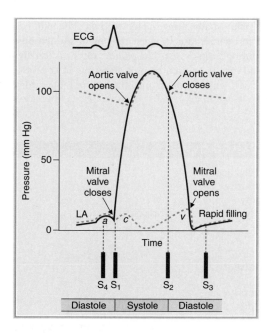

Figure 4-15 Cardiac sounds. S_1 is produced by opening of the atrioventricular valves. S_2 is produced by closure of the aortic valve. S_3 is heard during rapid filling in diastole in young persons. S_4 is the result of atrial contraction before the A-V valves close.

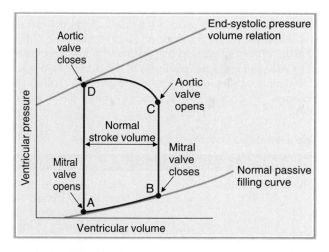

Figure 4-16 Pressure–volume loop of the heart during the contraction–relaxation cycle. The left ventricular pressure (ordinate) is plotted against the left ventricular volume (abscissa). A, Mitral valve opens and diastolic filling of the ventricles begins. A–B corresponds to diastolic filling. B, Mitral valve closes at the end of diastole and isovolumic contraction of the ventricles begins. B–C corresponds to isovolumic contraction of the ventricle. C, Aortic valve opens and the ejection of blood from the ventricle begins. C–D corresponds to the ejection phase of systole. D, Aortic valve closes and end-systolic volume is reached, whereupon the ventricles relax. D–A corresponds to isovolumic ventricular relaxation.

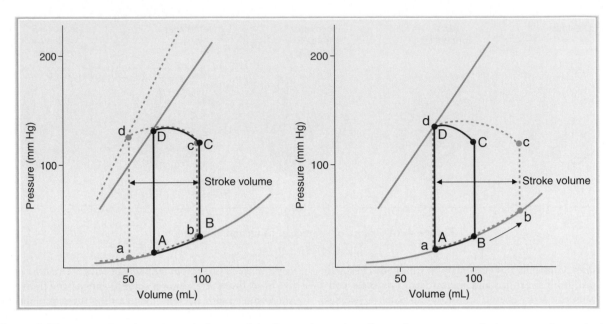

Figure 4-17 Increased stroke volume. Left part of the figure shows the effects of stronger ventricular contraction reducing the end-systolic ventricular volume (D–d). The right part of the figure shows the effects of increased diastolic filling, which also increase the stroke volume.

Ischemic cardiac pain originates from the myocardium that is not receiving enough oxygen for its needs. Typically this kind of pain is characteristic of ischemic coronary heart disease and is found in patients who have angina pectoris or who have had or are having a myocardial infarction (MI). Similar pain is experienced by patients who have aortic stenosis preventing normal perfusion of the coronary arteries.

Ischemic cardiac discomfort and pain are described as heaviness or pressure or squeezing behind the sternum (retrosternal pain). The pain has an epicenter over the sternum radiating to the arm, neck, and lower jaw. Most often it radiates into the left arm along the ulnar side (Fig. 4-18). Less commonly it may be bilateral, and occasionally it may radiate to the back, usually along the left scapula. The pain is usually related to exercise, but in MI it may be of sudden onset and occur during sleep or rest. The pain of angina is usually short-lived and can be relieved by nitroglycerine, in contrast to the pain of MI, which is often crushing and of longer duration.

Table 4-1 Risk Factors for Heart Diseases

TYPE OF RISK FACTOR	SPECIFIC DISEASES–RISK FACTOR ASSOCIATIONS
Hereditary factors	Hyperlipidemia: Coronary heart disease
	Familial hypertrophic cardiomyopathy
	Hemochromatosis: Cardiomyopathy
	Familial history of hypertension: Hypertensive heart disease
Social/nutritional factors	Smoking: Coronary heart disease
	Alcoholism: Cardiomyopathy
	Drug abuse: Endocarditis
Aging	Atherosclerosis: Coronary heart disease
Infections	"Strep throat": Rheumatic fever
	Systemic viral infection: Myocarditis
	Systemic viral infection: Pericarditis
Medical and surgical procedures	Sepsis: Endocarditis
Drugs/toxins	Adriamycin: Cardiomyopathy
	Alcohol abuse: Cardiomyopathy
External mechanical factors	Car accident: Rupture of the aorta
	Stabbing wound of the heart: Hematopericardium

Table 4-2 Major Causes of Chest Discomfort and Pain

Cardiac pain
  Angina pectoris
  Myocardial infarction
  Aortic stenosis
  Pericarditis
Chest wall syndromes
  Herpes zoster
  Myalgia of thoracic muscles
Gastrointestinal pain
  Esophageal disorders
  Peptic ulcer disease
  Gallstones and cholecystitis
Pulmonary pain
  Pneumonia
  Pleuritis
  Pulmonary embolism
Vascular pain
  Aortic aneurysm
  Aortic dissection

Pericardial pain is caused by pericarditis and is typically most intense behind the sternum or at the apex of the heart. It is described as stabbing, burning, or piercing. It lasts longer than ischemic pain and is unrelated to exercise. It may be aggravated by lying down, coughing, deep inspiration, or movement. It can be partially relieved by leaning forward or preventing chest movements. Pericardial pain is usually not radiating outside the chest.

Palpitation is a subjective feeling of heartbeating.

Patients typically complain that they feel their "heart beating fast" or "skipping beats." This very common symptom may be correlated with irregularities of the pulse. It may be caused by the following functional irregularities of heartbeat:

- **Atrial fibrillation.** The heartbeats are rapid and irregular.
- **Supraventricular or ventricular tachycardia.** The heartbeats are rapid and regular.
- **Premature atrial and ventricular contractions.** The patient complains of "skipped beats."

Cardiac dyspnea results from increased respiratory effort aimed at compensating for hypoxia.

Dyspnea is a sense of difficulty in breathing or shortness of breath. Note that it is a subjective feeling and reflects the patients' consciousness of increased respiratory effort. Furthermore, the sensation of shortness of breath is very common, and accordingly dyspnea is also a physiological phenomenon that occurs whenever there is a "hunger for air" due to strenuous exercise, a sudden rush of activity (e.g., a fast sprint), adjusting to high altitudes ("mountain sickness"), and even in anxiety states.

An important aspect of cardiac dyspnea is the sensation of chest tightness and shortness of breath. These symptoms result from impulses emanating from mechanoreceptors in the lungs, sensory stimuli from the chest wall, and those generated by the chemoreceptors reacting to the reduced concentration of oxygen in the blood. All these afferent signals act on the respiratory center to generate an adequate ventilatory response, perceived by the individual as a "respiratory effort" or "labored breathing" (Fig. 4-19).

Cardiac dyspnea must be distinguished from noncardiac dyspnea.

When a patient presents with dyspnea it is most important to establish whether it is acute or chronic and to decide whether it is of cardiac or noncardiac origin. The most common form of noncardiac dyspnea is respiratory dyspnea caused by a variety of bronchopulmonary diseases, such as bronchial asthma, chronic obstructive pulmonary

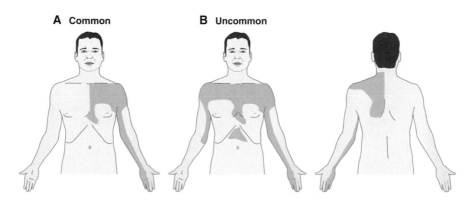

Figure 4-18 Ischemic cardiac pain. **A,** The pain most often radiates to the ulnar side of the left arm. **B,** Less often the pain radiates to the right side, the neck, and the face, or to the dorsal side of the chest.

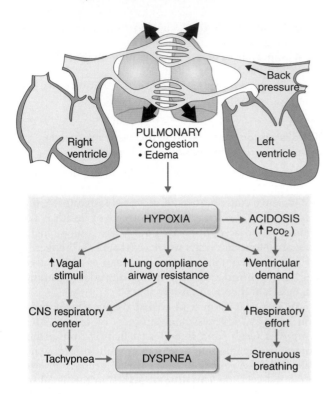

Figure 4-19 Cardiac dyspnea caused by left heart failure. CNS, central nervous system; Pco_2, partial pressure of carbon dioxide.

disease, and pneumonia (Fig. 4-20). Systemic diseases such as acidosis or neuromuscular diseases such as myasthenia gravis also may affect breathing and cause dyspnea. All these diseases can be excluded from the differential diagnosis by taking a thorough history, performing a complete physical examination, and conducting any necessary additional testing.

Once the pulmonary dyspnea has been excluded and cardiac dyspnea is suggested, it is important to decide whether the symptom is related to high-, normal-, or low-output heart failure. This determination allows the physician to decide whether the dyspnea is related to intrinsic heart failure presenting usually as low-output heart failure or some other condition, such as anemia or hyperthyroidism, which present with high-output failure. Obesity typically manifests with dyspnea with normal cardiac output.

Cardiac dyspnea is traditionally divided into two forms: dyspnea on effort and dyspnea at rest.

■ **Dyspnea on effort** may be the first sign of heart failure and is often associated with anginal pain. The patient typically complains of being short of breath after climbing up the stairs or strenuously walking. Usually it is progressive and can become incapacitating.

■ **Dyspnea at rest** is a common sign of heart disease and is usually related to pulmonary congestion and edema due to left heart failure. **Orthopnea** is a term used to describe breathing discomfort experienced while the patient is lying down that is relieved by sitting up in bed or using several pillows. **Paroxysmal nocturnal dyspnea** typically wakes the patient, who has a feeling of suffocation. It may be associated with wheezing or coughing and is occasionally called "cardiac asthma." A common cause of this form of dyspnea is tachyarrhythmia, which may be noticed by the patient. Acute heart failure, as in MI, can also cause nocturnal dyspnea.

Pulmonary edema is a sign of left heart failure, whereas peripheral edema is a sign of right heart failure.

Left heart failure causes increased pulmonary venous pressure, which in turn leads to transudation of fluid into the pulmonary interstitial spaces and alveoli (Fig. 4-21). This hydrostatic edema may be of acute onset, as in MI, or chronic, as in congestive heart failure (CHF). Chronic pulmonary edema is often associated with hydrothorax due to

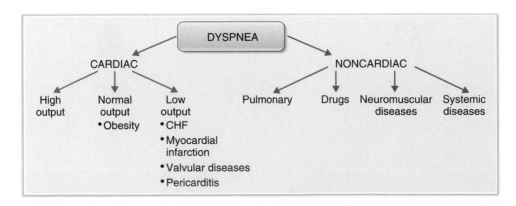

Figure 4-20 Differentiation of cardiac from noncardiac dyspnea. CHF, congestive heart failure.

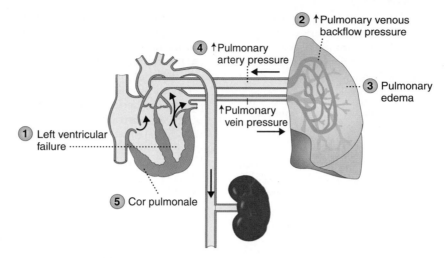

Figure 4-21 Left heart failure (1) leads to backflow pressure into the pulmonary system (2) and causes pulmonary congestion, edema (3). Consequently, increased pulmonary pressure (4) results in cor pulmonale (5).

the transudation of fluid into the pleural cavity. It is usually associated with dyspnea and may cause tachypnea. Pulmonary rales may be heard on auscultation.

Right heart failure leads to peripheral edema that typically manifests in the lower extremities ("pitting leg edema"). It is usually associated with chronic passive congestion, congestive hepatomegaly, and splenomegaly. As the heart failure progresses, edema becomes more generalized and includes ascites.

Since left heart failure is the most common cause of right heart failure, pulmonary edema is often associated with peripheral edema. Furthermore fluid retention in the kidneys, a common complication of heart failure, contributes to a fluid overload and generalized edema (anasarca)

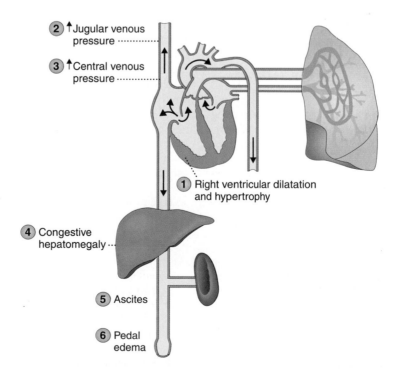

Figure 4-22 Right heart failure (1) leads to chronic passive congestion and peripheral edema (2–6).

(Fig. 4-22). Hence the patient complains of various forms of dyspnea, chest tightness due to pulmonary edema, generalized swelling and a feeling of "puffiness" pedal edema, epigastric fullness, pain in the liver or the spleen, or bulging abdomen and changes in bowel habits.

Cyanosis is a bluish discoloration of skin or mucosa caused by increased concentrations of reduced hemoglobin in arterial blood.

Cyanosis (derived from Greek word for dark blue) occurs when the concentration of unoxygenated hemoglobin exceeds the concentration of 5 g/dL. In practical terms that means the arterial saturation is 85% or less—a saturation level that is significantly less than normal (≥95%). Cyanosis occurs in two forms: central and peripheral.

- **Central cyanosis** presents as discoloration of lips or skin of the trunk. In adults it is most often a feature of pulmonary diseases, but it may occur in association with hemoglobin abnormalities (e.g., methemoglobulinemia) or among people living in high altitudes. In children it occurs as a manifestation of congenital heart diseases with right to left shunting of blood, as in the tetralogy of Fallot.
- **Peripheral cyanosis** presents with bluish discoloration of fingers and toes. It may occur on exposure to cold, but it may also be a manifestation of vaso-occlusive diseases, such as Raynaud's or Buerger's diseases, venous or arterial thrombi, and emboli. It is also found in patients with reduced cardiac output of any origin. In children it is usually a sign of congenital heart diseases with right to left shunting of blood.

Syncope is loss of consciousness due to the interruption of cerebral arterial blood flow.

Syncope, or a "fainting spell," is very common among healthy persons, but it may also be a sign of serious disease. The causes of syncope may be classified into four categories:

- **Reflex neurocardiogenic syncope.** It results from reflex-induced vasodilation or bradycardia. It may be induced by a variety of reflexes, such as the vasovagal, vasodepressive, or carotid sinus reflexes. These reflexes may be triggered by coughing, straining during micturition and defecation, or exercise. Such syncope is called **situational.**
- **Orthostatic hypotension.** It results from the effects on the autonomic nervous system and is classified as **hyperadrenergic** (e.g., volume depletion) or **hypoadrenergic** (e.g., due to autonomic dysregulation as in diabetes mellitus). Drugs affecting the autonomic nervous system, such as centrally acting hypotensive drugs (e.g., methyldopa), adrenergic neuron-blocking agents (e.g., guanethidine), various tranquilizers, antidepressants, and many others, can cause syncope. Orthostatic hypoten-

sion is the cause of **postprandial syncope** in the elderly. It is accompanied by hypotension after meals due to pooling of blood in the abdominal organs.
- **Neurologic disorders.** Transient ischemic attacks, attacks of migraine, or epileptic seizures may cause transient loss of consciousness.
- **Cardiac syncope.** It may be caused by **pump failure** in MI, **obstruction of blood flow** by valvular disease or atrial myxoma, **conduction disorders** (e.g., bradycardia or arrhythmia), and any other cardiac disease. Certain drugs that affect the coronary circulation, such as nitroglycerin, also can induce syncope.
- **Other causes.** Metabolic diseases (e.g., hypoglycemia), hyperventilation due to excitement, hysteria, and various psychiatric disorders may cause syncope, but in 30% of cases the cause remains unknown.

Pearl

> A mnemonic for remembering the causes of syncope are the first five letters of ORTHOstatic, which stands for **O**rthostatic, **R**eflex-related, **T**IA/seizure/epilepsy, **H**eart conditions, and **O**thers (after you have excluded the first four).

Cardiac murmurs can be caused by heart diseases but are often relatively "innocent" and caused by functional changes in the blood flow.

Cardiac murmurs may be a sign of heart disease, but more often such murmurs reflect changes in the blood flow through the heart. Such **functional murmurs** are typically related to fast blood flow and are most often found in children. They are heard during midsystole over the pulmonic area and along the left margin of the sternum. Elevated cardiac output in thyrotoxicosis or pregnancy is also accompanied by cardiac murmurs. Changes in the viscosity of the blood, as in anemia, also may cause cardiac murmurs.

Cardiac murmurs related to various heart diseases originate from turbulent flow of blood as it passes through abnormal cardiac chambers, valves, or shunts. Examples of cardiac diseases that may cause murmurs are as follows:

- **Endocardial diseases.** The murmurs may be caused by narrowing of the orifice by calcified valves in chronic rheumatic disease or calcific aortic stenosis. Irregularly shaped valves in floppy mitral valve disease, or irregular valvular surface in acute bacterial endocarditis may cause murmurs. The blood flow across prosthetic valves also causes murmurs.
- **Septal defects.** Left-to-right or right-to-left shunts through atrial and ventricular septal defects, or complex anomalies such as tetralogy of Fallot, produce cardiac murmurs.
- **Vascular diseases.** Congenital anomalies of the great vessels produce murmurs in the precordium. The best

known among these is the "machinery" murmur of patent ductus arteriosus. In the elderly the most common vascular "heart murmur" is that produced by supravalvular aortic stenosis related to atherosclerosis of the aorta.

■ **Myocardial disease.** Rupture of papillary muscle due to MI causes acute mitral insufficiency and a loud systolic murmur. Likewise, the turbulent blood flow in ventricular aneurysms and dilated cardiomyopathy may cause murmurs.

■ **Pericarditis.** Exudative pericarditis may cause a friction rub.

Diagnostically important cardiac murmurs are classified by their location, timing, duration, configuration, pitch, and intensity.

Auscultation of the heart is a very important technique for examining patients, but if a murmur is heard it may be also recorded by phonocardiogram. When describing and classifying heart murmurs one must take account of their physical properties as follows:

■ **Location.** It is important to determine the areas of the precordium where the murmurs are heard the best. The optimal auscultatory areas for each valve are shown in Figure 4-23. The murmur propagates in the direction of blood flow, which varies depending on the affected valve. For example, in aortic valvular stenosis the systolic murmur is maximal in the right intercostal space and radiates to the neck, reflecting the flow of the blood through the stenosed orifice.

■ **Timing, duration, and configuration.** Murmurs can be timed by simultaneous auscultation and monitoring of the heartbeat. This can be done by placing the

fingers over the apex of the heart or palpating the carotid or radial pulse. Murmurs are divided into three major groups: **systolic, diastolic,** and **continuous** (Table 4-3 and Fig. 4-24). Phonocardiography can precisely record the shape of the murmur and determine whether it changes intensity or is continuous at the same intensity. It is also possible to determine whether the murmur occurs during the entire systole (e.g., *pansystolic* or holosystolic) or is limited to midsystole or late systole. *Midsystolic* murmurs are also called *crescendo–decrescendo* murmurs because their intensity increases, reaches its peak at midsystole, and decreases thereafter.

■ **Intensity and pitch.** The intensity of a murmur is graded on a scale from 1 to 6. A grade 1 murmur is barely audible, whereas a grade 5 murmur is very loud. A grade 6 murmur is so strong that it can be heard without a stethoscope. The pitch of the murmur (i.e., its sound frequency) depends on the velocity of the blood as it passes through the pathologically altered part of the heart. The flow of blood across a stenotic mitral valve causes a low-pitched "rumbling" murmur. Regurgitation of the blood through a regurgitant aortic valve is accompanied by a high-pitched diastolic murmur.

Palpation of the pulse may provide information about the heart action.

Palpating the radial artery or carotid artery is the best and quickest way of assessing the pulse. One should record the frequency, regularity, volume, and contour of the pulse and also note the presence of palpable shudder or thrill and audible bruits.

The pulse can be measured and recorded by sphygmomanometry. In these tracings the normal pulse is **dicrotic** and consists of a primary systolic wave and a secondary

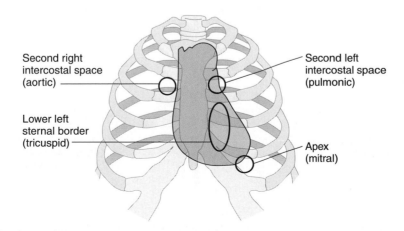

Second right intercostal space (aortic)

Second left intercostal space (pulmonic)

Lower left sternal border (tricuspid)

Apex (mitral)

Figure 4-23 Optimal positioning of stethoscope for the auscultation of cardiac murmurs. Aortic murmurs are heard best at the base to the right of the sternum. Tricuspid murmurs are heard best at the left lower sternal border. Mitral murmurs are heard best at the apex. Pulmonic murmurs are heard best at the base to the left of the sternum.

Table 4-3 Cardiac Murmurs

Systolic Murmurs
Mid-systolic (crescendo-decrescendo)
    Aortic stenosis
    Pulmonary stenosis
    Hypertrophic cardiomyopathy
Pansystolic
    Mitral regurgitation
    Tricuspid regurgitation
    Ventricular septal defect
Late-systolic
    Mitral valve prolapse

Diastolic Murmurs
Early diastolic
    Aortic regurgitation
    Pulmonary regurgitation
Mid-diastolic
    Mitral stenosis
    Tricuspid stenosis

Continuous Murmurs
    Patent ductus arteriosus

diastolic wave. These two waves are separated from each other by a *dicrotic notch* corresponding to the closure of the aortic valve at the end of systole (Fig. 4-25).

Recording of the pulse rate can be used to diagnose certain heart diseases as follows:

- **Fast or slow pulse.** These findings are typical of tachycardia or bradycardia, respectively.
- **Pulse deficit.** In this condition an absence of the palpable pulse is noted despite an audible heartbeat over the precordium. Typically, it occurs in atrial fibrillation; the contraction of the heart occurs and is audible by auscultation of the chest, but it is too weak to propel the blood into the aorta and arteries.
- **Anacrotic pulse** (also known by the Latin name *pulsus parvus et tardus*). It is typical of aortic stenosis. In this condition the initial upstroke is slow and the peak lower than normal and shifted to the right close to S_2, that is, the dicrotic notch.
- **Pulsus bisferiens** (also known by the Latin name *pulsus celer*). It is characterized by two systolic peaks

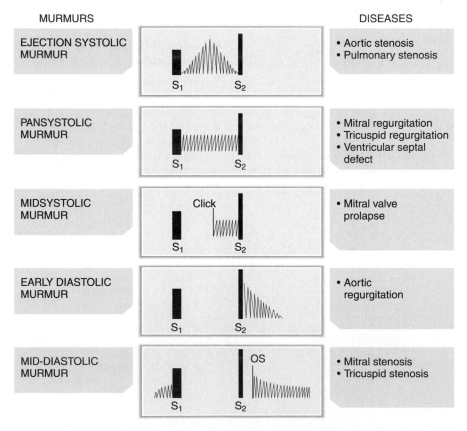

Figure 4-24 Cardiac murmurs. Murmurs heard in the interval between the first heart sound (S_1) and the second heart sound (S_2) are called systolic and those after S_2 and before the S_1 are diastolic. The intensity of the murmurs may vary, as is the case with the crescendo–decrescendo ejection systolic murmur, or they may be constant during the entire duration of the murmur as in pansystolic murmur. OS, opening snap.

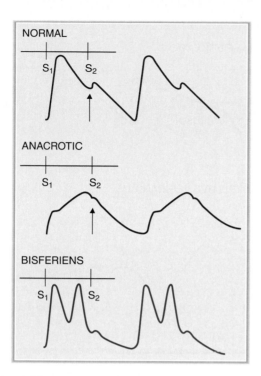

Figure 4-25 Carotid pulse tracings. A normal pulse has two peaks separated by a dicrotic notch (*arrow*). The anacrotic pulse has a slow upstroke, and its peak is lower than normal. Pulsus bisferiens has a fast upstroke and sharp downslope after the second wave. Both waves occur during the systole.

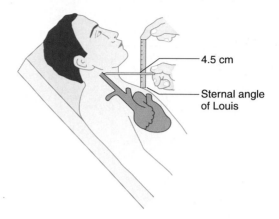

Figure 4-26 Measuring jugular venous pressure at the bedside. If measuring on a patient lying at an angle of 45 degrees, palpate the pulse at 4.5 cm above the sternal angle (*angle of Louis*).

> **Pearls**
>
> ➤ Use the right *external* jugular vein to measure venous pressure.
> ➤ Inspiration makes the jugular venous pulse more visible.

and it typically occurs in aortic regurgitation. The volume of such a pulse is larger than normal, and it has sharply rising contours.

■ **Pulsus paradoxus.** Normally the arterial pressure declines by 10 mm Hg during inspiration. In cardiac tamponade and constrictive pericarditis it declines more than that, and inspiration-induced decline can be noticed by palpation of the carotid or radial artery.

Jugular venous pulse measurements are useful for the assessment of central venous pressure and intravascular volume.

As Dr. S. Mangione of Jefferson Medical College, Philadelphia, memorably said, jugular vein pressure is a "poor man's monitor of right-heart hemodynamics." It can be measured at the bedside (Fig. 4-26). It might not always be precise and might be difficult to perform in some people, such as those with short fat necks, but still it gives a rough estimate of the central venous pressure. The jugular venous pulse can also be objectively measured and recorded.

In venous ECG tracings the jugular venous pulse consists of three positive waves (*a*, *c*, and *v*) and three negative descents (*x*, x_1, and *y*). The *a* wave is produced by **a**trial contraction. The *c* wave results from the bulging of the tricuspid **c**usps into the right atrium, but it is often not visible in most tracings. The *v* wave occurs during the end of **v**entricular systole and the early phase of ventricular diastole. The *x* descent reflects atrial relaxation during ventricular systole, and the much longer x_1 occurs due to retraction of the tricuspid valve into the dilated right ventricle in systole. The opening of the tricuspid valve in diastole produces the *y* descent (Fig. 4-27).

Abnormalities of the jugular vein pressure are found in many cardiac diseases but also occur in lung diseases and systemic conditions such as sepsis and shock. Three typical changes of the jugular venous pressure are given as illustrations:

■ **Absence of the *a* wave.** This is typically seen in atrial fibrillation. The *a* wave, which reflects the contraction of the atrium, is obviously missing because the atrium does not contract.

■ **Increased amplitude of the *a* wave with impaired y descent.** These findings are typically seen in tricuspid stenosis. The *a* wave reflects increased atrial strain, and the *y* descent is impaired because of the inability of the tricuspid valve to open completely.

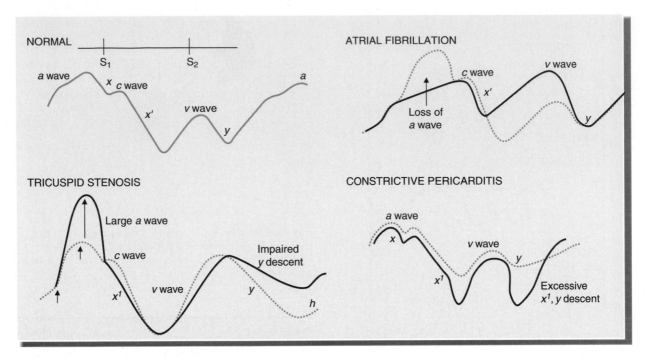

Figure 4-27 Jugular venous pulse tracing. Normal tracing has three peaks *a*, *c*, and *v*, and two down-slopes (*x* + *x*¹ and *y*). Atrial fibrillation is marked by a disappearance of the *a* wave. In tricuspid stenosis the *a* wave is large, and the *y* descent is impaired. In constrictive pericarditis a sharp and excessive descent occurs involving both the *x* and *y* part of the incline.

■ **Exaggerated *x* and *y* descent.** These changes occur in any condition with increased venous pressure but most prominently in constrictive pericarditis.

Arterial pressure changes are both the cause and the consequence of heart dysfunction.

Arterial hypertension is an extremely common disease that adversely affects the function of the heart. Uncontrolled, long-standing hypertension leads to cardiac hypertrophy and hypertensive heart disease, which is still a major cause of cardiac morbidity. In addition, hypertension is one of the major risk factors for atherosclerosis and accelerates the development of ischemic coronary heart disease. On the other hand low arterial pressure may be a sign of heart failure and is typically found in almost all forms of cardiogenic shock, such shock due to MI or CHF in acute viral myocarditis or acute cardiac block.

The cause of arterial hypertension is unknown in most instances (95%), and the disease is called *primary* hypertension. In the remaining 5% of cases the cause can be established, and the disease is called *secondary* hypertension. The causes of secondary hypertension are listed in Table 4-4. Also remember that pregnancy may be associated with secondary hypertension, which usually disappears after delivery.

Pearl
> The mnemonic for remembering the causes of secondary hypertension is RENAL: **R**enal **E**ndocrine **N**eurogenic **A**rterial **L**abile or **L**aboratory abnormalities

DIAGNOSTIC TESTS AND PROCEDURES

Some of the tests for cardiovascular diseases can be performed in outpatient clinics or doctors' offices, some are performed in general hospitals, but others can be performed only in specialized cardiac diagnostic centers. Understanding the purpose of these tests and why they are performed is vital to appreciating their diagnostic value as well their limitations. The most important diagnostic tests and procedures are listed here as follows:

■ Radiologic techniques
■ Electrocardiography
■ Stress testing

Table 4-4 Causes of Secondary Arterial Hypertension

Renal Diseases
Glomerulonephritis, acute and chronic
Diabetic nephropathy
Renal artery stenosis

Endocrine Diseases
Hyperfunction or tumors of pituitary, thyroid, parathyroid, adrenal cortex
Tumors of the adrenal medulla (pheochromocytoma)
Carcinoid tumors
Exogenous hormones (e.g., steroids)

Neurologic Diseases
Increased intracranial pressure (e.g., CNS tumors, infection)
Guillain-Barré syndrome
Sleep apnea

Arterial Diseases
Atherosclerosis
Coarctation of aorta
Aortitis

Labile/Temporary*
White coat hypertension
Psychogenic nervousness
Postoperative
Hypoglycemia
Sickle cell anemia
Drugs (e.g., cocaine, NSAIDs)
Pregnancy

---

*The term *labile* is used in clinics for "white coat hypertension." However, here we have included several other temporary and situational causes to fit them all under the mnemonic RENAL. CNS, central nervous system; NSAIDs, nonsteroidal anti-inflammatory drugs.

- Echocardiography
- Cardiac catheterization
- Laboratory testing

Routine chest radiography is part of the initial evaluation of cardiac patients and is a good source of information about the heart.

Routine chest radiographs are taken from an anteroposterior (AP) and lateral view. These films provide data about the following parameters:

- **Shape of the heart.** For example in the tetralogy of Fallot the heart has a "bootlike" shape.
- **Size of the heart.** Hypertension and various cardiomyopathies cause cardiac hypertrophy, which is easily recognized on radiographs.
- **Size of cardiac chambers.** For example the enlargement of the left ventricle may be recognized by the rounding of the apex and its downward and lateral displacement.

- **Pulmonary circulation.** Pulmonary congestion and edema that occur in left heart failure are easily recognized on radiographs.
- **Pulmonary disease.** Chronic obstructive pulmonary disease that may cause cor pulmonale is readily recognized on chest radiographs.
- **Aortic pathology.** Atherosclerosis and aneurysmal dilatations of the aorta can be also recognized on AP and lateral films.

Other radiologic techniques, such as **computed tomography (CT)** and **magnetic resonance imaging (MRI),** are widely used and could supplement or clarify the data obtained by routine radiographic examination. **Radionucleotide imaging** is widely used for assessing the thickness of the ventricles and evaluating cardiac functions.

Electrocadiography is the principal source of data about the electric activity of the heart.

An electrocardiogram (ECG) is the recording of the changes in the electric activity of the heart during the contractions cycle. ECG is routinely recorded from 12 leads placed on the body: six limb leads and six chest/precordial leads (Fig. 4-28) as follows:

- Bipolar leads
  - I—left arm-right arm
  - II—left leg-right arm
  - III—left leg-left arm
- Unipolar leads
  - aVL—left arm–indifferent electrode (right arm + right leg)
  - aVR—right arm–indifferent electrode (left arm + left leg)
  - aVL—left leg–indifferent electrode (left arm + right arm)
- Precordial chest leads
  - V_1—right sternal margin, fourth intercostal space
  - V_2—left sternal margin, fourth intercostal space
  - V_3—halfway between V_2 and V_4
  - V_4—fifth intercostal space in the left-midclavicular line
  - V_5—fifth intercostal spaces in the anterior axillary line
  - V_6— fifth intercostal space in the midaxillary line

The changes in the anterolateral part of the heart are reflected in the aVL lead and lead I. Inferolateral changes are reflected in leads II, III, and aVF. The pathology of the cavities is reflected in the aVR lead. V_1 and V_2 reflect changes in the right ventricle, V_3 and V_4 those in the septum, and V_5 and V_6 in the anterior and lateral wall of the left ventricle.

An ECG is recorded on calibrated paper that moves through the ECG machine at a preset speed of 25 mm/sec. The recording paper is subdivided into small (1 mm) and large (5 mm) squares. On the horizontal scale, which

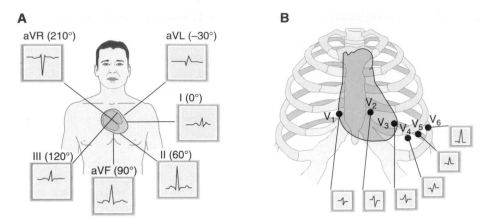

Figure 4-28 Tracing of ECG includes 12 standard leads. **A,** Unipolar and bipolar leads. **B,** Precordial leads V_1 to V_6. aVF, aVL, aVR, augmented limb leads.

records the time, each small square equals 0.04 second and each large square equals 0.2 second. In the vertical scale, which records the action potential, 10 mm equals 1 mV (Fig. 4-29).

The normal ECG is the summary of changes that occur from the initiation of the contraction potential in the SA node through the conduction of impulses through the conduction system, depolarization of the ventricles, and repolarization of the heart at the end of each cycle. The normal ECG has the following parts:

- **P wave.** This part reflects the depolarization of the atrium.
- **PR interval.** It lasts 0.12 to 0.20 second and represents the time needed for the impulse to pass through the AV node.

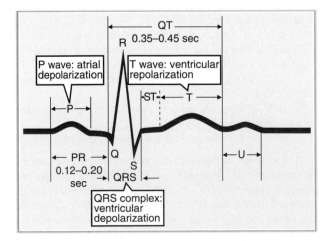

Figure 4-29 Standard ECG tracing consists of a P wave, QRS complex, and T wave and the corresponding intervals. The average duration of these ECG segments is given at a heart rate between 60 and 72 beats per minute.

- **QRS complex.** This bidirectional, high-amplitude complex lasts less than 0.10 second and consists of an initial downward deflection (Q), followed by an upward deflection (R), and a downward deflection (S). It corresponds to the depolarization of the ventricles.
- **ST segment.** This isoelectric segment follows the QRS complex. During that short period there is very little electric activity in the heart.
- **T wave.** This upward deflection corresponds to the repolarization of the ventricles. It is usually measured together with the time needed for the depolarization of the ventricles as the QT interval, which lasts normally 0.35 to 0.45 second.

ECG can detect disturbances in generation and conduction of electric impulses and myocardial contraction.

ECG is useful for assessing the electric currents through the heart as they are generated and transmitted through the conduction system and the cardiac myocytes. In general terms ECG can be useful for the evaluation of the following conditions:

- **Cardiac chamber abnormalities.** Both dilatation and hypertrophy of the ventricles or atria produce typical ECG changes. For example left atrial hypertrophy is accompanied by a widening of the P wave in lead II. Left ventricular hypertrophy is accompanied by widening of the QRS complex and a left-axis deviation.
- **Conduction abnormalities.** ECG is the method of choice for diagnosing various forms of arrhythmia, premature beats, and cardiac block.
- **Myocardial ischemia.** Myocardial ischemia typically causes repolarization of the ventricle and can be recognized in the ECG as ST segment depression and T wave inversion. The changes in the ECG make it also possible to localize the infarct.

Temporary ischemia caused by Prinzmetal's angina may produce reversible ST segment elevation.

■ **Disturbances in the heart caused by abnormal homeostasis of minerals.** The contraction and relaxation of the heart depends critically on the maintenance of homeostasis and is especially influenced by changes in the concentration of minerals in the blood and interstitial fluids. Both excess and deficiency of calcium and potassium may adversely affect the myocardium and produce typical changes in the ECG. For example, hyperkalemia makes the T wave symmetrically peaked, whereas hypokalemia leads to ST segment depression and flattening of T waves and the appearance of a terminal U wave (Fig. 4-30).

■ **Effects of drugs.** Many cardiotropic drugs produce typical changes in the ECG. Digitalis causes ST depression and T wave flattening and shortening of the QT interval. Quinidine prolongs the T wave, causing its flattening or inversion.

Stress testing is based on ECG monitoring of patients who are walking on a treadmill.

Placing a person on a treadmill and asking him or her to walk while the tester is increasing the speed of the treadmill tests how the heart responds to increased demand for greater effort. A normal heart responds to increased demand by increasing its rate, but the ECG remains normal. If the heart is not receiving enough blood due to coronary heart disease and ischemia develops, the ECG shows typical change such as up-sloping of the ST depression or down-sloping of the ST wave. Monitoring the action of the heart while gradually increasing

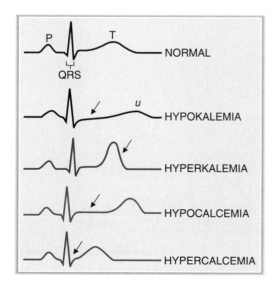

Figure 4-30 Effect of serum mineral disturbances on the ECG. Hypokalemia causes ST depression and T wave depression. Hyperkalemia causes symmetric peaking of the T wave. Hypocalcemia prolongs the QT interval. Hypercalcemia shortens the QRS and shortens the ST interval.

demand for oxygen can determine whether the heart is adequately supplied with blood and indirectly whether the coronaries are patent.

Stress testing is performed on patients who have signs of angina pectoris, exercise-induced arrhythmia, or other signs of early coronary insufficiency. Stress testing is also performed in the follow-up of patients who have undergone coronary bypass surgery to determine whether the surgery has improved the blood supply to the myocardium. Stress testing of patients who have recovered from an infarction can provide information about the extent of cardiac reserve after injury.

Echocardiography is useful for evaluating the cardiac chambers and blood flow through the heart.

Echocardiography is a noninvasive technique that includes two-dimensional ultrasound, Doppler echocardiography, and transesophageal echocardiography. With these techniques the following can be visualized:

■ Size of cardiac chambers
■ Thickness of the myocardium
■ Contractility of the myocardium and the foci of irregular contraction or akinesis
■ Integrity and function of the valves
■ Size and shape of the orifices
■ Velocity of blood flow
■ Direction of blood flow
■ Existence and size of septal defects

Echocardiography is useful for evaluating congenital heart defects, valvular diseases, complications of MI such as rupture of the papillary muscle or ventricular aneurysms, cardiomyopathy, and atrial tumors.

For example two-dimensional echocardiography is a relatively easy and fast way of visualizing akinesis or dyskinesis of the myocardium damaged by an acute MI. However, echocardiography cannot distinguish acute infarction from an old infarction or from "myocardial stunning," a temporary postinfarction ventricular dysfunction.

Doppler echocardiography is used for evaluation of possible cardiomyopathy. With this technique the size of the heart, the volume of the ventricles, and the thickness of the ventricular wall are assessed. Also the function of the heart during systole and diastole is evaluated and whether the problem is primarily systolic or diastolic is determined. Associated complications, such as mitral or tricuspid regurgitation, are also detected. Global akinesis, a common finding, is also documented, and the reduction of the total ventricular ejection fraction can be estimated.

Cardiac catheterization is useful for documenting the filling pressure in the cardiac chambers and the oxygen saturation in various parts of the heart.

Cardiac catheterization is performed by inserting a vascular catheter into thee heart chambers. This may be achieved by inserting the catheter through the femoral or brachial fossa veins to the right atrium and ventricle, or in a retrograde manner from the femoral artery through the aorta and through the aortic valve into the left ventricle. With these catheters the pressure in the cardiac chambers can be measured and thus the pressure gradients that develop across each valve can be calculated. Furthermore, blood from the cardiac chambers can be sampled and the degree of oxygen saturation determined.

Special pulmonary artery **balloon catheters** (Swan-Ganz catheters) can be inserted into the pulmonary artery to measure "pulmonary wedge pressure" and thus indirectly monitor the function of the left ventricle in patients who have suffered an MI (Fig. 4-31). Catheters can also be used to document the existence of septal defects and shunts, as well as the mixing of the venous and arterial blood across these defects.

Coronary catheterization is useful for establishing the site of coronary artery occlusion or narrowing.

Small-caliber coronary catheters can be used to inject the radiographic contrast media into the coronaries. Introduced through the femoral artery and the aorta these catheters are used for documenting the extent of coronary atherosclerosis and demonstrating areas of stenosis or complete occlusion. Coronary catheterization is also an emergency measure used in MI for localizing and treating thrombotic occlusion of the coronaries. If a thrombotic occlusion is found by injecting the contrast medium into the coronary through the catheter, the same routine can be used to inject thrombolytic substances used to dissolve the thrombus. Alternatively, angioplasty with an expandable intracoronary device can be used to reestablish the blood flow, remove the occlusion, and dilate the coronary enough so that a metal stent can be inserted. This procedure, called **percutaneous transluminal coronary angioplasty (PTCA),** is used more and more in the treatment of all coronary atherosclerotic lesions.

Laboratory testing is useful for the diagnosis of MI.

It has been known for some time that the cell membranes of damaged myocardial myocytes become more permeable and that the cell membranes of necrotic myocytes rupture, allowing many components from their cytoplasm to enter the circulating blood. Unfortunately, most of these macromolecules are found in other living cells as well, and thus a test measuring these substances would have low specificity. With time, nevertheless, several proteins unique to the myocardium have been identified, and reliable tests were developed for measuring them in the blood. The most useful tests are those that measure the blood concentration of myoglobin, creatine kinase, troponins, and lactate dehydrogenase (Fig. 4-32).

Myoglobin. This 17.8-kDa oxygen-binding heme protein is found in skeletal and cardiac muscles. In cardiac myocytes it accounts for only 2% of the total proteins. It is released from damaged myocytes within 2 hours after cell injury and peaks in the blood 6 to 9 hours later. It returns to normal levels within 24 to 36 hours; because of its small molecular weight myoglobin is mostly cleared from blood through the kidneys. Because myoglobin released from skeletal muscles cannot be distinguished from cardiac myoglobin this test is of low

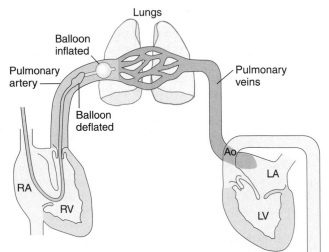

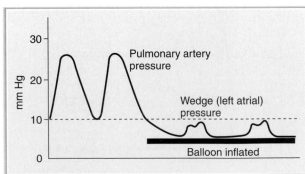

Figure 4-31 Measurement of pulmonary wedge pressure with a balloon catheter. When the balloon is inserted into one of the branches of the pulmonary artery its balloon is not inflated. Such an uninflated catheter measures the pulmonary artery pressure. An inflated balloon occludes venous blood flow through the vessels, and the pressure recorded corresponds to the backpressure from the pulmonary veins (i.e., the left atrium [LA]). LV, left ventricle; RA, right atrium; RV, right ventricle.

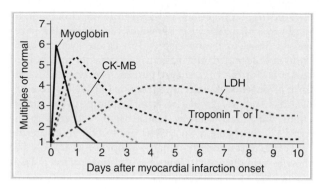

Figure 4-32 Markers of cardiac injury appearing in the serum after myocardial infarction (MI). Myoglobin appears first in the blood, but it is very nonspecific and its serum level drops to normal values within 24 to 30 hours. Troponin I and troponin T are sensitive markers that appear in serum within a few hours and persist for several days after MI. The myocardial muscle creatine kinase isoenzyme (CK-MB) is also a good marker of myocardial injury, but its serum level drops to normal within 3 days. LDH, lactate dehydrogenase.

specificity. Nevertheless, because myoglobin is released so fast after cell injury, it can be used as a marker for early myocardial cell necrosis in clinically defined conditions and when there is no evidence of skeletal muscle injury.

Creatine kinase (CK). CK is a cytosolic enzyme formed of two dimers, M and B, each of which has a molecular weight of 40 kDa. Three isoenzymes are formed from these dimers: MB, MM, and BB. The MB isoenzyme is found predominantly in the heart, where it accounts for 20% of total CK. The remaining 80% of the cardiac CK is of the MM type. In the skeletal muscle CK-MM predominates. CK-MB and CK-MM are released from injured cardiac myocytes 4 to 8 hours after injury. In clinical practice only the cardiac-specific CK-MB is measured. It peaks in serum within the

first 24 hours after the onset of the MI and returns to reference normal levels within 72 hours.

Troponins. Troponins are regulatory proteins forming a complex attached to tropomyosin, the principal regulator of actin contraction (Fig. 4-33). The troponin complex consists of three proteins:

- Troponin T (39 kDa). It links the troponin complex to **t**ropomyosin. It is also present in a free form in the cytosol.
- Troponin I (26.5 kDa). It acts as **i**nhibitor of actomyosin ATPase.
- Troponin C (18 kDa). This **c**alcium-binding protein regulates actin contraction.

Serum troponin T and I are derived from the heart or skeletal muscles. Highly specific tests have been developed for measuring the cardiac forms of troponin I and T and are available in most clinical laboratories. Elevation of serum troponins occurs 3 to 4 hours after infarction, reaching a peak during the second day. The serum concentration of troponins remains elevated for a few days and returns to normal reference values 5 to 6 days after the infarction. Troponins are currently used as the most specific markers for myocardial injury.

Lactate dehydrogenase (LDH). This ubiquitous enzyme is involved in the catalysis of lactate to pyruvate. Five isoenzymes are found in serum: LDH_1 is predominantly of cardiac origin, LDH_2 is from erythrocytes, LDH_3 from many organs, and LDH_4 and LDH_5 are mostly from the liver and skeletal muscle. Total serum LDH rises slowly after MI, reaching a peak 4 to 5 days after the onset of symptoms. It returns to a normal level 9 to 10 days after the onset of infarction. LDH is a relatively nonspecific marker of myocardial injury, which must be interpreted in context of other clinical and ECG findings. The specificity of the test may be improved by measuring the LDH isoenzymes and their ratio to one another in the serum. A ratio of LDH_1 to LDH_2 exceeding 1.0 is typical of MI.

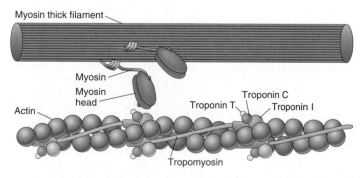

Figure 4-33 Troponins. Three troponins (Tn-C, Tn-I, and Tn-T) form a complex attached to tropomyosin in cardiac myocytes. Troponin C binds calcium and with Tn-I and Tn-T regulates the contraction of sarcomeres. (Modified from Boron WS, Boulpaep EL [eds]: Medical Physiology. Saunders, Philadelphia, 2003).

Clinicopathologic Correlations

ISCHEMIC HEART DISEASE

Ischemic heart disease is also known as coronary artery disease (CAD) and atherosclerotic coronary heart disease because in most cases it is caused by atherosclerotic narrowing of the coronary arteries. It is a very prevalent disease, accounting for significant morbidity and mortality in the United States and Europe.

Coronary heart disease has a multifactorial pathogenesis, including several modifiable and unmodifiable (fixed) risk factors.

Atherosclerosis, the principal cause of CAD, is a multifactorial disease that in most instances affects people older than age 50 years. The risk factors for CAD can be classified as *preventable* or modifiable or as *unavoidable* and *fixed* (Table 4-5).

Atherosclerosis is a disease of older people, and its prevalence increases dramatically after age 60 years. The progression of atherosclerosis can be retarded by dietary measures and healthy living, which includes adequate exercise, but it cannot be completely prevented. Atherosclerosis and CAD are more common in men, but after menopause the incidence of atherosclerosis increases in women, reaching the same rate as in men. Cigarette smoking, hypertension, hyperlipidemia, and diabetes all accelerate the progression of atherosclerosis and accordingly represent significant risk factors for CAD.

Hyperlipidemia is the most important metabolic risk factor for CAD.

Serum lipids play an important role in the pathogenesis of atherosclerosis, and thus it is worth reviewing some aspects of lipid metabolism and the genetic basis of hereditary hyperlipidemias.

Lipid metabolism. Lipids are absorbed into the body in the small intestine in the form of cholesterol, fatty acids, and mono- and diglycerides. In the intestines lipids are reconstituted into triglycerides and cholesteryl esters, which are packaged into chylomicrons and released into the lymphatics. From the lymphatics the lipids enter the bloodstream. Lipoprotein lipase, found on the surface of endothelial cells, removes the free fatty acids, whereas the chylomicron remnants are removed from the circulation by the liver. This pathway is known as the **exogenous pathway** of lipid circulation (Fig. 4-34). In the liver chylomicrons are degraded and various components metabolized separately, utilized for energy purposes, or excreted in the form of **very low density lipoproteins (VLDL).** This entry of VLDL into the circulation is the beginning of the endogenous circulation pathway, which begins and ends in the liver. The lipoprotein lipase acts on VLDL, transforming them into **intermediate-density lipoproteins (IDL),** and these in turn give rise to **low-density lipoproteins (LDL),** which have a half-life in plasma of 3 days. LDL are removed by endothelial cells that have LDL receptors, but also by other cells through nonreceptor pathways. **High-density lipoproteins (HDL)** are synthesized by the liver and the intestine and are important in the transport of lipids from the periphery into the liver.

Hyperlipidemias. From the pathogenetic point of view hyperlipidemias can be classified as primary, or genetic and secondary, if caused by some other disease. The most common causes of secondary hyperlipidemia are listed in Table 4-6.

For clinical purposes the genetic hyperlipidemias are classified into six major groups according to Fredrickson and the World Health Organization (WHO) (Table 4-7). As the genetic defects of various hyperlipidemias became evident, attempts were made to classify hyperlipidemia pathogenetically; unfortunately, the specific genetic entities cannot be readily and consistently grouped into the six categories of the Fredrickson and WHO classfication.

Atherogenesis. Atherosclerosis has a complex and multifactorial pathogenesis, which today is explained in the context of theories concentrating on the dysfunction and injury to the endothelium. Lipids play an important role and are considered essential for the formation of the main atherosclerotic lesions—**atheromas.**

As stated before lipids are transported through an exogenous and an endogenous pathway and metabolized in the liver, or are stored in peripheral fat stores and various tissues. The exogenous pathway can be regarded as the "food pathway," whereas the endogenous pathway can be regarded as the "metabolic" and "overflow pathways." Excess of lipid in the overflow pathways leads to atherosclerosis.

The total amount of lipid in the blood depends partly on the supply, partly on its metabolism, and partly on its removal from the blood. Excess intake and obesity increase the supply, and diabetes and other metabolic disturbances may impair the utilization of lipids. Impaired function of LDL receptors, as typically seen in familial hypercholesterolemia (type IIa hyperlipoproteinemia), also leads to an excess of lipids circulating in blood in the form of LDL. HDL, formed both in the exogenous and the endogenous pathway, accepts lipids from peripheral tissues and transports them back to the liver for further metabolism or utilization.

Table 4-5 Risk Factors for Coronary Artery Disease

FIXED (UNMODIFIABLE) RISK FACTORS	PREVENTABLE (MODIFIABLE) RISK FACTORS
Age	Cigarette smoking
Sex	Hypertension
Genetic and hereditary factors	Hyperlipidemia
	Diabetes mellitus

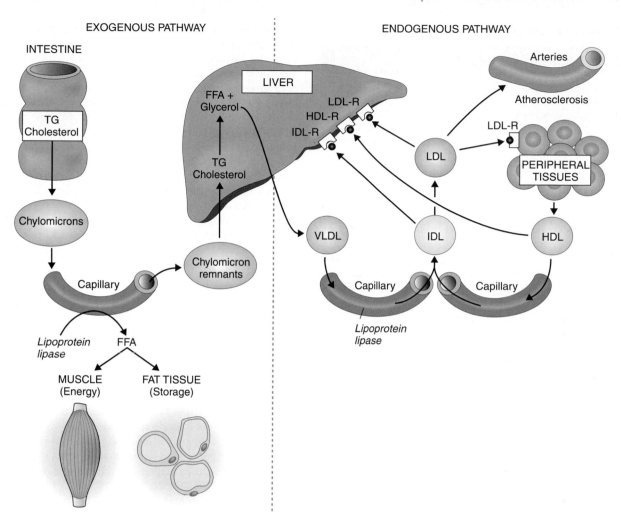

Figure 4-34 Exogenous and endogenous lipoprotein metabolic pathways. The exogenous pathway begins in the intestines. Triglycerides (TG) are partially broken down and then with cholesterol reassembled into chylomicrons. The lipoprotein lipase in the capillaries cleaves free fatty acids (FFA) from the chylomicrons, transforming them into chylomicron remnants, which are internalized into the liver. The FFA released from chylomicrons are used for energy in the muscle or stored in the peripheral fat cells. Some absorbed lipids are transported from the intestines in the form of high-density lipoproteins (HDL), which are not shown in the diagram for the sake of simplicity. Inside the liver the lipids are metabolized and used to generate energy, or reassembled into very low density lipoproteins (VLDL) and released into the circulation. This release of VLDL into the blood is the beginning of the endogenous pathway. Under the influence of lipoprotein lipase the VLDL become intermediate-density lipoproteins (IDL) and then low-density lipoproteins (LDL). LDL can be taken up by specific receptors of the liver (LDL-R) or other tissues. They can also enter arteries and are taken up by scavenger receptors on macrophages. This insudation of lipids into the vessels is the first step toward the formation of atherosclerotic lesions. The lipids stored in the peripheral tissues may be mobilized and transported by HDL directly to the liver, which has receptors for them (HDL-R). HDL can also transform into IDL, which are also taken up by liver receptors (IDL-R). The liver can also excrete some lipids into the intestines, most notably in the form of cholesterol and bile acids (not shown in the diagram).

Pearls

> High serum LDL and cholesterol have an adverse effect on arteries, promoting atherosclerosis.
> High HDL has a protective effect.

Lipids enclosed inside the chylomicrons and lipoproteins are protected from oxidation. However, once they enter the tissues they are exposed to oxidative stress and undergo lipoperoxidation. These oxidized lipids are a source of *free radicals*, which damage arterial endothelial cells, especially if hyperlipidemia is combined with other

Table 4-6 Secondary Hyperlipidemia

DISEASE	PREDOMINANT LIPOPROTEINS IN BLOOD
Diabetes mellitus	Triglyceride, VLDL, IDL
Hypothyroidism	Cholesterol, LDL
Nephrotic syndrome	Cholesterol, LDL
Alcohol abuse	Triglycerides, VLDL
Chronic renal failure	Triglycerides, VLDL
Drugs (e.g., thiazides)	Triglycerides, VLDL

IDL, intermediate-density lipoprotein; LDL, low-density lipoprotein; VLDL, very low density lipoprotein.

risk factors, such as hypertension and cigarette smoking and clotting abnormalities predisposing to thrombosis. *Oxidized lipids* may be ingested by macrophages or enter smooth muscle cells of the intima, transforming these cells into foam cells (Fig. 4-35). The lipid released from foam cells accumulates in the interstitial spaces, thereby contributing, together with the cell debris from damaged cells, to the formation of the porridge-like semiliquid contents of atheromas. Proliferation of smooth muscle cells and fibroblasts contributes to the plaquelike growth of atheromas, their fibrosis, and ultimately calcification.

Atheromas of the coronary arteries can be soft and prone to rupture or hard and causing fixed narrowing of the vessels.

Atheromas of the coronary arteries may be composed predominantly of semiliquid lipid-rich material or fibrotic and calcific connective tissue. Atheromas composed of semiliquid material and eccentrically bulging into the lumen of the coronary are called **soft.** They are covered on the luminal side by a thin fibrous cap (Fig. 4-36). This cap may rupture, and the contents of the atheroma may be discharged into the lumen of the coronary artery, causing instantaneous thrombus formation and complete occlusion of the artery and MI. Clinically it is customary to call them **"vulnerable atheromas,"** or "atheromas at risk."

Atheromas in which the lipid does not form large extracellular pools but rather stimulates proliferation of connective tissue cells tend to be solid and are prone to calcification. Such atheromas, called **hard,** are clinically also known as **stable atheromas.** They increase in size slowly, gradually narrowing the lumen of the coronary artery. The endothelium overlying these atheromas loses its normal function and cannot secrete nitric oxide or other vasodilatory substances. The fibrous tissue, which is rich in collagen and calcifications, replaces the smooth muscle cells and impairs the capacity of the coronaries to dilate, thus increasing the blood flow on demand. Such hard atheromas are typically associated with chronic ischemic heart disease and clinically manifest as angina pectoris.

Clinical manifestations of atherosclerotic heart disease depend on the nature and extent of anatomic lesions caused by the atherosclerosis of coronary arteries. Four major syndromes are recognized:

- Angina pectoris
- Myocardial infarction
- Chronic congestive heart failure
- Sudden cardiac death

Angina pectoris is caused by temporary cardiac ischemia.

Angina pectoris is a Latin term coined in the 18th century by the British physician William Heberden meaning "pain in the chest." It refers to chest pain caused by cardiac ischemia. In most instances it is related to narrowing of the coronary arteries by hard atheromas, but in variant, or Prinzmetal's, angina, it may be caused by a spastic constriction of the coronary arteries.

Fixed hard atheromas are found to be the cause of angina in most cases. Atheromas that cause more than a 70% reduction of the lumen may not be associated with myocardial ischemia at rest, but if the demand for oxygen is increased by exercise or additional effort, the narrowed artery cannot supply enough blood and ischemia results. The endothelium of atherosclerotic arteries does not function properly, and the reduced production of NO by endothelial cells impedes their dilatation. In some instances vasoconstriction triggered by the action of norepinephrine and epinephrine

Table 4-7 Classification of Primary Hyperlipoproteinemias

FREDRICKSON TYPE	PATHOGENETIC CLASSIFICATION	LIPID IN BLOOD	ELECTROPHORESIS (DOMINANT BAND)
Type I	Lipoprotein lipase deficiency Apo CII deficiency	Ch, TG	Chylomicrons
Type IIa	LDL-receptor deficiency	Ch (TG=N)	LDL
Type IIb	Single-gene defects	Ch, TG	VLDL, LDL
Type III	Apo E2 homozygosity	Ch, TG	VLDL remnants
Type IV	Familial combined hyperlipidemia	TG (some Ch)	VLDL
Type V	Familial hypertriglyceridemia	TG (some Ch)	VLDL

Ch, cholesterol; LDL, low density lipoprotein; N, normal; TG, triglycerides; VLDL, very low density lipoprotein.

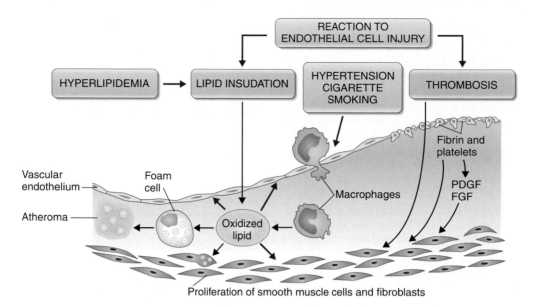

Figure 4-35 Pathogenesis of atherosclerosis. Risk factors, such as hyperlipidemia, hypertension, cigarette smoking, and thrombosis predispose to endothelial cell injury. Insudation of lipids leads to the formation of oxidized lipid derivatives into the wall of the vessels. These oxidized lipids are a source of free radicals, which damage the endothelial and smooth muscle cells. Ultimately they are phagocytosed by macrophages or enter into smooth muscle cells, thus transforming them into foam cells. Lipids accumulating in the extracellular spaces are admixed to cell debris and form atheromas. The proliferation of smooth muscle cells and fibroblasts contributes to the growth of atheromas and their fibrosis or calcification. FGA, fibroblast growth factor; PDGF, platelet-derived growth factor.

on α_1-adrenergic receptors may occur instead of vasodilatation. Calcification of the arterial wall and the loss of smooth muscle cells further impair their capacity for dilatation.

Pain is the hallmark of angina pectoris. It is usually described as discomfort associated with precordial pressure and "heaviness" or as a vague, gnawing, burning sensation. In some instances it may be severe and even crushing. Most often it is located behind the sternum, and the patient may place his or her fist over the chest to point where it is located. It tends to radiate into the left arm and less often to the neck and the right side of the chest and right arm. It is usually precipitated by physical activity and factors that increase oxygen demand of the myocardium. Thus it may be triggered by climbing stairs, short sprint, exercise, strong excitement, eating a meal, or peripheral constriction of arteries while walking in cold weather. The pain usually begins slowly, increasing over several minutes, and lasts less than 15 minutes. It can be relieved by nitroglycerin.

> ### Pearls
>
> > Sudden onset of severe chest pain is not caused by myocardial ischemia.
> > Ischemic cardiac pain is neither sharp nor stabbing.

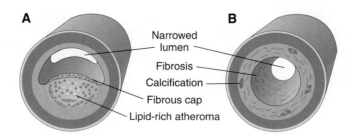

Figure 4-36 Atheroma of coronary arteries. **A**, A soft atheroma consists of a semiliquid, lipid-rich core covered on the luminal side by a thin fibrous cap. **B**, A hard atheroma consists of fibrous tissue, which is prone to calcification. It narrows the lumen and prevents normal dilatation of the artery.

Three forms of angina pectoris are recognized clinically: stable, unstable, and variant angina.

- **Stable angina.** It is characterized by pain that recurs predictably under identical conditions and at regular time intervals. Pathologically equivalent is an area of stenosis caused by a hard atheroma (Fig. 4-37). The narrowing of coronaries usually exceeds 70% of the luminal surface.
- **Unstable angina.** In this form of angina the quality and intensity of the pain tend to vary, usually increasing in severity, duration, or frequency. In some cases the symptoms worsen and pain appears even at rest (**rest angina**). Furthermore it may become unresponsive to nitroglycerin and may progress to MI. Hence, this form of angina is also known as **preinfarctional angina.**

The underlying pathology usually includes both a hard and a soft atheroma. The former may narrow the lumen of the coronary and contribute to unopposed vasoconstriction. The fibrous cap of soft atheromas may rupture, leading to focal intraluminal aggregation of platelets and formation of temporary nonocclusive thrombi. These thrombi contribute to the narrowing of the arterial lumen but do not lead to complete occlusion. They are dissolved through the action of circulating fibrinolytic substances in blood. Fibronolysis occurs fast after the onset of thrombosis, and thus ischemia of the myocardium is short-lived. Nevertheless ischemic changes may be detected in the ECG, such as ST inversion. Furthermore, myocardial ischemia can be documented by demonstrating ECG changes by a stress test.

- **Variant angina** (Prinzmetal's angina). Ischemia in this form of angina is caused by a spasm of the coronary arteries. The spasm usually involves arteries that contain hard atheromas, but in some cases there is no evidence of atherosclerosis. In ECG the spasm is associated with a transient ST segment elevation indicative of transmural ischemia. Typically the pain occurs at rest but may recur in a circadian manner (i.e., at a similar time every day). These episodes may be associated with arrhythmia and conduction abnormalities.

The diagnosis of angina pectoris is made on the basis of patient history and clinical findings, or a response to nitroglycerin. The importance of a careful history cannot be overemphasized. The diagnosis can be further documented by **ECG and additional cardiologic studies.** Resting ECG is normal in about 50% of cases, but many patients show electrocardiographic signs of myocardial ischemia, such as **down-sloping of the ST segment,** occasionally associated with new T wave inversion. ECG changes are more regularly found in **stress ECG,** which has a sensitivity of 70% and specificity of 90%. **Stress scintigraphy** with thalium-201 has even higher sensitivity and specificity since it may disclose areas of ischemic myocardial dysfunction. **Coronary angiography** is used to demonstrate coronary artery narrowing and serves as a preparation for insertion of coronary stents.

Myocardial infarction results from an occlusion of coronary arteries, causing ischemic necrosis of myocardium.

Myocardial infarction is usually caused by an occlusion of the coronary arteries with thrombi originating over a ruptured soft atheroma (Fig. 4-38). The MI is localized to a defined anatomic location corresponding to the anatomic supply area of the occluded artery (see Fig. 4-5). Less common causes of coronary occlusion are thromboemboli originating from endocarditic vegetations on the valves or mural thrombi in the fibrillating left atrium or left ventricle. Cocaine abuse can cause spasms of a coronary artery and is a rare cause of MIs.

Myocardial infarctions resulting from an occlusion of a coronary artery extend from the pericardium all the way to the subendocardial zone of the ventricular wall and are thus

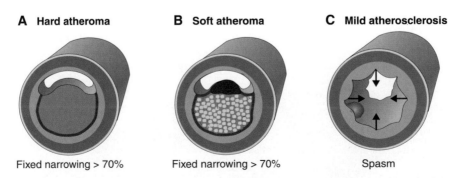

A Hard atheroma	**B** Soft atheroma	**C** Mild atherosclerosis
Fixed narrowing > 70%	Fixed narrowing > 70%	Spasm

Figure 4-37 Pathologic basis of angina pectoris. **A,** Classical angina pectoris is caused by hard atheromas that have narrowed the lumen of the coronary artery more than 70%. **B,** Unstable angina is caused by soft atheromas that narrow the lumen but are also prone to rupture, causing short-lived intraluminal thrombosis. **C,** Prinzmetal's angina is caused by coronary artery spasm. The artery may show mild or moderate atherosclerosis, but it may also be relatively intact.

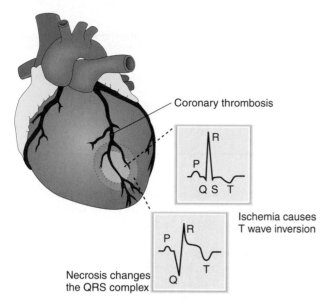

Figure 4-38 Transmural myocardial infarction. It is caused by thrombosis of a coronary artery and is localized to a specific anatomic area corresponding to the blood supply zone of that artery. The central area of necrosis is surrounded by a zone of ischemia that can be "salvaged" by reperfusion after the removal of the thrombus.

called **transmural** (Fig. 4-39). They are typically associated with inflammation that involves pericarditis. Necrosis of the entire myocardial wall can lead to rupture and hematopericardium. When large mural infarcts heal they can give rise to ventricular aneurysms. ECG abnormalities are found in 85% of such cases, but in a significant number of patients the ECG changes are nonspecific or even nonexistent. The typical changes in the leads that correspond to ischemic areas include the following:

- T wave inversion
- ST segment elevation
- Changes in the width and shape of the QRS complex
- Progressively deepening Q wave

As the infarct heals the ECG reverts to normal, but in many instances scarring that occurs during healing leaves permanent traces.

In contrast to a transmural infarct, infarcts that are not preceded by coronary thrombosis but occur due to hypoperfusion of the heart are limited to the subendocardial zone (see Fig. 4-39). These **subendocardial infarcts** are not limited to a specific anatomic region defined by the distribution of coronary arteries and may be **circumferential** or extend around a substantial portion of the left ventricle. Most often they occur in hypotensive shock. Since they do not form a Q wave they are called **non-Q wave infarcts.** In subendocardial infarcts the ST segment depression may be the only abnormality.

The differences between transmural and subendocardial infarcts are listed in Table 4-8.

Clinical symptoms and findings vary, but most MIs are characterized by sudden onset of **crushing chest pain** that lasts more than 30 minutes and is not relieved by nitroglycerin. In about 70% of patients premonitory signs occur, such as unstable angina pectoris, shortness of breath, and dyspnea. The pain usually occurs at rest but may be

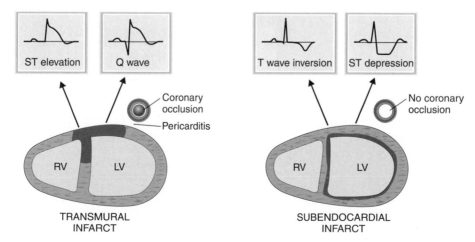

Figure 4-39 Transmural and subendocardial infarct. **A**, A transmural infarct is caused by coronary thrombosis. It is localized to an anatomic area and involves the entire thickness of the ventricular wall from the endocardium to the pericardium. It causes QRS changes and a deepening Q wave. **B**, A subendocardial infarct is not related to a coronary occlusion, but rather to generalized hypoperfusion. It extends circumferentially around the cavity of the left ventricle and does not produce a Q wave. LV, left ventricle; RV, right ventricle.

Table 4-8 Comparison of Subendocardial and Transmural Myocardial Infarction

FEATURES	TRANSMURAL INFARCT	SUBENDOCARDIAL INFARCT
Cause	Coronary thrombosis	Hypotension
Location	Single anatomic area corresponding to a specific coronary	Multiple foci may be circumferential
Echocardiogram	QRS changes with deep Q wave	ST depression, non-Q wave
Pericarditis	Yes	No
Rupture of ventricle	Yes	No
Aneurysm of ventricle	Yes	No

triggered by exercise and effort. It radiates the same way as in angina pectoris (Fig. 4-40).

Pearl

> Myocardial infarcts occur most often in the morning hours, probably due to a surge of catecholamines in blood on awakening.

Other important signs and symptoms include the following:

- Distress and agitation or fear of impending doom. Generally the patient appears apprehensive.
- Ashen pale skin with sweating due to a sympathetic response
- Tachycardia as a compensatory reaction to acute heart failure
- Hypotension due to pump failure
- Pulmonary rales due to left heart failure

- Elevation of neck vein pressure due to right heart failure, in response to left heart pump failure, dilatation, and consequent mitral regurgitation

Laboratory findings are important for the diagnosis of MI. Most useful is the elevation of serum concentration of troponins I and T, which becomes apparent 4 to 6 hours after coronary occlusion. CK-MB is also useful, and LDH is usually ordered, although in most hospitals troponins are used as the test of choice.

Complications of MI are very common and are a major cause of mortality.

Some patients with MI recover without any consequences, but in the majority of cases the infarct is accompanied by some complications. Subclinical or silent infarcts are rare and are most often seen in the elderly. The most important complications are as follows:

- Arrhythmia and conduction abnormalities
- Pump failure

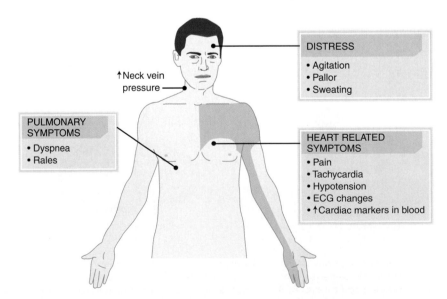

Figure 4-40 Clinical signs and symptoms of acute myocardial infarction. ECG, electrocardiograph.

- Mitral regurgitation
- Myocardial rupture
- Ventricular aneurysm
- Mural thrombosis
- Pericarditis
- Chronic heart failure
- Sudden death

Various complications occur at a different rate at various times after infarction. Some of these complications often occur in combination with others, or one complication is followed by another (Fig. 4-41).

Arrhythmia and conduction abnormalities represent the most common complications of MI.

Approximately 50% of all MI patients develop some arrhythmias and conduction abnormalities. In the early postinfarction period these abnormalities may be the cause of sudden death and are the main reason for admitting the patient to a coronary intensive care unit. Later these complications remain of considerable concern and contribute to late-term mortality.

Arrhythmias and conduction abnormalities develop due to ischemia of the SA or AV node or the conduction system fibers. Since the cardiac myocytes also conduct electric currents, any myocardial necrosis interrupts the normal electric cycle of the heart and thus causes electrophysiologic changes.

The electrophysiologic abnormalities that develop in MI patients can be classified as follows:

- Tachyarrhythmias
- Bradyarrhythmias
- Cardiac blocks

These changes can be further classified as **supraventricular** or **ventricular.**

The nature of these abnormalities can be explained in terms of the location of the infarction. For example an inferior (posterior) MI caused by the occlusion of the right coronary artery typically leads to sinus bradycardia or an AV nodal block because in 85% of patients the blood supply for the SA and AV node comes from the right coronary artery. Right and left bundle branch blocks occur in patients who have an anterior MI due to the occlusion of the LAD.

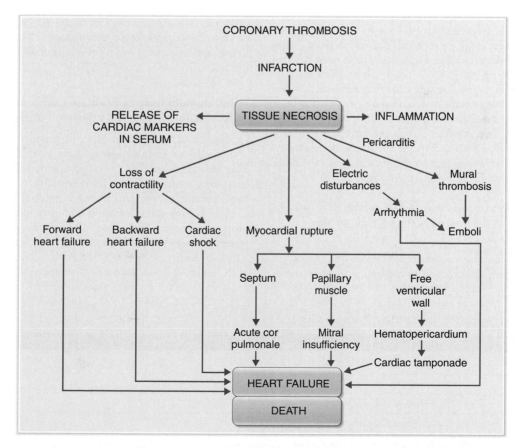

Figure 4-41 Pathogenesis of heart failure and other major complications of myocardial infarction.

Pump failure develops due to a loss of contractile myocardial cells.

Necrotic cardiac myocytes cannot contract, and pump failure is therefore proportional to the number of myocytes that have died. Note that ischemic myocytes **lose ATP** within minutes and that this functional change makes them inoperative even if they do not die immediately. Early pump failure is thus a result of myocardial necrosis, as is energy depletion in the surrounding **"stunned myocardium"** that is ischemic but not irreversibly damaged. These myocytes can be salvaged by reperfusion, and accordingly an early coronary angioplasty can substantially improve the initial pump failure.

One third of MI patients have no heart failure, another 40% have mild failure, 10% have frank pulmonary edema, and 20% have cardiogenic shock. Cardiogenic shock develops when more than 40% of the total myocardial mass has been destroyed. Such heart failure is characterized by reduced cardiac output, systolic pressure below 90 mm Hg, and low urinary output (<20 mL/hour). It is associated with a mortality rate of greater than 50%. The overall survival of MI patients depends on the severity of pump failure, which can be graded for prognostic purposes on a scale from I to IV. (Table 4-9).

Mitral regurgitation caused by left ventricular ischemia leads to pulmonary edema.

The inability of infarcted myocardium to contract leads to progressive dilatation of the ventricle. The concomitant dilatation of the mitral valve makes it insufficient, and since the valve cannot close completely systolic blood refluxes from the ventricle into the left atrium. Dysfunction of the ischemic papillary muscles is yet another cause of mitral regurgitation. In the most dramatic form, an infarction of one of the papillary muscles causes rupture of the papillary muscle and acute mitral insufficiency. The increased pressure in the left atrium is transmitted into the pulmonary veins and very soon causes transudation of fluid into the alveoli and massive pulmonary edema.

Rupture of the necrotic myocardial infarct may involve the free wall of the ventricle, the septum, or the papillary muscle.

Necrotic myocardium becomes infiltrated with neutrophils 1 to 3 days after the onset of infarction. These inflamma-

tory cells digest the necrotic myocytes and in that process die, forming an area of suppurative inflammation in the myocardium. Such softening of the myocardium causes local weakening of the ventricular wall that can be "blown out" by the pressure inside the ventricle. Rupture of the free ventricular wall leads to the formation of **hematopericardium** and **cardiac tamponade** (Fig. 4-42). Rupture of the interventricular wall causes a left-to-right shunting of blood and a sudden increase of right ventricular filling. The right ventricle transmits the extra blood into the lungs, causing acute pulmonary hypertension, but ultimately fails (**acute cor pulmonale**). The rupture of papillary muscles of the mitral valve leads to acute **mitral valve insufficiency,** regurgitation, and acute pulmonary edema.

Bulging of the fibrotic healed myocardial infarct leads to the formation of ventricular aneurysm.

Myocardial infarcts heal by fibrous scarring, a process during which the contractile myocytes are replaced with collagen-producing fibroblasts. Fibrous scars cannot contract, but respond to increased systolic pressure by stretching and bulging outward (Fig. 4-43).

Such a noncontractile bulging scar that irregularly expands the volume of the left ventricle is called a ventricular aneurysm. It weakens the strength of the left ventricle while posing an obstacle to the spread of electric impulses, thereby causing electrophysiologic disturbances. The flow of the blood inside the aneurysm is turbulent, thus predisposing to thrombosis.

Mural thrombi form in fibrillating atria or over the endocardial surface of the infarcted ventricular wall.

Intracardiac thrombi form often in patients with MI, and accordingly anticoagulation therapy is applied routinely. The thrombi form due to irregular blood flow related to irregularly contracting atria and ventricles. Arrhythmias are very common in the postinfarction period. Atrial fibrillation, one of the more common complications, is especially prone to thrombus formation. Thrombi may form in a dilated ventricle that predisposes it to turbulent blood flow. Thrombi form also over the infarcted portion of the ventricle, which is a rich source of thrombogenic substances.

Table 4-9 Classification of Cardiac Pump Failure

GRADE	TYPE	INCIDENCE (%)	MORTALITY RATE (%)
I	No heart failure	30	5
II	Mild failure	40	15
III	Pulmonary edema	10	40
IV	Cardiogenic shock	20	50–80

Modified from Killip T, Kimball JT: Treatment of myocardial infarction in a coronary care unit: A two year experience with 250 patients. Am J Cardiol 1967:20:457–464.

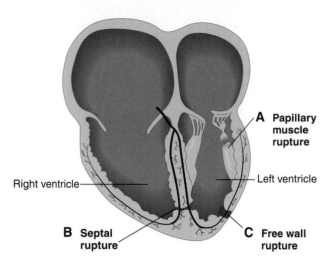

Figure 4-42 Rupture of the ventricle following myocardial infarction. **A,** Rupture of the mitral papillary muscle may cause acute mitral insufficiency. **B,** Rupture of the septum causes right ventricular overload and acute cor pulmonale. **C,** Rupture of the free wall of the left ventricle may cause hematopericardium.

Cardiac thrombi are an important source of **thromboemboli,** which, in previous times, were found in approximately 10% to 15% of all patients. Today, with the widespread use of anticoagulants, thromboemboli are less common. Those from the left heart cause arterial emboli to the brain, lower extremities, and many other organs. Emboli from the right ventricle are less common, but are to be considered in patients who develop signs of pulmonary embolism.

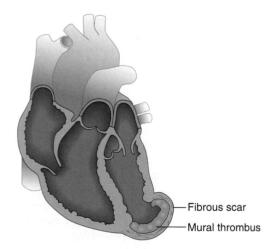

Figure 4-43 Ventricular aneurysm and mural thrombosis. The aneurysm forms at the site of the scar, replacing the myocardium destroyed by the infarction. The turbulent blood flow inside the aneurysm predisposes to thrombus formation.

Pericarditis results from the extension of the myocardial inflammation to the epicardial surface but may be also of an immune nature.

Myocardial cell necrosis elicits an inflammation. During the first few days the inflammatory area contains neutrophils, which are then replaced by macrophages and ultimately by fibroblasts. These inflammatory cells may involve the epicardium, leading to a localized **sterile pericarditis.** The roughening of the epicardial surface and the exudation of fibrin are typically associated with a **pericardial friction rub** that can be heard on auscultation. In most instances this form of pericarditis leaves no consequences, but it may cause fibrous adhesions between the visceral and parietal pericardium.

Necrosis of myocytes and the release of myocardial proteins into the circulation may cause an autoimmune reaction and result in the production of antibodies to cardiac antigens. These antibodies may attack the epicardial cells and cause an **immunologic pericarditis.** Clinically it presents as **Dressler's syndrome** in which the patient develops precordial pericarditic pain, pericardial friction rub, and pericardial effusion.

Pearl

> Dressler's syndrome responds favorably to steroid treatment, indicating that this complication of MI is immunologically mediated.

Myocardial infarctions are a common cause of chronic heart failure.

Pump failure related to MI may be acute or chronic. Chronic pump failure develops due to a loss of myocytes, electrophysiologic abnormalities, and valvular disturbances, but also may be related to ventricular aneurysm, intramural thrombi, and other complications of MI. Many infarcts tend to recur or expand, thus aggravating the patient's condition. Estimates are that the symptoms of left ventricular failure become clinically apparent following a loss of approximately 25% to 30% of the total myocardial mass. The most important clinical findings in patients with chronic heart failure are summarized in Figure 4-44.

Sudden cardiac death in adults is a complication of coronary atherosclerosis in 85% to 90% of cases.

Sudden cardiac death is defined as death that occurs without any preexisting or premonitory symptoms, or within 1 hour of onset of symptoms suggestive of coronary heart disease. It accounts for 300,000 to 400,000 deaths in the United States. In adults older than age 50 years it is in most instances associated with significant coronary atherosclerosis (narrowing of more that 75%). In the younger age groups cardiomyopathies are the leading cause of sudden death.

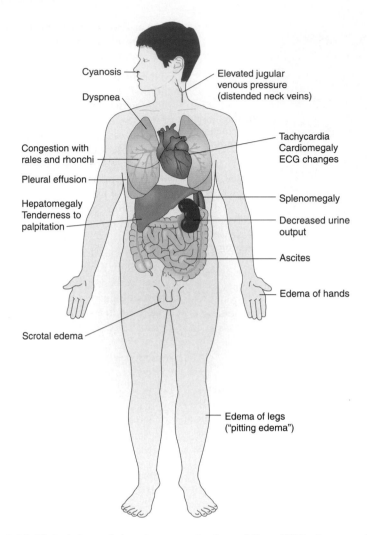

Cyanosis

Dyspnea

Congestion with
rales and rhonchi

Pleural effusion

Hepatomegaly
Tenderness to
palpitation

Scrotal edema

Elevated jugular
venous pressure
(distended neck veins)

Tachycardia
Cardiomegaly
ECG changes

Splenomegaly

Decreased urine
output

Ascites

Edema of hands

Edema of legs
("pitting edema")

Figure 4-44 Clinical signs of chronic congestive heart failure. ECG, electrocardiograph.

ARRHYTHMIA AND ELECTROPHYSIOLOGIC CARDIAC ABNORMALITIES

Arrhythmia, or "loss of normal rhythm," is a term traditionally used for electrophysiologic abnormalities in electrical impulse generation and conduction.

Pathogenetically arrhythmias can be classified as follows (Fig. 4-45):

■ Pacemaker abnormalities
■ Aberrant pacemaker function
■ Conduction blocks
■ Abnormal pathways for impulse conduction
■ Ectopic foci of impulse formation

Arrhythmia may result from organic and nonorganic disturbances.

Arrhythmia may result from structural pathologic changes in the heart or a variety of extracardiac influences (see Table 4-10).

Arrhythmias include supraventricular and ventricular arrhythmias.

Arrhythmias may result from disturbances at any step in the electric impulse formation or conduction. Accordingly, arrhythmias may be divided clinically into those that involve either the **atrial** or the **ventricular** part of the conduction system. In each category disturbances are marked by increased heart rate (**tachyarrhythmias**) or decreased heart rate (**bradyarrhythmias**).

Atrial tachyarrhythmia may be regular or irregular and may be either a normal physiologic response or a sign of underlying cardiac pathology.

Atrial tachyarrhythmias are associated with increased heart rate, but the ECG tracings of these disturbances show no change in the QRS complex, which in most instances remains narrow and of normal shape. Several forms of atrial tachyarrhythmia are recognized (Fig. 4-46) and are discussed briefly here.

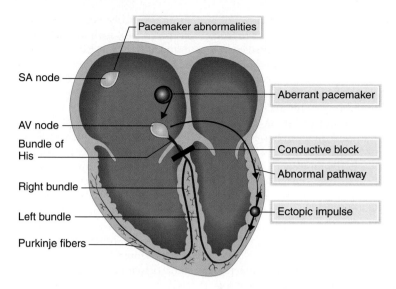

Figure 4-45 Causes of arrhythmia. It may be caused by abnormal pacemaker activity involving the sinoatrial (SA) node, aberrant pacemaker, conduction block, abnormal conduction pathways, or formation of ectopic impulses. AV, atrioventricular.

Sinus tachycardia. Characterized by an increased heart rate of over 100 beats per minute, sinus tachycardia may be a physiologic response to adrenergic stimuli. It typically occurs during exercise and the early stages of shock. Fever is also associated with sinus tachycardia caused by increased metabolism inside the SA node. The heart rate increases approximately 10 beats per degree Fahrenheit or 18 beats per degree Celsius. Sinus tachycardia occurs also in response to heart pump failure and is typically seen in MI. b-Blockers and calcium channel antagonists must be used under those conditions to reduce the heart rate.

Table 4-10 Causes of Arrhythmia

Cardiac Pathology
Congenital abnormalities of the SA and AV nodes or
   conduction system
Ischemic heart disease
   Myocardial infarction
   Chronic CAD
Mitral and tricuspid valve disease
Atrial septal defect
Myocarditis
Vasculitis involving the heart
Surgical injury of conduction system

Nonorganic Causes
Hypoxia
Electrolyte disturbances (e.g., Ca^{2+}, K^+)
Acid-base disturbances
Hormonal influences (e.g., hypothyroidism)
Drugs and toxins
Cardiac catheterization
Pacemaker insertion

AV, atrioventricular; CAD, coronary artery disease; SA, sinoatrial.

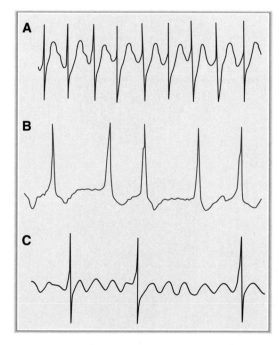

Figure 4-46 Atrial tachyarrhythmias. **A,** Atrial tachycardia is marked by the preservation of the normal rhythm, but the rate is abnormally fast. **B,** Atrial fibrillation is marked by rapidly occurring abnormal waves replacing the normal P wave. **C,** Atrial flutter appears as saw-toothed waves replacing the P wave. Ventricular depolarization occurs after several atrial waves.

Paroxysmal atrial tachycardia. It is characterized by sudden onset of tachycardia with a heart rate of 150 to 200 beats per minute. In most instances paroxysmal atrial tachycardia is secondary to reentry of electric currents around the AV node, as occurs in the presence of accessory conducting system bypass in Wolf-Parkinson-White syndrome. In orthodromic tachycardia the impulses pass normally through the AV node and reenter the atrium through an accessory pathway. In antidromic tachycardia the impulses enter the ventricle through the accessory pathway but reenter into the atrium through the AV node (Fig. 4-47).

Maneuvers that increase vagal tone, such as massage of the carotid sinus, Valsalva maneuver, or immersion of head in cold water, may stop the paroxysm, but sometimes drugs such as calcium channel blockers or digitalis must be administered.

Atrial flutter. It is characterized by an atrial contraction rate of 220 to 400 beats per minute. It is usually accompanied by an AV block at a rate of 2:1 so that the ventricular contraction rate is always less prominent. Atrial flutter al-

most invariably occurs in patients who have preexisting heart diseases, such as CAD, valvular heart disease, or cardiomyopathy. On ECG a typical saw-tooth pattern is usually evident. Atrial flutter requires medical treatment, but if the drugs do not help, direct current (DC) cardioversion is indicated.

Atrial fibrillation. Atrial fibrillation is an irregularly irregular arrhythmia in which multiple impulses are directed to the AV node without concomitant atrial contraction. The ECG contains multiple irregular flutter waves replacing the normal P wave. The ventricular rate depends on the extent of AV block. Atrial fibrillation is usually a sign of preexisting heart disease, but it may be caused by fever, stress, alcohol, and hyperthyroidism. Occasionally it is idiopathic and unrelated to other diseases. Hemodynamically unstable patients must be treated by DC cardioversion and given anticoagulation therapy.

Bradyarrhythmia may result from disturbances involving the SA node or be due to an AV block.

Bradyarrhythmias are characterized by heart rate below 60 beats per minute. They may result from disturbances in impulse generation or conduction. In most instances slow heart rate is of no clinical concern, except when the patient has low cardiac output. Several forms of bradyarrhythmia are recognized.

Sinus bradycardia. Athletes who are able to pump large quantities of blood under effort evidence **physiologic** sinus bradycardia. Blood entering the arterial system evokes reflexes that cause bradycardia when the athlete is at rest. **Vagal stimulation** also causes bradycardia because cholinergic stimuli reduce the heart rate. For example the pressure applied on the carotid body may reduce heart rate and even stop the heartbeat altogether. **Pathologic bradycardia** can occur in patients who have carotid sinus syndrome, which is caused by the entrapment of carotid baroreceptors stimulated by atherosclerotic coronary arteries. **Bradycardia due to ischemic heart disease or idiopathic SA node disturbances** (e.g., "sinus pause bradycardia") may cause symptoms once the heart rate drops below 35 beats per minute. These abnormalities require cardiac pacemaker implantation.

Atrioventricular block. It may manifest as an asymptomatic ECG abnormality or may cause clinical problems requiring medical or pacemaker treatment. **Mobitz type I block** is an example of asymptomatic blocks found in some persons for no obvious reasons. It is characterized by a progressive prolongation of the PR interval, until a P wave is not followed by a QRS complex (Fig. 4-48). In **complete block,** which is usually caused by underlying cardiac disease, the impulses do not pass from the atrium into the ventricle, and the ventricular contractions occur independently of the atrial contractions. Atropine and isoproterenol can remove the block, but complete block often requires a cardiac pacemaker.

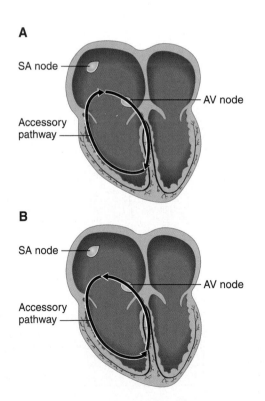

A

SA node

AV node

Accessory pathway

B

SA node

AV node

Accessory pathway

Figure 4-47 Paroxysmal atrial tachycardia in Wolf-Parkinson-White syndrome. **A,** Orthodromic tachycardia is characterized by the normal passage of the impulse through the AV node and a reentry through the accessory pathway. **B,** Antidromic tachycardia is characterized by initial passage of the impulse through the accessory pathway and the reentry of the impulse into the atrium through the AV node.

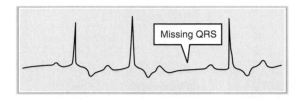

Figure 4-48 Atrioventricular block. In this Mobitz type I block the PR interval is gradually prolonged until the QRS complex completely disappears.

Ventricular tachyarrhythmias may occur concomitantly with atrial tachyarrhythmia or independently of atrial electric impulses.

Ventricular tachyarrhythmias typically cause changes in the ECG that present as alterations of the shape and duration of the QRS complex. Several forms are recognized.

Premature ventricular contraction. In this relatively benign condition the impulses arise inside the ventricle and do not pass through the His bundle and Purkinje fibers. The ECG shows temporary QRS abnormalities (Fig. 4-49). No therapy is required.

Ventricular tachycardia. This abnormality is characterized by an increased rate of the normal rhythm, exceeding 120 beats per minute. Typically it is a sign of severe cardiac disease. It is associated with atrioventricular dissociation, so that the atrial rhythm is not regularly linked to the ventricular beat. On the ECG, the QRS complex is widened and abnormally shaped and is not constantly related to the P wave. The QRS may be always of the same shape (*monomorphic*) or vary from one beat to another (*polymorphic*). Ventricular relaxation is impaired and the cardiac output reduced, causing hypotension. Ventricular tachycardia is a life-threatening condition that may progress to ventricular fibrillation and then death. It requires immediate treatment with antiarrhythmic drugs and DC cardioversion.

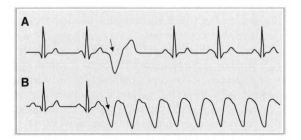

Figure 4-49 Ventricular arrhythmia. **A,** Premature ventricular contraction occurs at random, disrupting the normal rhythm. **B,** Ventricular tachycardia manifests with rapidly appearing widened QRS complexes of irregular shape.

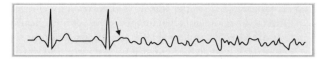

Figure 4-50 Ventricular fibrillation. In this tracing the fibrillatory waves are small and irregular, but they may be also larger and bizarrely shaped.

Ventricular fibrillation. This most severe form of ventricular dysfunction occurs typically in severe heart injury due to MI or the final stages of other cardiac diseases (Fig. 4-50). It results from irregular electric currents formed inside the damaged ventricles or transmitted in an abnormal way along the damaged conduction system. For example, fibrotic scars cannot transmit electric impulses and therefore the electric currents must pass around such scars, reentering with a slight delay into the myocytes downstream. Alternatively, the myocytes can be depolarized from two directions, or the impulse entering them cannot be further propagated because of the block by the fibrous tissue. Irregular contraction and relaxation of cardiac myocytes resulting from irregular electric currents are accompanied by a cessation of effective ventricular contractions. The cardiac output drops to zero and a loss of consciousness due to brain ischemia occurs within 4 to 5 seconds. Immediate cardiac resuscitation including electrical cardioversion is required, but the mortality is very high.

INFECTIVE ENDOCARDITIS

Infective endocarditis is a bacterial disease predominantly affecting the cardiac valves. Less often it may involve mural endocardium and the surface of cardiac defects in congenital heart diseases or artificial valvular prostheses. In some cases it is caused by fungi.

Bacterial endocarditis is most often caused by streptococci and staphylococci.

In the past infective endocarditis was classified as acute, usually related to infection with virulent bacteria such as *Staphylococcus aureus,* or subacute if more insidious and related to infection with less virulent bacteria such as *Streptococcus viridans.* Today, with the advent of antibiotic therapy, the distinction between acute and subacute endocarditis has become less obvious. In the evaluation of patients for possible infective endocarditis it is thus more important to accomplish the following:

- Identify the causative microorganism and establish its sensitivity to antibiotics
- Determine the source of infection and try to eliminate the source

■ Establish whether the infection involves a previously intact valve, previously damaged valve, or a surgically modified valve and a valvular prosthesis. Endocarditis involving valvular prosthesis accounts today for 10% to 15% of all endocarditides.

Streptococci account for approximately 60% to 70% of all infection. Viridans type streptococci, which live as commensals in the upper aerodigestive tract, are the cause of 30% to 40% of all endocardial infection. Other streptococci such as *S. fecalis* and *S. milleri* may enter the circulation from the bowel or the urinary tract. *Staphylococcus aureus,* originating from skin infections, vascular access sites, and intravenous drug abuse, is the cause of endocarditis in about 15% to 20% cases, which typically occurs in intact valves. Coagulase-negative *S. albus* is the most common cause of prosthetic valve infection.

Endocarditis more often affects the valves of the left than the right side of the heart.

Infective endocarditis more often affects mitral and aortic valves than the tricuspid and pulmonary valves. This is probably due to the higher blood pressure in the left heart, which can more easily damage the valves than the lower pressure on the right side.

The initial endothelial injury is covered with platelets and fibrin thrombi, which serve as the basis for bacterial infection. Previously damaged valves, such as those injured by rheumatic endocarditis, are more susceptible to infection than normal valves (Fig. 4-51). Rheumatic endocarditis is also more common on the left side than in the right heart. Congenitally abnormal valves, such as bicuspid aortic valves, found in 2% of all adults, and floppy mitral valves, are also injured much more easily than the normal valves and are thus more susceptible to infection. Highly virulent bacteria may, nevertheless, infect even structurally normal valves. Infection may start in the fibrin deposits forming the vegetations in marantic nonbacterial thrombotic endocarditis (NBTE).

The tricuspid valve is more often affected than any other valve by bacteria introduced into the venous circulation during intravenous drug abuse.

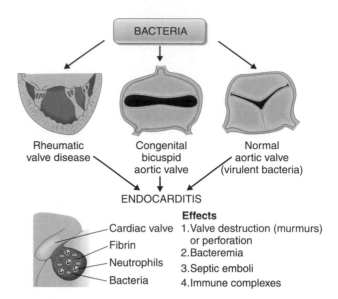

Figure 4-51 Endocarditis. Bacteria most often affect valves that have been damaged previously by rheumatic endocarditis or congenitally defective valves. Virulent bacteria may infect intact normal valves. Endocarditis leads to the formation of fibrin-rich vegetations containing bacteria and neutrophils. The infection may have local and distal effects and result in valve destruction, bacteremia, septic embolization, and formation of immune complexes.

Endocarditis manifests with systemic signs of infection, local cardiac symptoms, and distant symptoms related to peripheral septic emboli.

Endocarditis is primarily an infection, and thus it typically manifests with fever, night sweats, malaise, loss of appetite, weight loss, and weakness (Fig. 4-52). Besides these non-specific signs of infection, patients with endocarditis show symptoms related to the heart itself as well as some related to bacterial dissemination.

■ **Local cardiac signs and symptoms** include murmurs, found in approximately 80% to 90% of patients, signs of arrhythmia occur in up to 20%, and signs of heart failure are present in about 40% to 50% of patients. Cardiac murmurs result from the vegetations along the margins of the valves, as well as defects formed by more aggressive infection or rupture of the chordae tendineae. Since the infection may occur on previously abnormal valves, it is important to be aware of changes in murmur quality that occur as the vegetations form on previously damaged valves.

■ **Systemic symptoms** may be prominent but are often overlooked. Blood cultures are positive in over 90% of cases. **Bacteremia** is the cause of fever and other constitutional symptoms. The fragmentation of the valvular vegetations leads to **peripheral embolism,**

Pearls

> Noninfectious endocarditis may manifest with vegetations that may cause murmurs and may be confused with bacterial endocarditis.
> The most common form of noninfectious endocarditis is NBTE; Libman-Sacks endocarditis of SLE and acute rheumatic endocarditis also cause sterile vegetations.

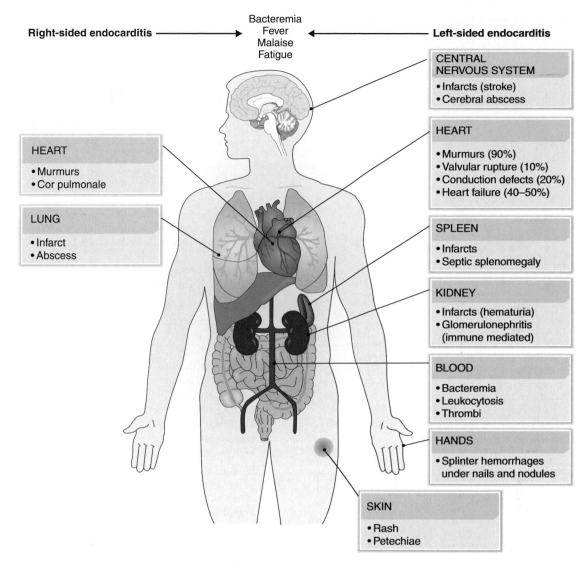

Figure 4-52 Clinicopathologic findings in bacterial endocarditis. Right-sided endocarditis and left-sided endocarditis have some common features (e.g., bacteremia) but differ in other respects.

which manifests with skin and mucosal petechiae, splinter hemorrhages under the finger or toe nails, swelling and small nodularity of the fingers *(Osler's nodes)*, and clubbing of fingers in later stages. The spleen is often enlarged and painful. Hematuria resulting from renal infarcts caused by thromboemboli is also present. **Immune complexes** formed from bacterial antigens and their resultant antibodies may cause symptoms of glomerulonephritis or vasculitis.

CHRONIC ENDOCARDITIS

Chronic endocarditis may be a consequence of rheumatic fever, healed bacterial endocarditis, or, less often, carcinoid syndrome. In some cases, such as aortic calcific stenosis, the causes of chronic changes are not obvious, and the disease is considered to be either mutlifactorial and related to atherosclerosis or idiopathic and of unknown origin. In some cases the degenerative changes and calcification involve congenitally abnormal valves, such as the bicuspid aortic valves or the floppy mitral valves.

Chronic endocarditis may involve any of the cardiac valves, but, like bacterial endocarditis, it more often affects aortic and mitral valves than the valves on the right side. Narrowing of the orifices manifests clinically as **valvular stenosis.** Dilatation of the ventricle and annulus fibrosus at the base of the valves or incomplete closure of the valves results in valvular **incompetence** (insufficiency) and **regurgitation** of the blood from the ventricle into atrium, or from the great arteries into the ventricle.

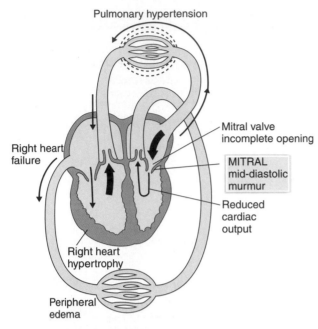

Figure 4-53 Mitral stenosis. Narrowing of the mitral orifice leads to backpressure into the left atrium, pulmonary circulation, and the right heart. Forward heart failure due to reduced cardiac output also occurs, and a mid-diastolic murmur is present.

Mitral stenosis impedes the blood flow from the left atrium into the ventricle.

Mitral stenosis is characterized by a narrowing of the inflow orifice of the left ventricle. It is caused by pathologic changes of the mitral valves, which, as a result, cannot retract completely during diastole. In most instances mitral stenosis is a late complication of rheumatic carditis, and for unknown reasons it occurs more often in women than in men.

Pathologic changes of the mitral valves represent a mechanical obstacle to the blood entering the left ventricle from the left atrium during diastole (Fig. 4-53). On auscultation mitral stenosis manifests with a **loud mid-diastolic murmur** radiating toward the axilla, accompanied by a loud first heart sound and an opening snap (Fig. 4-54).

The *left atrium dilates and becomes hypertrophic,* and the backpressure into the lungs causes both venous and arterial **pulmonary hypertension.** Ultimately the right ventricle becomes hypertrophic, and clinical signs of right heart failure **(cor pulmonale)** develop.

The pathologic changes involving the valves can be detected by echocardiography, which shows thickening of the valves, narrowing of the orifice, and reduced diastolic filling of the ventricle. The enlargement of the left atrium and right ventricle and pulmonary congestions and edema can be seen by radiograph. ECG, pulmonary pressure measurements, and pressure gradients recorded during cardiac catheterization are also abnormal and reflect the same pathologic changes.

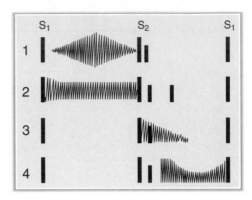

Figure 4-54 Cardiac murmurs. 1, Aortic stenosis. 2, Mitral regurgitation. 3, Aortic regurgitation. 4, Mitral stenosis. S_1 is the first heart sound, and S_2 is the second.

Clinical features of mitral stenosis can be readily understood in terms of the underlying pathology:

- **Diastolic murmur.** It results from the turbulent flow over the pathologically altered valve during diastole.
- **Opening snap.** It is related to the abnormal opening of the pathologically altered mitral valve.
- **Atrial fibrillation.** It is a complication of the dilatation and hypertrophy of the left atrium.
- **Fatigue.** It is related to hypoxia caused by diminished cardiac output.
- **Dyspnea.** It results from pulmonary venous congestion leading to pulmonary edema. It is often associated with cough and is more prominent while the patient is lying down.
- **Leg edema, hepatosplenomegaly.** These findings are a consequence of cor pulmonale (i.e., right heart failure).
- **Peripheral signs of infarction or hemorrhage in the brain, extremities, or kidneys.** These symptoms are related to arterial thromboemboli originating from the vegetations that form on the abnormal valves. These vegetations may become infected and are a common cause of septic infarcts and septicemia.

Mitral regurgitation is a result of incomplete closure of the mitral valve during systole.

Mitral regurgitation results from valvular incompetence (insufficiency)—the inability of the mitral valve to close completely during systole. It may be acute or chronic. In 40% of chronic cases it is a consequence of rheumatic carditis, in which case it is often associated with mitral stenosis. In the remaining 60% of cases it is caused by degeneration of congenitally floppy valves, damage to valves by endocarditis, or myocardial changes that lead to dilatation of the mitral valve ring. The last group includes patients who had an MI, myocarditis, or dilated cardiomyopathy. Acute mitral regurgitation occurs most often due to rupture of papillary muscle in MI or due to rupture of chordae tendineae in infective endocarditis.

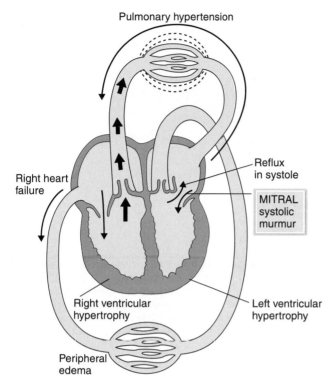

Figure 4-55 Mitral regurgitation. The incomplete closure of the mitral valve in systole leads to backflow of blood into the left atrium. Pulmonary hypertension and right heart failure develop. A systolic murmur is present.

Mitral regurgitation is characterized by a reflux of blood from the left ventricle into the left atrium during systole (Fig. 4-55). The reflux of blood during systole results in a **pansystolic murmur** with a maximum at the apex of the heart but that often radiates to the axilla. The first cardiac sound is soft.

The left ventricle pumps less efficiently and thus the patient exhibits signs of reduced heart output (**forward heart failure**). At the same time the blood flows backwards, causing dilatation of the left atrium and pulmonary venous and arterial hypertension. Ultimately cor pulmonale develops and signs of right ventricular failure, such as leg edema and hepatosplenomegaly, occur (**backward heart failure**). The strain imposed on the left ventricle causes left ventricular hypertrophy. Since the cardiac output is reduced, coronary filling is inadequate and ultimately the heart fails.

Clinical features of mitral regurgitation are distinct, yet many signs and symptoms are similar to those of mitral stenosis. Indeed in many cases of chronic rheumatic endocarditis signs of both stenosis and insufficiency coexist. The findings that favor mitral regurgitation are the pansystolic murmur and left ventricular hypertrophy. The final diagnosis is best documented by echocardiography, color Doppler, and cardiac catheterization.

Aortic stenosis impedes the outflow of blood from the left ventricle during systole.

Aortic stenosis is characterized by a narrowing of the outflow orifice of the left ventricle. The valves are deformed and often calcified and hence cannot open completely. In young persons the causes of stenosis are congenital valvular abnormalities. In middle-aged persons stenosis is related to the calcifications of congenital bicuspid valves or is a consequence of rheumatic carditis, which often concomitantly involves the mitral valve. In the elderly aortic stenosis may be related to the same conditions as in adults, but most often it is a sign of idiopathic calcification of aortic valves.

Aortic stenosis is characterized by a **pansystolic cardiac murmur** preceded by an ejection click and an accentuated first heart sound (Fig. 4-56). ECG shows signs of left ventricular hypertrophy. Echocardiography can detect the calcification of the cusps, and Doppler cardiography documents the existence of a gradient across the aortic orifice.

The strain imposed on the left ventricle may cause both **forward** and **backward heart failure.** Inadequate filling of coronary arteries, which originate from the sinus of Valsalva behind the calcified cusps, may cause signs of **angina.** These patients are also prone to **exertional syncope** and sudden death. The dilatation of the root of the aorta behind the stenotic orifice may cause widening of the aortic ring, and thus aortic regurgitation may become superimposed on stenosis.

Aortic regurgitation results from incomplete closure of the aortic valve during diastole.

Aortic regurgitation may be a consequence of valvular defects of various origin, including congenital bicuspid valves, or a result of rheumatic or infective endocarditis. Regurgitation can also develop due to dilatation of the aortic ring caused by atherosclerosis or syphilitic aortic aneurysm. It is also seen in association with aneurysms of Marfan's syndrome.

Aortic regurgitation is characterized by a **decrescendo diastolic murmur** and an **ejection systolic murmur,** which is best heard on the right side of the sternum when the patient is leaning forward holding his or her breath in expiration (Fig. 4-57). The diastolic murmur reflects the reflux of blood through the incompletely closed aortic valve. The systolic murmur is related to an increased stroke volume, and the additional work imposed on the left ventricle causes left ventricular hypertrophy.

Hyperdynamic heart action clinically manifests as a thrusting apex and causes the patient to feel the heartbeat or experience palpitation. The pulse has a large volume and is typically "collapsing" due to reflux of blood into the ventricle. **Pulsations** can be seen in the nailbeds, and in extreme cases even the entire head can be nodding in the rhythm of the pulse. The patient also may have **angina** because of inadequate filling of the coronary arteries.

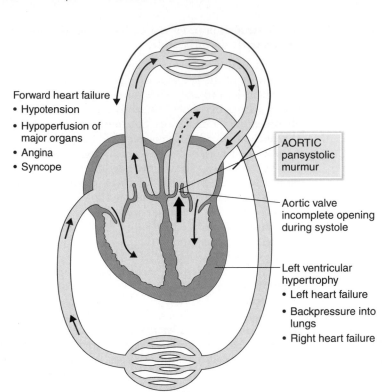

Forward heart failure
- Hypotension
- Hypoperfusion of major organs
- Angina
- Syncope

AORTIC pansystolic murmur

Aortic valve incomplete opening during systole

Left ventricular hypertrophy
- Left heart failure
- Backpressure into lungs
- Right heart failure

Figure 4-56 Aortic stenosis. The narrowing of the aortic valve poses a strain on the left ventricle, which undergoes hypertrophy. Forward heart pressure hypotension occurs along with left ventricle hypertrophy, leading ultimately to left heart failure, backpressure into the lungs, and right heart failure.

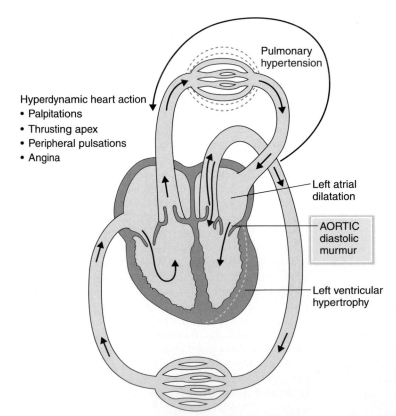

Pulmonary hypertension

Hyperdynamic heart action
- Palpitations
- Thrusting apex
- Peripheral pulsations
- Angina

Left atrial dilatation

AORTIC diastolic murmur

Left ventricular hypertrophy

Figure 4-57 Aortic regurgitation. Incomplete closure of the aortic valve during diastole leads to backflow of blood and left ventricular hypertrophy. A diastolic murmur is present, associated with a systolic murmur due to increased blood flow in the left ventricle.

Tricuspid stenosis and regurgitation manifest with increased central venous pressure.

Tricuspid stenosis is rare, but if found it is usually a component of complex rheumatic endocarditis and associated with the more common changes affecting the aortic and mitral valves. Tricuspid stenoses lead to an elevation of venous pressure in the venae cavae and peripheral chronic passive congestion in the liver, abdominal organs, and lower extremities. Jugular venous pressure tracing shows a prominent *a* wave and slow *y* descent, reflecting the obstruction to ventricular filling.

Tricuspid regurgitation is usually caused by right ventricular dilatation, but it may be also a consequence of rheumatic heart disease, bacterial endocarditis in intravenous drug abusers, or carcinoid syndrome. It manifests with venous reflux and increased central venous pressure. Jugular venous pulse shows a large *cv* wave replacing the normal *x* descent.

CARDIOMYOPATHY

Cardiomyopathies are classified as dilated, hypertrophic, or restrictive.

Cardiomyopathies are a diverse group of heart diseases caused by pathologic changes in the myocardium. On the basis of the underlying pathology these diseases are divided into three groups (Fig. 4-58):

- Dilated, characterized by a dilatation of both ventricles and an inability to contract during systole
- Hypertrophic, characterized by ventricular hypertrophy and an inability to dilate during diastole
- Restrictive, characterized by abnormally stiff myocardium that cannot dilate but that has a preserved capacity for contraction

In clinical practice the diagnosis is made by excluding coronary, valvular, hypertensive, or congenital heart diseases. Cardiomyopathies are lethal diseases that can be effectively treated only with cardiac transplantation.

Dilated cardiomyopathy is characterized by systolic failure.

Dilated cardiomyopathy is characterized by extensive dilatation of the ventricles, causing a weakening of ventricular function. It is classified as primary or idiopathic and occurs secondary to a variety of exogenous factors or diseases that damage the heart (Table 4-11).

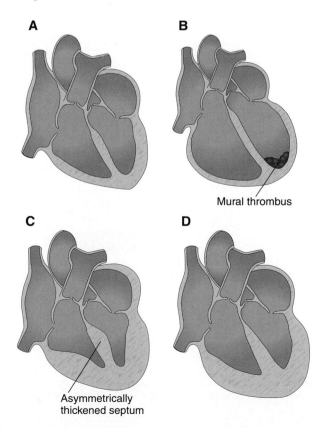

Figure 4-58 Cardiomyopathies. **A**, Normal heart. **B**, Dilated cardiomyopathy. **C**, Hypertrophic cardiomyopathy. **D**, Restrictive cardiomyopathy. (Modified from Roberts WC, Ferrans VJ: Pathologic anatomy of the cardiomyopathies. Hum Pathol 1975;6:289–342.)

Table 4-11 Causes of Dilated Cardiomyopathy

Idiopathic
Genetic
Infection
    Viral (e.g., coxsackievirus A and B)
    Parasitic (e.g., *Trypanosoma cruzi*)
Drugs and toxins
    Alcohol
    Anthracyclines
    Cobalt
Endocrine/metabolic
    Thyroid disorders (hyper- or hypothyroidism)
    Peripartum or postpartum cardiomyopathy
    Hemochromatosis
Nutritional
    Starvation
    Thiamine deficiency (beri-beri)
Immune
    Sarcoidosis
    Scleroderma
    Polymyositis

The heart is enlarged and weighs more than normal. However, the ventricles are disproportionately dilated, and thus the heart cannot contract forcefully enough to eject all the blood that has entered the ventricles during diastole. The left ventricular ejection fraction is reduced, usually below 45% (normal, 50–65%), and the volume-to-mass ratio is increased.

Patients present with signs of congestive heart failure. Mural thrombi form in the dilated ventricles, and thus embolic phenomena are quite common especially in the extremities, as well as in the supply zones of mesenteric and cerebral arteries (Fig. 4-59). Echocardiographic findings are consistent with poor systolic function. The ECG is almost always abnormal and shows QRS widening, arrhythmias, and conduction defects. Sudden death due to electrophysiologic disturbances is common.

Hypertrophic cardiomyopathy is characterized by diastolic failure.

Hypertrophic cardiomyopathy is characterized by an increased total cardiac mass without a corresponding increase in the size of the cavities. Hypertrophic cardiomyopathy is in most instances related to mutations of genes encoding cardiac proteins such as β-myosin heavy-chain, troponin, and α-tropomyosin, among others. The heart is enlarged, but the ventricles are not dilated. In some instances the ventricular septum is asymmetrically hypertrophic, causing a subaortic stenosis of the outflow tracts.

The heart action is hyperdynamic, and the stroke volume and the left ventricular ejection fraction are either high normal or increased (65–90%). The ventricular mass prevents normal

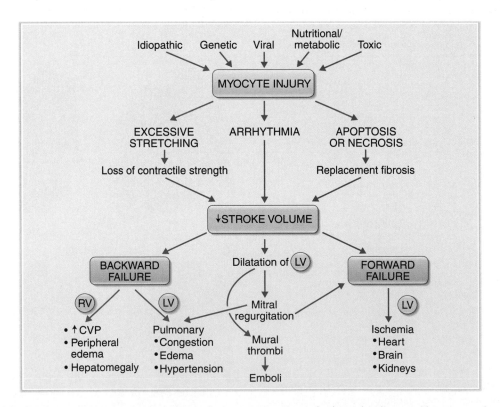

Figure 4-59 Dilated cardiomyopathy. The injury of myocytes weakens the heart leading to dilatation and systolic failure. CVP, central venous pressure; LV, left ventricle; RV, right ventricle.

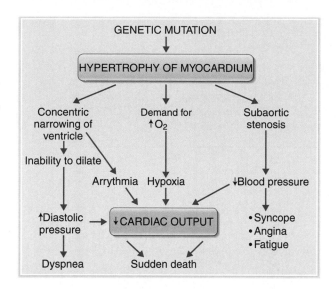

GENETIC MUTATION

HYPERTROPHY OF MYOCARDIUM

Concentric narrowing of ventricle → Inability to dilate

Demand for ↑O₂

Subaortic stenosis

Arrythmia   Hypoxia   ↓Blood pressure

↑Diastolic pressure → ↓CARDIAC OUTPUT

• Syncope
• Angina
• Fatigue

Dyspnea   Sudden death

Figure 4-60 Congenital hypertrophic cardiomyopathy. The hypertrophic heart cannot dilate and this leads to a diastolic failure. Subaortic stenosis of the septum contributes to the forward heart failure.

diastolic filling, and accordingly the end-diastolic intraventricular pressure is increased (Fig. 4-60). The volume-to-mass ratio is decreased, and the diastolic compliance is significantly reduced. The bulging septum may impede the outflow of blood from the left ventricle. Maneuvers that reduce the left ventricular volume, such as standing upright or Valsalva maneuver, or nitroglycerin may reduce the ventricular output and cause fainting. The echocardiogram shows the typical thickening of the interventricular septum and other parts of the ventricular wall. ECG shows increased QRS voltage, consistent with ventricular hypertrophy. Clinical symptoms vary and include dyspnea on exertion, syncope, palpitations, and angina. Sudden death and a history of sudden death in the family are common. β-Blockers and calcium channel blockers are used to slow down the heart rate and prolong diastole, and thus allow better diastolic filling of the ventricles.

Restrictive cardiomyopathy is characterized by slowly evolving diastolic failure combined in final stages with systolic failure.

Restrictive cardiomyopathy includes several diseases that decrease the compliance of the ventricles, thus impairing diastolic filling. The loss of compliance results from the infiltration of the myocardium with noncontractile inelastic material such as fibrous tissue, amyloid, or granulomas of sarcoidosis. The material infiltrating the myocardium makes it stiff, and clinically restrictive cardiomyopathy may mimic constrictive pericarditis.

Amyloidosis is the most common cause of restrictive cardiomyopathy. The total mass of the heart is enlarged, but the ventricles are of normal size. The left ventricular ejection fraction is initially within normal limits but then gradually decreases. Volume-to-mass ratio is markedly decreased, and the diastolic compliance is decreased. The ECG may be normal. Echocardiography may show increased ventricular thickness and foci of hypokinesis. The diagnosis is often made by endomyocardial biopsy.

HYPERTENSIVE HEART DISEASE

Arterial hypertension is a very widespread disease, and at least 50% of all adults in the United States are estimated to have a systolic pressure over 140 mm Hg and a diastolic pressure over 90 mm Hg, which qualifies them as hypertensive. Hypertension accelerates the progression of atherosclerosis and thus indirectly leads to heart failure. At the same time hypertension has a deleterious effect on several major organs, most notably the heart, brain, eyes, and kidneys (Fig. 4-61).

Hypertension is the most common cause of cardiac hypertrophy.

Hypertension increases the afterload, thus forcing the heart to work harder. Hypertrophy of the left ventricle is a common complication and is almost invariably found in all hypertensive patients who have not been treated. The hypertrophic heart requires more oxygen, and since the coronary arteries have a limited capacity, relative ischemia develops. Increased demand imposed by additional effort cannot be met, and, accordingly, hypertrophic hearts fail much faster than normal hearts. Left ventricular failure is accompanied by right ventricular hypertrophy. This cor pulmonale leads to backward heart failure and pedal edema, hepatosplenomegaly, and abdominal edema.

Hypertension damages vital organs.

Hypertension has a tendency to impair the vasculature in many organs, most notably the brain, eyes, and kidneys.

■ **Brain.** Hypertension accelerates the progression of coronary atherosclerosis and also produces changes in smaller intraparenchymal arteries and arterioles of the brain. Arterioles may form microscopic aneurysms, and the structural changes may cause foci of ischemia resulting in transitional ischemic attacks. Rupture of cerebral vessels may cause intracerebral hemorrhages, which are most often located in the basal ganglia–internal capsule region, pons, or cerebellum.

■ **Eye.** Hypertension has a tendency to damage the small arteries and arterioles of the retina, causing typical hypertensive changes visible by ophthalmoscopic examination of the fundus. Rupture and hemorrhages are common.

■ **Kidney.** Hypertension may damage renal arteries and arterioles and cause renal ischemia. Renal ischemia leads to a release of renin, which aggravates hypertension by acting on the angiotensin–aldosterone system. Sodium retention leads to a fluid overload in the cardiovascular system, further contributing to hypertension.

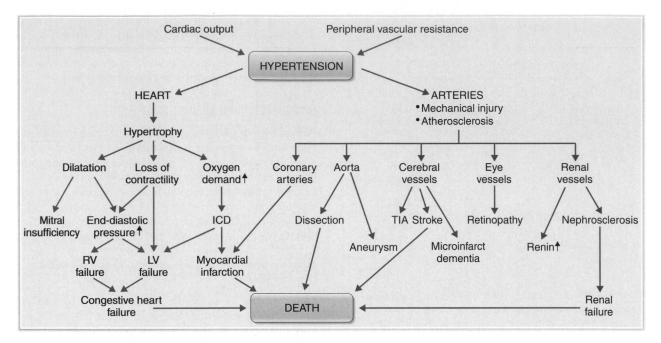

Figure 4-61 Hypertension. Hypertension causes hypertrophy of the heart and it affects arteries in most other organs. ICD, ischemic coronary disease; LV, left ventricle; RV, right ventricle; TIA, transient ischemic attack.

CASE STUDIES

Case 1 SUDDEN CHEST PAIN IN A 55-YEAR-OLD MAN WITH DIABETES

Clinical history   A 55-year-old man was brought to the emergency department by ambulance. He woke up at 6 AM feeling a crushing pain over his chest.[1] He has had previous attacks of precordial pain, mostly while walking outside in cold weather or when running with his dog. As of late the pain would appear while he was at rest as well, but it was never as severe as now.[2] He has diabetes and arterial hypertension for which he takes medication.[3]

He was given an aspirin and transferred to the coronary intensive care unit by 8 AM.[4]

Physical findings   He is obese, short of breath, sweating, and obviously in acute distress. His pulse rate is 90 and the blood pressure is 100/60 mm Hg.[5]

Laboratory and clinical findings   At the time of admission the serum levels of myoglobin, troponin I and T, and creatine kinase MB were within normal limits.[6] The ECG showed sinus tachycardia, but no other abnormalities.[7]

Outcome   He had a coronary angiography and a stent was inserted.[8] He was treated for a few days in the coronary care unit and recovered completely.

Questions and topics for discussion
1. What is the pathogenesis and what are the possible causes of chest pain of sudden onset?
2. What is the significance of precordial pain that occurs during effort in contrast to precordial pain that occurs at rest?
3. Is the history of diabetes and hypertension important for the understanding of the present illness of this patient?
4. Why was he given aspirin?
5. Why does he have tachycardia and hypotension?
6. Is it possible that this patient has an MI even though the laboratory findings do not support that diagnosis? When could one expect a rise of serum levels of myoglobin, troponin, and CK-MB?
7. Is ECG always abnormal in patients with acute MI?
8. What were the angiographic findings?

Case 2 STROKE IN A 45-YEAR-OLD WOMAN WHO HAD RHEUMATIC FEVER AS AN ADOLESCENT

Clinical history A 45-year-old woman experienced a stroke and was hospitalized.[1] As an adolescent she had rheumatic fever. During the last year she became more and more tired and would become short of breath when climbing stairs.[2]

Physical findings She was unconscious and was breathing heavily. Rales were heard above both lungs and the radiograph showed Kerley's B lines in the lower lung fields peripherally extending to the pleural surface.[3] The radiograph also revealed a dilated right atrium. Auscultation of the heart revealed a loud first heart sound, an opening snap best heard over the apex, and a diastolic rumble.[4]

Laboratory and clinical findings Erythrocyte sedimentation rate was increased and there was moderate leukocytosis. Blood culture revealed viridans streptococci.[5]

Outcome She was given antibiotics, but developed a brain abscess and died.[6]

Questions and topics for discussion
1. What are the possible causes of stroke?
2. Why would a person with a history of rheumatic fever become tired and short of breath?
3. What is the possible explanation for the heavy breathing associated with rales and Kerley's B lines seen on the radiograph?
4. Interpret and explain the pathogenesis of the auscultatory findings. Which valve is affected? Is the disease manifesting as stenosis or regurgitation?
5. What is the significance of positive blood cultures in a patient who has signs of chronic rheumatic heart disease and a stroke?
6. Explain the pathogenesis of the brain abscess in this patient.

Case 3 SYNCOPE AND HEART FAILURE IN A 20-YEAR-OLD MAN

Clinical history A 20-year-old student collapsed during a tennis game and was brought to the emergency department.[1] He had no previous cardiac symptoms, but his father died suddenly at age 33.[2] The patient regained consciousness spontaneously but was nevertheless admitted for complete examination.

Physical findings On admission radiographic examination revealed only a slightly enlarged heart. Echocardiography revealed thickening of ventricular walls with a bulge of the septum protruding into the left ventricle in the subaortic area. The ventricular ejection rate was 70%.[3]

Laboratory findings No laboratory findings were abnormal. Subsequent genetic testing revealed a mutation of the β-myoglobin heavy-chain gene.[4]

Outcome The patient was given β-blockers and was told to visit his cardiologist at regular intervals.[5]

Questions and topics for discussion
1. Define syncope and discuss some of its causes.
2. A family history of sudden death may be important for the understanding of syncope in a young man. Explain why.
3. Explain these echocardiographic findings.
4. What is the diagnosis? Is this a systolic or diastolic disorder? How is it inherited?
5. What is the rationale for giving β-blockers?

Case 4 SHORTNESS OF BREATH IN A MAN WITH LONG-STANDING HYPERTENSION

Clinical history A 60-year-old man known to have hypertension complained of shortness of breath and hemoptysis.[1]

Physical findings He had bilateral pulmonary rales and tachypnea. His blood pressure was 200/120 mm Hg.[2] He also had pitting edema of his legs and an enlarged liver and spleen.[3]

Laboratory findings No laboratory findings were indicative of a renal, endocrine, or neural basis of hypertension.[4]

Outcome He responded well to treatment with angiotensin-converting enzyme (ACE) inhibitors and diuretics.[5]

Questions and topics for discussion
1. Why does he have shortness of breath and hemoptysis?
2. Is this hypertension mild, moderate, or severe?
3. Do these findings suggest right or left heart failure?
4. What is the most likely cause of hypertension in this patient?
5. What is the rationale for this treatment?

Chapter 5

PULMONARY DISEASES

Introduction

The lungs are part of the respiratory system. As such they have a critical role in the exchange of gases—the inhalation of oxygen (O_2) and expiration of carbon dioxide (CO_2). Pulmonary diseases are a major cause of human morbidity and mortality as evidenced by the following clinical and epidemiologic facts:

- Respiratory infections, usually localized to the upper respiratory passages, account for most of the so-called common diseases of children and adults of all ages.
- The respiratory system is essential for sustaining life, and thus respiratory failure is one of the major causes of death in humans.
- Lungs are in contact with the external world and thus rather susceptible to deleterious exogenous influences. Most notably, lungs inhale living airborne pathogens, such as bacteria, viruses, and fungi. Organic and inorganic particles and fumes inhaled in the air also may adversely affect the lungs.
- The lungs are major "shock-organs" in humans and show pathologic changes in almost all forms of shock and terminal conditions preceding death.
- Changes in the lungs are seen during heart failure and in many metabolic and circulatory disorders affecting other vital organs such as the brain, liver, and kidneys. Pulmonary edema and acute respiratory distress syndrome (ARDS) are common findings in multiple organ failure.
- The lungs are affected by exogenous carcinogens and are the primary target for the carcinogens contained in tobacco smoke. Lung cancer is still the foremost cause of cancer-related death in both men and women.

Lung diseases can be classified according to their etiology. The relative clinical significance of various pulmonary diseases is presented graphically in Figure 5-1.

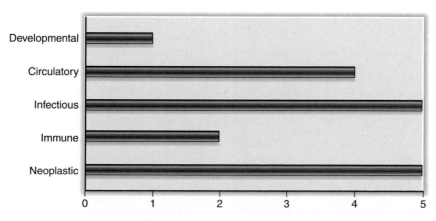

Figure 5-1 The relative clinical significance of various pulmonary diseases.

Anatomy and Physiology

Alveolus ("acinus") Small saclike part of the lungs forming the smallest respiratory unit of the lungs. It is lined by two cell types: pulmonary pneumocytes type I, which form the air–blood interface, and pneumocytes type II, which secrete surfactant.

Bronchioli Small bronchi that lack cartilage. They are interposed between the bronchi with the alveolar ducts and alveoli and further classified as terminal or respiratory bronchioli.

Bronchus Tubular part of the airways inside the lungs arranged into a branching tree of progressively smaller and smaller ducts connecting the trachea on the proximal side and bronchioli and alveoli on the distal side. Bronchi are lined with respiratory epithelium composed of ciliated and nonciliated cylindrical cells, mucus-secreting cells, and neuroendocrine cells. Their walls contain cartilage and smooth muscle cells.

Compliance Measure of the ability of the lungs to expand in response to increased pressure by the inhaled air.

Diffusion Movement of molecules across a gradient from areas of high concentration to ones of low concentration, until equilibrium is achieved.

Elasticity Ability of a material to return to its normal shape after a force has changed its shape. The elasticity of lungs is measured as a change of pressure in response to changes of the volume of intrapulmonary air.

Larynx Part of the respiratory tract between the pharynx and the trachea, which also acts as voice-generating organ.

Mucus Gel-like substance covering the surface of mucous membranes of air spaces, such as the nose, trachea, and bronchi.

Pharynx Part of the respiratory and alimentary systems connecting the nose with the larynx and the mouth with the esophagus.

Pleura External covering of the lungs composed of a mesothelial layer and underlying connective tissue. The visceral pleura covering the lungs is continuous with the parietal pleura covering the inside of the thoracic cage. The pleural cavity is the space between the visceral and parietal pleura. Normally it contains a few milliliters of serous fluid lubricating the pleural surfaces and allowing them to glide one over another during respiration.

Pulmonary surfactant Complex semiliquid surface-tension–generating material covering the surface of the alveoli. It is essential for keeping the alveoli open during inhalation. The deficiency of surfactant is the cause of neonatal respiratory distress syndrome and hyaline membrane formation in the lungs of premature babies.

Respiration (breathing) Process that includes external and internal respiration. External respiration refers to inhalation of air into the lungs and expiration of air out of the respiratory system, as well the gas exchange between inhaled air and the blood in the lungs. Inhalation provides oxygen, and expiration allows the elimination of carbon dioxide out of the body. Internal respiration refers to cellular processes allowing the transfer of oxygen from red blood cells through the capillary wall into the tissues and intracellular utilization of oxygen.

Trachea Air-conducting tube connecting the larynx with the bronchi.

Ventilation Movement of air in and out of the lungs.

Ventilation/perfusion rate ($\dot{V}/\dot{Q}$) Ratio of the overall alveolar ventilation to the overall pulmonary blood flow expressed in liters per minute, normally 0.8.

Clinical and Laboratory Findings and Procedures

Acidosis Decreased blood pH resulting from an abnormal accumulation of acids or a loss of bases from the body fluids. May be classified as respiratory or metabolic.

Alkalosis Increased blood pH resulting from an abnormal accumulation of bases or a loss of acids from body fluids. May be classified as respiratory or metabolic.

Allergy Generic term for many forms of hypersensitivity to foreign substances capable of inducing an immune response. Such substances are called allergens or immunogens.

Anoxia Condition in which the tissues do not receive oxygen. If partial, it is called hypoxia.

Cheyne-Stokes respiration Abnormal respiration characterized by periods of apnea and rapid breathing. Typically apnea lasts 10 to 30 seconds and is followed by a period of rapid and deepening respiratory movements, followed again by slowing down of respiration and apnea.

Cough Process resulting in the forceful expulsion of air from the respiratory tract. It may by mediated by a reflex or a voluntary expiratory effort.

Dyspnea ("shortness of breath") Sense of difficulty with breathing.

Expectoration Process that results in removal of mucus or tracheobronchial contents during coughing and spitting.

Forced vital capacity Maximum volume of gases that can be exhaled from the lungs as fast as possible over a specified short period of time.

Functional residual capacity Volume of air that remains in the lungs after a normal expiration. It can be calculated by adding the expiratory reserve volume and the residual volume.

Hyperinflation Excessive expansion of the pulmonary air spaces that occurs due to air trapping in asthma or because of the loss of alveolar walls in emphysema.

Hyperpnea Increased depth of respiratory movements without an increased number of respirations.

Hyperventilation Increased alveolar air exchange leading to increased exhalation of carbon dioxide and hypocapnia.

Inspiratory capacity Volume of air that can be inhaled after a normal exhalation. It can be calculated by adding the tidal volume to the inspiratory reserve volume.

Intubation Passage of a tubular instrument into the air spaces, typically through the nose or the larynx. It is used to facilitate or maintain the air flow into the lungs or administer inhalational anesthetics.

Kussmaul respiration Form of abnormal breathing characterized by increased depth and rate. It is typically encountered in acidosis, especially lactic acidosis of diabetes.

Rales ("crackles") Abnormal sounds heard over the regions of the thorax by auscultation during inspiration. These sounds result from the accumulation of fluid or exudates in the alveoli.

Shunting Process during which a stream of blood or air is diverted from its normal flow through expanded normal, newly formed or pathological passages.

Tachypnea Rapid breathing rate.

Pulmonary Diseases

Acute respiratory distress syndrome ("shock lung") Clinical syndrome caused by numerous exogenous and endogenous insults leading to diffuse alveolar-capillary unit damage (DAD). Most often caused by shock, airborne or blood-borne infections, chemical or physical injury of the lungs, or systemic metabolic disorders.

Asthma Inflammatory disease characterized by reversible obstruction of the air passages due to bronchospasm and oversecretion of mucus.

Atelectasis Process in which the lungs become airless and the alveolar spaces collapse.

Bronchiectasis Chronic lung disease characterized by irreversible dilatation of bronchi and bronchioli caused by inflammation, obstruction, or fibrosis, or various destructive changes in the peribronchial lung parenchyma.

Bronchitis Inflammation of bronchi that may be acute or chronic. It may be caused by viral or bacterial infection or chronic irritation, as seen in smokers. Clinically it presents with cough and expectoration of mucus or mucopurulent exudate.

Chronic obstructive pulmonary disease (COPD) Chronic lung disease caused by chronic bronchitis or emphysema or both. It is most often caused by smoking. Clinically it manifests as progressive dyspnea and signs of obstructive lung disease leading to respiratory insufficiency.

Emphysema Chronic condition caused by destruction of alveolar septa and dilatation of terminal air spaces. It occurs in several pathologic forms (e.g., centriacinar or panacinar), and clinically it manifests as chronic obstructive pulmonary disease. It may be a consequence of congenital α1-antitrypsin deficiency.

Empyema Localized accumulation of pus in the pleural cavity.

Hypersensitivity pneumonitis Group of lung diseases caused by a cellular immune reaction to exogenous organic allergens inhaled into the alveoli. These diseases are often related to the workplace and are known as farmer's lung, pigeon breeder's lung, and air conditioner lungs, among others.

Kartagener's syndrome Congenital ciliary dismotility disorder characterized by recurrent respiratory infections (sinusitis and bronchiectasis), situs inversus, and infertility in males (sperm immotility).

Lung cancer Group of malignant tumors originating from the bronchi or terminal bronchioli and pleura. Most often caused by smoking. Microscopically, lung cancer can be classified as squamous cell carcinoma, adenocarcinoma, or large- or small-cell undifferentiated carcinoma. Clinically these tumors are divided for practical purposed into two groups: small-cell carcinoma and nonsmall-cell carcinoma, including all the other microscopic variants.

Mesothelioma Malignant tumor of the pleura, often related to asbestos exposure.

Pleural effusion Accumulation of fluid in the pleural cavity. It may represent a transudate, as occurs in chronic heart failure, or generalized anasarca; or it may be an exudate, as is seen in infectious pleuritis. Tumors also cause pleural effusion ("malignant pleural effusion").

Pleuritis Inflammation of the pleura. It may be a complication of pneumonia or it may begin as a primary infection.

Pneumoconioses Group of chronic lung diseases caused by inhalation of inorganic and organic particles, chemical fumes, and vapors. Typical entities included under this heading are coal worker's pneumoconiosis, silicosis, asbestosis, and conditions such as farmer's lung, bagassosis, byssinosis, and various occupational lung disease caused by vapor inhalation.

Pneumonia Inflammation of the lungs. It can be acute or chronic and involve predominantly either the alveoli ("alveolar pneumonia") or alveolar septa ("interstitial pneumonia"). Pneumonia may be patchy ("lobular pneumonia" or "bronchopneumonia") or diffuse ("lobar pneumonia").

Pneumothorax Accumulation of air in the pleural cavity.

Pulmonary hypertension Increased pressure in the pulmonary circulation, typically reaching 25% of the systemic blood pressure. It may be primary, of unknown origin, or secondary, due to left heart failure and chronic lung disease or pulmonary emboli.

Restrictive lung disease Group of pathogenetically unrelated diseases characterized by reduced volume of terminal air spaces or an inability of the lungs to expand adequately during inspiration. Restrictive lung disease can be distinguished from obstructive lung disease by functional testing. This group of disease includes several forms of chronic interstitial pneumonia of unknown origin, dust-induced pneumoconioses, drug- and radiation-induced lung diseases, hypersensitivity pneumonias, and diseases of presumed immune origin such as sarcoidosis.

Sarcoidosis Systemic disease of unknown origin, characterized by the formation of noncaseating granulomas in the lungs, thoracic lymph nodes, and many other organs.

Usual interstitial pneumonia (UIP, idiopathic pulmonary fibrosis) Chronic restrictive lung disease causing irregular destruction of lung parenchyma associated with chronic alveolitis and patchy interstitial fibrosis ("honeycomb lungs"). In most instances the cause of UIP is unknown. The disease is incurable.

Normal Structure and Function

ANATOMY AND HISTOLOGY

The respiratory system is arbitrarily divided into two parts: (1) the upper respiratory system, comprising the nose, pharynx, and larynx, and (2) the lower respiratory system, comprising the tracheobronchial tree and the lungs (Fig. 5-2). In this chapter we concentrate on the lower respiratory tract, its functions, and diseases.

The respiratory tract is lined with specialized epithelia and encased by specialized support structures.

The main function of the respiratory system is to maintain external respiration. In other words, the respiratory system must enable the body to inhale and exhale air and make the exchange of gases between the blood and the air possible. Various parts of the respiratory system must thus be lined with specialized epithelia that support these functions.

The nasal and tracheobronchial mucosa. The epithelium of the nasal and tracheobronchial mucosa is pseudostratified and contains mucus-secreting and ciliated cells. The mucus-secreting cells produce mucus, which keeps the air spaces moist and also serves as a mechanical protective barrier and a receptacle for foreign particles and bacteria. The submucosa also contains larger mucous glands, which contribute mucus and fluid that covers the surface of the air spaces. Note that the epithelium of the mucosa also contains scattered neuroendocrine cells, the function of which has not been fully elucidated. Stem cells, which are important for the replacement of the more differentiated mucosal cells under both physiologic and pathologic conditions, are also scattered throughout the submucosa.

Because the nasal air spaces and the tracheobronchial tree need to be kept patent, their walls contain cartilage. Bony structures in the nasal air passages have the same protective functions. In the tracheobronchial tree the air spaces contain smooth muscle cells, which are thought to regulate the

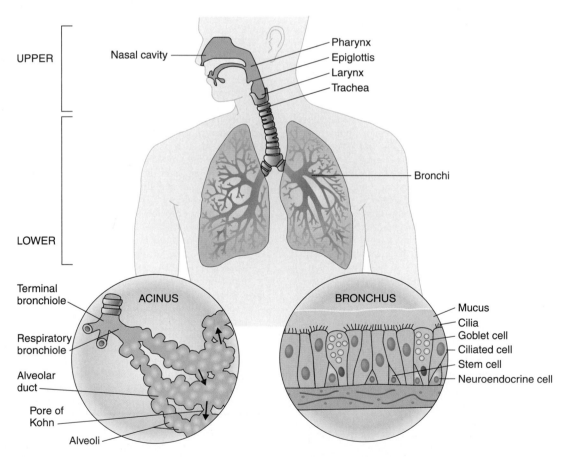

Figure 5-2 Normal respiratory system. The normal respiratory system consists of an upper and lower part and can also be divided into a conducting zone (comprising the nose, pharynx, larynx, trachea, bronchi, and bronchioli) and a respiratory zone (which includes the respiratory bronchioles, alveolar ducts, and the alveoli). The latter structures form the pulmonary acinus—the smallest functional unit of the lung.

contraction or dilatation of these air spaces designed for conductance and distribution of air in the lungs.

The caliber of the air spaces diminishes gradually, and as the air duct branches their diameter decreases. Their structure also changes. Most notably, as the bronchi become smaller and smaller they contain less and less cartilage, and ultimately they transform into bronchioli, which are devoid of cartilage. Finally, the smallest air ducts, called terminal bronchioli, transform into respiratory bronchioli, which open up into alveolar sacs and alveoli.

Alveoli. These terminal parts of the respiratory system are lined with type I and type II pneumocytes. Type II pneumocytes produce surfactant, a surface-active substance that maintains alveolar patency. Type I pneumocytes are in close contact with alveolar capillaries and form with them the *alveolar-capillary units,* the elementary respiratory functional units of the lung.

Lungs are enclosed in the thoracic cage, which protects them from external injury but also contributes to their rhythmic expansion and reduction in size.

The thoracic cage consists of bones and striated muscles (Fig. 5-3). It has two principal functions:

■ **Protection.** The sternum, ribs and vertebrae, clavicle, and scapula protect the lungs from external injury by providing a mechanical shield. The muscles of the chest and the back provide additional protection.

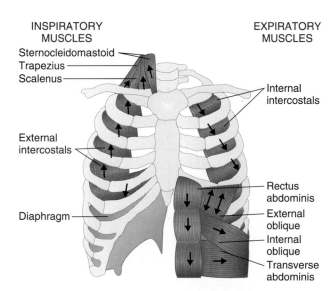

INSPIRATORY MUSCLES
EXPIRATORY MUSCLES

Sternocleidomastoid
Trapezius
Scalenus

Internal intercostals

External intercostals

Diaphragm

Rectus abdominis
External oblique
Internal oblique
Transverse abdominis

Figure 5-3 Chest wall and respiratory muscles. The lungs are enclosed in the chest wall, which consists of bones (ribs, sternum, clavicles, scapula, and the vertebral column) and muscles. The muscles include inspiratory and expiratory muscles of the thorax, neck, abdomen, and diaphragm.

■ **Respiration.** The striated muscles of the anterior and posterior surface of the chest wall, some neck and anterior abdominal wall muscles, and the diaphragm participate in the respiratory movements. These muscles could be divided into two groups: (1) **inspiratory muscles,** such as sternocleiodmastoid, trapezius and scalenus muscles, and the diaphragm, and (2) the **expiratory muscles,** such as the intercostals and the muscles of the anterior abdominal wall.

The lungs receive venous blood, which is oxygenated in the lungs and distributed through the arterial circulation.

The lungs receive the venous blood from the right heart, which in turn is the main confluence of the superior and inferior venae cavae. The blood enters the lungs through the pulmonary artery, which branches into progressively smaller branches. Ultimately the blood enters into capillaries, which are found in the alveolar septa, thus forming the alveolar-capillary units (Fig. 5-4). The red blood cells of the venous blood release CO_2, which enters the alveolar spaccs and is exhaled into the outside air. Oxygen inhaled from the air crosses the alveolar membrane that is formed from the attenuated cytoplasm of type I pneumocytes. Thereafter it passes through the capillary membranes, enters the blood, and binds to the hemoglobin of red blood cells. The oxygenated blood leaves the alveolar-capillary units and enters the pulmonary venules, from which it reaches the pulmonary veins, the left heart, and ultimately the arterial circulation.

Several cellular systems protect the lungs from airborne pathogens, allergens, and harmful particulate material.

The air inhaled through the nose or the mouth contains potentially noxious agents, including viruses, bacteria, and various organic and inorganic particles. The most important protective mechanisms (Fig. 5-5) are as follows:

Mucociliary clearance. The mucus produced by the goblet cells in the nasal mucosa or the tracheobronchial epithelium covers the entire surface of the air-conducting tubular part of the respiratory system. The bronchi also contain mucous glands. The mucus they secrete consists of glycosaminoglycans, glycoproteins, and complex carbohydrates. The mucus can bind living pathogens and other particulate matter. Bactericidal substances in the mucus, such as properdin, or immunoglobulin A, act on bacteria. Mucus also contains macrophages, which phagocytose or kill bacteria. These bacteria and other particulate matter are moved up the tracheobronchial tree through the ciliary movement of the columnar cells in the tracheobronchial epithelium. This mucociliary escalator system will, under normal circumstances, eliminate most of the particles that measure 2 to

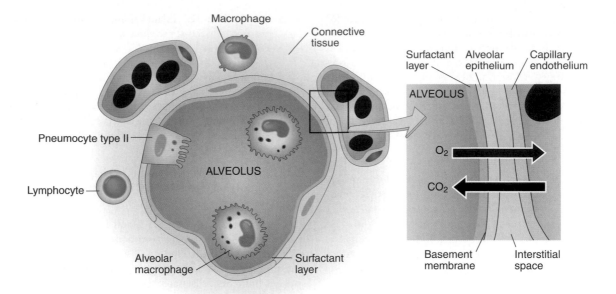

Figure 5-4 Alveolus and the alveolar-capillary unit. The alveolus is lined with type I and type II pneumocytes, lying on a basement membrane that separates them from the interstitial spaces around the alveolar capillaries. The interstitium contains a few fibroblasts and scattered lymphocytes and macrophages. Some macrophages, called alveolar macrophages, are also normally found inside the alveoli.

10 μm in diameter, but particles that are smaller than 2 μm may reach the alveoli. Such particles are usually taken up by alveolar macrophages and either are expectorated or enter into the interstitial spaces and ultimately are carried by the lymph into the local lymph nodes.

Pearls

> Kartagener's syndrome, a congenital ciliary motility disorder, is characterized by recurrent bronchopulmonary infections owing to reduced mucociliary clearance.
> Cystic fibrosis is characterized by a production of very viscous mucus that cannot be expectorated readily. Accumulation of mucus in the bronchi predisposes the patient to recurrent infections and formation of bronchiectases.

Lymphatic clearance. Foreign material taken up by the alveolar macrophages is transported by the lymphatics. Although the alveoli do not contain lymphatics, well-formed lymphatic channels are recognizable at the level of alveolar ducts. The lungs have an extensive lymphatic drainage system, which extends from the alveolar ducts, along the interlobular septa, to the connective tissue surrounding the blood vessels and bronchi. The lymph from both lungs, except for the left upper lobe, drains into the right lymphatic duct; the left upper lobe drains into the thoracic duct.

Pulmonary immune response. Along the intrapulmonary lymphatics and in the mucosae of the bronchi are aggregates of nonencapsulated lymphoid tissue that form the so-called **mucosa-associated lymphoid tissue (MALT).** These lymphoid follicles serve as mechanical barriers but are also the main source of immune cells that protect the lungs from bacteria and foreign allergens. The immune response typically includes both T and B cells. The lungs also contain numerous resident macrophages and antigen-presenting cells such as Langerhans cells. Hence some cell-mediated immune reactions, such as those that occur in response to exposure to *Mycobacterium tuberculosis* or fungi, result in granuloma formation.

Pearls

> Congenital immunodeficiency disorders are characterized by recurrent and often fatal pulmonary infections.
> Acquired immunodeficiency syndrome is often complicated by pulmonary infections. Pulmonary infection with *Pneumocystis jiroveci* is one of the opportunistic infections to which AIDS patients are vulnerable.

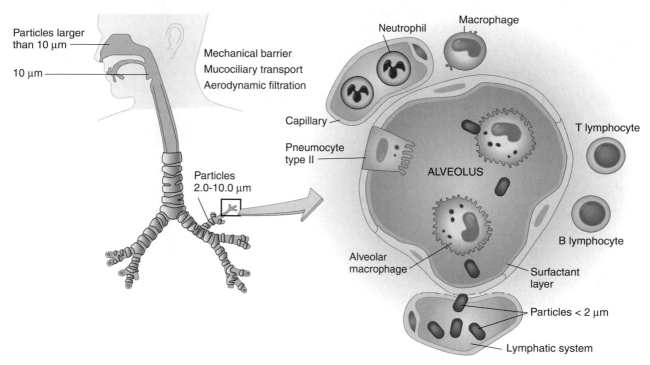

Figure 5-5 Defense mechanisms of the lungs. The airways protect the body from foreign particulate matter and bacteria. These defense mechanisms include a mechanical barrier, mucus, and mucociliary transport aided by the movement of cilia in the upper respiratory tact, trachea, and bronchi. Mobile phagocytic cells (macrophages) also protect the lungs by secreting cytokines. Lymphocytes of the mucosa-associated system include both B and T cells. Surfactant secreted by type II pneumocytes also protects the alveoli. White blood cells may enter the lungs from the alveolar capillaries to enhance the defense mechanisms.

PHYSIOLOGY

Ventilation is a process during which the air moves in and out of the lungs.

Oxygen enters the blood in the lungs from the inhaled air in the alveoli and is transported thereafter bound to the hemoglobin in red blood cells. At the same time carbon dioxide is released from venous blood and is exhaled through the lungs. Total ventilation (V_E) is expressed as the volume of air that enters and leaves the lungs in a minute, depending on the frequency of breath per minute (*f*) and the tidal volume of air inspired/expired per minute V_T:

$$V_E = f \times V_T$$

In normal adults the V_T is approximately 500 mL/min, and in children 3 to 5 mL/kg/min.

The air entering the lungs follows the basic physical laws defined by Boyle and Dalton. According to **Boyle's law** the pressure and volume of a gas are directly related if the temperature is constant. According to **Dalton's law** the partial pressure of a gas in a gas mixture equals the pressure that the gas would exert if it occupied the entire volume. Thus the sum of partial pressures of gases—which for the inhaled air is 21% oxygen and 79% nitrogen— must equal 100%. The tension of oxygen can thus be increased by increasing the pressure over the normal pressure under which the air enters the lungs (760 mm Hg at sea level) or by increasing the concentration of oxygen. This principle is used when applying machine-assisted artificial respiration. At high altitude, however, the total atmospheric pressure decreases and can thus result in hypoxia.

Partial pressure of gases is the key determinant of external and internal respiration.

External respiration takes place in the lungs. During this process the O_2 from the inhaled air is transferred to the blood and the CO_2 diffuses from blood into the air. *Internal respiration* refers to cellular processes that allow the transfer of O_2 from red blood cells through the capillary wall into the tissues and thereby for use within the cell. Both processes depend on the partial pressures of O_2 and CO_2 (Fig. 5-6). Note in Figure 5-6 that the consumption of O_2 leads to major fluctuations in the partial pressure of O_2, which drops from 100 mm Hg in the arterial blood to 40 mm Hg in venous blood. In contrast, the fluctuations of CO_2 are much smaller, from 40 mm Hg in arterial blood to 46 mm Hg in venous blood.

Transfer of gases in the alveolar-capillary unit occurs by simple diffusion.

The transition of O_2 from air into the blood and CO_2 from blood to the air occurs through diffusion across the alveolar lining and the basement membranes of the alveolar capillaries (Fig. 5-7). This process is governed by **Fick's law** as stated here:

$$V_{gas} = \frac{A \times D\,(P_1 - P_2)}{T}$$

where V_{gas} = volume of gas transferred per unit of time

D = diffusion coefficient of the gas

A = surface area of the diffusion membrane

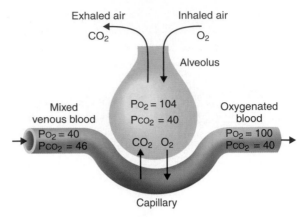

Figure 5-6 External and internal respiration. The lungs play a pivotal role in gas exchange between the air and the blood (external respiration). The oxygen (O_2) is transported to the periphery, where the internal respiration takes place in the tissues. The pressure of oxygen varies from 160 mm Hg in the inhaled air to 100 mm Hg in the terminal air spaces (alveoli). Note also that the air is humidified, which lowers the pressure of oxygen from 160 to 150 mm Hg. Carbon dioxide (CO_2) formed inside the tissues is carried by the blood from the tissues and exhaled in the lungs. P_{O_2}, partial pressure of oxygen; P_{CO_2}, partial pressure of carbon dioxide.

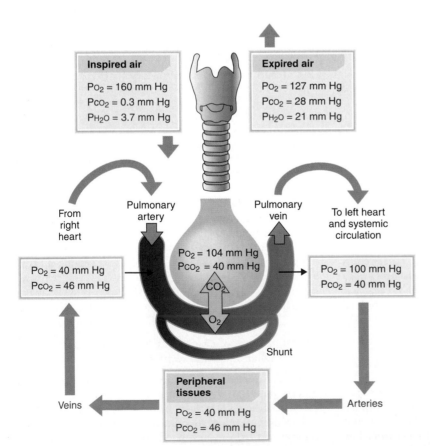

Figure 5-7 Alveolar-capillary unit. CO_2 from the venous blood is exhaled and O_2 from the inhaled air is taken up into the blood, which leaves the alveolar-capillary unit as oxygenated as arterial blood. P_{CO_2}, partial pressure of carbon dioxide; P_{H_2O}, partial pressure of water vapor; P_{O_2}, partial pressure of oxygen.

$P_1 - P_2$ = partial pressure of gas on each side of the diffusion membrane, which in the lungs includes two pressure gradients: one across the alveolar wall and the other across the capillary basement membrane

T = tissue thickness

Fick's law indicates that the diffusion of gases is directly proportional to the surface area of the alveoli and inversely proportional to the thickness of the tissue that prevents diffusion. In practice this diffusion rate is determined by measuring the inhalation efficiency of CO, a gas that has high solubility in blood and can be readily measured after inhalation in both the alveolar spaces and the blood.

Pearls

> In restrictive lung diseases the diffusion of CO_2 from alveolar air into the blood is reduced.
> In emphysema the alveolar surface area is reduced due to a loss of alveoli.

Oxygen pressure in inspired dry air is higher than in the humidified air in the trachea or the alveoli or the oxygenated arterial blood leaving the lungs.

Assuming that the air contains 21% O_2, at sea level the oxygen pressure in dry inhaled air is 160 mm Hg (760 × 0.21 = 160). This air is humidified during its passage through the nose and trachea, which brings down the oxygen pressure to 150 mm Hg (see Fig. 5-7). As the air passes into the alveoli, the oxygen pressure drops to 100 mm Hg. This is in part due to the fact that oxygen diffuses rather rapidly into the blood and is also diluted with CO_2 diffusing from the venous blood into the alveoli.

Theoretically the oxygen pressure in the alveoli should be the same as that in the pulmonary artery branches. However, the arterial oxygen pressure is lower than that in the alveoli, and thus the **ventilation/perfusion ratio ($\dot{V}/\dot{Q}$) is normally 0.8.** This defect results from the admixture of venous bronchial blood entering the pulmonary veins and a small amount of pulmonary venous blood that bypasses the alveoli through a **physiologic right-to-left shunt** and is not oxygenated. Approximately 2% of the normal cardiac output bypasses the alveoli. $\dot{V}/\dot{Q}$ ratio is reduced in many lung diseases.

Pearls

> Major right-to-left shunts occur most often in congenital cardiac defects rather than in the lungs.
> $\dot{V}/\dot{Q}$ defects can result from obstruction of the airflow passages (e.g., in obstructive lung disease) or from the obstruction of pulmonary blood flow (e.g., pulmonary embolism).

Breathing is an involuntary action that is under the control of the respiratory center in the brainstem.

Breathing is a vital function that is tightly controlled by the central nervous system, which receives impulses from the periphery and then sends efferent signals to the periphery (Fig. 5-8). The key anatomic foci of the respiratory control sensory and effector system are as follows:

■ Respiratory control centers in the medulla and the pons
■ Cerebral cortex
■ Central and peripheral chemoreceptors
■ Mechanoreceptors in the lungs, muscle, and joints
■ Inspiratory and expiratory muscles

Respiratory centers. Respiration is controlled by three centers in the brainstem: the medullary respiratory center, the apneustic center, and the pneumotaxic center. Automatic respiratory movements are under the control of the **inspiratory center** in the dorsal medulla, which receives the stimulatory impulses from the peripheral sensors, mostly through the glossopharyngeal and vagus nerves. Efferent signals are sent to the diaphragm through the phrenic nerve. The **expiratory center** located in the ventral medulla is dormant because expiration is normally a passive process. It becomes activated, however, during exercise. The inspiratory center also receives positive stimuli from the **apneustic center** in the lower pons. This center prolongs the inspiratory gaps ("apneusis") by prolonging the contraction of the diaphragm. The **pneumotaxic center** in the upper pons inhibits respiration by reducing the tidal volume, but it does not affect the rhythmicity of breathing.

Cerebral cortex. Respiration can be controlled to a certain extent by voluntarily cortical stimuli. Hyperventilation can be induced relatively easily, but once the arterial partial pressure of carbon dioxide (Pa_{CO_2}) falls below a critical level, the person loses consciousness and automatic respirations resume. Hypoventilation can also be induced but it does not last long because the reduction of the arterial partial pressure of oxygen (Pa_{O_2}) and increased Pa_{CO_2} are strong stimuli for the resumption of respiration.

Chemoreceptors. Chemoreceptors can be classified as central or peripheral.

■ **Central chemoreceptors** located in the brainstem act directly on the inspiratory center. They respond to changes in the pH of the cerebrospinal fluid; its acidity stimulates inspiration, whereas the increased pH slows down the respiratory movements.
■ **Chemoreceptors in the carotid and aortic bodies** respond to the Pa_{CO_2}, Pa_{O_2}, and pH, sending stimuli to the inspiratory center. Reduced P_{O_2}, decreased Pa_{CO_2}, and decreased pH increase the rate of respiration.

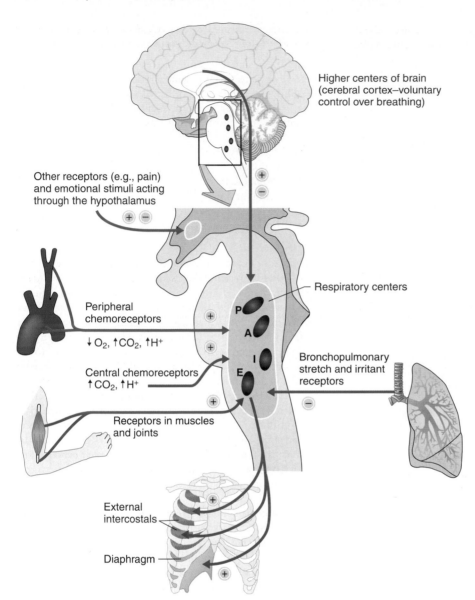

Higher centers of brain (cerebral cortex–voluntary control over breathing)

Other receptors (e.g., pain) and emotional stimuli acting through the hypothalamus

Peripheral chemoreceptors

$\downarrow O_2, \uparrow CO_2, \uparrow H^+$

Central chemoreceptors $\uparrow CO_2, \uparrow H^+$

Respiratory centers

P
A
I
E

Bronchopulmonary stretch and irritant receptors

Receptors in muscles and joints

External intercostals

Diaphragm

Figure 5-8 Neural control of respiration. Respiration is under the control of the medullary centers, which contain a sensitive area responding to chemical stimuli and receive impulses from the peripheral nervous system. The cortical centers also may influence respiration. The efferent stimuli from the respiratory center are transmitted to respiratory muscles, primarily the intercostals and the diaphragm. A, apneustic; E, expiratory center; I, inspiratory; P, pneumotaxic.

Pearl

> In metabolic acidosis the chemoreceptors respond to lowered pH by increasing the rate of respiration.

Mechanoreceptors. Receptors responding to stretch in the **smooth muscles** of the bronchi activate the **Hering-Breuer reflex,** which slows down respiration by prolonging the expiratory time. Stretch receptors found in the **skeletal muscles and joints** may also increase the respiratory rate.

Irritant receptors in the mucosa of the bronchi react to chemical stimuli and particles, causing bronchoconstriction, which also increases the rate of respiration. Irritant receptors

are important for initiating coughing, which can, however, also be triggered by the stimuli reaching the mechanoreceptors. Likewise, the irritant receptors in the nose are important for the initiation of sneezing. Irritant receptors are linked to C type nerve fibers, which also transmit pain.

The volume of air entering and leaving the lungs during inspiration and expiration can be measured objectively under controlled circumstances.

Normal breathing occurs in a cycle that includes four phases: rest, inspiration, a rest phase, and expiration. By measuring the volume of air entering the lungs during inspiration and leaving it during expiration the critical aspects of respiratory capacity can be defined as illustrated in Figure 5-9. By convention these **static lung volumes** are defined as follows:

- **Tidal volume** (V_T)—the amount of air entering and leaving the lung with each breath in a person who is breathing normally. In adults it measures approximately 500 mL.
- **Functional residual capacity** (FRC)—the amount of air remaining in the lungs after expiration in a person who is breathing normally. FRC cannot be measured by routine spirometry, but can be measured by the helium dilution method, the nitrogen washout technique, or whole-body plethysmography.
- **Expiratory reserve volume** (ERV)—the amount of air that can be exhaled from the lungs by forceful expiration.
- **Residual volume** (RV)—the amount of air remaining in the lungs after forceful expiration. RV is calculated by subtracting ERV from FRC (RV = FRC − ERV). In young adults it accounts for 20% of the total lung capacity. It increases by 1% per year and in older individuals it accounts for more than 60% of the total lung capacity.
- **Inspiratory reserve volume** (IRV)—the amount of air that can be forcefully inhaled in addition to the V_T.
- **Inspiratory capacity** (IC)—the amount of air that can be inhaled into the lungs in addition to the air accounting for the FRC (IC = V_T + IRV).
- **Vital capacity** (VC)—the amount of air expelled from the lungs during forceful expiration.
- **Total lung capacity** (TLC)—the total amount of air inside the lungs and the bronchial tree after maximal inspiration.
- **Forced vital capacity** (FVC)—the amount of air that can be expelled from the lungs if a person is told to exhale as fast as possible. Normally FVC does not differ from VC. However, FVC can be prolonged due to air trapping that occurs in persons who have emphysema.
- **Forced expiratory volume** (FEV_1)—the amount of air that can be expired in 1 second following maximal inspiration. FEV_1 in healthy young adults is normally 80% of the forced vital capacity (FEV_1/FVC = 0.8), but with aging FEV_1 is reduced to 65% to 70%. FEV_1/FVC is effort-dependent and is influenced by increased expiratory effort. In obstructive lung diseases FEV_1 is reduced (FEV_1/FVC < 70%). In restrictive lung diseases, both FEV_1 and FVC are reduced (FEV_1/FVC > 70%).
- **Forced expiratory flow rate** ($FEF_{25-75\%}$)—the rate of air flow over the middle (25% to 75%) half of the FVC. It is also called maximal midexpiratory flow rate and is considered to be the most sensitive parameter for identifying early obstruction. It reflects the status of small airways and it is effort-independent.

Pearl

> Vital capacity (VC), inspiratory capacity (IC), and expiratory reserve volume (ERV) can be measured with a spirometer, whereas the measurement of functional residual capacity (FRC) and total lung capacity (TLC) requires additional special studies.

Clinical and Laboratory Evaluation of Pulmonary Diseases

The evaluation of patients who may have lung diseases includes a complete history and physical examination, with special emphasis on symptoms that may be related to

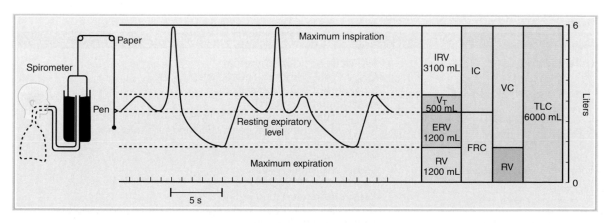

Figure 5-9 Respiratory volumes. The lungs have an enormous respiratory reserve and can increase their function when needed. The capacity of the lung to increase gas exchange can be measured and expressed as total lung capacity (TLC). Other lung volumes include vital capacity (VC), residual volume (RV), inspiratory capacity (IC), functional reserve capacity (FRC), inspiratory reserve volume (IRV), tidal volume (V_T), and expiratory reserve volume (ERV).

respiratory problems. In addition chest radiographs, laboratory test data, and acid–base balance must be reviewed. Spirometry and testing of respiratory function may be indicated. Bronchoscopy, thoracentesis, and fine-needle or tissue biopsy are required in certain conditions.

FAMILY AND PERSONAL HISTORY

A family history and a personal history are essential for identifying some of the major risk factors for lung diseases. Examples of such associations that can be discovered by carefully interviewing the patient or his family are given in Table 5-1.

SIGNS AND SYMPTOMS OF LUNG DISEASES

The most important signs and symptoms of lung diseases are as follows:

- Dyspnea
- Cough
- Hemoptysis
- Chest pain
- Altered breathing pattern
- Abnormal respiratory sounds
- Hypoxia, cyanosis, and respiratory acidosis

Dyspnea is a sensation of breathlessness out of proportion to the level of physical activity.

Dyspnea, also known as shortness of breath, is a subjective sensation of difficult breathing. The patients describe it as strained breathing or simply state that they are "short of breath." As stated by a famous pulmonary physician, "Dyspnea is not tachypnea, hyperpnea, or hyperventilation but difficult labored and uncomfortable breathing."

Elemental sensations include tightness in the chest, excessive ventilation, excessive frequency, and trouble breathing. These sensations have an *objective* aspect based on the integration of physiologic sensory impulses reaching the respiratory centers of the brainstem and a *subjective* aspect depending on the cortical perception of the efficiency of respiration. The objective impulses from central and peripheral chemoreceptors responding to blood oxygen levels, CO_2 content, and pH, and mechanoreceptors in the pulmonary parenchyma, airways, and respiratory muscles, can be measured. The subjective perception is, however, less quantifiable and varies from one person to another.

As discussed in Chapter 4, dyspnea can be classified as cardiac or noncardiac, acute or chronic. The most important causes of dyspnea are listed in Table 5-2.

Patients can usually grade their dyspnea as mild, moderate, or severe, and whether it is related to physical activity or also occurs at rest. The precipitating cause can often be identified.

Patients also can describe the time of onset and the duration of shortness of breath. The timing of dyspnea provides important diagnostic clues, as listed in Table 5-3.

Cough involves a reflex that can be triggered by a wide variety of stimuli.

Cough is a defense mechanism based on a reflex, which can be initiated by chemical or mechanical irritants or by voluntary action. The irritants, such as chemicals or foreign bodies reaching the larynx or the lower respiratory tract mucosa, act on mechanoreceptors and nociceptors. These receptors are connected to C type nerve fibers that serve as the conduit for pain impulses, leading them into the medulla oblongata through the vagus nerve. In the medulla the impulses trigger the efferent reaction that has three phases:

Table 5-1 Risk Factors for Lung Diseases

TYPE OF RISK FACTOR	SPECIFIC DISEASES–RISK FACTOR ASSOCIATIONS
Hereditary factors	AAT-deficiency: Emphysema
	Cystic fibrosis: Bronchiectasis/pneumonia
Social and work-related factors	Smoking: COPD, lung cancer
	Dust: Pneumoconiosis
	Exogenous allergens: Asthma, hypersensitivity pneumonitis
Infections	Viral and bacterial infections: URD and pneumonia
	Tuberculosis
	AIDS-related infections
Medical and surgical procedures	Sepsis and shock: ARDS
	Heart failure: Pulmonary edema
	Respirator-related lung injury
Drugs/toxins	Drug-induced lung diseases: Numerous drugs can cause lung diseases
External mechanical factors	Thoracic injury: Pneumothorax
	Brain injury: Injury of the respiratory center

AAT, α_1-antitrypsin; AIDS, acquired immunodeficiency syndrome; ARDS, acute respiratory distress syndrome; COPD, chronic obstructive pulmonary disease; URD, upper respiratory disease.

Table 5-2 Causes of Dyspnea

TYPE OF DYSPNEA	PATHOGENESIS	CLINICAL CONDITIONS
Pulmonary dyspnea	Obstruction of airways	Croup (acute laryngitis) Asthma Chronic bronchitis
	Alveolar filling	Pulmonary edema (e.g., toxic) Pneumonia
	Interstitial lung disease	Viral pneumonia Chronic pneumonitis
	Pulmonary artery obstruction	Pulmonary embolism Primary pulmonary hypertension
	Pleural disease	Pneumothorax Pleural effusion
Cardiac dyspnea	Left heart failure	Myocardial infarction
	Pericardial disease	Pericardial tamponade
	Endocardial defect	Chronic endocarditis
Other forms of dyspnea	Loss of RBC/Hb/O$_2$ transport	Bleeding Anemia CO poisoning
	Hypoperfusion of lungs	Multiple organ failure (shock)
	Psychogenic	Anxiety, panic attack
	Neuromuscular diseases	Myopathy/muscular dystrophy
	Thoracic deformities	Kyphoscoliosis

RBC/Hb/O$_2$, red blood cell/hemoglobin/oxygen.

Table 5-3 Classification of Dyspnea by Type of Onset

Hyperacute (minutes)
Strangulation
Airway obstruction (e.g., foreign body)
Pulmonary embolism
Pneumothorax

Acute (hours)
Cardiogenic pulmonary edema
ARDS, shock
Pneumonia
Asthma

Subacute (days)
Pleural effusion
Pulmonary disease (e.g., lung cancer, sarcoidosis)

Chronic (months/years)
COPD
Heart disease
Anemia, metabolic and systemic diseases

Intermittent (periodic/recurrent)
Asthma
Heart disease
Severe obesity

ARDS, acute respiratory distress syndrome; COPD, chronic obstructive pulmonary disease.
Data from Warrell DA, Cox TM, Firth JD (eds): Oxford Textbook of Medicine, 4th ed. Oxford, Oxford University Press, 2003.

- Deep inspiration leads to increased air content of the chest.
- Closure of the glottis concomitant with an expiratory effort results in increased intrathoracic pressure.
- Opening of the glottis while the expiratory muscles contract propels the air under high pressure into the oropharynx and into the atmosphere.

Pearl

> Forceful coughing may cause lightheadedness and syncope because increased intrathoracic pressure may compress the venae cavae and reduce the return of venous blood into the right heart.

Cough may be clinically classified as **acute,** lasting a few days or a week or two, or **chronic** if it last more than 3 weeks. It may be accompanied by bleeding or sputum production *(productive cough).* Some irritants that cause cough may also cause bronchospasm, and in such cases cough is associated with wheezing (e.g., in asthma). Cough may be the only complaint, but often it is just one of the symptoms of a complex disease such as asthma or bronchopneumonia. The most important causes of cough are listed in Table 5-4.

Table 5-4 Causes of Cough

Infections
Sinusitis ("postnasal drip")
Tracheobronchitis
Pneumonia

Environemental Irritants
Smoking
Dust and air pollutants
Pollen

Mechanical Irritants
Bronchial tumors
GERD with aspiration into lungs
Pulmonary edema (e.g., heart disease)

Chronic Inflammatory Conditions
COPD
Asthma
Sarcoidosis

Drugs
ACE inhibitors

ACE, angiotensin-converting enzyme; COPD, chronic obstructive pulmonary disease; GERD, gastroesophageal reflux disease.

Pearl

> Cough can be suppressed with drugs that anesthetize respiratory receptors (e.g., benzonatate or phenol-containing drugs) or by raising the threshold for the sensory impulses in the medullary cough center (e.g., dextromethorphan).

Hemoptysis may present as mild, in the form of blood-stained sputum, or massive and life-threatening.

Hemoptysis is defined as expectoration of blood from the respiratory tract. Most often it originates from the bronchial arterial circulation, but it may have other sources as well. Remember that the bronchial arteries are part of the greater arterial system, and the blood in these arteries circulates under much higher pressure than the blood in the pulmonary venous or arterial circulation, which are low-pressure systems. Hence, if these vessels rupture, the bleeding occurs under much higher pressure than if it stemmed from pulmonary arteries and veins. However, if the pressure inside the pulmonary circulation rises, as in pulmonary hypertension, bleeding may occur from other vessels as well. Tumors may cause bleeding by eroding into any blood vessel. Autoimmune diseases, such as Wegener's granulomatosis or Goodpasture's syndrome, may cause vascular lesions, leading to a rupture of various blood vessels from small capillaries to larger arteries and veins. The most important causes of hemoptysis are listed in Table 5-5.

Hemoptysis may be mild or severe; if the amount of expectorated blood is in the range of 100 to 500 mL/24 hours it is usually called *massive*. However, most patients are so frightened that the exact amount of blood often cannot be estimated from their description.

Pearl

> Hemoptysis must be distinguished from hematemesis of gastrointestinal origin. The blood expectorated from lungs is arterial and thus red and alkaline, whereas in hematemesis the blood is dark red and acidic due to the gastric contents.

Table 5-5 Sources and Causes of Hemoptysis

SITE	LESION/CAUSE	DISEASES
Bronchi	Tumors	Bronchial carcinoma
	Inflammation	COPD
		Bronchiectasis
Lung parenchyma	Infection	Pneumonia
		Abscess
		Tuberculosis
	Immune disease	Wegener's granulomatosis
		Goodpasture's syndrome
	Trauma	Rupture or gunshot wound
Pulmonary vessels	Thromboemboli	Pulmonary embolism
	Pulmonary hypertension	Mitral valve stenosis/insufficiency
		Left heart failure
		Primary pulmonary hypertension
Multifocal	Coagulopathy	Bleeding tendency
		Leukemia
	Shock/DIC	ARDS

ARDS, acute respiratory distress syndrome, COPD, chronic obstructive pulmonary disease; DIC, dismanianted intravascular coagulation.

Pain is of pulmonary origin in only 5% of patients who present with acute chest pain.

Most patients who present with acute chest pain have either an underlying gastroesophageal disorder (e.g., gastroesophageal reflux disease) or a cardiovascular disease (e.g., myocardial infarction or angina pectoris). The lungs are the source of pain in a minority of cases: 2% can be assigned to pleural or pulmonary inflammation, 2% to pulmonary emboli, and 1% to other causes including carcinoma.

Pain of pulmonary origin may be classified as visceral or pleuritic.

- **Visceral pain** is typically dull, deep-seated, and poorly localized. Such pain may be encountered in patients with pneumonia, cancer, or pulmonary emboli.
- **Pleuritic pain** is of variable intensity, intensifying during movements of the chest, and typically reaching its peak during inspiration or coughing. Pleuritic pain is a feature of pleuritis or pneumonia that has extended to the pleural surface. Pneumothorax may cause pleuritic pain that is typically of sudden onset and associated with dyspnea.

The automatic breathing pattern may be altered in several ways.

The normal breathing (**eupnea**) is under the control of medullary respiratory centers, which ensure its rhythmicity at a rate of 12 to 17 breaths per minute. The normal rhythm can be altered voluntarily through cortical input, but also in response to various impulses from the periphery and changes in the basic metabolism. Several clinically important respiratory patterns can be recognized, the most important of which are illustrated in Figure 5-10 and briefly described here.

Hyperpnea. This form of increased respiratory effort includes **tachypnea** (i.e., increased rate of respiration) and an increase of the tidal volume. Deeper than normal inspiration that occurs periodically in normal persons is called **sigh.** Extreme sigh is called **yawning.**

Hyperpnea occurs physiologically during exercise, it can be induced voluntarily, but it is also accompanied by fever in many diseases. Two forms of clinically important of hyperpnea occur:

- **Hyperventilation.** Due to forceful expiration of CO_2 this form of hyperpnea is characterized by low $PaCO_2$. Typically it occurs in pregnancy, panic attacks, and in patients who have cirrhosis or metabolic acidosis.
- **Kussmaul breathing,** characterized by very deep rapid breathing, is a feature of metabolic acidosis and is most often encountered in diabetic ketoacidosis.

Apnea. The term refers to the cessation of breathing that can be voluntary or involuntary. One may decide to stop breathing, but such voluntary apnea can last only for a short time, whereupon it resumes automatically. Respiration resumes when CO_2 accumulates in the blood and the PaO_2 reaches approximately 50 mm Hg. At that point the inspiratory stimulus overwhelms the voluntary effort to withhold the breath. If respiration does not resume, apnea results in respiratory arrest.

Apnea may occur under a variety of pathologic or otherwise poorly understood conditions as follows:

- **Depression or injury of the respiratory centers.** Brain edema or injury of the respiratory centers by trauma or stroke may depress the function of the respiratory centers and cause apnea.

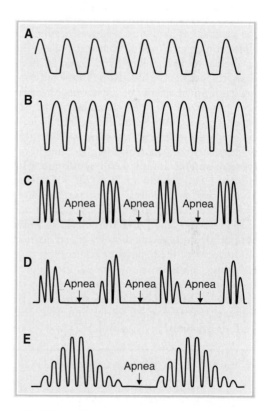

Figure 5-10 Breathing abnormalities. **A,** Eupnea. Normal breathing is characterized by regular rhythmicity. **B,** Kussmaul breathing. The breathing is fast and has a high amplitude. **C,** Cluster breathing. Spurts of respiration interchange with periods of apnea. The amplitude of respirations may vary, or the respirations may be of the same amplitude. If the amplitudes are uniform, the breathing is known as Biot's respirations. **D,** Ataxic respiration. The amplitude of respirations and their frequency vary. Periods of apnea occur at random. **E,** Cheyne-Stokes respiration is characterized by clusters of respiration that have waxing and waning amplitudes and are separated by periods of apnea.

- **Obstructed sleep apnea.** This rather common disease is characterized by an intermittent cessation of respiration during sleep. Typically it occurs in elderly men. Alcohol and obesity are considered to be among the risk factors, but the true pathogenesis of the apnea is not fully known. It is associated with a loss of muscle tone of pharyngeal muscles that occurs during the REM sleep and it is associated with snoring. The resulting hypoxia typically wakes up the affected person, thus disrupting the normal sleeping pattern. Accordingly such persons are chronically tired. Obstructed apnea may occur also in excessively obese patients. This condition is called **Pickwickian syndrome** in reference to Charles Dickens' novel *The Pickwick Papers,* in which the author described a constantly somnolent obese young man showing signs of periodic apnea.

- **Central (nonobstructed) sleep apnea.** In this disease, the central impulses that regulate breathing are lost. This condition may result from metabolic disturbances or alveolar hypoventilation syndromes. In these conditions Po_2 levels in the blood drop below the critical level needed for maintenance of respiration. Since the Po_2 is normally lower during wakefulness and in these patients it does not rise on falling asleep (as it normally does in healthy persons), apnea occurs during the onset of sleep. Central sleep apnea is also thought to be the cause of **sudden infant death syndrome (SIDS).** In affected infants respiration stops for 30 to 60 seconds, leading to a drop of Pao_2. These patients have apparently a decreased chemoreceptor sensitivity to oxygen tension in the blood and thus may die because the peripheral impulses are not generated to restart the automaticity of the respiratory center.

- **Gasping.** This form of apnea interrupted with bouts of respiratory effort typically occurs in dying patients. The inspiration is short and typically followed by prolonged expiration and prolonged periods of apnea.

Pearl

> Apnea, or cessation of breathing, must be distinguished from apneusis. Apneusis is a form of breathing in which prolonged and deep inspiratory movement is followed by a short and shallow expiration. Apneusis is under the control of the medullary apneustic center, which is activated when the lungs expand to a certain critical volume.

Periodic breathing. If the normal rhythmicity of respiration is disrupted, breathing becomes irregular. Such breathing typically occurs in patients who have medullary or pontine lesions. Several patterns can be recognized as follows:

- **Cluster breathing.** In this form of periodic breathing, groups of respiratory movements of variable amplitude are separated by prolonged periods of apnea.
- **Biot's respirations.** In this subtype of cluster breathing the amplitudes of respiration do not vary but are of equal size in each cluster.
- **Ataxic breathing.** In this form of breathing the amplitude of breaths varies greatly and respirations are followed by apnea at irregular intervals.
- **Cheyne-Stokes breathing.** This form is characterized by episodes of respiration showing a gradual increase and decrease in the tidal volume, followed by a gradual decrease and a period of apnea. Cheyne-Stokes breathing occurs in various conditions characterized by hypoxia, such as heart or lung disease, but also in patients with brain injury. Note that it can also occur in normal persons.

Respiratory sounds change in the course of various diseases and are of diagnostic importance.

The passage of air through the bronchi and the lungs generates sounds that can be auscultated during physical examination with the stethoscope. The same is true for the voice, which is formed in the larynx but is transmitted through the airways.

Normally aerated lungs transmit both high-pitched and low-pitched sounds to the chest wall (Fig. 5-11). High-frequency sounds are usually attenuated and thus barely

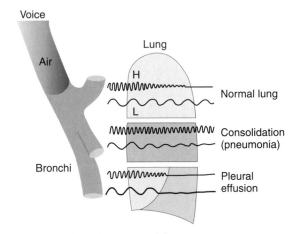

Figure 5-11 Sound transmission in the lungs. Air flow through the air passages generates high-pitched (H) and low-pitched (L) sounds that are transmitted to the chest wall and can be heard with the stethoscope. Consolidation of lungs in pneumonia filters the low-pitched sounds but does not affect the transmission of high-pitched sounds, which sound even more resonant. Pleural effusion reflects the sound and does not allow the sound to pass to the chest wall. (Modified and redrawn with permission from Brewis RAL: Lecture Notes on Respiratory Disease. Oxford, Blackwell Scientific, 1985, p. 52.)

heard during so-called normal **vesicular breathing.** In pneumonia, when the alveoli become consolidated, some low-pitched sounds are filtered, whereas the high-pitched sounds generated in the bronchi become more sonorous because of the filtering of the background noise. This phenomenon is called **bronchial breathing.** The same is true for vocal resonance while the patient is speaking. **Pleural effusion,** on the other hand, forms a barrier between the lungs and the chest wall, which does not allow transmission of bronchial sounds. Pleural masses and fibrosis or pneumothorax have the same effect. Hence no breath sounds can be heard, and vocal resonance is reduced.

Adventitious sounds include crackles and wheezes and pleural friction rub.

Adventitious sounds are signs of pulmonary pathology and are not heard over the normal lungs. Such sounds stemming from the lungs are classified as crackles and wheezes, whereas those originating from the pleura are called pleural friction rub.

Crackles. Previously known as "rales" or "crepitus," these sounds are nonmusical, explosive, discontinuous, and heard over a wide spectrum of frequencies. They result from the opening of small to medium-sized air spaces in an abnormally deflated part of the lung.

Crackles can be classified as early inspirational, late inspirational, and paninspirational (Fig. 5-12) as follows:

- **Early inspiratory crackles.** These low-pitched sounds, often associated with crackles in the late expiratory phase, are typically found in obstructive lung disease and severe congestive heart failure.

- **Late inspiratory crackles.** These sounds are characteristic of "stiffened lung" found in chronic interstitial disease or pulmonary fibrosis but may also be found in atelectasis and chronic heart failure.

- **Paninspiratory crackles.** These sounds are usually found in patients who have both cardiac and pulmonary disease.

Wheezes. These sounds are musical and can be heard through the stethoscope or at the mouth. Wheezes originate from the passage of air through narrowed medium and large airways (Fig. 5-13). The dynamics of the air flow cause back and forth vibrations of the bronchial wall and a flutelike musical sound that is recognized as high-pitched or low-pitched wheezes. Typically they are found in asthma.

Hypoxemia results from inadequate oxygenation of blood in the lungs.

Low oxygen level (hypoxemia) is often caused by lung diseases. It may result from the following disturbances:

- **Reduced concentration of oxygen in the air.** This typically occurs at high altitudes.
- **Obstruction of air spaces.** Typically this is found during strangulation or hanging, by inhalation of foreign bodies into the larynx and trachea, or by drowning.
- **Alveolar hypoventilation.** This occurs due to inadequate respiratory effort due to muscle weakness such as occurs in myasthenia gravis or muscular dystrophy, or in kyphoscoliosis.
- **Impaired diffusion of air into the blood in the alveolar capillary unit.** The diffusion of air into the

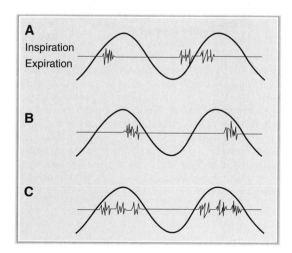

Figure 5-12 Crackles. **A,** Early inspiratory crackles, which are often associated with late expiratory crackles. **B,** Late inspiratory crackles. **C,** Paninspiratory crackles. (Modified from Glauser FL: Signs and Symptoms in Pulmonary Medicine. Lippincott Williams & Wilkins, Philadelphia, 1983.)

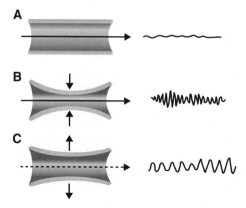

Figure 5-13 Wheezes. **A,** Normal passage of air does not cause any vibrations. **B,** If the bronchus is narrowed the air passes through faster than normal to maintain the same flow, leading to a high-pitched sound. **C,** Dilatation of the lumen slows the airflow, producing a lower pitched sound.

blood in the lungs could be impeded by edema, pneumonic infiltrates, or thickening of the alveolar walls in various chronic interstitial lung diseases.

■ **Ventilation/perfusion mismatch.** This occurs due to the obstruction of the terminal air spaces in COPD, loss of alveolar surfaces in emphysema, or inadequate perfusion of parts of the lungs due to pulmonary embolism (Fig. 5-14).

Cyanosis. Cyanosis is a bluish discoloration of the skin and mucosa resulting from the presence of deoxygenated or reduced hemoglobin in the capillary blood. It becomes clinically evident when the reduced hemoglobin reaches a concentration of 5 g/dL.

Respiratory acidosis. Hypoventilation leads to reduced removal of CO_2 from the blood and ultimately causes respiratory acidosis. The pathogenesis and consequences of respiratory acidosis were discussed in Chapter 2.

DIAGNOSTIC TESTS AND PROCEDURES

The most important tests and procedures used to evaluate cases of suspected pulmonary disease are as follows:

■ Auscultation and percussion
■ Radiologic techniques
■ Spirometry and lung function measurements
■ Laboratory testing

Auscultation and percussion of the chest provide the basic evidence of pulmonary status.

Auscultation is the most important part of the physical examination for detecting pulmonary abnormalities in a broad range from pulmonary edema to pneumonia and pleural effusions. Percussion is useful for detecting consolidations of pleural effusions, which manifest as a dull sound on percussion.

Chest radiographs are used to localize lung lesions and provide either the presumptive diagnosis or guidance for the differential diagnosis.

Chest radiographs taken in an anteroposterior (AP) or lateral position are most important for characterizing various lung lesions. Such lesions can be described as **opacifications, infiltrates, nodules,** or **masses.** Loss of pulmonary parenchyma in emphysema presents as increased **radiolucency. Pleural effusion** and masses can also be readily identified. The most important lesions are as follows:

■ Pulmonary edema
■ Atelectasis
■ Emphysema
■ Bronchiectases

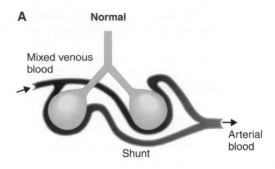

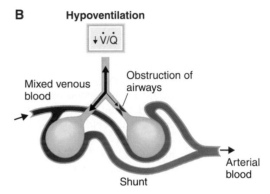

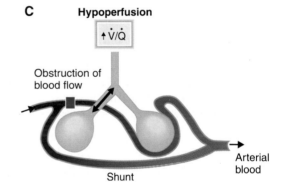

Figure 5-14 Ventilation/perfusion mismatch. **A,** Normal alveolar capillary units receive the air from the alveolar side. The air diffuses into the blood, transforming the venous blood into arterial blood. **B,** Obstruction of the airways reduces the ventilation-related oxygen supply, and thus the blood passing through this part of the lungs is not oxygenated. **C,** Occlusion of the pulmonary artery branches leads to hypoperfusion of parts of the lungs, again resulting in reduced oxygenation of pulmonary venous blood.

■ Lobar and lobular pneumonia (bronchopneumonia)
■ Interstitial pneumonia
■ Pulmonary fibrosis and chronic interstitial pneumonia
■ Pleuritis and pleural effusion
■ Tuberculosis and fungal diseases
■ Tumors

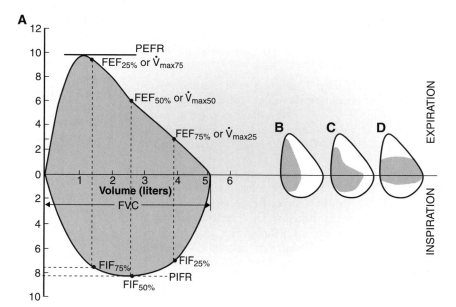

Figure 5-15 Expiratory flow rates. The flow is plotted on the y-axis and the volume on the x-axis. **A,** Normal. **B,** Restrictive lung disorder. **C,** Small airway obstruction. **D,** Fixed large airway obstruction. FEF, forced expiratory flow; FIF, forced inspiratory flow; FVC, forced vital capacity corresponding to the total lung capacity; PEFR, peak expiratory flow rate; PIFR, peak inspiratory flow rate.

Standard radiographs can be further supplemented with computed tomography (CT) scans and other radiologic techniques as well as radionucleotide imaging.

Spirometry and functional tests provide information about the functional status of the lungs.

Most of the pulmonary volumes can be measured using spirometry. The patient is asked to inhale and then forcefully exhale. Typical measurements include the following:

- FEV_1—forced expiratory volume of gas exhaled during the first second of expiration
- FVC—force vital capacity, or the total volume of gas exhaled
- MMF—maximal midexpiratory flow rate; that is, the rate of air flow in the 75% to 25% range of the FVC

These measurements indicate whether the lung volumes are within the normal range for the patient's age, or if they suggest obstructive or restrictive lung disease (Fig. 5-15). In asthma, characterized by reversible obstruction of the airways, the spirometric measurements may be combined with drug treatment to determine the extent to which drug treatment has improved pulmonary function and reduced the obstruction. The most important obstructive and restrictive lung diseases are listed in the Table 5-6.

The flow rate can also be plotted against lung volume, and if the maximal inspiratory effort is added a flow–volume curve can be generated (see Fig. 5-15). In obstructive lung disease the flow–volume curve shows reduced flow rates, and the entire curve is pushed to the left. In restrictive pulmonary diseases involving the lungs themselves ("parenchymal lung diseases") the vital capacity is reduced but the flow rates are normal. In extraparenchymal restrictive disease, such as pleural effusion or fibrosis, the volumes and the flow rate are reduced.

Table 5-6 Obstructive and Restrictive Lung Diseases

OBSTRUCTIVE	RESTRICTIVE	MIXED OR VARIABLE
Asthma	Interstitial pulmonary fibrosis	Congestive heart failure
COPD	Autoimmune lung disease	Pneumoconioses
Acute obstructive bronchitis	Extrinsic allergic pneumonitis	Carcinoma
Cystic fibrosis	Idiopathic lung diseases (UIP, DIP, LIP)	
Upper respiratory tract lesions (e.g., tumors)	Pleural diseases	
	Chest wall diseases	
	Neuromuscular disease	

COPD, chronic obstructive pulmonary disease; DIP, desquamative interstitial pneumonia; LIP, lymphocytic interstitial pneumonia; UIP, usual interstitial pneumonia.

Spirometry cannot be used, however, to measure residual volume (RV) or functional residual capacity (FRC). Therefore, to measure total lung capacity (TLC) other techniques must be employed as follows:

Gas exchange capacity. This aspect of lung pathology can be assessed by measuring the lung's diffusing capacity for carbon monoxide (D_{LCO}). The patient is asked to take a single breath of a gas mixture containing a known amount of CO and to exhale it. CO diffuses into the blood without any restrictions, so measuring the CO content in the exhaled gas indicates the amount of CO that has entered the blood. This test is abnormal in many diseases that hinder the gas exchange across the alveolar-capillary unit. The most important diseases that **decrease D_{LCO}** are pneumonia, interstitial pulmonary fibrosis, emphysema, and congestive heart failure (Fig. 5-16). Pulmonary vascular disorders and pulmonary embolism may also reduce CO diffusion.

Because CO binds to hemoglobin, **D_{LCO}** is increased in conditions associated with extravasation of red blood cells (RBCs) into the alveoli. The most important examples are ARDS, intra-alveolar hemorrhagic diseases such as Wegener's granulomatosis and Goodpasture's syndrome, and congestive heart disease.

Pearl

> Because CO avidly binds to hemoglobin in RBCs, the results of the CO diffusion test must be corrected for the values of hemoglobin in blood. Anemia is a common cause of decrease D_{LCO}.

Compliance curve. Compliance depends on the elasticity of the lung tissue, which can be assessed by plotting the lung volumes as they change during inspiration and expiration and the transpulmonary pressure—the difference between the pressure in the alveoli and the pleural space (Fig. 5-17). Under normal circumstances at the end of the expiration, corresponding to the FRC, the elastic recoil of the lungs pulling the lungs toward the hilum is counterbalanced by the elastic recoil of the chest wall exerting a pull in the other direction. At the point of maximal inspiration, when the TLC is reached, the lungs reach their maximal elastic recoil. The chest wall reaches its maximal elastic recoil at the point of maximal expiration, corresponding to the residual volume. The compliance curve for the entire respiratory cycle is determined from the ratio of the pressure–volume curve over the tidal–volume range. The compliance curve is left-shifted in emphysema, because the elastic recoil of the lungs has been diminished. In restrictive lung diseases the lungs are stiffer, TLC is decreased, and the compliance curve is shifted to the right and down. These and other respiratory parameters are summarized in Table 5-7.

Arterial blood gases and pH reflect lung efficiency.

Three main functions of the lungs (i.e., their ability to take in oxygen, remove carbon dioxide, and maintain blood pH) are monitored by measuring the partial pressures of oxygen ($Pa\{_2$) and carbon dioxide ($Pa\!\!\ae\{_2$) in arterial blood and its pH.

Partial arterial pressure of oxygen. $Pa\{_2$ provides an insight into the capacity of the lungs to oxygenate blood during

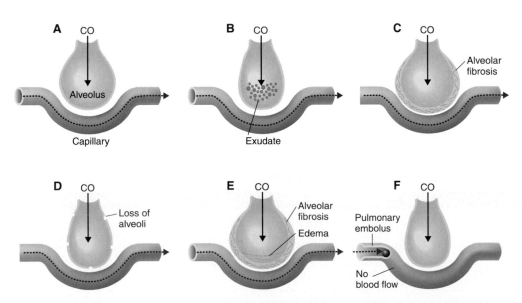

Figure 5-16 Conditions that reduce the diffusion capacity of the lungs. Normal (**A**), pneumonia (**B**), alveolar fibrosis (**C**), emphysema (**D**), congestive heart failure (**E**), and pulmonary vascular obstruction, such as pulmonary hypertension or pulmonary emboli (**F**).

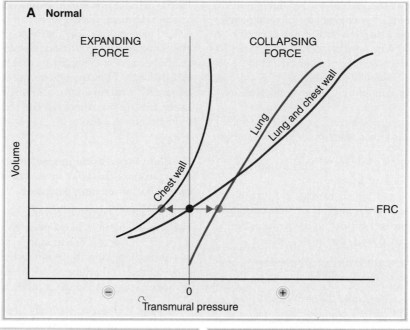

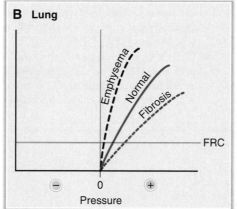

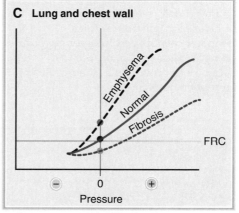

Figure 5-17 Compliance of the lungs. **A,** Normal compliance is reflected in the relaxation pressure curve, which is derived from the chest wall and lung pressure curves. **B,** Lung pressure curve, indicative of increased force needed to collapse the lungs, is up-shifted in emphysema. Loss of elasticity increases pulmonary compliance. It is reduced in pulmonary fibrosis (interstitial or restrictive lung disease). **C,** The equilibrium point indicative of functional residual capacity (FRC) is increased in emphysema and decreased in pulmonary fibrosis. (Redrawn with permission from Constanzo LS: *Physiology*. Philadelphia, Saunders, 1998.)

Table 5-7 Ventilatory Parameters in Obstructive and Restrictive Lung Diseases

LUNG DISEASE	PARAMETER				
	TLC	RV	C	FEV$_1$/FVC	COMPLIANCE
Obstructive	↑ or N	↑	↑	↓	↑
Restrictive-parenchymal	↓	↓	↓	N or ↑	↓
Restrictive-extraparenchymal	↓	↓	↓	N, ↓ or ↑	N or ↓

↑, increased; ↓, decreased; C, compliance; FEV$_1$, forced expiratory volume exhaled in 1 second; FVC, forced vital capacity; N, normal; RV, residual volume; TLC, total lung capacity.

respiration. Oxygen entering the blood in the lungs quickly enters the RBCs and binds to hemoglobin. In young adults $Pa\{_2$ is over 90 mm Hg, which leads to a 98% saturation of hemoglobin (Fig. 5-18). With age $Pa\{_2$ decreases to about 70 mm Hg, but hypoxemia is not present unless the $Pa\{_2$ drops below 60 mm Hg. As may be seen in Figure 5-18, even at $Pa\{_2$ of 60 mm Hg, the saturation of hemoglobin with oxygen is still 90%.

The oxyhemoglobin dissociation curve can be shifted either right or left by a number of factors. The most important influences are temperature, pH, and concentration of 2,3-diphosphoglycerate (2,3-DPG). This information is clinically important because it is impractical to measure PaO_2 directly in the arterial blood. Instead it is customary to estimate oxygenation by measuring oxygen saturation (SaO_2) with a pulse **oxymeter** clipped to the patient's finger. The PaO_2 can be calculated from the SaO_2.

Pearls

> Pulse oxymeter readings may be unreliable in patients who have heart failure and those who are treated with drugs causing peripheral vasoconstriction. In both conditions hypoperfusion of the extremities may affect oxymeter readings.

> The pulse oxymeter cannot used to determine SaO_2 in carbon monoxide poisoning because CO-hemoglobin cannot be distinguished by this method from oxyhemoglobin.

Partial arterial pressure of carbon dioxide. $Pa\mathrm{æ}\{_2$ provides a rough estimate of the capacity of the lungs to eliminated CO_2. Under normal circumstances $Pa\mathrm{æ}\{_2$ is 35 to 45 mm Hg. Since the CO_2 content of the blood affects blood pH, it should always be evaluated in context of the blood's acid–base balance. Hypercapnia of hypoventilation is typically associated with respiratory acidosis, whereas hypocapnia of hyperventilation is associated with respiratory alkalosis. For more details see Chapter 2.

Ventilation/perfusion mismatch is a common cause of hypoxemia that may be due to disturbances of ventilation or lung perfusion.

The normal $\dot{V}/\dot{Q}$ ratio is 0.8, indicating that even under optimal conditions not all blood passing through the lungs is oxygenated. This occurs due to a normal physiological shunting of venous blood directly into the arterial circulation.

If a part of the lung is not ventilated or inadequately perfused, $\dot{V}/\dot{Q}$ will change as follows:

- **Low $\dot{V}/\dot{Q}$ ratio.** Typically this results from the interruption of alveolar ventilation ($\dot{V}$), as in bronchial obstruction. This reduces oxygenation of the blood and increases right-to-left shunting of unoxygenated venous blood (Fig. 5-19).
- **High $\dot{V}/\dot{Q}$ ratio.** Typically the ratio is high when the perfusion ($\dot{Q}$) of parts of the lungs is interrupted, as in pulmonary embolism. $\dot{V}/\dot{Q}$ is reduced and the oxygen entering the alveoli is essentially unused.

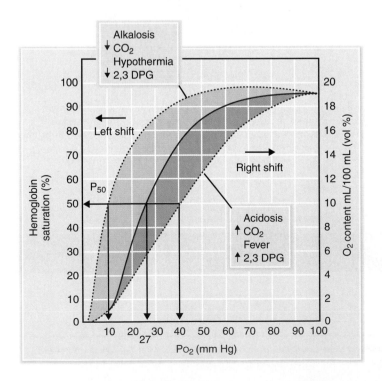

Figure 5-18 Oxygen saturation curve of hemoglobin. Note that hemoglobin is over 90% saturated even at PaO_2 of 60 mm Hg, but if the pressure of oxygen (PO_2) is reduced below 60 mm Hg, saturation drops precipitously. The oxygen saturation curve can be shifted right with increased temperature, acidosis, and high content of 2,3-diphosphoglycerate (2,3-DPG), indicating decreased affinity for oxygen. On the other hand, alkalosis, lower temperature, and low concentration of 2,3-DPG increase the affinity for oxygen and shift the curve to the left. P_{50}, oxygen half-saturation of hemoglobin.

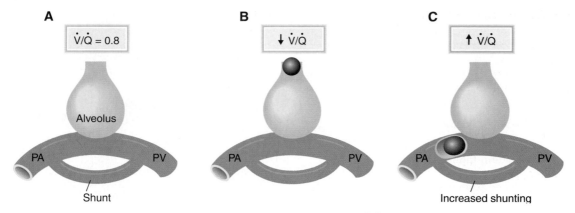

Figure 5-19 Ventilation/perfusion disturbances. Normal (**A**) and reduced (**B**) $\dot{V}/\dot{Q}$ due to inadequate ventilation of alveoli, and increased $\dot{V}/\dot{Q}$ (**C**) due to hypoperfusion of alveoli caused by a reduced influx of venous blood, as occurs in pulmonary embolism. PA, pulmonary artery; PV, pulmonary vein.

Clinicopathologic Correlations

ACUTE RESPIRATORY DISTRESS SYNDROME

Acute respiratory distress syndrome (ARDS), also known as adult respiratory syndrome, is a common form of hypoxemic respiratory failure caused by an injury of the alveolar-capillary membrane. The injury may begin at the endothelial or alveolar side of the alveolar-capillary unit (Fig. 5-20). Pathologically it characterized by diffuse alveolar damage (DAD), pulmonary edema and hemor-

rhage, and hyaline membrane formation. Typically ARDS does not respond to the administration of oxygen and is associated with high mortality. The most important clinical causes of ARDS are listed in Table 5-8.

Neutrophils play a key role in the pathogenesis of ARDS.

Neutrophils (polymorphonuclear neutrophils, PMNs) have been identified as the key players in the pathogenesis of lung injury in ARDS (Fig. 5-21). In early stages of

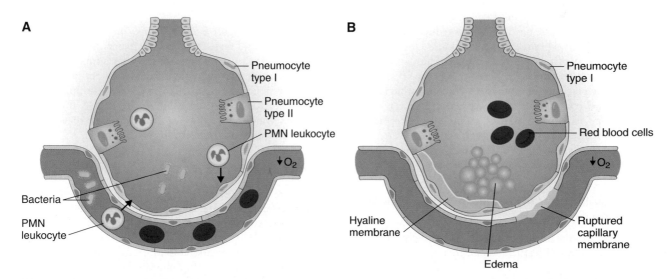

Figure 5-20 Acute respiratory distress syndrome. **A,** The injury of the alveolar-capillary unit may begin at either the endothelial or alveolar side of the unit. The polymorphonuclear neutrophils (PMNs), which may be inside the alveoli (as in pneumonia) or in the alveolar capillaries (as in sepsis) play a major pathogenetic role and mediate the injury of the alveolar-capillary unit. **B,** The injury leads to increased permeability of the alveolar-capillary membrane and pulmonary edema formation, often followed by intra-alveolar hemorrhage and deposition of fibrin (hyaline membranes). Destruction of alveolar-capillary units leads to hypoxia.

Table 5-8 Causes of Acute Respiratory Distress Syndrome

Endothelial Injury
Multiple organ failure (shock)
DIC
Sepsis
Trauma
Anaphylaxis, hypersensitivity reaction
Pancreatitis

Pulmonary (Alveolar) Injury
Viral pneumonia
Aspiration of gastric contents
Near drowning
Burns or smoke inhalation
Toxic fumes

Complex Injury of Alveolar Capillary Unit
Major surgery with anesthesia
Narcotic overdose
Heart failure
Metabolic injury (uremia)
Transfusion reaction

DIC, disseminated intravascular coagulation.

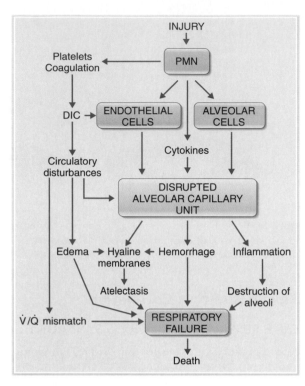

Figure 5-21 Pathogenesis of respiratory failure in acute respiratory distress syndrome (ARDS). Polymorphonuclear neutrophils (PMNs) have a pivotal role in the injury of the alveolar and endothelial cells in the alveolar-capillary units of the lung. Disseminated intravascular coagulation (DIC) aggravates the circulatory disturbances and contributes to the ventilation/perfusion disturbances ($\dot{V}/\dot{Q}$ mismatch).

pneumonia PMNs enter the alveoli in response to chemotactic pathogens inhaled from the air. In septicemia and other forms of shock PMNs aggregate in the pulmonary alveolar capillaries within hours of the onset of the disease. Both intra-alveolar and intracapillary neutrophils may damage the alveolar-capillary membrane because PMN granules contain lytic enzymes and cytokines. In animal studies, depletion of PMNs from the blood and administration of chemicals that inhibit the action of proinflammatory cytokines have been shown to reduce the intensity of ARDS under experimental conditions. Unfortunately, no efficient way of treating this condition has been discovered in clinical conditions.

PMNs release proinflammatory cytokines, which act on platelets and coagulation factors, promoting intravascular coagulation. The obstruction of pulmonary microvasculature disrupts the blood flow through the lungs. Part of the blood is shunted, leading to a $\dot{V}/\dot{Q}$ mismatch that cannot be corrected by administering oxygen.

Clinical findings in ARDS result from disruption of the alveolar capillary unit.

Irrespective of the initial insult ARDS usually manifests with classical clinical features, including:

- Severe dyspnea
- Hypoxia refractory to oxygen therapy
- Pulmonary infiltrates visible on radiographs
- Elevated pulmonary artery wedge pressure (>18 mm Hg)

As shown in Figure 5-21 the causes of respiratory failure are complex, and once the course of events is initiated it is hard to interrupt it. Treatment includes supportive measures to ensure that the patient survives the critical illness, but then should be primarily directed at eliminating the causes of ARDS. Patients who survive ARDS for several days are prone to infection, cardiac failure, or renal failure or succumb to sepsis that cannot be eradicated.

PNEUMONIA

The term *pneumonia* denotes pulmonary inflammation and does not indicate the cause of the inflammation. Every year approximately 4 million people suffer from pneumonia in the United States, and the disease is responsible for a considerable mortality, especially in the elderly and chronically ill. Pneumonia can thus be classified on the basis of several criteria:

- **Etiology.** The most common causes are bacteria, such as *Streptococcus, Staphylococcus,* or *Klebsiella,* and viruses such as influenza and parainfluenza, adenovirus, and

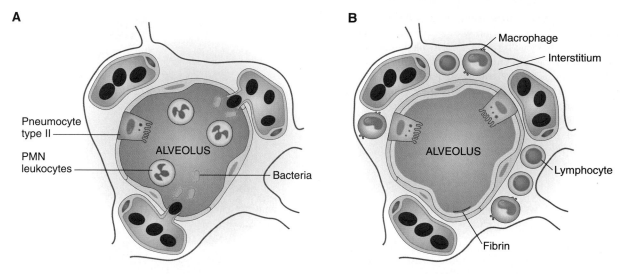

Figure 5-22 Microscopic features of pneumonia. **A,** Alveolar pneumonia is characterized by intra-alveolar exudates of polymorphonuclear neutrophils (PMNs). **B,** Interstitial pneumonia is characterized by infiltrates of lymphocytes in the interstitial septa.

picornavirus. *Mycoplasma pneumoniae* is a well-known cause of pneumonia. *Mycobacterium tuberculosis* is still a common cause of chronic pneumonia. Fungi, especially *Pneumocystis jiroveci,* are well-known causes of pneumonia in immunosuppressed persons, such as those suffering from AIDS.

- **Duration.** Pneumonia may be of acute onset or chronic. In patients with cystic fibrosis pneumonia is recurrent.

- **Pathology.** Pneumonias are classified pathologically according to the microscopic location of the inflammation

or the anatomic extent of infection. In **alveolar** pneumonia, typical of bacterial infection, the exudate is intra-alveolar (Fig. 5-22). In **interstitial** pneumonia, typical of viral of *Mycoplasma pneumoniae* infection, the infiltrate is predominantly interstitial. Alveolar pneumonia may be lobar or lobular (bronchopneumonia). Interstitial pneumonia is usually diffuse and bilateral (Fig. 5-23).

- The typical **complication** of interstitial pneumonia is bacterial superinfection. The most common complications of bacterial infections are related to the destruction of the lung, or spread into the adjacent structures

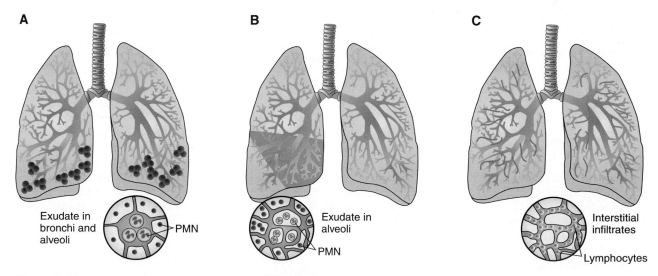

Figure 5-23 Anatomic distribution of various forms of pneumonia. **A,** Bronchopneumonia is characterized by focal infiltrates involving peribronchial lobules ("lobular" pneumonia). **B,** Lobar pneumonia involves lobes or large portions of the lungs. **C,** Interstitial pneumonia usually involves both lungs, which show radiologically visible reticular infiltrates corresponding to thickened alveolar septa.

such as pleura, mediastinum, or blood (septicemia) (Fig. 5-24). Lung infection with *Mycobacterium tuberculosis* usually spreads to the mediastinal lymph nodes, and it may disseminate through the respiratory passages, blood, or lymphatics (Fig. 5-25).

■ **Clinical setting.** Depending of the clinical setting in which pneumonias develop they may be classified as **community-acquired pneumonia** or **hospital-acquired pneumonia** (*nosocomial* pneumonia). The most important conditions that predispose to pneumonia are listed in Table 5-9.

Pneumonia manifests clinically with signs related to inflammation and lung injury.

In most instances pneumonia is an infectious disease, and as such it manifests with fever, leukocytosis, malaise, and fatigue. Due to the pulmonary infiltrates, blood ventilation is inadequate, and unoxygenated venous blood is shunted into the systemic circulation (reduced $\dot{V}/\dot{Q}$ ratio). Infection and deteriorating respiratory function cause dyspnea, tachypnea, rapid pulse rate, and cyanosis. In **severe pneumonia,** which is diagnosed when the patient is in severe respiratory distress (tachypneic over 30 respirations per minute and Pa$_2$ less than 60 mm Hg on a fraction of inspired oxygen [F*$_2$ > 0.30), there are signs of cardiovascular collapse and renal failure.

Dyspnea is a major symptom of pneumonia. It is in part related to infiltrates in the lungs and in part due to the shunting of blood that reduces the $\dot{V}/\dot{Q}$ ratio. The increased metabolic rate caused by infection typically increases the demand for oxygen, which cannot be met by the inflamed lungs. Dyspnea in bacterial infections is associated with **productive cough,** which results from the irritation of the nerve endings in the bronchi. Bronchial irritation leads to expectoration of **mucopurulent or hemorrhagic sputum (or both). Dry cough** without expectoration is characteristic of interstitial pneumonia caused by viruses or *Mycoplasma pneumoniae,* and thus these forms of infection are called **atypical pneumonia.**

Pulmonary infiltrates in the lungs cause typical radiologic and physical findings.

Inflammatory infiltrates in the lungs cause characteristic **radiologic changes** that make it possible to determine the extent of inflammation and complications in contrast to lobar and lobular pneumonia, which lead to consolidation of lung parenchyma. Interstitial pneumonia manifests with a reticular pattern of changes. Follow-up chest radiographic examination may reveal residual signs of pneumonia up to 3 months after acute infection, but this slow healing is usually of no clinical significance. Destruction of lung parenchyma, as seen in abscesses, manifests as areas of hyperlucent parenchyma in radiographs.

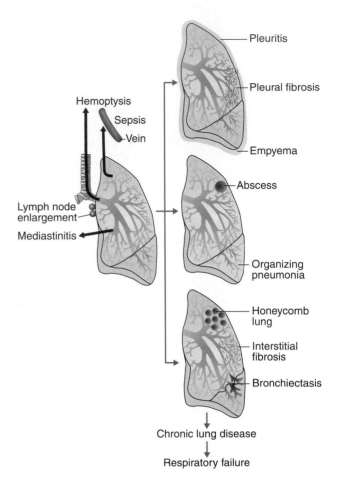

Figure 5-24 Complications of bacterial pneumonia. The infection may destroy portions of the lung (abscess, bronchiectasis) and evolve into chronic pneumonia. Destruction of lung parenchyma may cause hemoptysis (most notably in tuberculosis). Inflammation can also spread into the pleura and the mediastinum, or by invading the blood vessels cause septicemia.

Infiltrates in the lungs cause characteristic changes that can be recognized on auscultation or percussion of the chest. Since the sound travels much faster and easier through consolidated lungs the bronchial sounds are transmitted more readily—known as **bronchial respiration.** Infiltrates are also associated with **reduced resonance** to percussion. Pleural exudates, on the other hand, muzzle respiratory sounds. Pleural extension of inflammation is also associated with **pleuritic pain** (Table 5-10).

CHRONIC OBSTRUCTIVE PULMONARY DISEASE

Chronic obstructive pulmonary disease (COPD) refers to lung diseases characterized by airflow limitation, including the following two entities:

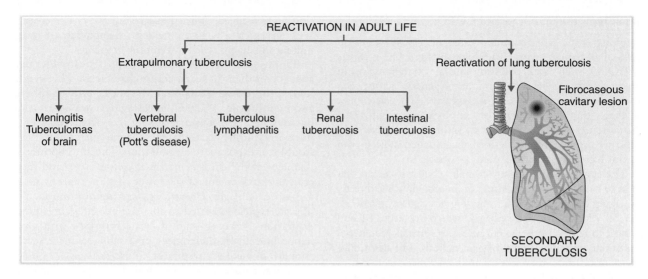

Figure 5-25 Pulmonary tuberculosis. Infection can spread through the lymphatics, blood vessels, or the air spaces. From the air spaces the *Mycobacterium tuberculosis* can be swallowed into the gastrointestinal tract and cause intestinal tuberculosis.

- **Emphysema.** It is defined pathologically as a dilatation and destruction of air spaces distant to the respiratory bronchioli.
- **Chronic obstructive bronchitis.** It is defined clinically as prolonged or recurrent productive cough that lasts at least 2 years and is symptomatic during that time for a duration of at least 3 consecutive months per year.

Most patients show signs of chronic bronchitis and emphysema, but for didactic purposes these two conditions are considered separately. Note that nonobstructive chronic bronchitis is not included under this rubric.

Table 5-9 Risk Factors Predisposing to Pneumonia

Respiratory tract diseases
  COPD
  Asthma
  Bronchiectasis
Workplace, social, and environmental factors
  Smoking
  Coal workers pulmonary disease
  Chronic alcoholism
Poor cough and gag reflex
  Drug overdose
  Stroke
  Neuromuscular diseases
Systemic diseases
  Immunosuppression (e.g., AIDS)
  Metabolic diseases (e.g., diabetes, cirrhosis, uremia)
  Sepsis
Heart diseases
  Congestive heart disease
  Chronic endocarditis
Diagnostic/therapeutic procedures
  Intubation and bronchial biopsy
  Mechanical ventilation
  Use of humidifiers

AIDS, acquired immunodeficiency syndrome; COPD, chronic obstructive pulmonary disease.

Table 5-10 Clinical Pathologic Findings in Pneumonia

PATHOLOGIC PROCESS	CONSEQUENCE
Infection	Fever, sweating, increased metabolic rate
	Leukocytosis, C-reactive protein ↑ in blood
	Malaise, weakness, fatigue
Pulmonary infiltrates	Dyspnea, tachypnea
	Hypoxia, $\dot{V}/\dot{Q}$ ratio ↓
	Cyanosis
	Radiologic findings
	Auscultation, percussion findings
Bronchial irritation	Coughing
	Mucopurulent or rusty sputum
Pleural exudates	Pleuritic pain
	Radiologic findings of fluid in the pleural space
Cardiorespiratory collapse*	Hypotension (<90/60 mm Hg)
	Oliguria (<20 mL/hr)

*Occurs in severe pneumonia.
$\dot{V}/\dot{Q}$, ventilation/perfusion.
Modified from Price SA, Wilson LM: Pathophysiology. Clinical Concepts of Disease Processes, 6th ed. St Louis, Mosby, 2003.

Smoking is the main cause of COPD.

Smoking is the most common cause of COPD—close to 90% of all patients with COPD are smokers. Other causes of COPD, such as air pollution and air contamination in the workplace, are less common. Some genetic factors, such as the autosomal recessive α_1-antitrypsin (AAT) deficiency, facilitate the development of emphysema. Emphysema therefore develops much faster in smokers who have a genetic predisposition than in normal age-paired subjects who do not have such a genetic predisposition.

The effects of smoking are complex, but it is known that tobacco smoke incites inflammation in bronchi while directly damaging the alveolar walls. Smoking has also an adverse effect on PMNs and macrophages, which are activated and primed to release histolytic enzymes (e.g., metalloproteinases and serine proteinases) and oxygen radicals. The destructive effects of inflammatory cells are under normal circumstances partially neutralized by the action of AAT. In genetic AAT deficiency these control mechanisms do not function, and the neutrophils and macrophages ravage the tissues, causing emphysema.

COPD patients are clinically classified as having either predominantly emphysema or predominantly chronic bronchitis.

Patients in whom chronic bronchitis predominates are in medical parlance called *blue bloaters,* and those who have mostly emphysema are called *pink puffers* (Fig. 5-26). In both conditions air flow (FEV_1) and functional residual capacity (FRC) are reduced, and residual volume (RV) is increased. $\dot{V}/\dot{Q}$ mismatch is relatively modest in emphysema but significant in patients who have chronic bronchitis.

Emphysema becomes clinically apparent in older persons (older than 60 years) and is characterized by **weight loss, progressive exertional dyspnea, mild hypoxia, and hypocapnia.** There is increasing dyspnea on exertion but dyspnea at rest is a relatively late occurrence. Dyspnea is typically exacerbated by viral infections, heart trouble, or exposure to air pollution. The anteroposterior diameter of the chest is increased *(barrel chest)* and there is inward movement of the lower ribs and narrowing of the subcostal angle *(Hoover's sign)* during inspiration. The lips are typically pursed to increase the pressure during expiration. Patients tend to lean forward, with their hands braced on their knees or a table to increase the strength of auxiliary respiratory muscles.

Chronic obstructive bronchitis becomes symptomatic in younger persons more often than emphysema. It is characterized by a **productive cough with expectoration of yellow-green purulent sputum.** Hemoptysis may occur, or the sputum may be blood-tinged. Due to respiratory problems, a mismatch in the $\dot{V}/\dot{Q}$ leads to **hypoxia, hypercapnia,** and **cyanosis.** Compensatory polycythemia may contribute to the bluish red appearance of the patient's face. Pulmonary hypertension leads to cor pulmonale, jugular vein distention, and pedal edema. Spirometry shows that all pulmonary volumes are reduced. The patient needs more time to exhale the air and the FEV_1 is less than 50% of the vital capacity (Fig. 5-27). FEV_1 can be improved by bronchodilators at least for some time. The clinical features of

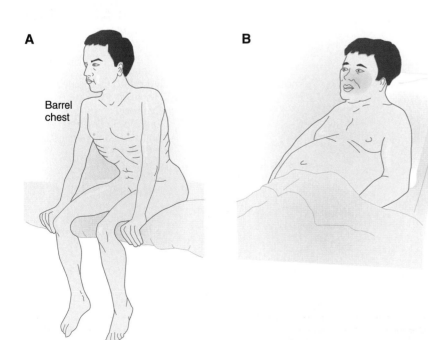

A

Barrel chest

B

Figure 5-26 Chronic obstructive pulmonary disease (COPD). **A,** Emphysema patients are asthenic pink puffers. **B,** Chronic obstructive bronchitis patients are blue bloaters. (Redrawn from Damjanov I: Pathology for Health Professions, 3rd ed. St. Louis, Saunders, 2005.)

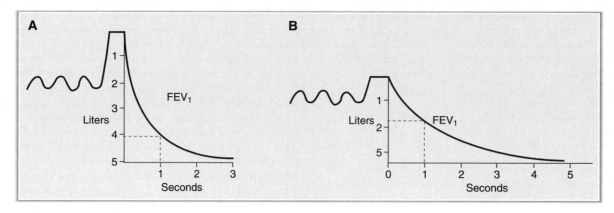

Figure 5-27 Spirometry in obstructive lung disease. Normal (**A**). **B,** Emphysema is characterized by reduced capacity to exhale air, and the forced expiratory volume in 1 second (FEV₁) is less than 50%.

chronic bronchitis and emphysema are listed comparatively in Table 5-11.

ASTHMA

Asthma is a chronic inflammatory respiratory tract disease characterized by increased irritability of the bronchi that leads to episodic reversible airway obstruction. It is marked by periodic attacks of bronchospasm that last from several minutes to several hours. Such attacks cease on their own or can be reversed by therapy with bronchodilators.

Asthma occurs in two forms: allergic (atopic) and idiosyncratic (nonatopic).

Asthma has a complex pathogenesis. In over 50% of cases it begins in childhood and is related to exogenous allergens. For unknown reasons it is much more common in boys than in girls. Such children have a family history of atopic dermatitis, hay fever, or asthma and are prone to secrete immunoglobulin (IgE) in response to a variety of exogenous allergens. This form of asthma, which has a genetic predisposition and is related to type I (IgE)–mediated hypersensitivity, is called **extrinsic, allergic,** or **atopic asthma.** Asthma that develops in adults is usually

Table 5-11 Chronic Obstructive Pulmonary Disease

FEATURES	EMPHYSEMA	CHRONIC BRONCHITIS
Age	>60 yr	45–50 yr
Appearance	"pink puffer"	"blue bloater"
Body build	Thin	Obese
Chest	Barrel shaped	N
Cigarette smoking	++	++
Genetic predisposition	+	−/+
Dyspnea	++ (exertional, progressive)	+ (episodic)
Cough	Dry, "hacking"	Productive, "deep"
Sputum	Scant, mucoid	Copious, mucopurulent
Respiration	Hyperventilation	Slow, shallow
Lung volumes	FEV₁ ↓	FEV₁ ↓ (improved by bronchodilators)
	RV ↑	RV ↑
	TLC ↑	TLC ↓
Pao₂	N, later ↓	↓ (<60 mm Hg)
Paco₂	N or ↓ (35–40 mm Hg)	↑ (50–60 mm Hg)
V̇/Q̇	Mild missmatch	Marked mismatch
Chest x-rays	Overinflation	Densities of bronchial tree
Hematocrit	N	↑ (50–55%)
Cyanosis	No	++
Cor pulmonale	No	++ → peripheral edema
Pneumonia	No	Common complication

FEV₁, forced expiratory volume in 1 second; N, normal; Paco₂, partial pressure of CO₂; Pao₂, partial pressure of O₂; RV, residual volume; TLC, total lung capacity; V̇/Q̇, ventilation/perfusion.

not related to identifiable allergens and is called **idiosyncratic,** or **intrinsic, asthma.**

In both forms of asthma bronchial inflammation provokes a number of pathologic and pathophysiologic responses (Fig. 5-28), including the following:

- Bronchoconstriction
- Vasodilatation, hyperemia, and edema
- Hypersecretion of mucus
- Chronic inflammation

In aggregate these changes lead to a narrowing of the bronchi, which are periodically accentuated by attacks of bronchospasm due to the constriction of smooth muscle cells in the wall of the bronchi.

Inflammation in allergic asthma is a chain reaction characterized by activation of several cell types and a secretion of multiple mediators.

In allergic asthma the complex inflammatory reaction begins by the inhalation of allergens. The initial events have all the hallmarks of a type I (atopic) hypersensitivity reaction, but then the inflammatory response is amplified and becomes self-sustaining. The reaction includes many inflammatory cells but most notably the following:

- Macrophages
- T helper cells
- B cells and plasma cells
- Eosinophils
- Basophils

Allergens are taken by macrophages, which act as antigen processing cells (APCs) (Fig. 5-29). Processed antigen is handed over to T lymphocytes, stimulating them to differentiate into T helper cells. T_H2 cells, critical for the interaction with the B cells, are stimulated preferentially, at the expense of T_H1 cells, which have a regulatory function and are capable of secreting interferon gamma. T_H2 cells secret the stimulatory cytokines (interleukins IL-3, IL-4, and IL-5), which act on IgE-secreting B cells and plasma cells, as well as on eosinophils. IgE secreted by plasma cells binds to the surface of basophils, stimulating a release of histamine and the secretion of slow-reacting substances of anaphylaxis—the leukotrienes. These mast cell products act on smooth muscle cells and blood vessels, producing their contraction and vasodilatation as well as increased permeability of vessels and edema. Eosinophils also release proinflammatory cytokines, enzymes, and chemotactic substances that are important for continuous recruitment of inflammatory cells into the bronchi.

Inflammatory mediators released in this chain reaction play a crucial role in the pathogenesis of bronchoconstriction, vasodilation and edema, hypersecretion of mucus, and maintenance of the chronic inflammation.

Asthmatic attacks can be provoked by many stimuli.

Once the bronchi become inflamed and hyper-reactive they can respond to a variety of stimuli. In allergic asthma these stimuli may be identical to those that have provoked the initial inflammation, but often, especially in idiopathic asthma, the stimuli of an asthmatic attack are unrelated to those that have evoked the disease. In principle asthmatic attacks can be produced by the following:

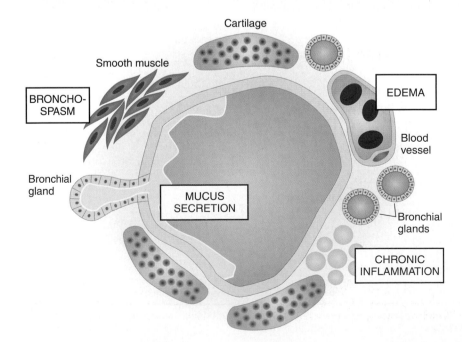

Figure 5-28 Pathology of asthma. The wall of the bronchus is thickened due to edema, infiltrates of inflammatory cells, hyperplasia of mucous glands, and hyperplasia and hypertrophy of smooth muscle cells. The lumen is narrowed by the thickened wall, but it also contains plugs composed of mucus and inflammatory cells.

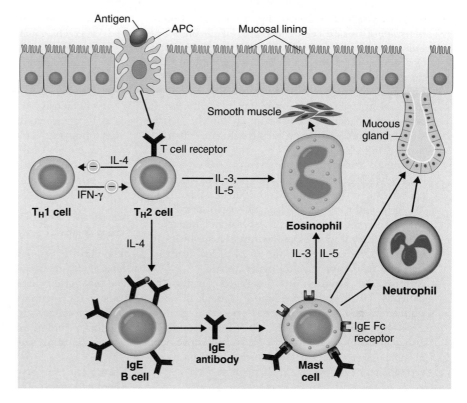

Figure 5-29 Cellular basis of asthma. Antigen processed by the antigen-presenting cells (APCs) is passed on to the helper lymphocytes (T$_H$2). T$_H$2 act on T$_H$1 and B lymphocytes, and eosinophils. Immunoglobulin E (IgE) released from B lymphocytes that have transformed into plasma cells (not shown in this diagram for sake of simplicity) binds to mast cells, stimulating them to release histamine and synthesize leukotrienes, which act on mucous glands and smooth muscle and other structures in the bronchial wall. Fc, crystallizable fragment; IL, interleukin.

- **Allergens.** They may be seasonal (e.g., pollens) or year-round (e.g., mites and house dust).
- **Air pollution.** Asthmatic attacks occur more often when air pollution peaks. Such attacks are mostly provoked by ozone, nitrogen dioxide, or sulfur dioxide.
- **Occupational air contamination.** These include a variety of dusts, chemicals, plastics, and biologic enzymes used for industrial purposes or in the household.
- **Infections.** Most notably, asthmatic attacks can be provoked by respiratory viruses.
- **Drugs.** Certain drugs, such as aspirin or β-adrenergic antagonists, can cause bronchospasm and asthmatic attacks.
- **Exercise.** Exercise-induced asthma occurs especially during cold weather.
- **Psychological factors.** Emotions and excitement can induce bronchospasm and probably play a modifying role during attacks induced by other factors.

Clinical symptoms of asthma reflect the extent of bronchial inflammation and obstruction.

Asthma is a chronic disease characterized by episodic exacerbations of bronchospasm and bronchial obstruction. The most important symptoms are as follows:

- **Cough.** It is usually episodic and related to bronchial inflammation. It may be dry or result in expectoration of viscous mucus.
- **Abnormal breathing pattern.** Most patients exhibit **tachypnea** with prolonged expiration. It is related to the partial obstruction of the bronchi with mucous plugs and narrowing caused by bronchial constriction. Abnormal breathing typically results in **overinflation** of the chest.
- **Wheezing.** It is typically high-pitched and most pronounced during expiration (Fig. 5-30). It is related to

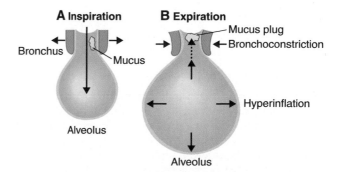

Figure 5-30 Wheezing in asthma. Inspiration (**A**). Expiration (**B**). During expiration the bronchus contracts causing wheezing because the air is exiting the terminal air spaces (alveoli) under pressure and passing through a narrowed cylinder.

the narrowing of the bronchi due to the contraction of the smooth muscle cells, thickening of the bronchial wall caused by edema, and chronic inflammation and hypersecretion of mucus from bronchial glands and the goblet cells.

■ **Dyspnea.** Shortness of breath is usually noticed by the patient, who also complains of tightness of breath or a feeling of constraint in the chest. It is usually accentuated by progressive mucous obstruction or bronchospasms.

■ **Asthmatic attacks.** These attacks of severe dyspnea, loud wheezing, and distress are caused by vehement contraction of hypertrophic smooth muscle cells in the wall of the bronchi. They are usually associated with tachypnea. Severe bronchospasm and impaction of mucus may lead to **status asthmaticus,** which can be fatal. Hypoventilation due to bronchial obstruction may cause hypoxia and hypercapnia.

■ **Respiratory fatigue.** In prolonged attacks the patient's breathing becomes more labored. In addition to tachypnea, the patient experiences profuse sweating and distress, and the blood Po_2 becomes elevated. **Abdominal paradox,** an inward movement of the anterior abdominal wall during inspiration, is a typical sign of fatigue of the diaphragm.

Pulmonary function testing shows obstructive changes during asthmatic attacks, but these changes can be reversed by bronchodilator drugs.

For many patients who have asthma no functional deficits are detected on spirometry. During asthmatic attacks FEV_1, FEV_1/FVC, and peak flow are reduced. These abnormalities can be reversed with bronchodilators. A peak flow of less than 100 L/min or an FEV_1 reduced below 1 L are signs of severe obstruction.

Bronchial obstruction with mucus may lead to overinflation, which manifests with increased TLC, RV, and lung compliance. Because of increased lung volumes D_{LCO} can be reduced. Hypoxia is common due to $\dot{V}/\dot{Q}$ mismatch. $Paco_2$ is usually low (i.e., below 36 mm Hg). Hypercapnia, on the other hand, develops only in severe obstruction and is typically found in status asthmaticus.

RESTRICTIVE LUNG DISEASES

Pulmonary diseases that manifest as a restrictive respiratory failure can be subdivided into two major groups: acute and chronic parenchymal lung diseases. **Acute restrictive lung diseases** are characterized by diffuse alveolar damage (DAD) and are clinically grouped under the heading of ARDS. **Chronic restrictive lung diseases** comprise a heterogeneous group of disorders such as:

■ Inorganic dust-related diseases (pneumoconioses), such as silicosis, berryliosis, and asbestosis

■ Hypersensitivity pneumonitis due to exogenous allergens, such as organic dusts

■ Pulmonary autoimmune diseases such as Wegener's granulomatosis, Churg-Strauss syndrome, and Goodpasture's syndrome

■ Diseases of presumptive immune etiology, such as sarcoidosis

■ Drug-related lung diseases

■ Idiopathic pulmonary diseases, grouped under the name of usual interstitial pneumonia (UIP), desquamative interstitial pneumonia (DIP), or idiopathic interstitial pulmonary fibrosis

Restrictive lung diseases can be the consequence of many forms of lung injury.

The initial lung injury in various interstitial lung diseases is typically followed by destruction of normal lung parenchyma and prolonged repair reactions. Since the lungs have a limited capacity for regeneration, the repair results in the replacement of the respiratory surfaces with fibrous tissue or granulomas and foci of chronic inflammation. Several pathogenetic mechanisms can be recognized (Fig. 5-31).

Direct injury of alveolar lining cells. Toxic fumes, various **chemicals** that give off toxic oxygen radicals, ozone, and even pure oxygen itself can injure the cells of the alveolar lining. Alveolar injury is known to occur on inhalation of hot fumes and smokes in fire; insecticides; and chemicals such as ammonia, sulfur dioxide, and nitrogen oxide. Likewise, injury can result from **bacterial and viral infections.**

Activation of macrophages. Intra-alveolar macrophages can be activated by organic antigens or various exogenous inorganic substances that are inhaled into the alveoli. The best examples are silica particles, which are taken up by macrophages. Silica particles processed by the macrophages then initiate a chronic inflammation accompanied by fibrosis. These changes account for the nodular fibrosis that typically develops in **silicosis. Sarcoidosis,** a disease of unknown origin, is characterized by nodular infiltrates of macrophages and T lymphocytes arranged into noncaseating granulomas.

Immune injury. Antigens inhaled into the lungs stimulate an immune response, which may include production of cytotoxic antibodies (type II hypersensitivity reaction) or formation of granulomas (type IV hypersensitivity reaction). In many instances there is evidence of both cell-mediated and antibody-mediated hypersensitivity reaction, but the inciting antigen cannot be identified. Many of the pulmonary **adverse drug reactions** involve immune mechanisms. Immune mechanisms play a role in **organic dust hypersensitivity reactions** such as farmer's lung, bagassosis, byssinosis, and many others.

Vascular injury. Immune injury of pulmonary vessels, and especially injury of capillaries, which are part of the alveolar

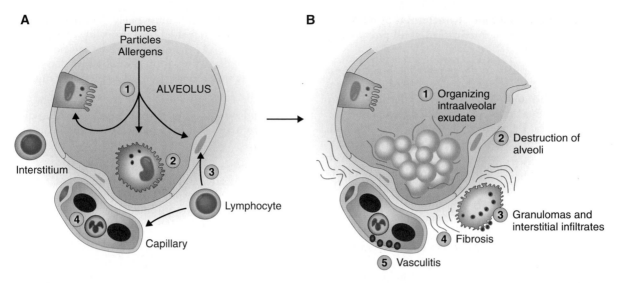

Figure 5-31 Pathogenesis of parenchymal lung injury leading to restrictive lung disease. **A,** Injury can occur due to the entry of fumes, irritant particles, or allergens, which may directly damage the alveoli (1), stimulate macrophages to secrete cytokines and growth factors (2), or activate the lymphocytes to mount an immune reaction (3). The injury could also be initiated by endogenous factors, such as antibodies or neutrophils, or by lymphocytes entering the lungs from the capillaries (4). **B,** The reaction to injury can result in organizing pneumonia (1), destruction of alveoli (2), formation of granulomas (3), fibrosis (4), or vascular injury such as necrotizing or granulomatous vasculitis (5).

capillary units, may lead to parenchymal lung injury. Restrictive lung disease due to the destruction of lung parenchyma is thus typically found in Wegener's granulomatosis, which is characterized by pulmonary granulomatous arteritis and capillaritis, Goodpasture's syndrome, which is characterized by immune injury of alveolar walls and intra-alveolar bleeding, or Churg-Strauss syndrome, which is characterized by vasculitis, asthma, and eosinophilia. Systemic immune diseases, such as systemic lupus erythematosus, or dermatomyositis and systemic sclerosis (scleroderma) also affect the lungs.

> **Pearl**
>
> > Cryptogenic fibrosing alveolitis, also known as idiopathic pulmonary fibrosis, is the most common form of parenchymal lung disease. As its name implies, the origin of this disease is unknown, and the diagnosis is made by excluding other possibilities.

Restrictive lung diseases are characterized by injury of alveolar-capillary units and small bronchioli, followed by repair in the form interstitial fibrosis or chronic inflammation.

Restrictive lung diseases are characterized by a major destruction of lung parenchyma and a loss of alveolar-capillary units. Major bronchi are typically spared, but the terminal bronchioli and respiratory bronchioli are also frequently involved. A common form of alveolar-bronchiolar-alveolar injury is known as **bronchiolitis obliterans organizing pneumonia (BOOP).** Pulmonary fibrosis of uneven distribution combined with foci of inflammation is a feature of **usual interstitial pneumonia (UIP),** a common pathologic finding in these patients. If the alveolar fibrosis is accompanied by desquamation of pneumocytes and exudation of macrophages, the pathologic features of **desquamative interstitial pneumonitis (DIP)** predominate. Radiologic findings of focal fibrosis combined with cystic loss of parenchyma are also a common finding known as **honeycomb lungs.**

Chronic restrictive lung diseases often begin as pneumonia that has not resolved completely or as diffuse alveolar damage in ARDS that could not be repaired completely. Acute lung injury often leads to destruction of alveoli. However, even if the alveoli are preserved, the distance between the air that is inhaled into the terminal air spaces and the blood is increased due to the formation of **hyaline membranes** and **organizing intra-alveolar exudates,** as well as **fibrosis,** between the alveolar cells and the capillaries. The infiltrates of inflammatory cells and **granulomas** interposed between the alveoli and the capillaries also impede gas exchange. Destruction of capillaries, as typically seen in Wegener's granulomatosis, leads to the same functional consequences. In Wegener's granulomatosis, **vasculitis** involving large pulmonary vessels is also present.

Restrictive lung diseases are characterized by a loss of respiratory capacity and a reduction of all pulmonary volumes.

Loss of alveolar-capillary units results in a loss of respiratory surfaces, and the gas exchange is consequently markedly reduced. **Total lung capacity, vital capacity, and functional residual capacity** are all reduced proportionately (Fig. 5-32). **Expiratory flow rates** remain normal and even slightly increased because the air spaces remain open due to the rigidity of the fibrotic lungs. Since the lungs resist expansion during inspiration and exhibit higher elastic recoil, pulmonary fibrosis is typically accompanied by a reduction of **pulmonary compliance.** Accordingly, even if strained breathing is trying to expand the lungs during each inspiration by increasing transpulmonary pressure, the volume of the lungs does not increase proportionately.

As the pulmonary fibrosis advances the gas exchange leads to a progressively diminished diffusion of oxygen into the blood. The difference between the **oxygen pressure** in the inhaled air and in the blood is pronounced, as evidenced by an increased alveolar-arterial pressure difference ($P_{(A-a)}O_2$). **Diffusing capacity** is impaired and can be documented by showing reduced D_{LCO}. **Hypoxemia** first occurs only during exercise but with time it is evident even at rest. It most likely develops due to a $\dot{V}/\dot{Q}$ mismatch and impaired diffusion of oxygen in the fibrotic alveoli. On the other hand there is no **hypercapnia,** and the $Paco_2$ is within normal limits. Hypercapnia occurs only in terminal stages of respiratory failure.

Signs and symptoms of chronic restrictive lung disease result from a loss of lung parenchyma and ensuing hypoxia.

The symptoms of chronic restrictive lung disease may evolve slowly after a bout of pneumonia or ARDS, but in most instances they evolve insidiously and are unrelated to an acute insult. In most instances the diagnosis is based on clinical findings and is further documented by pulmonary function testing or lung biopsy. The most important clinical findings are as follows:

■ **Dyspnea.** Initially it is found only on effort, but as the disease advances it becomes evident at rest as well. Respiration is fast and shallow, and the patient does not strain, having learned that by increasing the respiratory effort he or she will not reduce dyspnea. Dyspnea may be frightening, and the patient may require constant oxygen administration.

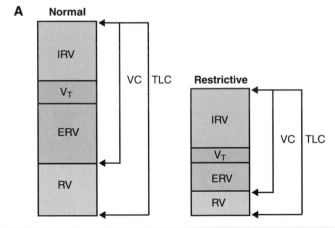

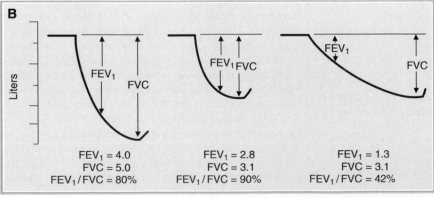

Figure 5-32 Pulmonary volumes in restrictive lung disease. **A,** All pulmonary volumes are reduced proportionately. **B,** Both forced expiratory volume in 1 second (FEV_1) and forced vital capacity (FVC) are reduced. The normal and obstructive patterns are included for comparison. ERV, expiratory reserve volume; IRV, inspiratory reserve volume; RV, reserve volume; TLC, total lung capacity; VC, vital capacity; V_T, tidal volume.

- **Cough.** Shallow and nonproductive cough is common.
- **Auscultatory findings.** Fine crepitus is the most common finding.
- **Chest radiographic findings.** These findings are typical and reflect the underlying pathology. Fibrosis, focal nodularity, and ultimately the features of honeycomb lung are evident. Superinfections are common. Specific diseases, such as Wegener's granulomatosis, show unique features, which can also be documented by lung biopsy.
- **Cyanosis and clubbing of fingers.** These findings are seen in over 60% of patients.
- **Cor pulmonale.** Signs of right heart failure develop in later stages of pulmonary fibrosis.

PULMONARY EMBOLISM

Pulmonary emboli are venous thromboemboli that most often develop in the leg veins and lodge in the lungs. Every year in the United States approximately 700,000 persons develop major pulmonary emboli, 20% to 25% of which are lethal. The most important predisposing risk factors are listed in Table 5-12.

Pearl

> The mnemonic SITCOM covers over 90% of all causes of pulmonary embolism:
> **S**urgery
> **I**mmobilization
> **T**rauma
> **C**ongenital thrombophilia
> **O**bstetrical conditions
> **M**alignant tumors

Signs and symptoms of pulmonary embolism depend on the size of emboli.

Pulmonary emboli can be classified as massive, medium-sized, or small (Fig. 5-33).

- **Massive emboli.** These emboli obstruct the main pulmonary artery ("saddle emboli") and its branches, causing major circulatory disruption. Typically they are accompanied by sharp chest pain of sudden onset, respiratory distress, dyspnea, and hyperventilation. The blockade of blood flow into the lungs causes sudden hypotension often accompanied by collapse and loss of consciousness, and even death.
- **Medium-sized emboli.** Smaller emboli lodge in the lobar or segmental branches of the pulmonary artery. In some instances such emboli cause no clinical symptoms ("silent emboli"), or they may be accompanied by pulmonary infarctions. In such cases patients present with pleuritic pain, cough and hemoptysis, and signs of lung necrosis (e.g., fever and leukocytosis). The patient may be short of breath and is in distress depending on the extent of vascular occlusion.
- **Small emboli.** A few small emboli that lodge in the small arteries and arterioles usually do not produce symptoms. However, such emboli often manifest in showers that recur, causing obstruction of the pulmonary circulation and ultimately leading to pulmonary hypertension. Such patients have dyspnea due to pulmonary hypoperfusion. Even though the lungs are properly ventilated, there is a $\dot{V}/\dot{Q}$ mismatch because the blood cannot reach the alveolar-capillary units. Pulmonary hypertension leads to cor pulmonale and impedes venous return to the heart from the periphery.

Table 5-12 Risk Factors Predisposing to Pulmonary Embolism

- Immobilization and prolonged bed rest (e.g., chronic disease)
- Surgery (1% of major surgeries!)
- Trauma with fractures (especially legs and pelvis)
- Malignant tumors (especially pancreatic, gastrointestinal, and breast cancer)
- Chronic heart failure with venous stasis
- Childbirth (especially with eclampsia and amniotic fluid embolism)
- Drugs (e.g., intravenous drug abuse, oral contraceptives)
- Congenital thrombophilia (e.g., factor V Leyden, protein C and S deficiency)
- Venous diseases (e.g., phlebothrombosis, varicose veins)

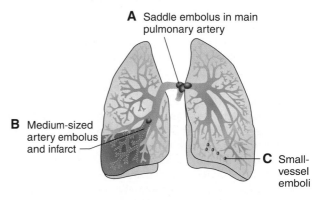

Figure 5-33 Pulmonary embolism. **A,** Massive embolism occludes the pulmonary artery or its major branches and may cause death. **B,** Medium-sized embolism may cause pulmonary infarcts. **C,** Recurrent small emboli may cause pulmonary hypertension due to small-vessel occlusion.

Pulmonary emboli cause complex changes in the pulmonary vasculature but also in the other parts of the lungs.

The effects of pulmonary emboli are to a great extent mechanical, and the obstruction of the pulmonary artery leads mostly to hemodynamic disturbances. Remember, however, that pulmonary emboli also act directly or indirectly on nerve endings, eliciting several adaptive reflexes. Biologically active substances released from the platelets and inside the thromboemboli and the endothelial cells of the occluded pulmonary vessels also contribute to the chain of events that follows pulmonary embolization. These events include the following:

- **Increased pulmonary artery pressure.** Mechanical obstruction of the pulmonary artery increases pressure within it. In response to the obstruction the right heart contracts more forcefully, but if it fails an acute cor pulmonale develops.
- **Vasoconstriction of the pulmonary artery and its branches.** The pulmonary artery has a wider caliber than the leg veins from which the emboli have originated. The emboli usually twist and form a bundle, thus creating a much larger mass. However, even small emboli may have profound obstructive effects, which are most likely related to the reactive vasoconstriction of the pulmonary arterial system. In part it is related to the mechanical stimuli of the nerve endings and in part it is mediated by the vasoconstrictors released from the platelets in the thromboemboli. Vasoconstriction of the smaller branches of the pulmonary circulation contributes to the dyspnea by causing $\dot{V}/\dot{Q}$ mismatch.
- **Alveolar hyperventilation.** Hyperventilation, a typical sign of pulmonary embolism, results from the stimulation of irritant receptors and a central nervous system response to hypoxia. "Hunger for air" is accompanied with dyspnea and anxiety, indicating that the central respiratory centers are also involved.
- **Bronchoconstriction.** Hypoperfusion of the lungs causes a reflex constriction of smooth muscle cells in the bronchi as an adaptation to reduced blood flow through the alveolar capillaries. Ischemia and acidosis and mediators released from the platelets contribute to the bronchospasm.
- **Cough.** Cough reflex is initiated by the stimulation of irritant receptors in the lungs. Contributory factors are edema and intra-alveolar hemorrhage, which may occur at the site of infarction. In such cases cough may be accompanied by hemoptysis.
- **Syncope.** Loss of consciousness results from hypoxia and is a consequence of pulmonary artery obstruction, reflex vasoconstriction, changes in the perfusion of the lungs, and $\dot{V}/\dot{Q}$ mismatch. Massive emboli occluding more that 60% of the pulmonary vascular system may be lethal.

Diagnosis of pulmonary embolism is not straightforward, and many cases remain undiagnosed.

None of the clinical signs and symptoms encountered in patients with pulmonary embolism are pathognomonic of this disease. The diagnosis is usually established "in context," and by excluding other conditions that could present with the same symptoms. It is most important to include this diagnosis in the differential, especially under circumstances that predispose to pulmonary embolism.

Dyspnea and tachypnea of sudden onset in a patient who had surgery or trauma are highly suggestive of pulmonary embolism. Pleuritic pain, hemoptysis, and fever may develop, but in elderly patients these symptoms are not always present. Likewise, pulmonary emboli may be easily missed in previously healthy young men who often do not express any of the classic symptoms of pulmonary embolism or infarction. The diagnosis may be confirmed by a variety of tests. Most specific tests include noninvasive and invasive radiologic techniques, such as venous **ultrasonography, pulmonary perfusion scan, and pulmonary angiography.** These techniques are time-consuming and expensive, and, unfortunately, the results are often obtained too late for effective treatment.

The plasma fibrin D-dimer test is a good indicator of intravascular coagulation and is positive in almost all patients with pulmonary embolism. However, this test cannot distinguish between pulmonary embolism and peripheral venous thrombosis, which is present in most patients.

Pearl

> A normal chest radiograph in a person who has dyspnea of sudden onset is highly suggestive of pulmonary embolism.

LUNG CANCER

Lung cancer is the leading cause of cancer-related death in the Unites States and Europe. Even though it is more common in men than women, the incidence of lung cancer in women is on the rise. In both men and women it is related to tobacco smoking. Other risk factors, such as exposure to radon, asbestos, and radioactive minerals, are significantly less important than smoking.

More then 90% of all lung cancers originate from the bronchial epithelium and are thus called bronchogenic. Accordingly, most lung cancers are located in the central hilar area. Peripheral carcinomas, such as adenocarcinomas of bronchiolar origin and mesotheliomas originating from the pleura, are less common.

Lung cancers are microscopically subclassified into two groups: small-cell carcinoma and nonsmall-cell carcinomas. The latter group comprises several microscopic variants, such as squamous cell carcinoma, adenocarcinoma, and large-cell carcinoma, which often occur intermixed with one another.

Lung cancer was discussed in greater detail in Chapter 3. Lung cancer is also mentioned in this chapter in the differential diagnosis of dyspnea, hemoptysis, bronchiectasis, chest pain, and pleural effusion.

PLEURAL DISEASES

The pleural space is delimited on one side by the parietal pleura and on the other by the visceral pleura covering the lungs. It contains only a few milliliters of serous fluid, approximately 10 mL on each side, which keeps its surface moist, allowing the parietal and visceral pleura to remain closely apposed and yet freely movable. The fluid film also contributes to the negative pressure in the pleural cavity that keeps the lungs from collapsing. It may be -25 to -35 cm H_2O at the end of deep inspiration. At the end of expiration it is in the range from -2 to -5 cm H_2O (Fig. 5-34). Even though the capillary force of the pleural film is relatively small when compared with the outward pulling pressure exerted by the chest wall and the elastic forces of the lung parenchyma pulling the lung toward the hilum, the pleural fluid is essential for keeping the lungs expanded.

Pleural effusion forms when more fluid enters the pleural fluid than is removed.

Under normal circumstances the small amounts of fluid in the pleural spaces are constantly exchanged by the fluid coming in from the systemic capillaries. At the same time the fluid is drained from the pleural space entering into the pulmonary lymphatics and the venous system of the lungs.

Pleural effusion forms if more fluid enters the pleural space than is drained. The most important pathogenetic mechanisms are as follows:

- **Increased pulmonary venous pressure.** Typically this occurs in left heart failure. Congestive heart failure is the most common cause of pleural effusion.
- **Lymphatic obstruction.** Obstruction of lymphatics by granulomas or tumor cells may cause pleural effusion.
- **Increased permeability of pleura.** Pleural effusions of this type typically occur as a complication of pneumonia extending to the pleura. In pulmonary tuberculosis, pleural effusion is in part due to inflammation and in part related to the obstruction of lymphatic drainage.
- **Decreased intrapleural pressure.** This occurs following a collapse of the lungs due to pneumothorax or atelectasis.
- **Decreased oncotic pressure of the plasma.** Hypoalbuminemia due to chronic liver disease or nephritic syndrome is associated with generalized edema (anasarca), which usually includes pleura effusions.
- **Complex changes related to malignancy of the pleura.** Malignant tumors mechanically disrupt the pleural surface and also cause irritation, leading to transudation of the fluid from the newly formed blood vessels. The immune response to tumors is accompanied by an increased permeability of pleura and accumulation of fluid in the pleural cavity. Tumor cells occlude the lymphatics and prevent normal drainage of the fluid from the pleural cavity.

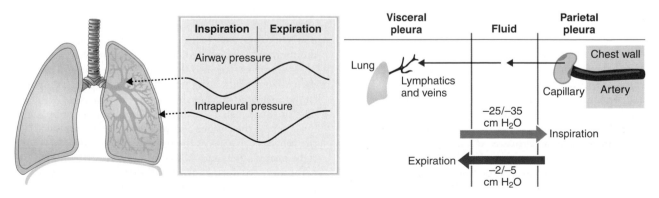

Figure 5-34 Pleural space. The fluid is formed through ultrafiltration from capillaries on the arterial side, mostly in the parietal pleura. The fluid is absorbed into the pulmonary lymphatics and pulmonary veins. The film formed by the fluid keeps the parietal and visceral pleura juxtaposed, thus contributing to the negative pressure in the pleural spaces. This negative pressure is formed as the difference between the expansile forces of the thoracic cage during inspiration and the elastic recoil of the lungs pulling the lungs toward the hilum. At inspiration the negative pressure is -25 to -35 cm H_2O, but it drops down to -2 to -5 cm H_2O at the end of expiration.

Pleural effusions are classified as transudates or exudates. A **transudate** is formed due to altered hydrostatic pressure gradients, whereas an **exudate** is a sign of increased permeability of the pleural surfaces caused by inflammation or neoplasia. The features of pleural transudates and exudates are compared in the Table 5-13.

Additional studies may be performed to determine the nature of the pleural effusion. Accumulation of pus is a typical feature of **empyema**, which develops in bacterial infections. Red blood cells are found in pleural effusions that accompany pleural malignancy, trauma, or pulmonary embolism. Whereas most bacterial infections are accompanied by an exudate that contains mostly neutrophils, tuberculosis is accompanied by an exudation of lymphocytes and macrophages. Likewise, pleural fluid found in the course of autoimmune diseases such as rheumatoid arthritis or systemic lupus erythematosus contains lymphocytes and macrophages. Thus cytologic examination is routinely performed on pleural effusions. Cytologic examination is essential for the diagnosis of malignant tumors of the pleura.

Table 5-13 Pleural Transudate and Exudate

FEATURE	TRANSUDATE	EXUDATE
Appearance	Clear	Turbid
Specific gravity	<1.012	>1.020
Protein	<3 g/dL	>3 g/dL
Protein PF/S	<0.5	>0.5
LDH	<200 U/L	>200 U/L
LDH PF/S	<0.5	>0.6
White blood cells	<1000 µL	>1000 µL

LDH, lactate dehydrogenase; PF/S, pleural fluid/serum ratio.

Pearls

> Chylothorax is characterized by an accumulation of lymph (lipid-rich fluid), resulting from the rupture of the thoracic duct due to trauma or its obstruction by tumor.

> On routine chest radiograph fluid exceeding 250 mL on one side can be detected. Such an accumulation of fluid represents a space-occupying mass compressing the lungs. Consequently, it decreases the lung volume and causes restrictive ventilatory abnormalities. Unilateral effusion causes mediastinal shift toward the opposite side.

Pneumothorax is air in the pleural space.

Under normal circumstances the pleural space does not contain air. Accumulation of air in the pleural space is an abnormality called **pneumothorax.** The air may enter under several of the following conditions:

■ **Spontaneous rupture of lung parenchyma.** In young men it may be related to solitary subpleural bullae, possibly of developmental origin. Pleural rupture may also occur in lungs affected by emphysema,

tuberculosis, following infarction, or as a result of interstitial fibrosis.

■ **Trauma.** Penetrating chest wounds caused by gun shot or stabbing allow air to enter into the thoracic cavity.

Iatrogenic causes. All thoracic interventions requiring opening of the chest cage cause pneumothorax. After surgery the air is reabsorbed and the symptoms of pneumothorax disappear. Air may enter the pleural spaces during transthoracic needle biopsy, subclavian central line placement, or thoracentesis of the pleural fluid. Positive pulmonary ventilation may cause rupture of the lung parenchyma and also cause pneumothorax.

If the pneumothorax develops due a penetrant thoracic cage injury, the wound allows air to enter the thorax and will, due to the increased pressure, dislocate the lung to the opposite side. This dislocation is seen on radiograph as tracheal deviation (Fig. 5-35). If the wound is gaping, air can pass in and out **(open pneumothorax).** If the wound is tight, it may act as a ball-valve allowing the entry of the air during inspiration but not its exit during expiration. Such a **tension pneumothorax** results in very high intrathoracic pressure, which must be relieved clinically to prevent further complications. Pneumothorax that develops due to a rupture of the lung parenchyma without a hole in the thoracic cage is called **closed pneumothorax.**

The entry of air into the pleural space causes pain, and the collapse of the lung leads to dyspnea. The radiograph shows increased translucency of the thorax filled with air. The pressure inside the affected chest causes contralateral deviation of the trachea and mediastinum. Compression of the venae cavae reduces the return of venous blood into the right heart. Since both respiration and heart function are compromised during pneumothorax, it is important to perform decompression as soon as possible.

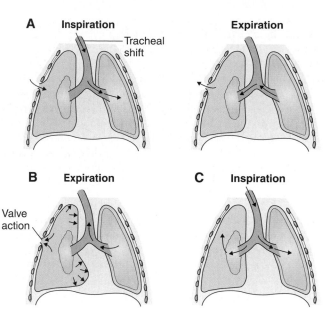

Figure 5-35 Pneumothorax. **A,** Open pneumothorax—the air enters and exits the pleural space in equilibrium with the air in the environment. **B,** Tension pneumothorax—the air enters during inspiration and cannot exit from the pleural space during expiration. Thus the pressure increases, progressively compressing the venae cavae and pushing the mediastinum to the contralateral side. **C,** Closed pneumothorax—there is no chest wall defect. The air enters the pleural space through a defect of visceral pleura during inspiration.

CASE STUDIES

Case 1 WHEEZING AND SHORTNESS OF BREATH IN A 5-YEAR-OLD BOY

Clinical history A 5-year-old boy was brought to the emergency department at 10 PM. Prior to that he had had an uneventful day and went to sleep around 9:30 PM. Soon thereafter he woke up and came to the living room coughing and wheezing.[1] He was breathing rapidly and was short of breath.[2] The parents became scared and brought the child to the hospital.

Family and past history His father has hay fever. Since early childhood the boy has had eczema.[3]

Physical findings The boy was obviously short of breath, agitated, and in a state of acute distress. He was breathing fast and was constantly coughing. He did not expectorate. The auscultation of the chest revealed rhonchi and rales and wheezing during the prolonged expiratory phase.[4] The chest radiograph appeared normal. He was tachycardic, but no other abnormalities were noticed. The boy was treated with a β_2-agonist given through an inhaler and his symptoms improved.[5]

Clinical course During the next month the boy had several similar attacks of coughing and shortness of breath. Thus he was brought to the medical center for further studies.

Laboratory data Eosinophilia in peripheral blood and increased levels of serum IgE were found.[6]

Pulmonary function tests (PFTs) Spirometric studies were performed during one of the attacks. He was found to have an obstructive pattern which could be corrected by administering a β_2-agonist bronchodilator.[7]

He also had undergone skin hypersensitivity tests, which showed allergy to house dust.[8]

Outcome He was given medical treatment but with time his coughing spells became less common.

Questions and topics for discussion
1. What are the possible causes of cough of sudden onset associated with wheezing in a child?
2. What are the technical terms for rapid breathing and for shortness of breath? Explain the pathogenesis of these clinical findings.
3. What is the significance of the father's history of hay fever and the child's long-standing eczema? Do these diseases have a genetic basis?
4. What is the pathogenesis of rhonchi and rales, and why was the expiration prolonged?
5. How did β_2-agonist treatment relieve the symptoms?
6. Interpret eosinophilia and elevated IgE in the context of other clinical findings.
7. What is the significance of spirometric data?
8. Do all patients with bronchospasm have allergies?

Case 2 CHRONIC COUGH AND EXPECTORATION IN A SMOKER

Clinical history   A 55-year-old, who has been smoking two packs of cigarettes a day for 30 years, complains of progressive shortness of breath especially while walking, prolonged cough, and increased expectoration.[1] For the last 3 years he has had similar episodes of prolonged coughing and expectoration during the winter months that lasted at least 2 to 3 months. He has noticed episodes of fever as his sputum became yellow-green and occasionally tinged with blood.[2]

Physical findings   The patient appeared bloated and dark red in his face. He was short of breath and was using his respiratory muscles while breathing. Auscultation revealed coarse crackles, expiratory wheezes, and rhonchi.[3] Both hands showed clubbing of fingers. He had distended jugular veins and pedal pitting edema.[4]

The chest radiograph showed increased lung markings and right heart enlargement. No nodules or solid masses were identified.[5]

Laboratory findings   Arterial blood gas (ABG) analysis showed hypoxemia and increased $Paco_2$, associated with mild acidosis.[6]

Pulmonary function tests (PFTs)   The FEV_1/FVC percentage and forced expiratory flow ($FEF_{25-75\%}$) were reduced. His FEV_1 was reduced to 0.6 L. Bronchodilators had no effect on the pulmonary function test.[7]

Outcome   He was given antibiotics, and his condition improved. Nevertheless he remained short of breath and was thus given oxygen on a regular basis.

Questions and topics for discussion
1. What are the possible causes of chronic cough and expectoration in a smoker?
2. What is the importance of the duration of the coughing episodes and the color of the sputum? What is the most likely diagnosis in the present patient?
3. Explain the pathogenesis of these auscultatory findings.
4. What is the significance of distended jugular veins and pedal edema? Are these findings related to the clubbing of fingers?
5. Interpret the chest radiographic findings in the context of the other findings. Why is it important to note no nodules or masses were visible on radiograph?
6. What are the consequences of these ABG abnormalities?
7. Does this patient have an obstructive or restrictive lung disease?

Case 3 FEVER, PRODUCTIVE COUGH, AND SHORTNESS OF BREATH IN A CHRONIC ALCOHOLIC

Clinical history   A 50-year-old malnourished chronic alcoholic was hospitalized for fever and exhaustion. At the time of admission he had high fever and was sweating profusely. He was short of breath and had chest pain accentuated by each inspiration.[1] He was short of breath and was constantly coughing and expectorating large amount of rusty yellow sputum.[2]

Physical findings   He had a temperature of 39.2°C, respiratory rate of 30/min, and pulse rate of 120/min. Blood pressure was 110/70 mm Hg. The lips were bluish red and the face was swollen. On percussion of the chest bilateral basal diminished resonance was evident. Auscultation revealed bronchial breath sounds in both lower part of the lungs. A pleural friction rub could be heard on the right midfield of the chest.[3] Chest radiograph disclosed opacities in both lower lobes and pleural effusion on the right side.[4]

Laboratory findings   Blood analysis revealed leukocytosis, with a left shift of neutrophils and elevated erythrocyte sedimentation rate (ESR).[5] ABG analysis showed Pao_2 of 80 mm Hg, $Paco_2$ of 30 mm Hg, HCO_3^- of 23 mEq/L.[6]

Bacteriological studies   *Streptococcus pneumoniae* was isolated from the sputum.[7]

Outcome   The patient was treated with antibiotics and recovered completely.

Questions and topics for discussion
1. Discuss the possible causes of chest pain in this man.
2. What is the significance of a rusty yellow sputum in a patient who has fever and is short of breath?
3. Interpret the physical findings in the context of the other clinical data.
4. What is the pathogenesis of the pleural effusion? Which one of the listed symptoms is related to pleural effusion?
5. What is the significance of leukocytosis and the left shift of neutrophils? What is the significance of the elevated ESR?
6. Interpret the ABGs and blood pH changes. Does the patient have acidosis or alkalosis? What is the role of hyperventilation in the pathogenesis of these changes?
7. Is this an alveolar or interstitial pneumonia? Community-acquired or nosocomial?

Case 4 SLOWLY EVOLVING
PROGRESSIVE SHORTNESS OF BREATH
IN A 45-YEAR-OLD MAN

Clinical history A 45-year-old computer engineer notice shortness of breath on exertion.[1] He did not smoke, and had no workplace exposure to any known harmful gases or particulate matter. The cardiologic examination disclosed no abnormalities.

Physical findings Inspiratory crackles were heard over both lungs. Chest radiographic examination revealed bilateral reticular opacification and some changes suggestive of focal honeycomb changes. High-resolution CT showed changes consistent with interstitial lung disease.[2]

Laboratory findings Pao_2 55 mm Hg, $Paco_2$ 55 mm Hg, HCO_3^- 30 mEq/L, and pH 7.45.

Pulmonary function tests (PFTs) TLC 75% of expected, FEV_1 2.2 L, FVC 2.65 L, FEV_1/FVC % 75. Carbon monoxide diffusion test (D_{LCO}) gave results that were 40% of the predicted value.[3]

Pathology findings Open lung biopsy was interpreted as consistent with usual interstitial pneumonia.[4]

Outcome His condition progressively deteriorated and he finally had a lung transplantation.

Questions and topics for discussion

1. What are the most common causes of progressive dyspnea? The mnemonic **HEART** could help you discuss this question.

    It stands for **h**eart failure, **e**xogenous lung disease (smoking-related COPD, **a**sthma, pneumoconiosis, extrinsic allergic alveolitis), **r**estrictive lung diseases of autoimmune or unknown origin (e.g., UIP, DIP), and **t**hromboemboli (i.e., pulmonary thromboembolism).

2. What are the possible causes of chronic interstitial lung disease?

3. Explain the significance of a relatively normal TLC, reduced FEV_1 in proportion with a loss of FVC, and reduced D_{LCO}? Do these data favor an obstructive or restrictive pattern of lung injury?

4. What is the prognosis for this disease?

Chapter 6

Blood, Bone Marrow, and the Lymphoid System

Introduction

Bone marrow and the lymphoid system contribute cells to the circulating blood, and thus all three are traditionally included under the heading of hematology. The study of blood and blood-forming, or lymphoid, organs is an important aspect of internal medicine and many surgical specialties as illustrated by the following facts:

- Some of the blood diseases, such as anemia or thrombosis, are extremely common and are encountered daily by medical specialists of any profile, including primary care physicians and general practitioners.
- Blood abnormalities are found by means of laboratory testing not only in persons who have hematologic diseases per se, but also those who have many other systemic or organ-centered diseases. For example, hematologic abnormalities, such as high white blood cell (WBC) count, are encountered in the course of many infections. In such cases the hematologic abnormalities are more a symptom of other diseases than diseases in their own right.
- Hematologic tests are routinely performed on both healthy and sick people, and essentially all who are hospitalized or prepared for surgery.
- Malignant tumors of the bone marrow and lymphoid organs are important causes of morbidity and mortality. Every year approximately 65,000 new cases of lymphoma and 25,000 cases of leukemia are diagnosed in the United States.
- The incidence of non-Hodgkin's lymphoma increases with age from 2.4 cases per 100,000 persons in the 20- to 24-year age group to more than 100 cases per 100,000 persons in those older than 75 years.

The relative clinical significance of various diseases involving the blood, bone marrow, and the lymphoid organs is presented graphically in Figure 6-1.

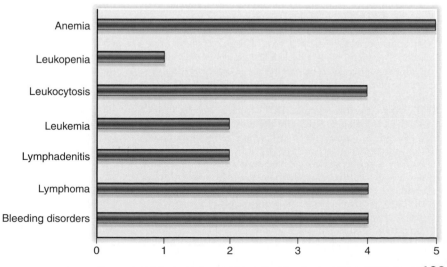

Figure 6-1 Relative clinical significance of hematologic diseases.

KEY WORDS

Anatomy and Physiology

Antibody   Immunoglobulin produced by plasma cells in response to immunization with a specific antigen.

Basophil (basophilic leukocyte)   Mononuclear white blood cell that contains abundant basophilic granules (stains blue with the Giemsa stain). Like mast cells, to which it is related, it participates in inflammatory reactions and atopic hypersensitivity reactions.

Bone marrow   Central part of the bones, composed of trabecullar bone, fat cells or hematopoietic cells, and stroma. The hematopoietic bone marrow occupies the medullary part of most bones in neonates and infants, but in adults it is mostly limited to flat or short bones, such as the sternum, ilium, or vertebrae.

Clot (coagulum)   Semisolid mass made up of a meshwork of polymerized fibrinogen (i.e., fibrin) and other coagulation proteins activated in the intrinsic or extrinsic coagulation pathway. In vivo formed clots also contain blood cells enmeshed in the strands of fibrin.

Cluster of differentiation (CD) antigens   Cytoplasmic and cell surface molecules differentially expressed during the development and differentiation of various subsets of white blood cells and their bone marrow precursors. CD antigens are recognized immunohistochemically with monoclonal antibodies and named by consensus of an international committee. They carry numerical designations (e.g., CD4 as marker or helper T cells). CD antigens are also expressed on malignant cells and are important for the diagnosis of lymphomas and leukemias by immunohistochemistry and flow cytometry.

Coagulation factors   Group of plasma proteins that participate in the coagulation cascade and the formation of the fibrin clot. Coagulation factors are numbered from 1 to 13, but most of them also have assigned names. Calcium is also a coagulation factor and is also known as factor IV. Protein coagulation factors are mostly synthesized by the liver. The activation of factors II, VII, IX, and X occurs only in the presence of the vitamin K-dependent carboxylase.

Coagulation pathway   Physiologic process that leads to the formation of a fibrin clot. It can proceed through an intrinsic and an extrinsic pathway, which converge into a common terminal pathway.

Eosinophil (eosinophilic leukocyte)   Nucleated cell that in its mature form has a bilobed nucleus and numerous eosinophilic cytoplasmic granules. It participates in the defense of the body against infections and plays a prominent role in allergic reactions and the body's response to parasites.

Erythrocyte (red blood cell, RBC)   Nuclear blood cell containing hemoglobin. RBCs are the most abundant cells in the blood, accounting for its red color. Their primary function is oxygen transport.

Erythrocyte precursor cells   Nucleated ancestors of mature red blood cells that are derived in the bone marrow from erythroid progenitor cells in the erythroid burst-forming unit (BFU-E). As they differentiate sequentially, erythrocyte precursor cells can be recognized cytologically in bone marrow aspirates as pronormoblasts, normoblasts, and reticulocytes.

Erythropoietin   Growth/differentiation factor produced primarily by kidneys, stimulating the growth and differentiation of erythrocyte precursor and progenitor cells.

Fibrinolysis   A physiologic process that leads to a controlled dissolution of the fibrin component of the clot. It is principally mediated by plasmin, a zymogen derived from the plasma protein plasminogen under the influence of tissue plasminogen activator (TPA). Plasmin acting on fibrin forms fibrin degradation products (FDPs), which may be found in plasma or urine during fibrinolysis.

Hematopoietic growth factors   Polypeptides that act on hematopoietic progenitor and precursor cells, promoting their proliferation or differentiation (or both). This group of polypeptides includes erythropoietin; thrombopoietin; granulocyte colony-stimulating factor (G-CSF); macrophage colony-stimulating factor (M-CSF), interleukin-3; and related cytokines produced by stromal cells, macrophages, T lymphocytes, and many others.

Hemoglobin   Main protein in erythrocytes enabling them to carry oxygen. Biochemically it is a heterodimeric tetramer composed of four globin polypeptide chains and four heme moieties linked to an iron. Several forms of hemoglobin are recognized on the basis of their globin composition. In adult red blood cells the most abundant is hemoglobin A, which is composed of two alpha and two beta globin chains ($\alpha_2\beta_2$).

Lymphocyte   Mononuclear white blood cell with a round nucleus and scant cytoplasm. Lymphocytes are subdivided into two major groups: T and B lymphocytes. They are derived from precursors located in the bone marrow, lymph nodes, spleen, thymus, and mucosa-associated lymphoid tissue. Lymphocytes participate in inflammatory reactions and are essential for immune reactions.

Megakaryocytes   Multinucleated cells in the bone marrow acting as a precursor of platelets that form by budding of its cytoplasm.

Monocyte   Mononuclear cell containing only a few cytoplasmic granules that are not visible under light microscopy. It participates in inflammatory reactions and can differentiate into tissue macrophages.

Multipotent bone marrow stem cell   Developmentally pluripotent cell, which can differentiate into progenitor cells, giving rise to myeloid or lymphoid lineages.

Myeloblast   Mononuclear poorly granulated precursor of neutrophils that has a relatively large nucleus.

Neutrophil (neutrophilic granulocyte or polymorphonuclear leukocyte (PMN)   Motile phagocytic white blood cell (WBC) derived from precursors in the bone marrow. In its mature form it has a segmented nucleus and abundant cytoplasmic granules, which are neither acidophilic (as in eosinophils) nor basophilic (as in basophils). Neutrophils are the most numerous WBC, even though only 10% of neutrophils are found in circulating blood at any one time. Neutrophils can migrate through the vessel wall in response to chemotactic stimuli and participate in acute inflammatory reactions.

Neutrophil precursor cells   Nucleated ancestors of mature neutrophils derived from the pluripotential stem cell, which gives rise to the myeloid stem cell. This multilineage precursor cell also gives rise to the precursors of monocytes, eosinophils, basophils, platelets, and erythrocytes. In the lineage giving rise to neutrophils it differentiates consecutively into myeloblasts, promyelocytes, metamyelocytes, and band neutrophils prior to becoming mature neutrophils.

Normoblast Bone marrow precursor of red blood cells, characterized by a bluish cytoplasm that contains small amounts of hemoglobin and a round, relatively large nucleus.

Plasma cell Immunoglobulin producing terminally differentiated cells derived from B lymphocytes. Typically found in tissues in chronic inflammation.

Platelet (thrombocyte) Small (2–4 μm) anuclear cell, derived from the fragmentation of the cytoplasm of bone marrow megakaryocytes. It contains many biologically active substances and participates in blood coagulation and inflammation.

White blood cells (WBCs) Nucleated blood cells including neutrophils, eosinophils, basophils, monocytes, lymphocytes, and platelets. WBCs can be seen as a buffy coat on the interface between centrifuged red blood cells and plasma.

Clinical and Laboratory Findings and Procedures

Activated partial thromboplastin time (aPTT) Laboratory test based on measuring the time needed for the in vitro formation of a clot under conditions most favorable for estimating the intrinsic and common coagulation pathway.

Agranulocytosis (granulocytopenia) Reduced number of granulated WBCs (neutrophils, eosinophils, and basophils) in peripheral blood. Typically it is caused by the reduced production of blood cells in the bone marrow and is a feature of aplastic anemia.

Anemia In laboratory medicine it is used as a designation for a reduced red blood cell mass. It is characterized by a reduced volume of RBCs (low hematocrit), a reduced RBC count, or a reduced concentration of hemoglobin.

Bleeding time Clinical test based on measuring the duration of bleeding that follows a needle prick. It is a rough measure of the integrity of the vessel wall and platelet function.

Bone marrow biopsy Sampling of tissue from the bone marrow with a needle. The tissue may be prepared for histologic examination, or the aspirated cells can be smeared and stained for microscopic examination (bone marrow smear).

Coagulopathy Any disturbance of coagulation characterized by either increased coagulability of blood (hypercoagulability or thrombophilia), or a bleeding tendency (hemorrhagic diathesis) related to inadequate clotting of blood. Coagulopathies can be acquired (e.g., vitamin C and K deficiencies) or congenital (e.g., hemophilia).

Disseminated intravascular coagulation (DIC—consumption coagulopathy, or defibrination syndrome) Condition characterized by widespread clotting in the peripheral circulation. It is accompanied by the formation of microthrombi in arterioles, capillaries, and venules (microangiopathy), hemolytic anemia, and a tendency for uncontrolled bleeding due to the consumption of coagulation factors. It may be triggered by many diseases and is a common feature of shock.

Eosinophilia (hypereosinophilia) Increased number of eosinophilic leukocytes in blood or tissues. It is often induced by allergies or parasitic infections.

Fibrin degradation products (FDPs or fibrin split products) Cleaved fragments of fibrin formed through the enzymatic action of fibrolytic enzymes such as plasmin. Since FDPs are relatively small, they pass in urine and can be detected there in DIC.

Hematocrit Measure of the packed red blood cell volume, obtained by separating the red blood cells from plasma by centrifugation in a calibrated tube.

Hemolysis Lysis of red blood cells, which may occur in vivo in circulation or in tissues or in the test tube in vitro. A feature of various hemolytic anemias, lysis also occurs due to aging of RBCs or following bleeding. In vitro it may be induced by toxins, antibodies, or exposure to hypotonic fluid.

Leukocytosis Increased number of WBCs in the circulation. Most often it is a reaction to infection or other diseases, but it may also be a sign of leukemia.

Leukopenia Reduced number of WBCs, usually due to bone marrow failure or bone marrow suppression by some adverse influences, such as toxins or viruses.

Lymphadenopathy Enlargement of lymph nodes of unknown origin. Most often it represents lymph node hyperplasia in response to infection, due to a neoplastic process involving the lymph nodes (e.g., lymphoma or metastatic carcinoma).

Lymphocytosis Increased number of lymphocytes in the peripheral blood. It may be a reaction to infection or immune stimuli, but it is also a sign of lymphocytic leukemia.

Lymphopenia Reduced number of lymphocytes in the peripheral blood. Usually caused by viral infections, as in AIDS.

Monoclonal gammopathy Increased concentration of immunoglobulin gamma, presenting in serum electrophoresis as a sharp ("monoclonal") peak. Typical of multiple myeloma, a neoplastic disorder characterized by monoclonal proliferation of malignant plasma cells that all secrete the same immunoglobulin. Monoclonal gammopathy is also found in monoclonal gammopathy of unknown significance (MNGUS), which may progress to multiple myeloma.

Peripheral blood smear Microscopic specimen prepared by spreading a thin film of peripheral blood on a glass slide and staining it with a metachromatic stain such as Giemsa stain. It used for microscopic examination of the morphology of RBCs and WBCs.

Prothrombin time Clinical test designed to measure the rate at which thrombin is formed in vitro under optimal conditions for estimating the function of factors II, V, VII, and X. It is thus used for assessing the extrinsic and common coagulation pathways. Clinical laboratories report it as standardized to external test values, such as the international normalized ratio (INR).

Thrombocythemia Increased number of platelets in peripheral blood, often a sign of myelodysplastic disorders or leukemia.

Thrombocytopenia Reduced number of platelets in peripheral blood. It may be caused by bone marrow failure or increased destruction of platelets in the spleen or during a coagulopathy, such as DIC.

Thrombosis Formation of clots inside the blood vessels or the heart. Thrombi form due to increased coagulability of the blood, damaged blood vessels, or abnormal circulation.

Hematopathology

Anemia Group of diseases characterized by a decreased number of circulating RBCs or hemoglobin content of blood. It can be classified pathogenetically as anemia due to defective RBC production in the bone marrow or increased blood loss and hemolysis.

Bleeding tendency Group of congenital or acquired disorders characterized by uncontrollable or recurrent bleeding usually from more than one site.

Hemophilia Congenital bleeding disorder characterized by a deficiency of factor VIII (hemophilia A) or factor IX (hemophilia B). Clinically it is characterized by uncontrollable bleeding following trauma or surgery.

Leukemia Group of clonal neoplastic disorders involving the stem cells and precursors of myeloid and lymphoid cells, in which the peripheral blood contains an increased number of neoplastic leukocytes. It can be classified as myelogenous or lymphocytic, and acute or chronic. Each of these groups comprises several distinct clinicopathologic subsets, which can be distinguished from one another by their unique cytogenetic, immunocytochemical, and molecular biologic features.

Lymphoma Malignancy involving the lymphoid system. It includes Hodgkin's lymphoma and non-Hodgkin's lymphoma, which in turn can be subclassified into several clinicopathologic entities. Each of these subtypes has unique histopathologic, immunocytochemical, cytogenetic, and often molecular biologic features, which must be taken into account when choosing proper chemotherapy.

Multiple myeloma Malignancy involving neoplastic proliferation of plasma cells, characterized by monoclonal gammopathy.

Myelodysplastic syndrome Group of clonal hematologic disorders affecting maturation of erythroid, myeloid, and megakaryocytic precursors, with consequent trilineage cytopenia (pancytopenia) in the peripheral blood. It may be hereditary (genetic), primary (idiopathic), or secondary (treatment-related). This group of disorders includes several variants of refractory anemia (e.g., with ring sideroblasts or with an excess of blasts) and chronic myelomonocytic leukemia.

Myeloproliferative disorders Group of neoplastic hematopoietic stem cell disorders characterized by clonal expansion of the bone marrow or ineffective hematopoiesis and the appearance of neoplastic cells and their descendants in the peripheral blood. This group of disorders includes clinicopathologic entities such as chronic myelogenous leukemia, polycythemia vera, essential thrombocythemia, and agnogenic myeloid metaplasia (myelofibrosis).

Polycythemia vera Form of neoplastic clonal myeloproliferative disorder characterized by panmyelocytic hypercellularity of the bone marrow and an increased red blood cell mass. It must be distinguished from secondary polycythemia, in which the increased production of red blood cells is related to exogenous factors evoking oversecretion of erythropoietin.

Purpura Group of bleeding disorders characterized by widespread bleeding into the skin and internal organs. It results from diseases affecting the small blood vessels, platelets, or the entire coagulation system. It comprises a variety of diseases such as vascular, thrombotic, thrombocytopenic, or idiopathic purpura. Etiologically it may be classified as genetic, immune, drug-induced, viral, or idiopathic.

von Willebrand's disease Genetic disease characterized by a bleeding tendency due to a congenital defect in the production of von Willebrand's coagulation factor.

Normal Hematopoiesis

The blood consists of plasma and cells suspended in it. The red blood cells (RBCs) and most of the white blood cells (WBCs) are formed in the bone marrow. The lymphoid system, including the lymph nodes, the thymus, the spleen, and the mucosa-associated lymphoid tissue (MALT), contribute some of the lymphocytes.

In the adults most blood cells are derived from the bone marrow.

During prenatal life, the first signs of embryonic hematopoiesis are found in the **yolk sac** 4 weeks after conception. During the second trimester the **liver** and the **spleen** become the primary sites of fetal hematopoiesis, to be gradually relocated to the bone marrow inside the developing skeleton. In adults, the hematopoietic bone marrow is confined to the **axial skeleton,** including the sternum, ribs, vertebrae, and pelvic bones (Fig. 6-2).

The hematopoietic bone marrow comprises **hematopoietic cells** and **bone marrow stroma,** which form the microenvironment essential for the growth and differentiation of the hematopoietic cells (Fig. 6-3). It also contains blood vessels, mostly in the form of sinusoids. These **sinusoids** have fenestrated walls so that the newly formed blood cells can easily enter the circulation. The bone marrow also contains thin bone trabeculae, which provide mechanical support and protection, and fat cells. With aging the hematopoietic elements decrease in number, and the fat cells become more numerous, replacing up to 70% of the total hematopoietic bone marrow in the elderly.

Blood cells develop from pluripotent hematopoietic stem cells under the influence of growth and differentiation factors.

The formation of blood cells is a highly regulated process that occurs in several steps involving both cell multiplication and differentiation. Several **cell lineages** are formed, ultimately giving rise to mature RBCs, platelets, and several distinct types of WBCs: neutrophils, eosinophils, basophils, monocytes, and lymphocytes (Fig. 6-4).

All hematopoietic cell lineages can be traced to a common ancestor—the **pluripotent hematopoietic stem cell.** Even though these cells account for less than 1% of all

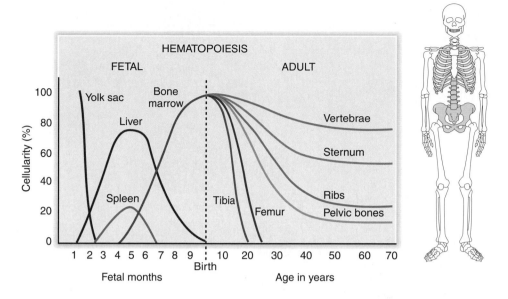

Figure 6-2 Blood-forming and lymphoid organs.

hematopoietic bone marrow cells, the adult bone marrow contains 25 to 500 million pluripotent stem cells. Some of these stem cells also enter into the circulating blood, from where they can be harvested for bone marrow transplantation. The pluripotent hematopoietic stem cells resemble small lymphocytes and can be identified only immunocytologically or by flow cytometry using labeled antibodies to their cell membrane marker—CD34.

Like all stem cells the totipotent hematopoeitic stem cells have a capacity for self-renewal but can also differentiate into two types of **multilineage progenitor cells:** lymphoid and myeloid progenitor cells. These progenitor cells give rise to **unilineage progenitor cells,** which in turn differentiate into **committed precursor cells** of mature lymphocytes,

RBCs, neutrophils, monocytes, eosinophils, basophils, and platelets.

The replication of stem cells and progenitor cells and the differentiation of precursor cells depend on the action of **growth** and **differentiation factors** produced by the stromal cells, macrophages, and T lymphocytes. Numerous growth and differentiation factors have been isolated and characterized; many of these have been synthesized using recombinant DNA technology and are used in clinical practice to stimulate and or regulate hematopoiesis. **Erythropoietin** acts on the precursors of RBCs, **thrombopoietin** stimulates platelet production, and **granulocyte colony-stimulating factor** (G-CSF) acts on the differentiation of neutrophil precursors. **Interleukin 3** (IL-3) behaves as a nonlineage-specific growth

Figure 6-3 Bone marrow. The hematopoietic cells are located between the bone trabeculae. Cells of a single lineage tend to form groups, most prominent of which are the myeloid and erythroid nests. Megakaryocytes stand out because of their large size and multilobed nuclei. Blood vessels occur mostly in the form of sinusoids, which have fenestrated walls. RBC, red blood cell; WBC, white blood cell.

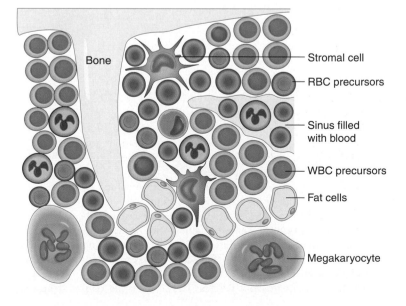

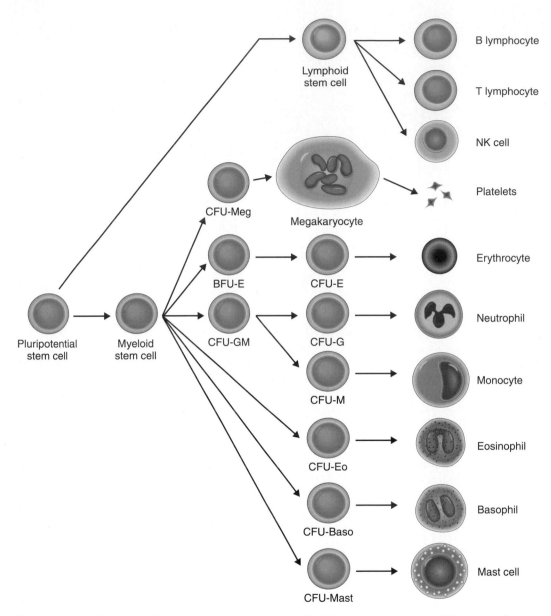

Figure 6-4 Cell lineages of hematopoiesis. Baso, basophil; BFU, burst-forming unit; CFU, colony-forming unit; E, erythrocyte; Eo, eosinophil; GM, granulocyte/macrophage; M, monocyte; Meg, megakaryocyte; NK, natural killer.

factor, acting on both myeloid and lymphoid lineages. Note that the terminal stages of lymphocyte maturation and differentiation are **antigen-dependent** and can be significantly amplified during immune reactions.

The differentiation of precursor cells is accompanied by the appearance and disappearance of specific cell surface molecules. Cell surface molecules known as **clusters of differentiation (CD)** have been especially useful for monitoring the maturation and differentiation of myeloid and lymphoid cells. For example CD34 is a marker of stem cells, CD4 is a marker for T helper cells, and CD8 is a marker for T cytotoxic cells, whereas CD20 is marker of B

cells. Over 200 CD markers have been identified today, and many of them are used for diagnostic purposes in clinical hematopathology and immunology.

Normal hematopoiesis requires an adequate supply of energy, nutrients, and vitamins.

Formation and maturation of hematopoietic stem cells are tightly controlled by growth and differentiation factors. This process is also critically dependent on the normal supply of energy, nutrients, and vitamins. The most important among these are as follows:

- **Proteins.** Proteins are essential ingredients of food, and a protein-deficient diet adversely affects hematopoiesis. This is most prominent in persons who have unusual dietary habits, suffer from eating disorders, or have intestinal malabsorption syndromes. Increased demand for proteins during pregnancy or childhood also may affect hematopoiesis, especially if combined with other nutritional deficiencies, such as an iron or vitamin deficiency.
- **Iron.** A normal diet contains adequate amounts of iron, which is essential for the formation of hemoglobin (Hb). Inadequate intake or abnormal absorption in malabsorption syndromes, or an increased loss of RBCs (e.g., during heavy menstruation), may cause iron deficiency.
- **Vitamin B_{12}.** This vitamin complex includes several cobalamines, which are normally present in meat and animal products. Vitamin B_{12} binds to the intrinsic factor secreted by gastric parietal cells and is absorbed in the small intestines. Dietary deficiency or abnormal absorption may adversely affect the synthesis of DNA during hematopoietic cell growth and maturation. Vitamin B_{12} is crucial for the formation of tetrahydrofolate, which plays the role of an essential coenzyme in the synthesis of DNA (Fig. 6-5). A lack of vitamin B_{12} typically results in megaloblastic anemia.
- **Folic acid.** Normally present in green leafy vegetables, folic acid together with cobalamin is essential for normal DNA synthesis. Deficiency may result from inadequate intake, absorption, or utilization (i.e., as in

patients treated with folic acid antagonists). Clinically it also manifests as megaloblastic anemia.

The life span of normal blood cells varies.

The blood cells can be divided into three groups: RBCs (erythrocytes), WBCs (leukocytes), and platelets, or thrombocytes. The RBCs and platelets do not have nuclei, whereas the WBCs do. On the basis of the shape of their nuclei the WBCs can be further divided into segmented cells (neutrophils and eosinophils) and nonsegmented, or mononuclear, cells (monocytes and lymphocytes).

The normal life span of blood cells varies. The process of formation of blood cells and their maturation inside the bone marrow varies, and the duration the mature cells remain in the bone marrow is also cell lineage-specific. Likewise, the half-life of cells in the circulation varies. Remember that mature RBCs spend all their life inside the blood vessels, whereas WBCs can exit into the tissues and live there as well.

Red blood cells. Erythrocytes live in the circulation the longest—on average 120 days. This is important because RBCs can be removed from the blood and stored a few days or even a week or two for transfusion. Old and damaged RBCs are mostly lyzed by the splenic macrophages, but a small portion of them are hemolyzed inside the blood vessels. Thus we can distinguish between extravascular and intravascular hemolysis.

- **Extravascular hemolysis.** Lysis of RBCs in the splenic macrophages results in an efflux of **bilirubin** that is bound to albumin ("unconjugated bilirubin") and transferred for further processing and excretion into the liver (Fig. 6-6). In the liver bilirubin is conjugated and made water-soluble and excreted into the intestine. Most of the intestinal bilirubin is recirculated and reused, but part of it is excreted in the urine as **urobilinogen.**
- **Intravascular hemolysis.** Under normal circumstances intravascular hemolysis affects only a small percentage of RBCs, but under certain abnormal conditions it may take major proportions. The fragmented RBCs release free Hb, mostly in the form of Hb dimers, which bind to a plasma protein called **haptoglobin.** It serves as a carrier for free Hb dimers and transports them to the liver. A part of Hb is oxidized into methemoglobin, which is degraded into globin and oxidized heme (**ferriheme**). Ferriheme binds to **hemopexin,** which carries it to the liver. After hemopexin is exhausted, excess oxidized heme can also bind to albumin and thus form **methemalbumin,** which is also taken up by the liver. Hemoglobin dimers that are not bound to plasma proteins are excreted in the urine. Hence, intravascular hemolysis is accompanied by **hemoglobinuria, hemosiderinuria,** and **urobilinuria.**

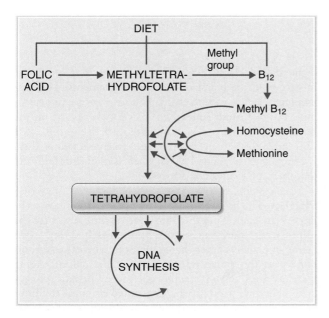

Figure 6-5 The role of vitamin B_{12} and folic acid in DNA synthesis. Vitamin B_{12} is essential for the formation of tetrahydrofolate (THF) from folic acid. THF in its methylated form acts as a coenzyme for DNA synthesis.

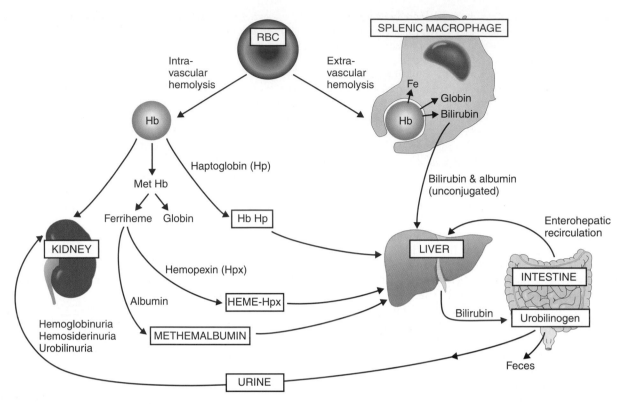

Figure 6-6 Lysis of senescent red blood cells (RBCs). Extravascular hemolysis occurs in the spleen and results in the formation of bilirubin, which is processed in the liver. Intravascular hemolysis leads to the formation of hemoglobin degradation products, which bind to specific plasma proteins carrying them into the liver. Unbound hemoglobin dimers are excreted in the urine, accounting for hemoglobinuria and hemosiderinuria. Both forms of hemolysis are associated with an increased excretion of urobilinogen in urine. Met Hb, methemoglobin.

Iron released in extravascular or intravascular hemolysis is reused to synthesize Hb. Globin is also reused.

Granulocytes. White blood cell precursors in the bone marrow form two compartments: a proliferative compartment and a maturation-storage compartment. In the first the cells remain for less than one day. It has been estimated that the maturing neutrophils remain in the maturation-storage department of the bone marrow for 7 to 10 days. Eosinophils remain there 2.5 days and basophils for only 12 hours.

Neutrophils enter the circulation from the bone marrow pool maturation-storage compartment, which contains the equivalent of neutrophils in reserve for 4 to 8 days. The half-life of neutrophilic granulocytes in circulation is 6 to 12 days. Neutrophils enter the blood in the form of segmented neutrophils or band cells. In the circulation they form two distinct sets: the marginating pool (storage portion) and the circulating pool. Neutrophils also can enter into the tissue, where they live, on average, for 2 to 3 days (Fig. 6-7).

Approximately 6% of all circulating WBCs are nonsegmented (band cells), whereas all others undergo nuclear segmentation. As they age their nuclei become more segmented, and the oldest ones have five segments. This segmentation can be used to estimate the average age of neutrophils in the **Arneth index,** which is a curve based on the number of segments of neutrophilic nuclei (Fig. 6-8). Left shift indicates that fewer nuclei are segmented; that is, there is a prevalence of young PMNs, whereas right shift indicates that there are more aging PMNs.

Platelets. The half-life of platelets in circulation is 8 to 10 days. Platelets leaving the bone marrow initially enter the spleen where they remain for approximately 2 days. Two thirds of platelets enter the circulation, whereas one third remain as the active reserve pool of the spleen. Aging platelets are phagocytosed by splenic or hepatic phagocytic cells but may also be consumed at sites of minor endothelial cell injury, thereby activating intravascular coagulation.

Lymphocytes. These cells are long-lived, and their life span may be measured in months or years.

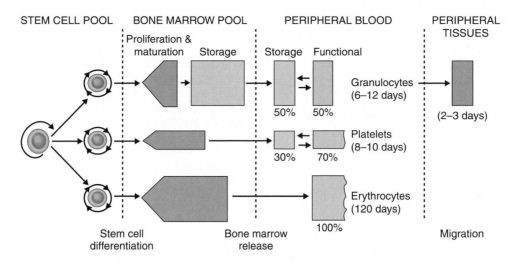

Figure 6-7 Typical life span of neutrophils, platelets, and red blood cells and their bone marrow precursors. As shown in the diagram, all these cells originate from stem cells, but their life span in the bone marrow and outside of it varies. In the bone marrow the neutrophils are found in a proliferation–maturation compartment and a storage compartment. Platelets and erythrocytes are released as soon as they are formed and do not form a storage compartment. In peripheral blood the neutrophils and platelets form two compartments: a storage pool and a functional compartment. All red blood cells are in circulation and there is no red blood cell storage compartment. Under normal circumstances only neutrophils (and other leukocytes) emigrate into tissues.

Normal Functions of Blood Cells

The blood cells have many functions. Nevertheless, each type has a highly specialized primary function as follows:

- **Red blood cells**—Oxygen transport. Red blood cells also serve as the primary transport vehicle for carbon

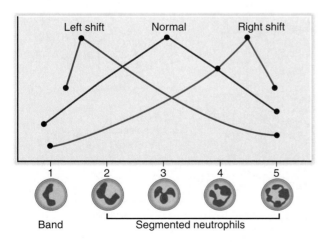

Figure 6-8 Arneth index. The blood contains young neutrophils (band cells) and old neutrophils (cells with five segmented nuclei), but most neutrophils have nuclei with three segments. Left shift of the curve indicates more young neutrophils in the circulation, and right shift more aging neutrophils.

dioxide, carrying it from the tissues into the lungs, where it is excreted. They also bind other gases and some other chemicals and act as part of the buffer system of the blood.

- **Granulocytes**—Defense against infectious pathogens. **Neutrophils, eosinophils,** and **basophils** form the primary line of defense against bacteria, and eosinophils act against parasites. All WBCs secrete cytokines and other biologically active substances that are important for the inflammatory reactions and also may contribute to the metabolic response to infections.

- **Monocytes**—Defense against pathogens and particulate matter. Monocytes are precursors of some tissue **macrophages,** and together they form the body's phagocytic system. Tissue derivatives of monocytes act as **antigen-presenting cells** and participate in antigen uptake and presentation to lymphocytes; hence, they are an important part of the immune response. Macrophages produce **cytokines** and many other biologically active substances. They also participate in tissue repair, as in wound healing or healing of fractures.

- **Lymphocytes**—Immune response. **B lymphocytes** differentiate into antibody-secreting **plasma cells,** whereas the **T lymphocytes** participate in the cell-mediated immune reactions. These cells also participate in the defense against viral infections. Lymphocytes are a major source of **cytokines,** which regulate many body functions in health and disease.

■ **Platelets**—Coagulation. Platelets are essential components of blood clotting, but they also secrete **mediators of inflammation** and participate in many inflammatory and some immune reactions.

The primary function of red blood cells is transport of oxygen.

Erythrocytes, or **red blood cells (RBCs),** are highly specialized cells that do not have nuclei. In contrast to RBCs in the peripheral blood, their precursors in the bone marrow are nucleated. As the erythroid precursors mature, their nuclei become smaller and smaller and are finally extruded from the cytoplasm. The anucleated RBCs that still have residual RNA and a few cytoplasmic organelles may be also released into the circulation. These cells, called **reticulocytes,** account for less than 1% of all RBCs under normal circumstances.

The primary function of RBCs is transport of oxygen from the lungs into the peripheral tissues, but they also can bind other gases and also act as buffers. These functions are accomplished primarily through Hb, which accounts for 98% of their total weight.

Hemoglobin is a complex protein composed of globin and heme (Fig. 6-9). Globin is a tetramer composed of two α chains and two β chains or their equivalents γ and δ. The most abundant form of Hb is Hb A composed of two α and two β chains ($\alpha_2\beta_2$). During fetal life the most predominant Hb is fetal hemoglobin (Hb F), which contains two α chains and two γ chains ($\alpha_2\gamma_2$), but its level drops precipitously after birth, and by the age of 6 months it accounts for only 1% of the total Hb. Adult blood also contains Hb A_2, which is composed of two α and two δ chains ($\alpha_2\delta_2$), accounting for less than 3.5% of total Hb. The concentration of Hb in the blood is lower in females than in males and also lower in adults than in newborns (Table 6-1).

Table 6-1 Normal Values of Hemoglobin (Hb) in Blood

Adults	Hb A ($\alpha_2\beta_2$) >95%
Males 14.0–18.0 g/dL (140–180 g/L)	Hb A_2 ($\alpha_2\delta_2$) <3.5%
	Hb F ($\alpha_2\gamma_2$) 1–2%
Females 12.0–15.0 g/dL (120–150 g/L)	
Newborns 16.5–21.5 g/dL (165–215 g/L)	Hb F ($\alpha_2\gamma_2$) 60–90%
	Hb A ($\alpha_2\beta_2$) 10–40%

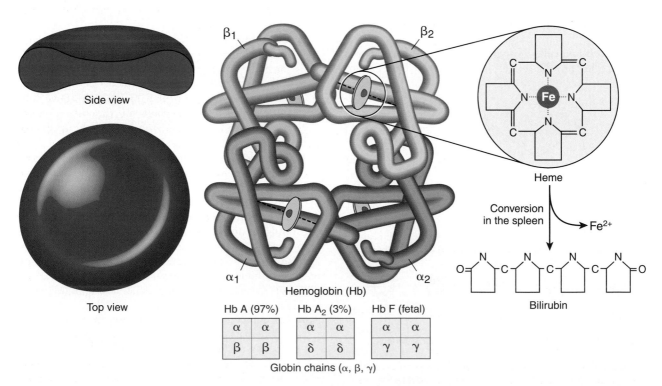

Figure 6-9 Hemoglobin structure. (Reproduced with permission from Damjanov I: Pathology for Health Professions, 3rd ed. Philadelphia, Elsevier, 2005.)

Affinity of hemoglobin for oxygen varies and depends on several factors.

Hemoglobin has a high affinity for oxygen, but it also binds carbon dioxide and carbon monoxide. The affinity of Hb for oxygen depends on the pH of the blood, temperature, and concentration of 2,3-biphosphoglycerate (2,3-BPG), and the presence of variant hemoglobins that have a higher affinity for oxygen. The affinity for oxygen can be determined by measuring the oxygen pressure needed to achieve 50% saturation of Hb (P_{50}) (Fig. 6-10). In a normal person at pH 7.35 this saturation can be achieved at a Po_2 of 27 mm Hg. The oxygen saturation curve can be left-shifted, meaning that a P_{50} can be achieved at lower partial pressure by changing the following variables:

- Increasing the pH of blood into the alkaline range
- Reducing the Pco_2
- Reducing the temperature
- Decreasing the concentration of 2,3-BPG
- Increasing the concentration of Hb variants that have high oxygen affinity, such as Hb F, or decreasing the amount of low-affinity Hb, such as Hb S in sickle cell anemia.

Variant and abnormal hemoglobins influence oxygen binding and its release in tissues as follows:

- **Fetal hemoglobin (Hb F)** binds weakly with 2,3-BPG, thus shifting the curve to the left. In fetal or neonatal blood a P_{50} can be achieved at a Po_2 of 19 to 21 mm Hg.

This has an advantage before birth because it enables the fetus to "steal" oxygen from the mother. However, since the release of oxygen is also slower, in postnatal life the persistence of Hb F does not serve the affected person well.

- **Hemoglobin S (Hb S).** In sickle cell anemia the RBCs containing Hb S tend to bind oxygen with high affinity, thus shifting the curve to the right.
- **Methemoglobin.** Instead of the ferrous iron (Fe^{2+}) present in the normal Hb, methemoglobin contains ferric iron (Fe^{3+}). Normal blood contains less than 1% of Hb in this form, which is produced due to spontaneous oxidation of Hb. Methemoglobin has an increased affinity for oxygen, and it cannot release it in tissues as efficiently as normal Hb. Increased amounts of methemoglobin, caused by drugs and toxins may result in cyanosis, especially in infants whose normal methemoglobin-reducing capacity has not been fully developed. It leads to a left shift of the oxygen dissociation curve.
- **Carboxyhemoglobin.** Carbon monoxide (CO) is formed in small amounts in the healthy body. It binds to Hb, forming carboxyhemoglobin, which in normal persons accounts for 0.2 to 0.8% of total Hb in blood. In smokers it may be elevated from 4% to 15%. Since Hb has approximately 200 times higher affinity for CO than for oxygen, large amounts of carboxyhemoglobin are formed in CO poisoning, as after suicide by inhaling car exhaust gases or kitchen oven gas. Death results from CO preventing oxygenation of Hb, which ultimately leads to lethal hypoxia.

Granulocytes participate in the defense against infection.

Granulocytes respond to infection by entering the circulation and moving toward the site of infection (Fig. 6-11). At the site of infection the neutrophils marginate, adhere to the endothelial cells of capillaries and venules, and undergo activation. In addition to surface changes and changes in motility, activated neutrophils secrete biologically active substances that act on other cells in the tissues, most notably endothelial cells, macrophages, and lymphocytes. In concert with the activated neutrophils these cells secrete cytokines and growth factors, such as interleukins, tumor necrosis factor (TNF), platelet-activating factor (PAF), and many others. These substances act on the bone marrow, stimulating it to release new neutrophils into circulation and to proliferate stem cells and the precursors of granulocytes. All these events lead to neutrophilia—an increase in the number of neutrophils in circulation.

Neutrophils phagocytose and kill bacteria.

Neutrophils (also known as polymorphonuclear leukocytes—PMNs) form the first line of defense against bacterial infection. PMNs are so efficient at fighting bacteria because of the following properties:

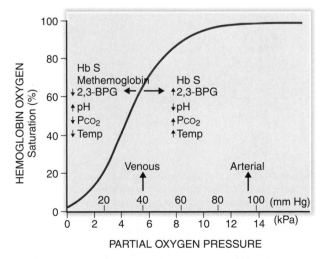

Figure 6-10 Oxygen dissociation curve. Alkalization of the blood, low temperature, low partial pressure of CO_2 (Pco_2), and a low concentration or availability of 2,3-biphosphoglycerate (2,3-BPG) cause a left shift, whereas acidity of the blood, high temperature, and a high 2,3-BPG cause a right shift. Fetal hemoglobin (Hb F) has a higher affinity for oxygen than adult hemoglobin, thus causing a left shift. Hb S found in sickle cell disease shifts the curve to the right.

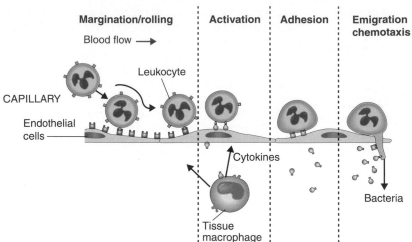

Figure 6-11 Reaction of neutrophils to infection. The neutrophils become marginated, adhere to the endothelium, and are activated in that process. Neutrophils respond to chemotactic stimuli and migrate toward the bacteria in the tissue. Cytokines and other biologically active substances produced at the site of inflammation act on the bone marrow, causing a release of neutrophils into the circulation (neutrophilia) and increased production of neutrophils in the bone marrow.

- **High mobility.** The PMNs are capable of amoeboid movement, allowing them to exit blood vessels and reach the site of infection much faster than any other cell.
- **Sensitivity to chemotactic stimuli.** PMNs respond to chemotactic substances generated by bacteria and injured tissue cells.
- **Phagocytic capacity.** PMNs readily form phagocytic vacuoles and are thus capable of ingesting bacteria and any other fragments found at the site of infection. Bacterial ingestion is facilitated by **opsonins,** such as complement fragment C3a and immunoglobulin G.
- **Bactericidal activity.** PMNs can kill phagocytosed bacteria by oxygen-dependent and oxygen-independent enzymatic mechanisms (Fig. 6-12).

Loss of phagocytic cells, such as occurs in agranulocytosis caused by cytotoxic drugs and various disorders affecting the basic functions of the neutrophils, results in increased susceptibility to bacterial infections. These disorders can be congenital or acquired. The most important examples of deficient function of neutrophils are listed in Table 6-2.

Neutrophil dysfunction may be induced by drugs and alcohol and is typically found in many metabolic diseases, such as diabetes or end-stage kidney disease. Autoimmune diseases and HIV infection also cause neutrophil dysfunctions.

Eosinophils play a role in defending the body against parasites.

Eosinophils participate in the body's defense against bacteria. However, eosinophils are less numerous and migrate much slower than neutrophils, and thus they contribute significantly less in the fight against bacteria than PMNs. If the infection is long-lasting eosinophils become more prominent. Eosinophils are most prominently involved in the reaction to parasites. Eosinophilia is also found in patients who have allergies, autoimmune diseases, and skin diseases and is present in response to certain malignancies, such as Hodgkin's disease.

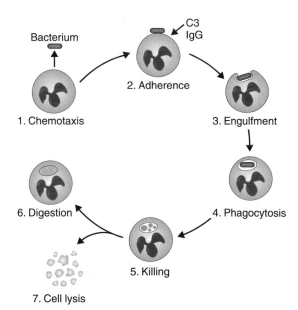

Figure 6-12 Phagocytosis of bacteria. Several phases can be recognized. (1) The bacterium acts chemotactically, attracting the neutrophil. (2) Adherence of bacteria to the surface of leukocytes is facilitated by opsonins such as complement fragments (C3) or IgG. (3) The bacterium is engulfed in the pseudopodia formed by the elongation of the cytoplasm of the neutrophil. (4) Phagocytosis of the bacterium includes formation of a phagosome from the phagocytic vacuoles and lysosomes. (5) Phagocytosed bacteria are killed by oxygen-dependent and oxygen-independent mechanisms. (6) Killed bacteria are digested. (7) During the interaction with the bacterium the leukocyte may be killed, releasing its cytoplasmic contents into the extracellular space. The exudate composed of dead and dying leukocytes and lyzed tissue components is called pus.

Table 6-2 Congenital Disorders of Leukocyte Function

DEFECTIVE MECHANISM	DISEASE
Defective adhesion	Leukocyte adhesion deficiency I and II
Decreased motility	Lazy leukocyte syndrome
Decreased phagocytosis	Chediak-Higashi syndrome
Decreased bacterial killing	Chronic granulomatous disease
	Myeloperoxidase deficiency

Lymphocytes are involved in the immune reactions.

Like all other WBCs and RBCs, lymphocytes originate from a common hematopoietic stem cell, which gives rise to developmentally restricted stem cells, populating the bone marrow and the peripheral lymphoid tissues. Three cell lines develop from this common lymphocytic precursor: T lymphocytes, B lymphocytes, and natural killer (NK) cells. In the circulating blood approximately 70% to 80% lymphocytes are B cells, 10% to 15% T cells, and 10% to 15% NK cells.

The differentiation of lymphocytes occurs gradually and is characterized by the appearance and disappearance of cell surface molecules known as **clusters of differentiation** (CD).

- **T cells** mature by passing through the thymus, which typically occurs during fetal life and childhood. Inside the thymus the T cells differentiate into CD4$^+$ **T helper cells** and CD8$^+$ **T cytotoxic cells.** T cells are primarily involved in cell-mediated immune reactions, but they also regulate the functions of B cells.
- **B cells** also differentiate stepwise and finally give rise to plasma cells—terminally differentiated cells involved in the production of immunoglobulins. Like T cells, the B cells interact with antigen-presenting cells, such as macrophages, Langerhans cells, or dendritic cells, but also among themselves.
- **NK cells** differ from T and B cells in that they do not have immunologic memory, but act without priming against tumor cells and virus-infected cells.

Platelets are involved in coagulation of the blood.

Platelets are derived from the fragmentation of the cytoplasm of megakaryocytes in the bone marrow. This process is primarily regulated by **thrombopoietin,** a cytokine produced by the liver. The platelets released from the bone marrow are carried to the spleen, which serves as their primary reservoir. From the spleen the platelets periodically enter the circulation and are dispatched to areas of endothelial injury.

Platelets are small membrane-bounded particles measuring 2 to 4 μm. They do not have nuclei and are barely visible under light microscopy. The cytoplasm of platelets contains several components that are essential for their function (Fig. 6-13). Thus, it contains the following organelles:

- **Mitochondria.** These organelles generate energy, which is used to support all the essential functions of platelets. **Glycogen** stored in the cytoplasm serves as a source of energy.
- **Granules.** The platelets contain several forms of granules. The most abundant are the **alpha granules,** which contain numerous proinflammatory and procoagulant and even anticoagulant proteins. Among other substances, alpha granules contain von Willebrand's factor, fibrinogen, factor V, platelet-derived growth factor (PDGF), transforming growth factor-β (TGF-β), and the anticoagulant protein S. **Dense granules** contain energy-rich compounds such as adenosine diphosphate (ADP) and vasoactive substances such as serotonin. **Lysosomes** are important for lytic functions.
- **Cytoskeleton.** The principal components of the cytoskeleton are the **microtubules,** composed of tubulin, and **microfilaments,** composed of actin and myosin. These fibrils are important for the maintenance of the shape of the platelets, their contraction, and the movement of other organelles and extrusion of granules.
- **Plasma membrane.** This complex membrane is important for maintaining the integrity and the shape of

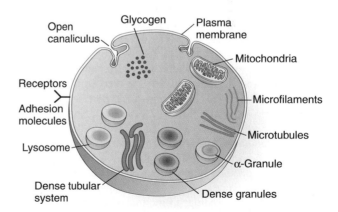

Figure 6-13 Ultrastructure of the platelet. The external plasma membrane is studded with receptors and adhesion molecules (cannot be seen by electron microscopy). The plasma membrane invaginates, forming a canaliculus. Cytoskeletal fibers (microtubules and microfilaments) are important for the changes in the shape of platelets and the excretion of preformed substances sorted in various granules (alpha granules, dense granules, dense tubular system, lysosomes). Glycogen forms pools and is an important source of energy, which is produced primarily by the mitochondria.

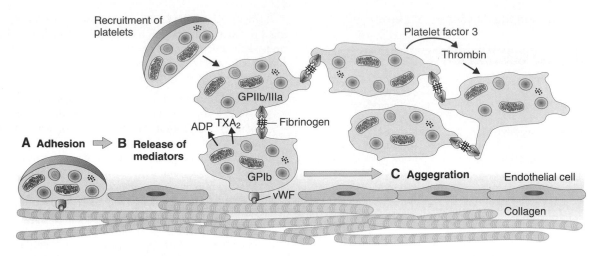

Figure 6-14 Formation of the platelet plug. **A,** Adhesion of platelets to the collagen in the vessel wall denuded of endothelial cells is mediated by von Willebrand's factor (vWF), which binds to collagen and the platelet adhesion molecule GPIb. **B,** Adhesion is followed by a change in the shape of platelets accompanied by a release of various procoagulants, most notably adenosine diphosphate (ADP) and thromboxane A_2 (TXA_2), and fibrinogen. **C,** The procoagulants released from the activated platelets recruit additional platelets to the site of endothelial injury and also promote their aggregation, leading to the formation of the primary hemostatic plug.

platelets. It invaginates into the cytoplasm in the form of open canaliculi; it also contains numerous cell surface **receptors** and **adhesion molecules.** These complex glycoproteins are part of the cell membrane and are essential for the adhesion of platelets to surfaces and the initiation of the coagulation process. For example, the adhesion molecule **GP IIb-IIIa** binds to fibrinogen, and **GP Ib** binds to von Willebrand's factor and collagen. Surface receptors also bind activators of platelets such as ADP or thromboxane A_2 (TXA_2).

Circulating platelets readily adhere to damaged endothelial cells and fill the endothelial defects in disrupted or damaged blood vessels. The **hemostatic platelet plug** that forms under such conditions is a hallmark of **primary hemostasis** (Fig. 6-14). It leads to the activation of the coagulation cascade and formation of the **fibrin clot** known as **secondary hemostasis** (Fig. 6-15).

Defective primary hemostasis manifests as bleeding from capillaries and venules. Clinically skin bruises (petechiae and ecchymoses) or bleeding from mucosae of the mouth (gingival bleeding), nose (epistaxis), or intestine (hematochezia) may be evident. Bleeding usually results from vascular defects or platelet abnormalities, such as thrombocytopenia. The bleeding time is prolonged.

Defective secondary hemostasis is associated with bleeding from small arteries and arterioles and is often related to trauma, surgical procedures, or tooth extraction. It may result in the formation of large intramuscular or retroperitoneal hematomas, or hemarthrosis. Bleeding is usually related to a congenital deficiency of clotting factors, as occurs in hemo-

philia, or acquired abnormalities of the coagulation pathway, as occurs in chronic liver disease. Prothrombin time (PT) and activated partial thromboplastin time (aPTT) are prolonged.

The typical features of defective primary and secondary hemostasis are compared in Table 6-3.

Clinical and Laboratory Evaluation of Hematologic Diseases

Family and personal history may provide important diagnostic clues.

Family and personal history can point to some important risk factors that play a role in the pathogenesis of hematologic diseases. A few examples of such links and associations are given in Table 6-4.

Physical examination is important for evaluating hematologic disorders.

Symptoms and signs of hematologic diseases usually result from a loss or disturbance in the formation and function of RBCs, WBCs, or platelets and coagulation proteins. In some patients the hematologic problems dominate the clinical picture, whereas in others they are of secondary importance. Most manifestations of hematologic disorders are nonspecific and linked to a specific disturbance of blood-forming organs only with the judicious use of laboratory examinations. The following list includes some signs and symptoms that illustrate how these findings could point to a hematologic disease.

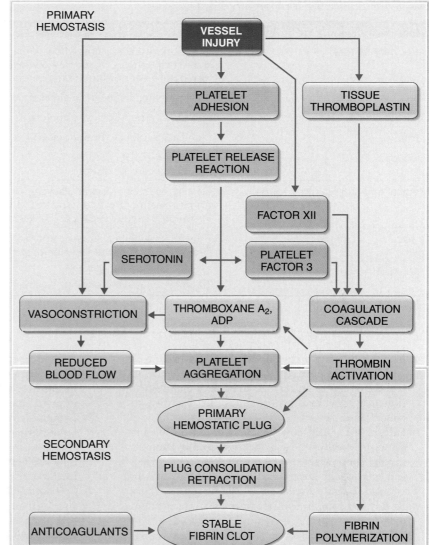

Figure 6-15 Primary and secondary hemostasis. As shown in Figure 6-14, vessel injury leads to the formation of the platelet adhesion, followed by the release of procoagulants and platelet aggregation. These events, leading to the formation of the primary hemostatic plug, are known as primary hemostasis. Substances released from platelets also cause vasoconstriction (thereby reducing blood flow to the damaged vessels) and activate the coagulation cascade and the formation of thrombin. Thrombin acts on platelets, promoting platelet aggregation, consolidation of the primary hemostatic plug, and its retraction. It also promotes polymerization of fibrin and thus contributes to the formation of a stable fibrin clot. These events are called secondary hemostasis. The fibrin clot is the substrate for several anticoagulants and fibrinolytic proteins, the most important of which is plasmin. ADP, adenosine diphosphate.

Table 6-3 Disturbances of Primary and Secondary Hemostasis

PARAMETER	PRIMARY HEMOSTASIS	SECONDARY HEMOSTASIS
Cause	Vessel wall, platelets	Coagulation factors
Source of bleeding	Capillaries, venules	Arteries and arterioles
Mode of bleeding	Spontaneous	Trauma/surgery-related
Site of bleeding	Skin and mucosae	Intramuscular hematomas, hemarthrosis, surgical wounds
Screening tests	Platelet count	Prothrombin time
	Bleeding time	Activated partial thromboplastin time

Table 6-4 Risk Factors for Hematologic Diseases

TYPE OF RISK FACTOR	SPECIFIC DISEASES–RISK FACTOR ASSOCIATIONS
Hereditary factors	Sickle cell disease: Hemolytic anemia Hereditary spherocytosis: Hemolytic anemia Hemophilia A or B: Bleeding disorder
Nutritional factors	Folate or vitamin B_{12} deficient diet: Megaloblastic anemia
Gastrointestinal bleeding	Iron deficiency: Microcytic anemia
Cirrhosis	Bleeding tendency: Prolonged PTT or thrombocytopenia
Infections	Malaria: Hemolytic anemia Anemia of chronic disease
Medical and surgical procedures	Gastric resection: Megaloblastic anemia Cancer treatment with antifolates: Megaloblastic anemia Radiation therapy for cancer: Leukopenia
Drugs	Bone marrow injury: Aplastic anemia Drugs acting as haptenes: Hemolytic anemia
External mechanical factors	Trauma-related shock: DIC Traumatic massive bleeding: Anemia due to blood loss

DIC, disseminated intravascular coagulation; PTT, prothrombin time

- **Easy fatigability.** Fatigue is a common symptom of anemia and is related to the reduced capacity of blood to carry oxygen. It may also manifest as shortness of breath, drowsiness, or inability to concentrate.
- **Pallor.** A reduced concentration of Hb in anemia causes paleness of the mucosae best seen by examining the conjunctiva or oral mucosa. Previously when leukemia could not be treated, excess of WBCs in circulation also caused a white complexion.
- **Ruddy red face.** In contrast to anemia, which causes pallor, polycythemia is typically associated with a ruddy red face. Sluggish flow of the hyperviscous blood in these patients also leads to prominent dilatation of the retinal blood vessels, which can be seen with the ophthalmoscope.
- **Jaundice.** Hemolytic anemia is typically associated with jaundice. Excess bilirubin released from hemolyzed RBCs predisposes to the formation of gallstones.
- **Tachycardia.** Anemia is associated with compensatory tachycardia and audible cardiac murmurs.
- **Oral mucosal changes.** Deficiency of iron may cause angular cheilitis, whereas vitamin B_{12} and folate may produce a velvety red tongue typical of glossitis.
- **Recurrent infection.** Skin and nasopharyngeal infections occur at an increased rate in patients who have leukopenia, aplastic anemia, or functional disorders affecting leukocytes.
- **Excessive bleeding.** Bleeding from the gums or nose or into the skin are signs of thrombocytopenia caused by bone marrow failure, which occurs in aplastic anemia or in various forms of leukemia. Hemophilia presents with post-traumatic bleeding, hemarthrosis, or prolonged bleeding after surgical interventions.
- **Lymphadenopathy.** Lymph node enlargement may be the first sign of lymphoma, but it could also be related to infections or autoimmune diseases. Clinically it is best to consider lymphadenopathy as either localized or generalized (Table 6-5).
- **Splenomegaly.** Enlargement of the spleen may be a sign of increased hemolysis in some forms of anemia, such as hereditary spherocytosis. Splenic enlargement is found in many forms of leukemia and lymphoma. Other causes of splenomegaly are listed in Table 6-6.

Table 6-5 Causes of Lymphadenopathy

TYPE OF DISEASE	EXAMPLES
Acute infection	Strep throat, viral pharyngitis, syphilis, cat scratch disease
Chronic infection	Tuberculosis, histoplasmosis, chronic dermatitis
Autoimmune disease/ unknown origin	SLE, sarcoidosis, erythema nodosum
Lymphoma	Non-Hodgkin's lymphoma, Hodgkin's lymphoma
Carcinoma	Metastatic carcinoma

SLE, systemic lupus erythematosus.

Table 6-6 Causes of Splenomegaly

TYPE OF DISEASE/ MECHANISM	EXAMPLES
Hemolytic anemia	Spherocytosis, thalassemia
Leukemia/lymphoma	CML, CLL, hairy-cell leukemia
	B-cell and T-cell lymphoma
	Hodgkin's lymphoma
Infections	Sepsis, endocarditis, malaria
Immune disorders	Rheumatoid arthritis, SLE, sarcoidosis
Storage diseases	Gaucher's disease, Niemann-Pick disease
Portal hypertension	Cirrhosis, cardiac failure

CLL, chronic lymphocytic leukemia; CML, chronic myelogenous leukemia; SLE, systemic lupus erythematosus.

Pearl

> A mnemonic for remembering the causes of splenomegaly is **SPLENIC:** **s**plenitis (inflammation, especially sepsis), **p**ortal hypertension, **l**eukemia/ lymphoma, **e**rythrocyte disorders causing hemolysis, **n**eonatal disorders due to inborn genetic errors, **i**mmune disorders, **c**ardiac failure.

Laboratory studies are essential for the exact diagnosis of hematologic disorders.

Laboratory studies used in the work-up of hematologic disorders range from routine tests, such as complete blood count (CBC), to specialized tests for assessing the function of WBCs or platelets, to cytogenetic analysis of bone marrow cells and molecular analysis of specific genes known to be mutated in certain diseases. These tests are essential for the proper diagnosis of all hematologic diseases.

We discuss only the most commonly performed tests, however, as they are used for evaluating RBC, WBC, and coagulation disorders. The most important hematologic values used in general clinical practice are listed in Tables 6-7 to 6-9.

Red blood cell indices and parameters of RBC production or destruction are used to diagnose RBC disorders.

Red blood cell indices are calculated automatically by cell counters taking into account the number of RBCs in a given volume of blood, their average size, and the concentration of Hb. Reduced amounts of Hb and a reduced number of RBCs are called **anemia,** whereas increased numbers of RBCs are called **polycythemia** (erythrocytosis). Peripheral blood smears are used to obtain additional data on the changes in the morphology of RBCs.

Table 6-7 Normal Red Blood Cell Indices in Adults

Hemoglobin	Male: 14.0–17.5 g/dL
	Female: 12.3–15.3 g/dL
Hematocrit	Male: 41.5–50.4%
	Female: 35.9–44.6%
Red blood cell (RBC) count	Male: 4.5–$6.5 \times 10^6/\mu L$
	Female: 4.1–$5.1 \times 10^6/\mu L$
Mean corpuscular hemoglobin	27–33 pg/cell
Mean corpuscular hemoglobin concentration	33–35%
Mean corpuscular volume	80–96 μm^3 (fL)
Red cell distribution width	11.5–14.5%
Reticulocyte count	0.5–2.5% of all RBCs
Iron	Male: 65–175 $\mu g/dL$
	Female: 50–170 $\mu g/dL$
Ferritin	Male: 20–250 ng/mL
	Female: 10–120 ng/mL

Table 6-8 Normal White Blood Cell Indices in Adults

White blood cell count	4.5–$11 \times 10^3/\mu L$
Differential blood count	
Neutrophils	45–75%
Bands	0–5%
Eosinophils	0–8%
Basophils	0–3%
Monocytes	4–11%
Lymphocytes	16–46%

Table 6-9 Normal Platelets and Coagulation Parameters

Platelet count	150–$450 \times 10^3/\mu L$
	$(150$–$450 \times 10^9/\mu L)$
Bleeding time	2–9.5 min
Prothrombin time	11–13 sec*
Activated partial thromboplastin time	22–35 sec*
Thrombin time	17–25 sec*
Fibrinogen	200–400 mg/dL
Fibrin degradation products in serum	<10 $\mu g/mL$
Fibrin D-dimers in plasma	<200 ng/mL

*The duration of these tests varies from one laboratory to another and depends on the activator used or the concentration of thrombin used.

On the basis of the mean corpuscular volume (MCV), the anemias can be classified as

■ Microcytic
■ Normocytic
■ Macrocytic

The variation in size of RBCs and the presence of several populations of cells are best detected by calculating the red blood cell distribution width (RDW), which is a measure of **anisocytosis** of RBCs (Fig. 6-16).

On the basis of the mean corpuscular hemoglobin (MCH) and mean corpuscular volume (MCV), anemias can be further subclassified as **hypochromic, normochromic,** or **hyperchromic.** For example, iron deficiency anemia is typically microcytic (low MCV), hypochromic anemia (low MCH and MCHC) with pronounced anisocytosis (high RDW). Examination of peripheral blood smears may reveal **poikilocytosis** (i.e., marked variation in the shape of RBCs). If the bone marrow is adequately responding to a loss of blood, the number of **reticulocytes,** immature RBCs that are recognized in smears as **polychromatic macrocytes,** will be increased. The cytoplasm of these larger than normal RBCs contains ribosomes, imparting them a bluish tinge.

White blood cell count and differential counts are simple tests used for routine evaluation.

White blood cell count is routinely performed by laboratory machines and is part of the complete blood count (CBC). A differential count can be obtained at the same time, which delineates how many WBCs are neutrophils, eosinophils, basophils, monocytes, and lymphocytes. An increased number of WBCs is called leukocytosis, and a reduced number of WBCs is called leukopenia. Since the neutrophils account for more than two thirds of all WBCs, leukocytosis is most often caused by neutrophilia. Neutropenia (i.e, reduced number of neutrophils) is also called agranulocytosis. *Lymphocytosis* and *lymphopenia* are terms used for an increased or decreased number of lymphocytes in blood, respectively. *Eosinophilia, basophilia,* and *monocytosis* are terms used for an increased number of eosinophils, basophils, or monocytes, respectively.

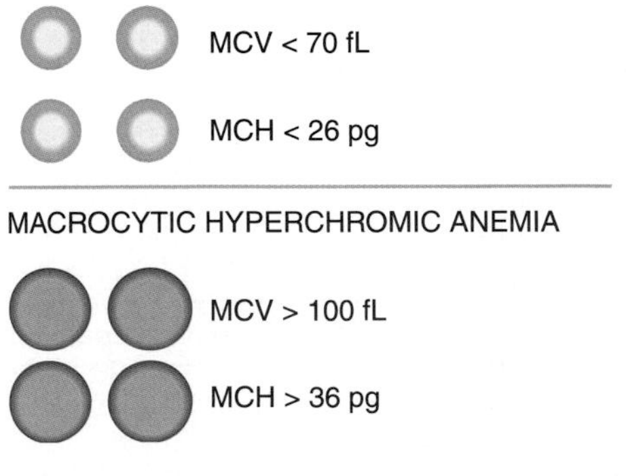

Neutrophilia (leukocytosis), defined as a WBC count over 12×10^9/L, is one of the most common hematologic abnormalities. It may be a sign of infection, but it may be also caused by many other noninfectious forms of inflammation as well as in response to cell injury and necrosis. The increase in the number of neutrophils may be due to several mechanisms such as:

- Increased bone marrow production of neutrophils
- Accelerated maturation process
- Increased release of neutrophils from the bone marrow
- Redistribution of neutrophils in circulation ("demarginalization")
- Decreased splenic trapping

The most important causes of neutrophilia are listed in Table 6-10.

Note that neutrophilia occurs not only in acute but also in chronic suppurative infections. Localized suppurative inflammation associated with tissue destruction is called an **abscess,** and such abscesses can be acute or

NORMOCYTIC NORMOCHROMIC ANEMIA

MCV 90 fL

MCH 32 pg

MICROCYTIC HYPOCHROMIC ANEMIA
WITH ANISOCYTOSIS AND POIKILOCYTOSIS

MCV < 70 fL

MCH < 26 pg

MACROCYTIC HYPERCHROMIC ANEMIA

MCV > 100 fL

MCH > 36 pg

Figure 6-16 Morphologic classification of anemias. Normocytic normochromic anemia is contrasted with microcytic anemia (small red blood cells) and macrocytic anemia (large red blood cells). Microcytic anemia shows anisocytosis (variation in size) and poikilocytosis (variation in shape). MCH, mean corpuscular hemoglobin; MCV, mean corpuscular volume.

Table 6-10 Causes of Neutrophilia (Leukocytosis)

DISORDERS	EXAMPLES
Acute bacterial infection	Acute appendicitis, pneumonia
Chronic bacterial infection	Chronic suppurative osteomyelitis
Autoimmune diseases	Dermatomyositis, SLE, vasculitis
Tissue injury/necrosis	Myocardial infarction, trauma
Metabolic disorders	Uremia, gout, acidosis
Decreased trapping of WBCs	Splenectomy
Therapy	Steroids, growth factor therapy (G-CSF)
Myeloproliferative disorders	Polycythemia vera, myelofibrosis, chronic myeloid leukemia
Neoplasms	Lymphoma, melanoma, necrotic tumors of any kind

G-CSF, granulocyte colony-stimulating factor; SLE, systemic lupus erythematosus; WBCs, white blood cells.

chronic. Infections in enclosed spaces that prevent proper drainage, such as suppurative chronic osteomyelitis or empyema of the pleural cavity, are yet another example of chronic infections characterized by neutrophilia.

Neutropenia (agranulocytosis) is a neutrophil count below 2.5×10^9/L. Most often it is caused by reduced granulocytopoiesis and bone marrow injury, but occasionally it can be related to increased removal of WBCs in an enlarged spleen or autoimmune destruction of WBCs by antibodies, as occurs in systemic lupus erythematosus (SLE). The most important causes of neutropenia are listed in Table 6-11.

Eosinophilia is defined as an increased number of eosinophils above 0.4×10^9/L. Most often it is related to allergies or parasitic infections, but in many cases the cause of eosinophilia remains undetermined (Table 6-12). Mild eosinophilia is harmless, but eosinophilia in excess of 5000/µL may cause endocardial fibrosis and heart failure. Severe eosinophilia in idiopathic hypereosinophilic syndrome or eosinophilic leukemia may cause multiple organ failure.

Pearl

> A mnemonic to remember the causes of eosinophilia is **PARASITE: p**arasitic infection, **a**llergy, **r**x (drug reaction), **a**utoimmune disorders, **s**kin diseases, **i**nfections (nonparasitic), **t**umors, **e**osinophilic syndromes of unknown origin.

Lymphocytosis is an increased number of lymphocytes in the circulation above 5000/µL. It is found in various acute and chronic infections, but may be also a consequence of thyrotoxicosis and several other conditions, even smoking. Chronic lymphocytic leukemia presents also with lymphocytosis (Table 6-13).

Lymphocytopenia is defined as fewer than 1000 lymphocytes/µL. Most often it is caused by treatment, and bone marrow failure may be caused by radiation or chemotherapy. Low lymphocyte counts are seen in patients who had bone marrow transplantation. Corticosteroids may reduce the total lymphocyte count and also depress their normal functions, causing immunosuppression. Infections with viruses such as HIV, cytomegalovirus (CMV), or herpes zoster may induce lymphocytopenia. Other causes of lymphocytopenia are listed in Table 6-14.

Approximately 65% of all lymphocytes in the peripheral blood are CD4$^+$ T helper cells. Accordingly, most patients with lymphocytopenia have a reduced number of T helper cells. Symptoms of immunodeficiency become apparent when the helper T-cell count drops below the low limit of normal, which is 300 cells/µL.

Table 6-12 Causes of Eosinophilia

Parasitic infections
    Protozoan infections (e.g., amebiasis, toxoplasmosis)
    Metazoan infections (e.g., intestinal worm, or echinococcus infestation)
    Other fungal or bacterial infections (e.g., aspergillosis, scarlet fever)
Allergic disorders
    Bronchial asthma
    Hay fever
    Eczema
Autoimmune diseases
    Pemphigus vulgaris
    Churg-Strauss syndrome
Neoplastic diseases
    Hodgkin's lymphoma
    Non-Hodgkin's lymphoma
    Myeloproliferative disorders
    Eosinophilic leukemia
    Squamous cell carcinoma of lung, mouth, etc.
Hypereosinophilia of unknown origin
    Hypereosinophilic syndrome
    Loeffler's syndrome

Table 6-11 Causes of Neutropenia

MECHANISM	EXAMPLES
Drug-induced bone marrow injury	Antibiotics, chlorpromazine, antimitotic cancer drugs
Infection	HIV, parvovirus infection
Autoimmune diseases	SLE, Felty's syndrome
Idiopathic trilineage bone marrow failure	Aplastic anemia
Cyclic interruption of granulocytopoiesis	Idiopathic cyclic neutropenia
Bone marrow infiltrates	Leukemia, myelofibrosis

HIV, human immunodeficiency virus; SLE, systemic lupus erythematosus.

Table 6-13 Causes of Lymphocytosis

Acute infections
    Viral infection: rubella, mumps, infectious mononucleosis
    Bacterial infection: pertussis, β-streptococcal infection
Chronic infections
    Viral infection: chronic viral hepatitis
    Bacterial infection: tuberculosis, syphilis, brucellosis
    Protozoan infection: toxoplasmosis
Noninfectious causes
    Hyperthyroidism
    Smoking
    Immunization
    Drug reaction
Neoplasia
    Chronic lymphocytic leukemia

Table 6-14 Causes of Lymphocytopenia

Therapy-related
    Radiation
    Cytotoxic drugs
    Corticosteroids
    Bone marrow transplantation
Infections
    Human immunodeficiency virus
    Cytomegalovirus
    Herpes zoster
Autoimmune diseases
    SLE
    Myasthenia gravis
Dietary deficiency and metabolic disorders
    Alcohol abuse
    Chronic renal failure
Congenital immunodeficiency disorders
    Ataxia–telangiectasia
    Wiskott-Aldrich syndrome
    Severe combined immunodeficiency

SLE, systemic lupus erythematosus.

Table 6-15 Causes of Thrombocytopenia

Reduced production
    Aplastic anemia
    Radiation or cancer chemotherapy
    Leukemia and myelodysplastic syndrome
    Myelofibrosis
    Vitamin B_{12} or folate deficiency
    HIV infection
Dilutional
    Massive hemorrhage
    Massive blood transfusion
Distributional
    Splenomegaly
Immune destruction
    Drugs: heparin, quinidine
    Idiopathic thrombocytopenic purpura
    Systemic lupus erythematosus
Consumptive
    Disseminated intravascular coagulopathy
    Thrombotic thrombocytopenic purpura
    Eclampsia-HELLP syndrome
    Malignant tumor related coagulopathy

HELLP, hemolysis, elevated liver enzymes, low platelet count; HIV, human immunodeficiency virus.

Pearl

> The blood of adults contains 1000 to 5000 lymphocytes/μL, but children younger than age 2 years have more lymphocytes and the normal range is 3000 to 9500/μL. Accordingly lymphocytopenia in neonates and infants is defined as a lymphocyte count under 3000/μL. In 6-year-old children the lower limit is 1500/μL.

Pearl

> Heparin-induced thrombocytopenia is the most common drug-induced immune thrombocytopenia. It occurs in approximately 5% of patients receiving bovine heparin, and 1% of those receiving porcine heparin.

Platelet count and coagulation parameters are important for the evaluation of bleeding disorders.

In general terms bleeding disorders can be classified as related to diseases affecting the blood vessels, platelets, or the coagulation factors of the plasma. The following tests have been designed for evaluating these components of the coagulation system.

Platelet count. The normal blood contains 150,00 to 400,000 platelets/μL. Even though it is customary to call platelet count below 100,000/μL **thrombocytopenia,** adequate hemostasis can be achieved even with 50,000/μL. Bleeding disorders begin when the platelet count drops below that level, but spontaneous bleeding is encountered only when the platelet count is in the range of 10,000 to 20,000/μL. The causes of thrombocytopenia are listed in Table 6-15.

Bleeding time (BT). This test is performed by making a small incision on the skin and measuring the time until the blood stops flowing, normally within 4 to 6 minutes. Thrombocytopenia, or structural/functional platelet disorders, prolongs bleeding time. BT is usually prolonged only after the platelet count drops below 100,000/μL.

Pearl

> Bleeding time is prolonged in von Willebrand's disease, the most common inherited bleeding disorder. Activated thromboplastin time (aPTT) is also prolonged, but PT is normal.

Prothrombin time (PT). This test measures the adequacy of the coagulation factors of the extrinsic and common coagulation pathways. The test is performed by adding a commercially prepared mixture of phospholipids and tissue factor

(factor III) and calcium to citrated plasma (Fig. 6-17). Prothrombin time is prolonged due to a deficiency of fibrinogen (factor I), thrombin (factor II), and factors V, VII, and X. The presence of an inhibitor of these factors also may prolong the PT. Normal PT is 10 to 14 seconds, but the PT test shows considerable variation from one laboratory to another, and thus the results must be standardized and are expressed as an **international normalized ratio (INR).**

> ### Pearl
>
> > Prothrombin time is used as a clinical test to monitor anticoagulant therapy, for evaluating the function of the liver, and as a screening test for coagulation deficiencies.

Activated partial thromboplastin time. This test measures the adequacy of coagulation factors of the intrinsic and common coagulation pathways (Fig. 6-18). The test is performed by adding kaolin to citrated plasma, and thus activating Hageman factor (XII). After the intrinsic pathway is activated one adds phospholipids and calcium, and the time from that point until fibrin clot formation is measured. This process lasts normally 25 to 38 seconds. The aPTT may be prolonged due to a deficiency of factors I, II, V, VIII, IX, X, XI, and XII.

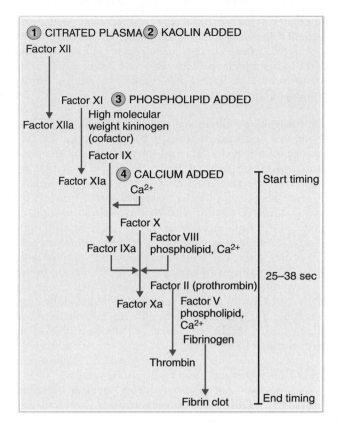

Figure 6-18 Activated partial thromboplastin time. (1, 2) Kaolin is added to citrated plasma and incubated for 3 to 5 minutes. (3) Phospholipid is then added and the entire mixture recalcified. (4) The timing begins when calcium is added.

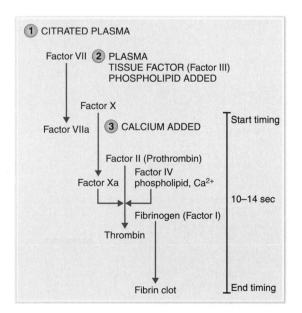

Figure 6-17 Prothrombin time. (1) Citrated plasma is used. (2) A commercial mixture of phospholipids and tissue factor is added and mixed. (3) Calcium is then added, and the stopwatch is started to determine the time till the clot is formed.

> ### Pearl
>
> > Activated partial thromboplastin time is a test of choice for monitoring heparin therapy and is also used as a screening test for hemophilia, other clotting factor deficiencies, and inhibitors of these factors.

Thrombin time. This test is performed by adding thrombin to plasma, thus leading directly to fibrin clot formation. Normally it takes 14 to 16 seconds for the clot to form. Thrombin time is prolonged in the presence of heparin or due to quantitative or qualitative fibrinogen deficiencies.

Mixing test. An abnormal PT or aPTT may be caused by a deficiency of a coagulation factor or the presence of an inhibitor. To exclude the latter possibility, the patient's plasma is mixed with normal plasma to replenish the deficiency. If the test is still abnormal, we conclude that the patient's plasma contains an **inhibitor.** The inhibitors may be directed to a specific coagulation factor (e.g., **anti-factor VIII** in hemophilic patients who have received numerous transfusions), or it may be nonspecific, such as **lupus anticoagulant** in SLE.

Fibrinogen, or fibrin degradation products (FDPs). Coagulation cascade activation has two results: the formation of fibrin thrombi and the activation of the plasmin fibrinolytic pathway (Fig. 6-19). These two pathways constantly interact. Thrombin cleaves fibrinogen into fibrin monomers, which are stabilized into fibrin clot by factor XIIIa. Thrombin also promotes the formation of factor XIIIa from factor XIII. At the same time plasmin cleaves fibrinogen into fibrin degradation products X, Y, D, and E. These FDPs may bind to soluble fibrin monomers, helping them to form an unstable fibrin clot, prone to easy dissolution. FDPs also bind to platelets, causing their dysfunction. Plasmin generates the same FDPs from insoluble fibrin in the clot. Simultaneously plasmin mediates major fibrinolysis, leading to the formation of fibrin D-dimers.

In contrast to the large molecular weight of fibrinogen and fibrin, FDPs and fibrin D-dimers are small and are excreted in the urine. Normal blood contains less than 10 μg/mL FDPs, but in hypercoagulable states and disseminated intravascular coagulation (DIC) the FDP concentration may increase more than 10 times. The highest concentration of FDPs is found in patients in whom the intravascular coagulation is associated with renal failure, preventing the excretion of FDPs.

> **Pearls**
>
> > The concentration of FDPs in plasma is elevated in many hypercoagulable states but most notably in DIC, deep vein thrombosis, pulmonary embolism, and preeclampsia during pregnancy.
>
> > Fibrin D-dimers are also elevated in DIC, but not in patients with deep vein thrombosis or pulmonary emboli. In the latter group of patients the concentration of plasma fibrin D-dimers increases, however, following thrombolytic therapy.

Special coagulation tests. In addition to the routine tests listed earlier, specialized coagulation tests must be performed in some cases. These include the following:

- **von Willebrand's factor (vWF).** This test, based on an immunoassay, measures the concentration of vWF in blood.
- **von Willebrand's multimer composition.** The test is used for subtyping of von Willebrand's disease.
- **Platelet aggregation.** The test measures the ability of platelets to respond to normal stimuli and is used for demonstrating hereditary or acquired platelet disorders.
- **Clot stability.** This test is used to detect excessive fibrinolytic activity.
- **Anticoagulant proteins S and C.** The concentration of these procoagulant proteins is reduced in some forms of congenital thrombophilia.

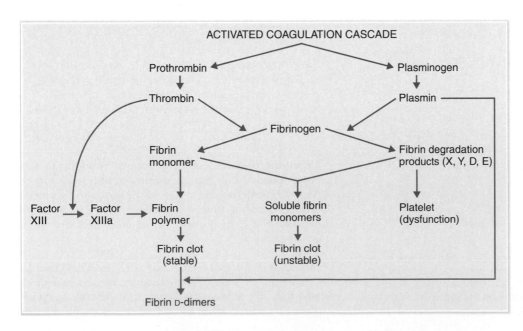

Figure 6-19 The relationship of coagulation and fibrinolysis.

- **Concentration of fibrin and other coagulation factors**. Each of these factors can be quantitated in blood.
- **Plasmin activity.** Genetic studies of specific mutations accounting for abnormalities of certain clotting factors (e.g., clotting factor V Leyden).

Clinicopathologic Correlations

ANEMIA

Anemia is used to describe a group of diseases characterized by decreased Hb concentration or reduced RBC volume. Pathogenetically it can be a consequence of inadequate or defective RBC production, or excessive RBC loss and destruction (Fig. 6-20).

Anemia is not a single disease, and in most instances it is more often a sign and consequence of some other disease than a pathologic entity in itself. In clinical practice the first step toward elucidating the etiology and pathogenesis of anemia includes laboratory measurement of Hb concentration and RBC count. On the basis of these data one can classify anemias as microcytic, normocytic, or macrocytic (Table 6-16). These data are then paired with the reticulocyte count to provide a quick estimate of RBC production in the bone marrow and the capacity of the bone marrow to compensate for the loss of RBCs.

Iron deficiency is the most common cause of microcytic anemia.

Iron deficiency anemia develops after the iron stores are depleted below the physiologic levels needed for adequate synthesis of Hb. It can develop due to inadequate intake, increased demand, or excessive chronic blood loss (Table 6-17). In Western countries heavy menstrual bleeding is the most common cause of iron deficiency anemia in women; chronic gastrointestinal bleeding is the most common cause of iron deficiency anemia in men.

The normal human body contains approximately 4000 mg of iron, 65% of which is found in RBCs incorporated in Hb (Fig. 6-21). The remaining iron is predominantly stored in the macrophages of the bone marrow, spleen, and liver, and to a lesser extent in extracellular connective tissue of

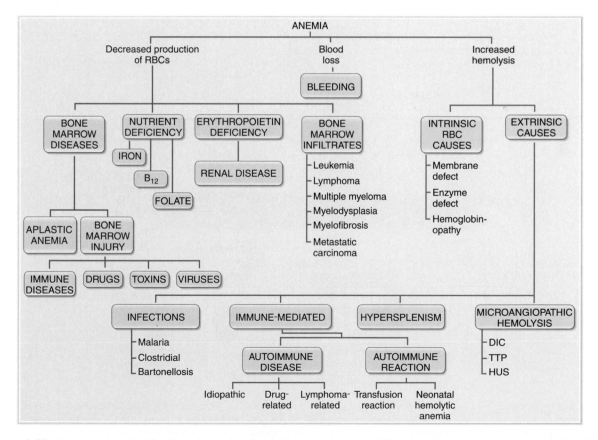

Figure 6-20 Pathogenetic classification of anemias. Anemias can result from defective or inadequate hematopoiesis or from excessive loss or destruction of erythrocytes. DIC, disseminated intravascular coagulation; HUS, hemolytic uremic syndrome; TTP, thrombotic thrombocytopenic purpura.

Table 6-16 Classification of Anemia According to the Red Blood Cell Size and the Hematopoietic Capacity of the Bone Marrow

RETICULOCYTE COUNT	MICROCYTIC	NORMOCYTIC	MACROCYTIC
<2	Iron deficiency Thalassemia	Chronic disease Aplastic anemia Myelofibrosis Chronic renal disease	Vitamin B_{12} deficiency Folate deficiency Liver disease
>2	—	Hemolytic anemia	Massive blood loss

Table 6-17 Causes of Iron Deficiency

INADEQUATE IRON INTAKE	INCREASED IRON DEMAND	EXCESSIVE BLOOD LOSS
Dietary deficiency (rare) Gastrectomy Malabsorption syndromes	Infancy–adolescence Pregnancy	Menstrual bleeding Chronic bleeding Tumors

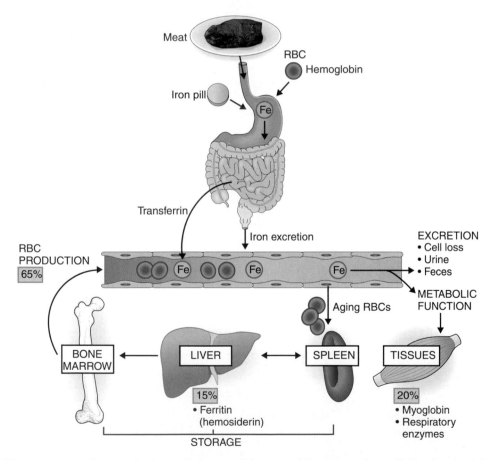

Figure 6-21 Distribution of iron in the body. Only a small fraction of the ingested iron (Fe) is absorbed. In the blood it is transported as ferritin or bound to transferrin and mostly utilized for new red blood cell production in the bone marrow. Most of the iron is found in the erythrocytes. Iron is stored in the macrophages of the spleen, liver, and bone marrow. It is also found in almost all living cells as part of the oxidative enzymes. Normal loss is in the range of the amount absorbed. The loss occurs due to excretion in the urine, bile, and feces, and as a result of the desquamation of skin and mucosal cells. RBCs, red blood cells.

the bone marrow. Approximately 15% of iron is found in myoglobin of the muscle and cellular respiratory enzymes in somatic tissues. Less than 1% of body iron is found in serum in the form of ferritin or bound to transferrin, a serum transport protein that carries iron in the circulating blood. Excretion of iron in the urine, bile, and feces, and through the desquamation of skin cells, is approximately equivalent to the amount absorbed. Menstrual bleeding is a significant cause of iron loss in women.

Serum iron is a measure of iron bound to transferrin, which normally has a concentration in serum of 50 to 150 µg/dL. Additional iron is found in the form of serum **ferritin** in concentrations from 30 to 300 ng/mL. Ferritin concentration in the blood is tightly regulated and is a very sensitive indicator of the total iron stores. Reduced serum ferritin (<12 ng/mL) is a reliable sign of iron deficiency. It correlates with low total serum iron concentration and reduced **transferrin saturation.** These biochemical findings correlate with the reduced amount of Hb in RBCs and reduced amounts of **hemosiderin** in bone marrow macrophages.

Typical biochemical findings in iron deficiency anemia are listed in Table 6-18. These findings are useful for distinguishing iron deficiency anemia from thalassemia, another common form of microcytic anemia.

Thalassemia is caused by a globin gene mutation that adversely affects Hb synthesis. Iron stores are normal, however, and may be even larger than normal because the body contains more iron than it can use for Hb synthesis.

Anemia of chronic disease, which may be normocytic or microcytic, must be also taken into consideration in the differential diagnosis. This anemia is most likely mediated by cytokines produced in chronic infections and in response to cancer. The bone marrow is also refractory to erythropoietin, and the life span of RBCs is reduced. Iron utilization is impaired, and the iron remains stored in the macrophages. High iron stores are reflected in the elevation of serum ferritin. Transferrin saturation is normal or even increased, but the total amount of iron in serum is lower than normal. All these data indicate that the body contains enough iron but it cannot use it for Hb synthesis nor can it properly recirculate it.

> **Pearl**
>
> > Low serum ferritin is the most reliable sign of iron deficiency. A normal level of ferritin, however, does not exclude iron deficiency. Ferritin is an acute-phase reactant and thus may be elevated even in the presence of iron deficiency in patients who have infection, tumors, or acute liver disease.

In peripheral blood smears of patients with iron deficiency anemia the RBCs appear pale (**hypochromic**) and vary in size (**anisocytosis**) and shape (**poikilocytosis**). Polychromatic reticulocytes are not visible, but the number of platelets is often increased. The bone marrow biopsy shows an increased number of erythroid precursors, which contain scarce amounts of Hb in their cytoplasm. Prussian blue stain shows decreased amounts of hemosiderin in bone marrow macrophages.

Clinical findings. Iron deficiency anemia shares the same clinical features of other forms of anemia, reflecting the blood's decreased capacity to carry oxygen from the lungs to the tissues. Some clinical findings seem to be unique to iron deficiency and are probably related to a lack of intracellular iron in some tissue. Some symptoms cannot be readily explained. The clinical findings depend on the extent of anemia, but in general the patient complains of symptoms related to:

■ **Hypoxemia.** These include fatigue, palpitations, shortness of breath, dyspnea on exertion, and, in severe cases, even heart failure.

Table 6-18 Laboratory Findings in Common Microcytic Anemias

PARAMETER	TYPE OF ANEMIA		
	IRON DEFICIENCY	CHRONIC DISEASE	THALASSEMIA
MCV	↓ to ↓↓↓	→ or ↓	↓↓ to ↓↓↓
RBC count	↓ to ↓↓↓	↓ to ↓↓	↓
Hemoglobin	↓ to ↓↓↓	↓	↓ to ↓↓↓
Serum iron	↓ to ↓↓	↓	→ or ↑
Serum ferritin	↓ to ↓↓	↑	→ or ↑
Transferrin saturation	↓ to ↓↓	→ or ↑	→
Bone marrow iron	↓ to ↓↓	↓ to ↑↑	→ or ↑
Electrophoresis of hemoglobin	—	—	Abnormal

↓, reduced slightly; ↓↓, moderately reduced; ↓↓↓, severely reduced; →, normal; ↑ to ↑↑, slightly to moderately increased; MCV, mean corpuscular volume; RBC, red blood cell.

■ **Epithelial changes.** These include atrophy of the epithelium of the oral mucosa causing redness of the tongue and rhagades in the corners of the mouth *(angular cheilitis)*. Dysphagia may be caused by esophageal webs *(Plummer-Vinson syndrome)*. Dyspepsia achlorhydria may be related to atrophy of the gastric mucosa.

■ **Koilonychia.** Spoon-shaped nails may be seen in severe iron deficiency anemia, but their pathogenesis is not understood.

■ **Pica syndrome.** Some patients develop strange cravings, such as an urge to eat ice, paint, or dirt (geophagia). There is no explanation for the pica syndrome.

Vitamin B_{12} and folate deficiency produce megaloblastic macrocytic anemia.

Vitamin B_{12} and folate are essential for DNA synthesis. A deficiency of these nutrients interferes with the maturation of hematopoietic cell precursors, resulting in anemia, leukopenia, and thrombocytopenia.

Vitamin B_{12}. This water-soluble vitamin is present in many animal tissues and is found in more than adequate amounts in the normal American diet to meet the daily requirement of 1 mg/day. Dietary deficiency thus rarely develops except in strict vegetarians or persons on fad diets. Most often vitamin B_{12} deficiency results from problems pertaining to its absorption (Fig. 6-22). Ingested vitamin B_{12} binds to the intrinsic factor (IF) and is then carried to the terminal ileum where it is absorbed. Deficiency of IF in atrophic gastritis and diseases of the small intestine that interfere with the absorption of the B_{12}–IF complex may cause vitamin B_{12} deficiency. Other causes of vitamin B_{12} deficiency are listed in Table 6-19.

Pearl

> The normal liver contains 1000 μg of vitamin B_{12}. Since the daily requirement is only 1 μg, it takes 1000 days for a deficiency to develop.

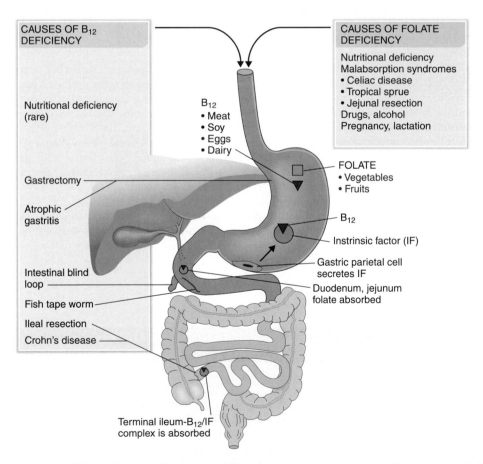

CAUSES OF B_{12} DEFICIENCY

Nutritional deficiency (rare)

Gastrectomy

Atrophic gastritis

Intestinal blind loop

Fish tape worm

Ileal resection

Crohn's disease

CAUSES OF FOLATE DEFICIENCY

Nutritional deficiency
Malabsorption syndromes
• Celiac disease
• Tropical sprue
• Jejunal resection
Drugs, alcohol
Pregnancy, lactation

B_{12}
• Meat
• Soy
• Eggs
• Dairy

FOLATE
• Vegetables
• Fruits

B_{12}

Instrinsic factor (IF)

Gastric parietal cell secretes IF

Duodenum, jejunum folate absorbed

Terminal ileum-B_{12}/IF complex is absorbed

Figure 6-22 Vitamin B_{12} and folate deficiency. Vitamin B_{12} deficiency requires gastric intrinsic factor (IF), which binds to B_{12} and carries it to the terminal ileum, where both of them are taken up by the intestinal mucosal cells. Vitamin B_{12} deficiency is most often caused by diseases that interfere with its absorption. Folate deficiency is most often related to dietary deficiency, but it may also be due to intestinal malabsorption. Many drugs interfere with folate utilization.

Table 6-19 Causes of Deficiency of Vitamin B$_{12}$ and Folic Acid

MECHANISM	VITAMIN B$_{12}$	FOLIC ACID
Dietary deficiency	Vegetarian diet Fad diet Total parenteral nutrition	Diet lacking raw or slightly cooked food Alcoholism
Abnormal/reduced absorption	Atrophic gastritis Celiac disease Blind loop syndrome Crohn's disease Tape worm infection	Celiac disease Blind loop syndrome Drugs (e.g., antiepileptics)
Interference with utilization	Liver disease Drugs	Drugs (e.g., folic acid antagonists) Alcoholism
Increased demand (physiologic)	Infancy	Pregnancy, lactation, infancy
Increased utilization (pathologic)	Hyperthyroidism Thalassemia	Lymphoma and other malignancies Thalassemia Hypermetabolism
Increased excretion/loss	Liver disease Kidney disease	Renal dialysis

Folate. This water-soluble vitamin is present in many leafy green vegetables and fruits, but it may be destroyed by cooking. The daily requirement is 50 μg, and since the body stores of folate are relatively small, a deficiency caused by dietary factors may develop in 2 to 4 months. Folate is absorbed in the duodenum and jejunum. Its absorption is affected by malabsorption syndromes and diseases affecting the small intestine. Certain drugs (e.g., antiepileptics) may interfere with absorption, and others may interfere with its utilization. Increased requirements for folate occur during pregnancy, lactation, and infancy. Other causes of folate deficiency are listed in Table 6-19.

Laboratory findings. Interference with DNA synthesis results in the formation of **megaloblasts**—the cells that are much larger than normal erythroblasts (Fig. 6-23). In contrast to normal erythroblasts whose nuclei progressively diminish in size, the megaloblasts retain their large nuclei and their cytoplasm remains filled with RNA. These cells ultimately mature into **macro-ovalocytic RBCs.** Inefficient erythropoiesis results in an increased intramedullary hemolysis and subsequent hyperbilirubinemia and hyperuricemia. The number of reticulocytes in the blood is reduced, reflecting sluggish hematopoiesis. The abnormal neutrophils often appear hypersegmented, and the formation of platelets from abnormal megakaryocytes results in thrombocytopenia.

The hematologic findings of vitamin B$_{12}$ deficiency are indistinguishable from those of folate deficiency. A deficiency of vitamin B$_{12}$ and folate should be suspected in all patients who have megaloblastic anemia. Serum levels of vitamin B$_{12}$ or folate can be measured to confirm the diagnosis, but the currently available tests are not always reliable. Thus one must use clinical clues to decide about the most likely cause of megaloblastic anemia. Antibodies to IF or parietal cells are often found in patients who have vitamin B$_{12}$ deficiency.

Folate deficiency should be suspected if the diet is inappropriate or the patient is being treated for cancer. Symptoms may be corrected by vitamin B$_{12}$ or folate therapy.

Clinical findings. Most of the symptoms of vitamin B$_{12}$ and folate deficiency anemia are nonspecific and similar to those seen in other forms of anemia. In vitamin B$_{12}$ deficiency, also known as **pernicious anemia,** approximately 40% of patients have neurologic symptoms indicative of posterior and lateral spinal column demyelination. These symptoms include abnormal gait, disturbances of proprioception, and a sense of vibration. The disease may progress to spastic paraparesis. In severe cases personality changes occur and even overt psychosis.

Pearl

> To remember the key aspects of **p**ernicious anemia note that many of them begin with the letter **p**: parietal cells of the stomach (produce IF and are destroyed by antibodies), posterior columns of the spinal cord, proprioception, paraparesis, psychosis.

Aplastic anemia is a term used for bone marrow failure involving all three myeloid cell lineages.

Aplastic anemia is a synonym for bone marrow failure characterized by anemia, leukopenia, and thrombocytopenia. It may result from hematopoietic stem cell injury or an injury to the hematopoietic microenvironment in the bone marrow. Clinically it is classified as primary (idiopathic) if no obvious causes can be identified, or secondary (Table 6-20). The causes of secondary bone marrow injury include cytotoxic drugs, radiation therapy, hypersensitivity to identifiable antigens, and

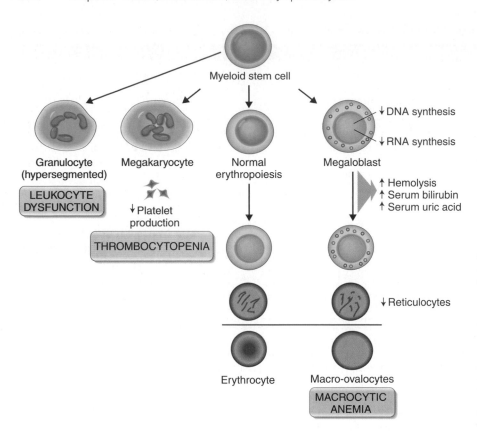

Myeloid stem cell

Granulocyte (hypersegmented)

LEUKOCYTE DYSFUNCTION

Megakaryocyte

↓ Platelet production

THROMBOCYTOPENIA

Normal erythropoiesis

Megaloblast

↓ DNA synthesis

↓ RNA synthesis

↑ Hemolysis
↑ Serum bilirubin
↑ Serum uric acid

↓ Reticulocytes

Erythrocyte

Macro-ovalocytes

MACROCYTIC ANEMIA

Figure 6-23 Megaloblastic anemia. Vitamin B_{12} deficiency affects the maturation of myeloid stem cells and their derivatives, resulting in hypersegmentation of neutrophils, thrombocytopenia, and macrocytic anemia. Inadequate maturation of RBC precursors leads to increased hemolysis, hyperbilirubinemia, and hyperuricemia. The number of reticulocytes in the blood is low. Folate deficiency produces similar changes.

viral infections. Rare genetic forms of aplastic anemia (e.g., Fanconi's anemia) also exist. In most cases of aplastic anemia the cause cannot be identified, and the disease is considered to be idiopathic.

Clinically aplastic anemia has an insidious onset and manifests with generalized weakness related to anemia, recurrent infections related to leukopenia, or bleeding due to thrombocytopenia. The peripheral blood count shows pancytopenia. The RBCs are normocytic and normochromic, and the reticulocyte count is low. Bone marrow biopsy typically shows depletion of blood cell precursors, which are replaced by fat or fibrous tissue.

Hemolytic anemia is a group of diseases characterized by increased destruction of RBCs.

Diseases classified as hemolytic anemia can be classified according to several criteria as follows:

- **Duration of hemolysis.** Hemolysis may be acute, as occurs in a mismatched blood transfusion, or chronic, as occurs in sickle cell anemia. In malaria, acute bouts of hemolysis recur over regular intervals for many years.
- **Location.** Depending on where the hemolysis occurs it may be classified as **intravascular** or **extravascular.**

Under normal conditions 90% of old or damaged RBCs are lyzed extracellularly, and likewise, increased hemolysis is more often extravascular than extracellular.

- **Nature of the defect.** The causes of hemolysis can be classified as **intrinsic,** when the hemolysis occurs due to structural defects of the RBCs, or it may be **extrinsic** to the RBCs.
- **Inheritance.** The conditions leading to hemolysis can be **hereditary,** as in sickle cell anemia, or **acquired,** as in immune-mediated hemolytic anemia.

Table 6-20 Etiologic Classification of Aplastic Anemia

Primary (idiopathic) (>80%)
Genetic (e.g., Fanconi's anemia)
Secondary
Drugs (cytotoxic drugs, chloramphenicol, indomethacin)
Radiation therapy
Toxic chemicals (e.g., benzene, insecticides)
Viral infections (e.g., hepatitis virus C, Epstein-Barr virus, HIV, parvovirus B19)
Immune disorders (e.g., graft-versus-host reaction, thymoma-related anemia)
Myelofibrosis

HIV, human immunodeficiency virus.

Hemolytic anemias are mostly caused by chronic extravascular hemolysis. The prevalence of various forms of hemolytic anemia varies geographically and according to the genetic background of populations. For example sickle cell anemia typically affects people of African background, but in Europe hereditary spherocytosis is the most common hemolytic hereditary anemia. Malaria is endemic in Africa and is an important cause of hemolytic anemia in that part of the world.

Clinical and laboratory findings. Hemolytic anemias have many clinical manifestations in common with other anemias, but they also have some unique features. These clinical findings could be related to the following pathophysiologic mechanisms:

- **Hypoxia.** Reduced capacity of blood to deliver oxygen causes fatigue, dyspnea, palpitation, and in severe cases even heart failure. Prolonged hypoxia in severe hereditary hemolytic anemias, such as sickle cell anemia, may adversely affect the developing brain in children and cause lethargy and impair mental development.

- **Acute hemolysis.** Lysis of RBCs is associated with a release of enzymes and proteins from their cytoplasm. Elevated serum **lactated dehydrogenase** (LDH) is a sensitive marker of hemolysis. Free Hb in the plasma accounts for its red color (**hemoglobinemia**). Free Hb binds to **haptoglobin** and is carried to the splenic and hepatic macrophages, where it is degraded into bilirubin and released into circulation, causing **hyperbilirubinemia** and jaundice (Fig. 6-24). Heme from Hb is oxidized into ferriheme and binds to albumin, forming **methemalbumin,** which gives the plasma a brown color. The binding of free Hb to haptoglobin reduces haptoglobin concentration in

blood for 2 days or even longer. Once haptoglobin is depleted from circulation, free Hb is filtered in the glomeruli and appears in the urine (**hemoglobinuria**). Renal tubular cells take up some Hb from the primary filtrate and transform it into hemosiderin. Shedding of these tubular cells subsequently results in **hemosiderinuria.**

- **Chronic hemolysis.** The release of bilirubin from hemolyzed RBCs causes **jaundice.** Bilirubin is bound to albumin and is not conjugated and thus does not appear in the urine. Prolonged hyperbilirubinemia predisposes to the formation of pigmented **biliary stones.** Lactate dehydrogenase remains elevated in serum.

- **Splenomegaly.** The spleen is the principal place for the removal of damaged RBCs, and typically it is enlarged in most forms of hemolytic anemia. In sickle cell anemia, the sickling episodes tend to occlude splenic blood vessels and cause infarctions, which ultimately reduce the size of the spleen to a small nubbin (*"autosplenectomy"*).

- **Reduced life span of RBCs.** Dynamic clinical studies using tagging of RBCs with radioactive chromium (^{51}Cr) show that the half-life of RBCs is significantly reduced and that these cells preferentially sequester into the spleen or the liver.

- **Increased erythropoiesis.** To compensate for the loss of RBCs, the bone marrow expands its erythropoietic capacity. This is reflected in the increased number of **reticulocytes** in the peripheral blood, usually in the range of 3% to 5%. The myeloid-to-erythroid (M:E) ratio, which is normally 1:4, may be increased to 1:1,

- **Expansion of hematopoiesis** may replace the fatty bone marrow. Bone growth stimulated by expanded hematopoiesis may produce visible **deformities of**

Figure 6-24 Acute hemolysis. Hemolysis is associated with a release of lactate dehydrogenase (LDH) into serum, depletion of haptoglobin, and the appearance of hemoglobin in serum. Depletion of haptoglobin is followed by hemoglobinuria. Methemalbumin is elevated in serum. Bilirubin is elevated in the blood causing jaundice. It is unconjugated, however, and thus bilirubinuria does not occur. Hemoglobin transformed into hemosiderin in the kidneys is also excreted in the urine, usually with some delay after hemoglobinuria.

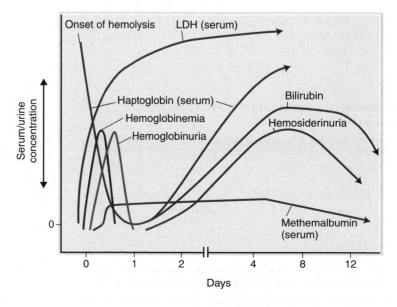

short bones, especially in children (e.g., *"hemolytic facies"* due to broad cheek bones and maxillae, and the *"crew-cut"* appearance of calvaria on radiographs of children with thalassemia).

■ **Extramedullary hematopoiesis.** It may be recognized histologically in the spleen or liver, but occasionally it may even form nodules outside of the bone marrow.

Etiologic studies. The cause of hemolytic anemia can be usually determined by specialized laboratory studies as listed in Table 6-21.

Many of the hemolytic anemias are associated with altered RBC morphology. The most important morphologic abnormalities are illustrated in Figure 6-25 and listed in Table 6-22.

MYELOPROLIFERATIVE DISORDERS

Myeloproliferative disorders (MPDs) result from clonal proliferation of bone marrow stem cells, which may differentiate along granulocytic, erythrocytic, or thrombocytic lineages or cause myelofibrosis (Fig. 6-26). Clinically MPDs may manifest as:

■ Polycythemia vera (PV), characterized with erythrocytosis
■ Chronic myelogenous leukemia (CML), characterized with granulocytosis
■ Essential thrombocythemia (ET), characterized by an increased number of platelets
■ Primary myelofibrosis (MF), characterized by granulocytosis and increased platelet count with replacement of the bone marrow with fibrous tissue

Interconversion of these diseases into one another is common, and all of them may ultimately transform into acute myelogenous leukemia (AML). All of these conditions can transform into myelofibrosis. The rate of this transformation varies from 80% in CML to 15% in PV, 10% in MF, and as low as 1 to 2% in ET.

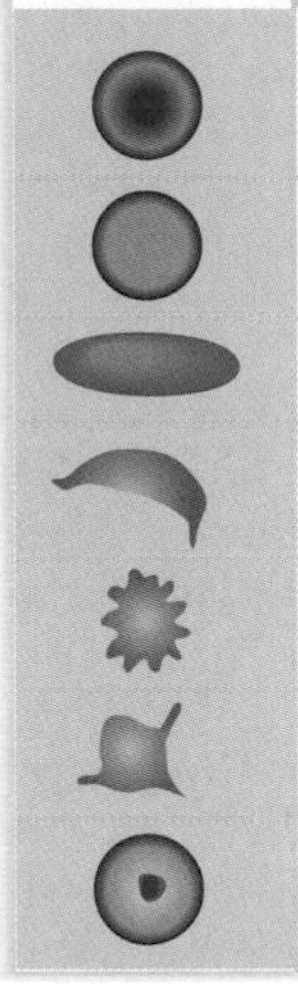

	MORPHOLOGY OF RBC	DISEASES
	Normal RBC	
	Spherocyte	Hereditary spherocytosis
	Elliptocyte	Hereditary elliptocytosis
	Schistocyte	Microangiopathic hemolytic anemia, DIC
	Echinocyte	Renal failure, malnutrition
	Acanthocyte	Abetalipoproteinemia, cirrhosis
	Target cell	Thalassemia

Figure 6-25 Peripheral blood abnormalities in some hemolytic anemias. DIC, disseminated intravascular coagulation; RBC, red blood cells.

Polycythemia vera is characterized by an increased RBC mass.

Polycythemia vera is a myeloproliferative disorder in which the predominant disturbance is erythrocytosis. It is a relatively uncommon disease with an incidence of 2 to 3 million, affecting people in the older adult age group, and a peak between 50 and 60 years. It is characterized by the following features:

■ **Increased RBC count.** Erythrocytosis typically exceeds $6 \times 10^6/\mu L$ in men and $5.7 \times 10^6/\mu L$ in women.

Table 6-21 Special Tests Used in the Study of Hemolytic Anemias

TEST	DISEASE
Hemoglobin electrophoresis	Sickle cell anemia Thalassemia
Osmotic fragility of RBCs	Hereditary spherocytosis
Enzymatic tests	G6PD deficiency
Genetic tests	Hemoglobinopathies
Immunologic tests (e.g., Coombs' test)	Autoimmune hemolytic anemia

G6PD, glucose-6-phosphate dehydrogenase; RBCs, red blood cells.

Table 6-22 Morphology or Red Blood Cells in Hemolytic Anemias

MORPHOLOGY OF RBCs	DISEASES
Spherocytes	Hereditary spherocytosis Autoimmune hemolytic anemia
Sickle cells	Sickle cell anemia
Target cells	Thalassemia, hemoglobin C or SC disease
Elliptocytes	Hereditary elliptocytosis
Acanthocytosis	Cirrhosis, abetalipoproteinemia
Fragmented RBCs, burr cells, helmet cells	DIC, TTP, HUS

DIC, disseminated intravascular coagulation; HUS, hemolytic uremic syndrome; RBCs, red blood cells; TTP, thrombotic thrombocytopenic purpura.

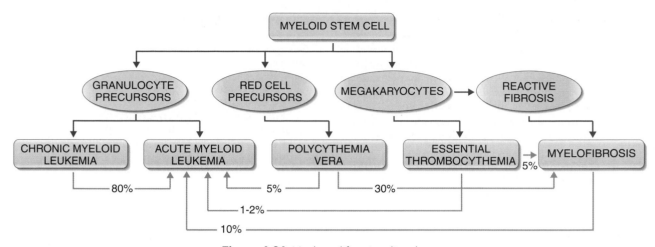

Figure 6-26 Myeloproliferative disorders.

- **High hematocrit values.** Hematocrit is typically high in more than 54% of women and 59% of men with PV.
- **High Hb values.** Values are typically over 17.5 g/dL in men and 15.5 g/dL in women.
- **Increased total RBC mass.** Radioactive chromium labeling of RBCs typically shows a RBC mass increased over 36 mL/kg in men and over 32 mL/kg for women (normal values are 25–31 mL/kg for men and 23–28 mL/kg for women).
- **Increased WBC count.** Leukocytosis is found in over 60% of patients. Typically, these WBCs are differentiated and express neutrophil alkaline phosphatase (NAP) like normal leukocytes. The differential count shows an increased number of basophils.
- **Increased platelet count.** The peripheral blood contains usually 400,000 to 800,000 platelets/mL.

The neoplastic stem cells form erythroid colonies in the bone marrow, which proliferate autonomously and do not require erythropoietin stimulation. Serum level of erythropoietin is thus undetectable, in contrast to secondary polycythemia, in which erythropoietin concentration in the blood is markedly increased. Vitamin B$_{12}$ and vitamin B$_{12}$-binding capacity are often elevated. The bone marrow is hypercellular, showing not only erythroid but also granulocytic and megakaryocytic hyperplasia. Marrow contains no hemosiderin-laden macrophages, because all the iron is utilized for Hb synthesis.

Clinical findings. The clinical features of PV can be related to the primary pathologic changes in this disease as follows (Fig. 6-27):

- **Increased RBC volume.** The increased number of RBCs accounts for the ruddy plethoric complexion. Headaches due to increased blood volume related

intracranial pressure and dyspnea due to congestion of the lungs are common. High-output heart failure is found in long-standing disease.

- **Hyperviscosity of the blood.** Sluggish blood flow through the retinal blood vessels causes visual problems. Neurologic symptoms, such as paresthesias and transient ischemic attacks, also occur.
- **Thrombosis.** Thrombi occur due to sluggish circulation and hyperviscosity of the blood, and the number of

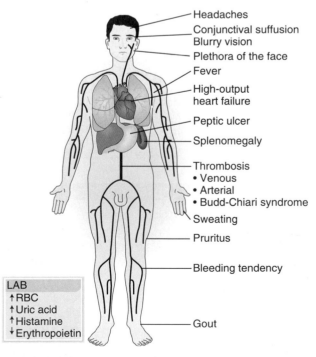

Headaches
Conjunctival suffusion
Blurry vision
Plethora of the face
Fever
High-output heart failure
Peptic ulcer
Splenomegaly
Thrombosis
• Venous
• Arterial
• Budd-Chiari syndrome
Sweating
Pruritus
Bleeding tendency
Gout

LAB
↑RBC
↑Uric acid
↑Histamine
↓Erythropoietin

Figure 6-27 Clinical features of polycythemia vera. RBC, red blood cells.

platelets is increased. Thrombosis has been reported in 30 to 60% of all patients and is a major cause of death in this cohort. Thrombi may form anywhere, including the large veins of the abdominal and thoracic cavity or the brain. Note that PV is the most common cause of hepatic vein thrombosis and Budd-Chiari syndrome.

- **Bleeding tendency.** Bleeding is clinically evident in one third of all patients. The reasons for the bleeding tendency are complex and include ischemic damage of the blood vessel wall caused by thrombi, a weak clot formation due to an excess of RBCs, distention of the blood vessels by the increased volume of the blood, and platelet dysfunction, among others.
- **Splenomegaly.** Pooling of RBCs, WBCs, and platelets in the spleen is associated with splenomegaly in over 75% of patients.
- **Hyperuricemia.** Uric acid is generated in the hyperactive bone marrow. Deposits of monosodium urates in the joints may cause attacks of gout and tophi.
- **Histamine excess.** It is found in 90% patients. Histamine is released from platelets and basophils circulating in the blood. Excess of histamine is the most likely explanation for frequent **pruritus** and formation of **peptic ulcers.** Patients typically complain of itching when entering a hot bath. Peptic ulcers occur five times more often in PV patients than in age-matched controls.
- **Hypermetabolism.** The patients complain of sweating, low-grade fever, and weight loss.

Polycythemia vera must be distinguished from **secondary polycythemia,** which typically develops due to hypoxemia or excessive stimulation of the bone marrow with erythropoietin, and from **relative polycythemia (erythrocytosis),** which is caused by a loss of plasma and hemoconcentration during dehydration. The most important causes of polycythemia are listed in Table 6-23.

Table 6-23 Classification of Polycythemias

Polycythemia vera (myeloproliferative disorder)
Secondary polycythemia
   Hypoxia
     High altitude
     Chronic lung diseases
     Right to left shunt in congenital heart diseases
   Hemoglobinopathies affecting oxygen affinity
     Congenital (e.g., 2,3-bisphosphoglycerate deficiency)
     Carboxyhemoglobin in smokers
   Erythropoietin overproduction
     Renal tumors
     Renal ischemia (e.g., cysts, renal artery stenosis)
     Postrenal transplantation
     Hepatocellular carcinoma
     Cerebellar hemangioblastoma (von Hippel-Lindau syndrome)
     Androgen excess (e.g., exogenous or Leydig/adrenal cell tumor-derived)
Relative polycythemia
   Dehydration
   Stress polycythemia

In contrast to secondary polycythemia, which is characterized by reduced oxygen saturation and increased erythropoietin concentration in blood, in PV the oxygen saturation is high (over 92%) and erythropoietin is undetectable. The features that help in the differential diagnosis of PV and secondary polycythemia are listed in Table 6-24. The main features distinguishing true polycythemia from relative polycythemia are the red cell mass and plasma volume. In relative polycythemia the red cell mass is normal, but the plasma volume is decreased, in contrast to PV in which the volume of RBCs is increased and the plasma volume normal.

Table 6-24 Clinical and Laboratory Findings Useful for Distinguishing Primary from Secondary Polycythemia

FINDINGS	POLYCYTHEMIA VERA*	SECONDARY POLYCYTHEMIA
Obvious causes of hypoxia (e.g., heart, lung disease)	−	+
Splenomegaly	+ (>75%)	−
Hepatomegaly	+ (35%)	−
Arterial O_2 saturation	>92%	<75%
Leukocytosis	+ (>70%)	−
Thrombocytosis	+ (50%)	−
Erythropoietin (serum)	−	+
Vitamin B_{12} (serum)	>950 pg/mL	<900 pg/mL
Bone marrow cytogenetic abnormalities	+	−

*The median survival of patients who have polycythemia vera is 16 years. Myelofibrosis develops in approximately 30%, and acute myelogenous leukemia develops in 5% of all patients.
Plus sign indicates the finding is present in some patients; the percentage of patients is listed in parentheses.

Chronic myelogenous leukemia is characterized by a proliferation of bone marrow precursors of granulocytes.

Chronic myelogenous leukemia (CML) is a form of MPD characterized by the clonal proliferation of granulocytic precursors that are still capable of differentiating into granulocytes. It accounts for approximately 15% of adult leukemias, and it most often affects adults.

It is the first hematopoeitic malignancy in which a chromosomal abnormality, known as the Philadelphia (Ph) chromosome, was identified. It results from a translocation of a portion of chromosome 9 to chromosome 22. In that process the c-*abl* proto-oncogene from chromosome 9 is translocated next to the *bcr* cluster on chromosome 22, resulting in an abnormal *bcr–abl* fusion product that presumably plays a role in the pathogenesis of this disorder (Fig. 6-28).

Chronic myelogenous leukemia usually has an insidious onset and is often discovered accidentally in older persons who have so-called **constitutional symptoms**; that is, they complain of fatigue and weight loss, or night sweats and low-grade fever. Other symptoms include discomfort because of

enlarged spleen or a bleeding tendency (Fig. 6-29). The disease is characterized by the following laboratory findings:

- **Elevated WBC count.** Leukocytosis exceeds 50×10^9/L, and the usual range varies in the 50 to 300×10^9/L range. The differential count shows a complete spectrum of granulocytic cells from myeloblasts to mature neutrophils. Basophils and eosinophils are usually increased in number.
- **Reduced neutrophil alkaline phosphatase (NAP).** This enzyme is not expressed on the cell membrane of neoplastic cells and thus it cannot be demonstrated enzyme-histochemically in WBC smears. This important finding distinguishes CML from leukemoid reactions and polycythemia vera, in which the NAP is elevated.
- **Reduced RBC count.** Anemia is usually mild, but in later stages of the disease it may be pronounced.
- **Variable platelet counts.** The platelet count may be normal or markedly increased or decreased.
- **Hyperuricemia.** Hyperuricemia results from increased breakdown of neoplastic WBCs.
- **Splenomegaly.** Splenomegaly may be associated with pain or a feeling of heaviness and hepatomegaly.
- **Hypercellular bone marrow.** The bone marrow contains an increased number of cells, most of which are precursors of granulocytes. The M:E ratio is elevated and may be as high as 20:1.

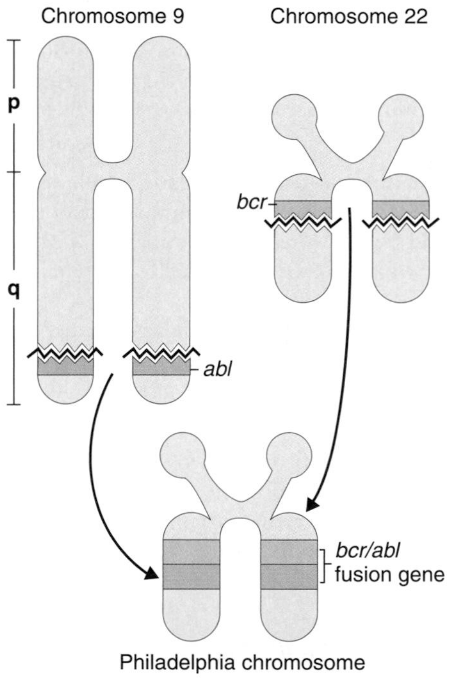

Figure 6-28 Philadelphia chromosome. The shortened chromosome 22 (22q−) is formed by reciprocal translocation of a portion of the short arm of chromosome 9 to chromosome 22 and vice versa. The translocation results in the juxtaposition of the *bcr* and *abl* genes, which in tandem produce a chimeric fusion protein that has strong tyrosinase activity and is important in the malignant transformation of myelogenous cells.

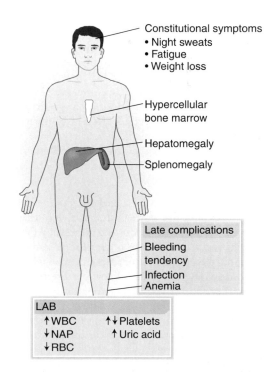

Figure 6-29 Clinical features of chronic myelogenous leukemia. NAP, neutrophil alkaline phosphatase; RBC, red blood cells; WBC, white blood cells.

The disease has typically three phases: A **chronic stable phase** lasting 1 to 5 years, an **accelerated,** or **transformation, phase** characterized by the appearance of blast cells and reduced RBC and platelet counts, and a **blast crisis,** during which the number of blasts in the bone marrow exceeds 30%. A blast crisis is equivalent to **transformation into acute myeloblastic leukemia (AML),** and it occurs in over 80% patients with CML. Typical clinical findings include signs of progressive anemia, increased incidence of bacterial infections, and a progressively worsening bleeding tendency.

ACUTE LEUKEMIA

Acute leukemia is a clonal proliferation of bone marrow stem cells that spill into the circulation and are readily identifiable in peripheral blood smears. Depending on the stem cell or precursor cell that is affected, it may be classified as AML or acute lymphoblastic leukemia (ALL). These diseases may develop:

- **Acutely without any preexisting conditions.** Both AML and ALL can develop as the first sign of clonal proliferation of transformed stem cells.
- **By blastic transformation of a preexisting myeloproliferative disorder.** Leukemia, which is usually of the AML type, is preceded in such cases by CML, primary myelofibrosis, polycythemia vera, or essential thrombocythemia.
- **By blastic transformation of a preexisting myelodysplastic syndrome.** Myelodysplastic syndromes are clonal diseases of the bone marrow characterized by abnormal hematopoiesis and cytopenia involving erythroid, myeloid, and megakaryocytic lineages. Leukemia developing in myelodysplastic syndromes is of the AML type. It is preceded by refractory anemia, with or without sideroblasts or excess blasts.
- **By blastic transformation of a preexisting lymphoma or lymphocytic leukemia.** Some lymphomas may transform into leukemia.
- **As a complication of treatment.** Both AML and ALL can develop as late complications of treatment of another malignancy.

The classification of AML is based on cytogenetic data, morphologic analysis of the degree of dysplasia, and determination of whether the disease is associated with therapy (Table 6-25). Leukemias that do not show recurrent chromosomal rearrangements, multilineage dysplasia, or are not therapy-related are then classified according to a system known as the revised French-American-British (FAB) classification. According to this system, AML can be classified into eight major groups labeled as FAB M0 to FAB M7. Some of these groups have subgroups identified morphologically, cytogenetically, or clinically in response to treatment (e.g., "good risk," "standard risk," or "poor risk"). The pretreatment karyotype seems to be one of the most important prognostic parameters. The ALLs are morphologically classified into three groups, but these may be further subclassified on the basis of molecular biology data.

Table 6-25 WHO Classification of Acute Myeloblastic Leukemia (AML)

1. AML with recurrent chromosomal rearrangements
2. AML with multilineage dysplasia
3. AML therapy related
4. French-American-British (FAB) classification of acute leukemias, NOS

M0	Undifferentiated
M1	Weak differentiation (>90% blasts)
M2	Differentiated (30–90% blasts)
M3	Promyelocytic, granular
M4	Myelomonocytic
M5a	Monocytic with differentiation
M5b	Monocytic without differentiation
M6	Erythroid
M7	Megakaryoblastic

NOS, not otherwise specified; WHO, World Health Organization.

Clinical findings. Symptoms of **AML** result from the uncontrolled proliferation of neoplastic myeloid cells in the bone marrow. According to the World Health Organization (WHO) criteria, the diagnosis of AML is made if blasts account for more than 20% of all cells in the bone marrow. The neoplastic cells destroy the normal precursors of RBCs, WBCs, and platelets in the bone marrow, causing the following set of findings:

- **Anemia.** The reduced number of RBCs causes easy fatigability, shortness of breath, weakness, and somnolence. The skin and the mucosae tend to be pale.
- **Leukopenia.** A reduced number of WBCs is associated with reduced resistance to bacterial infections. Fever is a common finding.
- **Thrombocytopenia.** A reduced number of platelets is associated with increased bruising and bleeding from various sites, such as gums or skin or during menstruation.

ALLs can be classified into two clinical subgroups: those with good prognosis and those with poor prognosis (Table 6-26). The central nervous system is commonly involved. Over 70% of all children with ALL are cured, but only 40% of adults.

CHRONIC LYMPHOCYTIC LEUKEMIA

Chronic lymphocytic leukemia (CLL) is a clonal proliferation of well-differentiated B lymphocytes. The leukemic form, in which the clonal proliferation of lymphoid cells is limited to lymph nodes, is called small lymphocytic lymphoma (SLL). Both CLL and SLL may involve the bone marrow, spleen, and other tissues that normally contain lymphoid tissues, such as the mucosa-associated lymphoid system of the gastrointestinal and respiratory tracts.

Table 6-26 Clinical and Laboratory Findings Determining the Prognosis of Acute Lymphoblastic Leukemia

FEATURES	GOOD PROGNOSIS	BAD PROGNOSIS
Age	Children (2–9 yr)	Adults
Sex	Female	Male
White blood cells	Low ($<10 \times 10^9$/L)	High ($>50 \times 10^9$/L)
Chromosomes	Hyperdiploid	—
Translocations	t(12;21) (p12;q22) t(4;11) (q21;q23)	t(9;22) (q34;q11)
Extramedullary infiltrates	Yes	No
Induction of remission	4 wk	>4 wk
Disappearance of blasts from peripheral blood	1 wk	> 1 wk
Disappearance of blasts from bone marrow	1–3 mo	>3 mo

CLL is a disease of older age (mean age at diagnosis is 70 years); it is two times more common in males than females. It represents the most common form of leukemia in the United States. Many patients are asymptomatic or have only nonspecific symptoms and are diagnosed only after extensive hematologic studies. The disease typically has a prolonged course, lasting 10 years or even more. A progression into a more aggressive form of lymphoma occurs in terminal stages of the disease and it occurs in approximately 5% of all cases (Richter's syndrome).

Clinical features of CLL are a consequence of excessive proliferation of functionally subnormal neoplastic lymphocytes.

Most clinical signs and symptoms can be related to an increased number of neoplastic lymphocytes. Cells infiltrating the bone marrow may suppress normal hematopoiesis or displace the precursors of normal blood cells. Because of the sheer volume of this neoplastic cell compartment, hypermetabolism and a sense of weakness usually occur. The CLL lymphocytes may appear normal cytologically, but the cytogenetic and molecular biology analysis shows that they are actually abnormal. Likewise their function may be altered; for example, they produce less immunoglobulins than normal cells and hypogammaglobulinemia is a common feature. Aberrant activation of immunoglobulin genes may occasionally cause production of monoclonal immunoglobulins. Dysregulation of antibody production may lead to the production of autoantibodies and a variety of autoimmune disorders (Fig. 6-30).

In many patients the disease has an insidious onset and manifests with nonspecific **constitutional symptoms,** such as night sweats, low-grade fever, weight loss, and fatigue. The most notable clinical and laboratory features of CLL are as follows (Fig. 6-31):

■ **Lymphocytosis.** It may vary, but in most instances it is greater than 5×10^9/L.

■ **Clonal proliferation of lymphocytes.** This can be demonstrated by flow cytometry or fluorescent in situ hybridization (FISH) analysis. Flow cytometry typically shows that the lymphocytes express either kappa or lambda light chains of immunoglobulin G and express some antigens that are not normally present on B cells (e.g., CD5, a T-cell marker aberrantly expressed on CLL cells).

■ **Chromosomal abnormalities.** CLL cells do not divide readily in culture and thus chromosomal anomalies cannot be documented easily. FISH analysis can be used instead to analyze interphase nuclei and show the typical cytogenetic abnormalities. Excess of cytogenetic anomalies is associated with adverse prognosis.

■ **Depressed serum immunoglobulins.** It may be an isolated biochemical finding or it may be associated with immunosuppression. In some patients, however, there could be a monoclonal spike of an abnormal immunoglobulin (so-called M protein).

■ **Anemia and thrombocytopenia.** In about 15% of cases antibodies to RBCs and platelets are present. Apparently these autoantibodies are produced by normal lymphocytes and are a sign of immune dysregulation related to the clonal proliferation and abnormal immunoglobulin secretion of transformed lymphocytes. Bleeding and weakness due to anemia have major adverse effects in prolonged disease.

■ **Lymphadenopathy and splenomegaly.** Enlarged lymph nodes are present in 50 to 60% of all CLL patients. Neoplastic lymphocytes infiltrate typical B-cell areas of lymph nodes and spleen. In classical SLL, which manifests as a small-cell diffuse lymphoma, the normal architecture of lymph nodes is diffusely effaced.

■ **Signs of hypermetabolism.** These include fever, night sweats, weight loss, and fatigue.

■ **Elevated serum LDH, uric acid, and β_2-microglobulin.** These laboratory findings reflect increased cell mass and increased rate of lysis of abnormal lymphocytes.

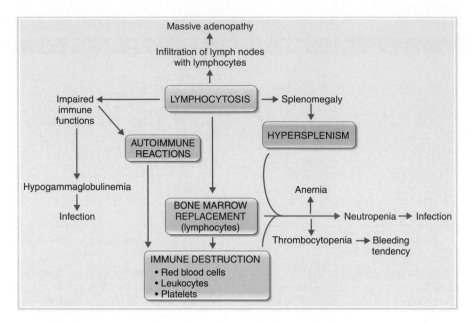

Figure 6-30 Pathogenesis of clinical signs and symptoms in chronic lymphocytic leukemia.

The prognosis depends in general terms on the stage of the disease and the biologic properties of tumor cells. Stage 0 CLL has the best prognosis, whereas stage IV has the worst (Table 6-27).

> **Pearl**
>
> > Poor prognosis is also predicted by the following findings: Blood lymphocyte count in excess of 300×10^9/L, diffuse lymphadenopathy, short lymphocyte doubling site, more than one cytogenetic abnormality, and large tumor burden (high serum LDH, β_2-microglobulin, urate).

Table 6-27 Staging of Chronic Lymphocytic Leukemia

STAGE	FEATURES
Stage 0	Peripheral lymphocytosis and BM involvement
Stage 1	Stage 0 + enlarged lymph nodes
Stage 2	Stage 0 or 1 + enlarged spleen or liver
Stage 3	Stage 1 or 2 + low hemoglobin (<11 g/dL)
Stage 4	Stage 1, 2, or 3 + low platelet count (<100 × 10⁹/L)

BM, bone marrow.
Modified from Rai KR, Peterson BL, Appelbaum FR, et al: Fludarabine compared with chlorambucil as primary therapy for chronic lymphocytic leukemia. N Engl J Med 2000;343:1750–1757.

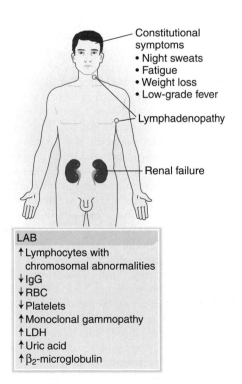

Constitutional symptoms
• Night sweats
• Fatigue
• Weight loss
• Low-grade fever

Lymphadenopathy

Renal failure

LAB
↑ Lymphocytes with chromosomal abnormalities
↓ IgG
↓ RBC
↓ Platelets
↑ Monoclonal gammopathy
↑ LDH
↑ Uric acid
↑ β_2-microglobulin

Figure 6-31 Clinical features of chronic lymphocytic leukemia. IgG, immunoglobulin G; LDH, lactate dehydrogenase; RBC, red blood cells.

LYMPHOMA

Lymphoma is a clonal proliferation of neoplastic lymphoid cells. It may begin within the lymphoid tissues of the lymph nodes, bone marrow, spleen, thymus, or the mucosa-associated lymphoid tissue (MALT), and less commonly in other anatomic sites.

Pathologically lymphomas are divided into two major groups: Hodgkin's lymphoma and non-Hodgkin's lymphoma. Each of these categories is further subdivided into several clinicopathologic entities, which are further subclassified by taking into account the following features:

- Histopathology of the lymph node or other tissue biopsy
- Immunophenotype, microscopic morphology, and size of tumor cells as seen in histology section, smears, or by flow cytometry
- Cytogenetic or molecular characteristics of tumor cells submitted for chromosomal analysis, FISH, or genetic studies

The most widely accepted and most up-to-date classification of lymphomas adopted by the World Health Organization divides lymphomas into four groups:

- **Neoplasms of immature B and T cells.** This group consists predominantly of ALL/lymphoma cases (see Acute Leukemia section).
- **Neoplasms of mature B cells.** This is the largest group of lymphomas. The most prevalent in this group are low-grade follicular lymphoma (20%) and high-grade diffuse large B-cell lymphoma (30% to 40%). Small lymphocytic lymphoma, mantle cell lymphoma, and marginal zone B-cell lymphoma account for approximately 20% of all non-Hodgkin's lymphomas. This group also includes Burkitt's lymphoma, which is relatively rare in the United States but is endemic in sub-Saharan Africa.
- **Neoplasms of mature T or NK cells.** Peripheral T-cell lymphomas, a rather heterogeneous group of neoplasms, accounts for approximately one half of these neoplasms. **Mycosis fungoides** is a dermatotropic T-cell lymphoma.

Sezary's syndrome presents with neoplastic T cells circulating in peripheral blood.
- **Hodgkin's lymphoma.** It accounts for 30% of all lymphomas. Epidemiologically, pathologically, and clinically this form of lymphoma differs significantly from all others and it thus represents a separate clinicopathologic entity. With modern therapy over 80% of all patients can be expected to live a normal life after therapy.

All these pathologic data are summarized and correlated with the clinical data, the extent of tumor spread, and the general assessment of the patient's health condition to prescribe the proper treatment.

Some lymphomas are etiologically linked to environmental causes or preexisting diseases.

Lymphomas are malignant diseases and as such their etiology and pathogenesis remain incompletely understood. Epidemiologic and clinical studies have pointed out several very important links between certain forms of lymphoma and some potentially carcinogenic environmental or morbid conditions (Table 6-28).

Lymphomas involve primarily lymph nodes but may be also extranodal.

Most lymphomas begin with lymph node enlargement in any of several major anatomic areas (Fig. 6-32).

In contrast to these primary nodal lymphomas, some lymphomas begin outside of the lymph nodes and are thus called **extranodal lymphomas.** Most often the extranodal lymphomas may be found in the gastrointestinal tract, but they may occur in other sites such as the skin, lung, central nervous system, or eyes, just to mention a few. It is not uncommon to have a lymphoma first diagnosed as extranodal, only to discover later on that the lymph nodes or spleen are also involved. Some lymphomas are limited to certain regions, such as hepatosplenic lymphoma involving the liver and the spleen only, or central nervous system lymphoma in persons with AIDS.

Table 6-28 Linkage Between Certain Forms of Lymphoma and Potentially Important Exogenous and Endogenous Factors

TYPE OF LYMPHOMA	ASSOCIATED CONDITION
T-cell CLL	HTLV-1 infection (in Japan and Caribbean islands)
Burkitt's lymphoma	Epstein-Barr virus infection (in sub-Saharan Africa)
Large-cell lymphoma of CNS	HIV infection
Lymphoma at an early age	Congenital immunodeficiency
MALT lymphoma	*Helicobacter pylori* gastritis

CLL, chronic lymphocytic leukemia; CNS, central nervous system; HIV, human immunodeficiency virus; HTLV-1, human T-cell lymphoma virus; MALT, mucosa-associated lymphoid tissue.

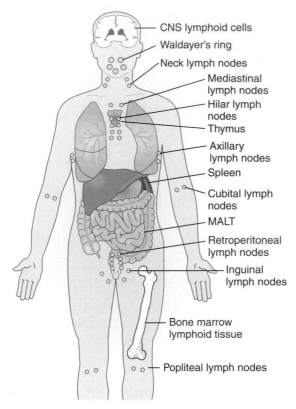

- CNS lymphoid cells
- Waldayer's ring
- Neck lymph nodes
- Mediastinal lymph nodes
- Hilar lymph nodes
- Thymus
- Axillary lymph nodes
- Spleen
- Cubital lymph nodes
- MALT
- Retroperitoneal lymph nodes
- Inguinal lymph nodes
- Bone marrow lymphoid tissue
- Popliteal lymph nodes

Figure 6-32 Lymph nodes in major anatomic regions. In addition to lymph nodes, lymphoid tissue occupies parts of the thymus, spleen, and bone marrow. Lymphoid cells are found in the central nervous system (CNS), peripheral blood, and in the mucosa-associated lymphoid tissue (MALT) of the gastrointestinal and respiratory tracts.

Lymphomas most often manifest with lymph node enlargement.

Lymph node enlargement (often referred to as **lymphadenopathy,** i.e., "disease of lymph glands") is the most common presenting sign of lymphoma. It is, however, important to realize that lymph node enlargement is not always a manifestation of lymphoma and that other disease may case lymphadenopathy (Table 6-29). Note also that lymph node enlargement can be localized or diffuse, painless or painful. All these findings must be taken into consideration during the diagnostic work-up.

The pattern of evolving lymphadenopathy in Hodgkin's lymphoma varies from that in non-Hodgkin's lymphoma (Table 6-30). In non-Hodgkin's lymphoma lymphadenopathy may be accompanied by extranodal involvement, which is uncommon in Hodgkin's lymphoma. Other signs and symptoms also vary, as shown in Table 6-30.

Clinical symptoms of lymphoma vary from one case to another, yet several patterns of presentation are recognized.

Malignant lymphomas are a group of diseases, and their symptoms vary from one subset to another. Several disease patterns are recognized depending on the type of lymphoma, the extent of the disease, the presence or absence of extranodal involvement, and the presence or absence of local or systemic symptoms. Several patterns of clinical presentation are listed here as follows:

- **Lymphadenopathy.** The painless enlargement of lymph nodes may be the only sign of the disease. This pattern is typically seen in well-differentiated SLL or follicular lymphoma.
- **Constitutional symptoms.** In some patients the enlargement of lymph nodes may be accompanied by fever, night sweats, loss of appetite, and weight loss.

Table 6-29 Causes of Lymphadenopathy

CAUSES	EXAMPLES
Local infection	
Viral	Rubella, viral pharyngitis
Bacteria	Strep throat, otitis media, genital syphilis
Mycobacterial	Pulmonary tuberculosis
Fungal	Pulmonary histoplasmosis
Systemic infection	Infectious mononucleosis, HIV infection, toxoplasmosis, bacterial endocarditis
Autoimmune or unknown origin	Sarcoidosis, SLE, RA, Kikuchi's disease
Drug reaction	Hydantoin hypersensitivity reaction
Neoplasia	
Lymphoma/leukemia	Hodgkin's lymphoma, non-Hodgkin's lymphoma, CLL, ALL
Metastatic carcinoma	Axillary lymph nodes in breast carcinoma

ALL, acute lymphoblastic leukemia; CLL, chronic lymphocytic leukemia; HIV, human immunodeficiency virus; RA, rheumatoid arthritis; SLE, systemic lupus erythematosus.

Table 6-30 Comparison of Hodgkin's and Non-Hodgkin's Lymphoma

FINDING	HODGKIN'S LYMPHOMA	NON-HODGKIN'S LYMPHOMA
Presentation	Localized LN enlargement	Localized or multiple LN enlargement
Primary site involved	Neck LN	Any LN
Spread	Contiguous groups of LN	At random
Pharyngeal/mesenteric LN	Uncommon	Often involved
Extranodal involvement	Uncommon	May occur
Bone marrow involvement	Rare, except in stage IV	Common
Leukemic phase	No	20–40%
Anemia	No, until later	30% at presentation → 90% later
T-cell immunity	Depressed (most)	Variable
B-cell immunity	Depressed in advanced stage	Depressed in 30–50%
Systemic symptoms (fever, night sweat, weight loss)	Yes (25%)	Yes (70%)
Pruritus	Yes (25%)	Not common
Signs of organ obstruction (e.g., vena cava, bile ducts)	Rare	Common in late stages
Recurrence rate after therapy	20%	>50%
Cure rate	80%	Variable (10–60%). Depends on the type of lymphoma, age, stage II, etc.

LN, lymph node.

These symptoms are related to **hypermetabolism.** Occasionally the symptoms may precede lymph node enlargement. Itching (pruritus) is common in Hodgkin's lymphoma, but the exact pathogenesis of this symptom is unknown.

■ **Immunologic disturbances.** Lymphomas are often accompanied by immune disturbances involving either T- or B-cell functions. These abnormalities vary and may include loss of **delayed hypersensitivity, hypogammaglobulinemia,** or **monoclonal globulin production.** Immune dysregulation may result in the production of autoantibodies, leading to hemolytic anemia. Antibodies against immunoglobulins may cause deposition of these immune complexes in blood vessels, most notably in cold **(cryoglobulinemia).** Reduced immune response is the most important cause of **recurrent infections** in many lymphoma patients.

■ **Rapidly evolving lymphadenopathy with involvement of extranodal sites.** Extranodal spread is seen in highly aggressive lymphomas that form neoplastic masses. **Mass effect** may cause **obstruction** of some organs (e.g., ureter) or compression of the vena cava. Extranodal involvement of the stomach and intestines causes mass effects that are indistinguishable from other tumors.

■ **Extranodal masses.** Some forms of lymphoma manifest primarily in extranodal sites. **Mycosis fungoides** is a T-cell lymphoma that manifests with skin lesions that vary from erythroderma to widespread skin nodularity. *T-cell lymphoma of the nasal cavity* leads to local-

ized destruction of the septum and was previously called lethal midline granuloma. **Burkitt's lymphoma** is well known for frequent extranodal manifestation, involving the jaw or internal organs.

MULTIPLE MYELOMA AND RELATED DISORDERS

Multiple myeloma (MM) is a clonal proliferation of neoplastic plasma cells or their precursors committed to plasmacytic differentiation. Most often it involves the bone and forms multiple foci of plasma cell proliferation. However, it may also be extramedullary and it may be solitary. It may develop de novo, or it may be preceded by a nonmalignant condition known as **monoclonal gammopathy of unknown significance (MGUS).**

Multiple myeloma is a disease of old age, and the median age at the time of presentation is 70 years. It accounts for 15% of all lymphoid malignancies, and for unknown reasons it is more common in blacks than in whites. Multiple myeloma is incurable with conventional chemotherapy, but most patients live 4 to 6 years after diagnosis.

Clinical signs and symptoms of multiple myeloma are a consequence of uncontrolled proliferation of neoplastic plasma cells.

The diagnosis of MM is made on the basis of clinical and laboratory findings, which are all directly or indirectly related to the lytic bone lesions formed from neoplastic plasma cells (Fig. 6-33). The most important clinical and laboratory findings include the following:

- **Lytic lesions of the bones.** Punched out lesions are readily visible on radiograph. Bone lesions may cause pain, and back pain or skeletal chest pain is found in about 70% of patients. These lesions may lead to pathologic fractures and **hypercalcemia. Alkaline phosphatase** is not elevated, indicating that the bone lysis does not occur due to the activation of osteoclasts.

- **Monoclonal gamma globulin in serum.** Because all the neoplastic plasma cells are descendants of a single cell that has undergone malignant transformation, they all secrete the same immunoglobulin. This manifests in the form of a monoclonal spike in electrophoresis. Most often this immunoglobulin is IgG (70%), and less often IgA (20%), whereas other immunglobulins are less commonly involved. Monoclonal gammopathy contributes to the increased concentration of γ-globulins in the serum **(hypergammaglobulinemia).** It also contributes to **hyperviscosity** of the blood mostly due to RBC rouleaux formation and increased "stickiness." Monoclonal IgM spike **(macroglobulinemia)** is typically associated with clinical signs of hyperviscosity. It is a feature of lymphoplasmacytic lymphoma known as **Waldenström's disease.**

- **Urinary paraproteins.** Incomplete assembly of light and heavy chains of immunglobulins in the cytoplasm of neoplastic plasma cells leads to an excess of free light or heavy chains in serum. These proteins may be excreted in urine as Bence Jones protein.

- **Amyloid formation.** Light-chain deposition in tissues may lead to their transformation into amyloid fibers. Amyloidosis damages the kidneys, but may also affect the liver, adrenal glands, and the gastrointestinal tract.

- **Kidney failure.** Renal failure is the most common cause of death in MM patients. It may be related to chemical injury to the tubules by paraproteins or hypercalcemia. Hypercalcemia is associated with increased **urinary stone** formation. Amyloid deposits also damage the kidneys.

- **Decreased resistance to infection.** Proliferation of neoplastic plasma cells leads to a suppression of normal plasma cells, and thus the immune response to infections is reduced.

- **Anemia.** Anemia, often associated with leukopenia and thrombocytopenia, is due to the suppression of the bone marrow. Reduced RBC counts associated with disturbances in the albumin:globin ratio accelerate the sedimentation of RBCs, and thus the erythrocyte sedimentation rate (ESR) may be markedly elevated.

DISORDERS OF HEMOSTASIS

Disorders of primary hemostasis include several forms of vascular purpura.

As mentioned in the review of normal coagulation (see page 208), three screening tests are routinely used in the initial evaluation of patients with a bleeding tendency: bleeding time (BT), PT, and aPTT.

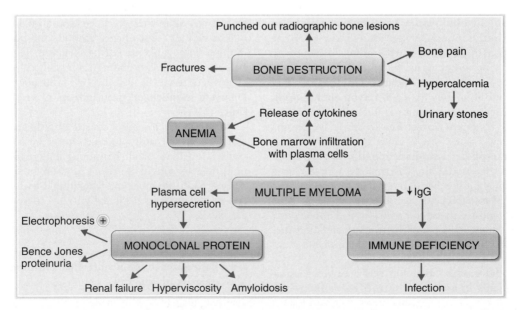

Figure 6-33 Clinical features of multiple myeloma. Most signs and symptoms are related to the clonal proliferation of neoplastic plasma cells and their secretion of immunoglobulins and cytokines.

Patients who have prolonged BT are considered to have a disturbance of hemostasis related to either blood vessels or platelets.

Vessel wall abnormalities. Vascular abnormalities associated with a bleeding tendency result in purpura and mucosal hemorrhages. Typically they are caused by a weakness of blood vessel walls and are classified as either hereditary or acquired (Table 6-31).

The salient features of the most common vascular purpuras are summarized as follows:

- **Hereditary hemorrhagic telangiectasia.** Also known as Rendu-Osler-Weber disease, this autosomal dominant disease is characterized by the appearance of pinpoint dilation of the skin and mucosal venules. It is related to the mutation of a gene on chromosome 9q encoding the cell adhesion protein endoglin.
- **Ehlers-Danlos syndrome.** It includes several disorders characterized by hyperelasticity and fragility of skin, joints, and vessels. The most common form is autosomal dominant and is related to a mutation of a gene encoding collagen V.
- **Marfan's syndrome.** This autosomal dominant disease is characterized by loose joints, aortic aneurysms, subluxation of the lens of the eye, and fragility of blood vessels. It is caused by mutations of the gene encoding *fibrillin,* a protein that serves as glue for filaments of the connective tissue.
- **Scurvy.** It is caused by vitamin C deficiency. Since vitamin C is essential for the synthesis of the intercellular matrix of blood vessels, a deficiency of the vitamin causes fragility of blood vessels and widespread bleeding from gum, oral mucosa, conjunctiva, and skin.
- **Senile purpura.** The cause of this very common form of purpura, associated with increased fragility of blood vessels in the elderly, is unknown.
- **Immune purpura.** Hypersensitivity vasculitis (pathologically often called "**leukocytoclastic vasculitis**") affects venules and other small blood vessels of the skin

and mucosa. It is associated with *"palpable purpura"* because the immune deposits cause vessel wall inflammation and rupture with bleeding into the tissue that can be palpated as small nodules. Similar vascular lesions can be induced by a **hypersensitivity reaction** to drugs and are a constant feature of an IgA-mediated hypersensitivity disease called **Henoch-Schönlein** purpura. In **bacterial endocarditis** and **sepsis** purpura can also be related to a deposition of immune complexes in dermal venules, but can be also due to the direct toxicity of toxins acting on endothelial cells.

Pearl

> The most common form of vascular purpura is called *purpura simplex.* It is also called idiopathic purpura because the characteristic easy bruisability has no obvious causes. It affects women more often than men. The condition is not serious and does not require any treatment.

Platelet disorders, which may be qualitative or quantitative, cause a hemorrhagic diathesis similar to vascular purpura.

Platelet disorders causing a bleeding tendency may be classified as congenital or acquired, and further subclassified as numerical (thrombocytopenia) or functional (qualitative platelet disorders). The causes of thrombocytopenia were listed in Table 6-15, and the causes of most important functional platelet disorders are listed in Table 6-32.

Congenital platelet disorders are relatively rare and of limited clinical significance. The only disease in the group

Table 6-31 Vascular Purpuras

Hereditary vascular purpura
   Hereditary hemorrhagic telangiectasia
   Genetic mutation affecting connective tissue
   (e.g., Ehler-Danlos syndrome, Marfan's syndrome)
Acquired vascular purpura
   Vitamin C deficiency (scurvy)
   Senile purpura (aging)
   Sepsis
   Drugs
   Amyloidosis
Hypersensitivity vasculitis
   Henoch-Schönlein purpura
Idiopathic

Table 6-32 Functional Platelet Disorders

Congenital Disorders
Membrane defects (e.g., Glanzmann's thrombasthenia, Bernard-Soulier syndrome)
Storage pool disorders (e.g., dense granule deficiencies, "gray platelet syndrome")
Genetic deficiencies of plasma proteins (e.g., von Willebrand's disease, afibrinogenemia)

Acquired Disorders
Drug induced (e.g., aspirin, NSAIDs)
Uremia
Cyanotic heart disease
Myeloproliferative disorders and leukemia
Dysproteinemia (e.g., monoclonal gammopathy in multiple myeloma or cryoglobulinemia in viral hepatitis or lymphoma)
Intravascular coagulation syndromes (e.g., DIC, ITP)
Cardiovascular surgery

DIC, disseminated intravascular coagulation; ITP, idiopathic cytopenic purpura; NSAIDs, nonsteroidal anti-inflammatory drugs.

that is commonly encountered in medical practice is von Willebrand's disease.

von Willebrand's disease. This disease is the most common bleeding disorder, affecting 1% to 2% of the population. The bleeding tendency varies from mild to severe. It may be caused by a quantitative deficiency of vWF (type 1, mild form, and type 3, severe form, of von Willebrand's disease) or a qualitative defect of vWF (type 2 von Willebrand's disease). Type 1 disease, inherited as an autosomal dominant disorder, accounts for 70% of all cases. Type 2, which is inherited the same way, accounts for 20% of all cases.

vWF is a multimeric protein produced by endothelial cells and megakaryocytes. It is stored in Weibel-Palade granules of the endothelial cells and in platelet α-granules. Since the vWF is essential for the proper function of platelets and also serves as a carrier of coagulation factor VIII, the disease manifests with signs and symptoms of a hemorrhagic diathesis similar to those for thrombocytopenia or hemophilia A. Prolonged bleeding following trauma or surgery and spontaneous mucosal bleeding in the mouth or nose or during the menstrual period are the most likely presenting signs.

The laboratory findings typical of von Willebrand's disease are as follows:

- Bleeding time—prolonged
- MCH and platelet count—normal
- Activated thromboplastin time—prolonged
- Factor VIII and vWF—reduced
- Platelet aggregation (with ristocetin)—abnormal
- DNA analysis for mutation of vWF—positive in type 2 and 3 (gene for type 1 has not been identified yet)

It should be noticed that asymptomatic normal persons of blood group 0 may have markedly reduced levels of vWF in their blood.

Pearl

> Desmopressin (an analogue of vasopressin) stimulates the release of vWF from endothelial cells and is useful in type 1 von Willebrand's disease, but is of no use in type 2 with disease. Suppression of fibrinolysis with ε-aminocaproic acid may also be used in the treatment of bleeding in these patients.

Acquired disorders of platelet functions are common. The most common causes of platelet dysfunction are aspirin and NSAIDs. Use of extracorporeal circulation during cardiothoracic surgery also makes platelets dysfunctional. Platelet transfusions are thus given to bleeding patients after surgery even if the platelet count is within normal limits. The reasons for platelet abnormalities in uremia, myeloproliferative disorders, and MM are complex and not fully understood.

Intravascular coagulation may cause consumption of disseminated intravascular coagulation (DIC) platelets.

This common complication of shock and septicemia is a prototype of consumptive thrombocytopenia. Procoagulants entering the bloodstream lead to the formation of microthrombi in the peripheral circulation. As a consequence of increased coagulation in small blood vessels, platelets and coagulation factors are consumed and bleeding ensues. Activation of plasmin leads to fibrinolysis, resulting in fibrin split products, which adversely affect the function of platelets, further contributing to the bleeding tendency. The typical laboratory findings are as follows:

- Platelet count—reduced
- MCH—prolonged
- aPTT—prolonged
- Fibrinogen concentration—reduced
- Fibrin degradation products—increased
- D-dimer—present

Thrombotic thrombocytopenic purpura (TTP). This clinical syndrome is related to an uncontrolled coagulation of blood in small blood vessels. It is related to the excessive formation of procoagulant vWF multimers, known in clinical laboratories as unusually large von Willebrand's factor (ULvWF) multimers. They can be demonstrated in early stages of TTP, but if the disease lasts a few days they may not be demonstrable in blood.

Thrombotic thrombocytopenic purpura may be related to a viral infection, which often precedes by a few days the onset of the disease. In most cases the real cause cannot be identified. It is not known why TTP occurs more often in women than in men. In some instances it may result from a genetic deficiency of a vWF multimer-cleaving enzyme called ADAMTS13 (also known as vFW metalloprotease) or the presence of inhibitors of this enzyme.

The underlying enzyme deficiency permits the formation of ULvWF multimers, which promote aggregation of platelets and formation of platelet thrombi in small blood vessels **(thrombotic microangiopathy).** Microthrombi cause ischemia and tissue injury, accounting for most clinical symptoms. RBC passage through partially occluded small blood vessels leads to **microangiopathic hemolytic anemia.** Blood smears contain fragmented RBCs and deformed RBCs (e.g., schistocytes, keratinocytes, "helmet cells," etc.). The typical clinical findings include:

- Thrombocytopenia
  Bleeding
- Evidence of hemolysis
  Microangiopathic anemia (fragmented RBCs, helmet cells, etc.)
  Low RBC count, hematocrit, Hb
  Increased serum bilirubin and jaundice
  LDH concentration increased in serum
  Reticulocytosis

- Fever
- Signs of tissue ischemia
  - CNS—neurologic signs and symptoms
  - Renal injury—proteinuria, hematuria
  - Heart—cardiac contraction irregularities

A syndrome similar to TTP may develop in children following infection with enterohemorrhagic *Escherichia coli* O157. Because it is dominated by marked hemolysis and renal failure it is called **hemolytic uremic syndrome (HUS)**, but pathologically it shows the same changes as TTP and related conditions listed in Table 6-33.

In most patients the onset of the TTP is sudden, and the cause of the disease is not apparent. Associated mortality is high, but with plasma exchange 85% of patients can be saved.

Hemophilia is caused by factor VIII or factor IX deficiency.

All 13 coagulation factors participating in the coagulation cascade, except factor IV (calcium), are proteins. Like all other proteins these factors are encoded by genes, which may be mutated and inherited in an abnormal form. Such mutations are typically associated with hereditary coagulopathies.

The most common hereditary bleeding tendency is hemophilia A. It results from the mutation of the gene for factor VIII, which is located on the X chromosome. Hemophilia B is caused by the mutation of the gene for factor IX.

Hemophilia A. Accounting for 80% of all hemophilias, hemophilia A is caused by changes of the factor VIII gene on the X chromosome and thus it is inherited as an X-linked trait. In about 30% of patients there is no family history and thus it is a new mutation.

The genetic changes involve point mutations, deletion, or inversion of the gene. The last change accounts for approximately 50% of all *severe* cases of hemophilia; that is, those who have less than 1% of normal factor VIII activity.

Table 6-33 Causes of Thrombotic Thrombocytopenic Purpura

TTP (idiopathic, virus-related, or familial)
HUP due to infectious enterocolitis
Escherichia coli O157
Shigella dysenteriae
Toxemia of pregnancy
Preeclampsia
HELLP
Drug-related TTP (e.g., cytotoxic drugs)
Bone marrow transplantation
Malignant tumor-related TTP

HELLP, hemolysis, elevated liver enzymes, and low platelet count; HUP, hemolytic uremic syndrome; TTP, thrombotic thrombocytopenic purpura.

These patients bleed following minor injury, surgery, or dental extraction. Traumatic hemarthrosis is a typical complication, which after several bleeding episodes may become crippling. The bleeding tendency is *mild* when the factor VIII activity is 5% of normal. These patients do not have post-traumatic bleeding, but may bleed profusely during surgery. Patients who have 10% to 30% of factor VIII activity have a *very mild* form of hemophilia evidenced by prolonged bleeding after surgery.

Hemophilia B. It is less common than hemophilia A, from which it cannot be distinguished clinically. Patients suffering from this form of hemophilia either produce inadequate amounts of factor IX or synthesize a functionally inactive form of factor IX.

The laboratory findings in hemophilia are as follows:

- Platelet count—normal
- Bleeding time—normal
- MCH—normal
- aPTT—prolonged
- Factor VIII—C activity reduced in hemophilia B (<30% of normal)
- Factor IX—C activity reduced in hemophilia B
- Genetic studies—positive for abnormal gene for factor VIII or IX

THROMBOTIC DISORDERS

Predilection to thrombosis (**thrombophilia**) may be congenital or acquired. In most instances thrombi form due to the effects of more than one factor. For example atherosclerosis predisposes to the formation of arterial thrombi, chronic venous stasis in heart failure predisposes to deep vein thrombosis of lower extremities, polycythemia vera predisposes to thrombosis in the portal system, and malignant tumors predispose to thrombosis of large veins.

Congenital predisposition to thrombosis is usually a consequence of a reduced level of normal anticoagulant factors or resistance to their activity.

A congenital predisposition to thrombosis is found in 25% to 50% of persons who have recurrent thrombi, and it should be especially considered in persons who have thrombosis at young age or have a family history of thrombosis.

Under normal circumstances the formation of thrombi is counteracted by the action of anticoagulants. The most important among these plasma proteins are:

- **Antithrombin III.** This serum protease inhibitor is the most important and most potent anticoagulant. It disrupts the coagulation cascade by acting on all coagulation factors that have serine protease activity (i.e., thrombin and activated factors IX, X, and XI).
- **Protein C.** When activated by thrombin and thrombomodulin, protein C becomes a serine protease,

which disrupts the coagulation cascade by acting on factors Va and VIIIa. It also participates in fibrinolysis by preventing the degradation of plasminogen activator. Protein C is normally under the control of a protein C inhibitor.

■ **Protein S.** It acts as a cofactor for protein C. Note that protein S binds to complement C4-binding protein (BP), an acute-phase reactant. Since only the free protein S is available as an anticoagulant, excessive binding to C4-BP may cause a functional deficiency of S protein and a tendency for thrombosis during inflammation.

■ **α_2-Macroglobulin.** It is a potent inhibitor of several enzymes including the coagulation factors.

Once the thrombi are formed they are dissolved through the action of **fibrinolytic proteins.** The most important among these is **plasmin,** which is formed from plasminogen through the action of tissue plasminogen activator (TPA). Exogenous activators of plasminogen such as synthetic TPA and streptokinase are used for therapeutic purposes.

The most common congenital causes of thrombophilia are as follows:

■ **Factor V Leyden.** This disorder is found in 5% of the population. It is related to a mutation of the gene encoding factor V. The altered factor V is resistant to the action of factor C, a protein that normally prevents excessive thrombus formation.

■ **Deficiency of antithrombin III.** It occurs as an autosomal dominant disorder at a rate of 1:2000. The affected patients usually develop thrombi in early adulthood, usually in the veins of the legs, upper extremities, or the abdomen. In severe forms of deficiency, the patient is resistant to heparin, a drug whose effectiveness depends on the presence of antithrombin III.

■ **Protein C deficiency.** It occurs as an autosomal dominant disorder affecting 1 in 300 persons. Episodes of venous thrombosis begin early in life and may present even in the neonatal period as purpura fulminans neonatalis.

■ **Protein S deficiency.** It resembles protein C deficiency but occurs much less often.

Acquired thrombotic disorders are related to the Virchow triad: disturbances of blood flow, abnormalities in vessels, or hypercoagulability of blood.

The 19th-century German pathologist Rudolf Virchow posited that thrombosis occurs due to disturbances of the blood flow, abnormalities of the vessel wall, or hypercoagulability of blood. These tenets still hold true and are important for assessing the risk for thrombosis. The most important risk factors for venous, arterial, and intracardiac thromboses are listed in Table 6-34.

Table 6-34 The Most Common Acquired Risk Factors for Thrombosis

ABNORMAL BLOOD FLOW	VASCULAR PATHOLOGY	COAGULATION DISORDERS
Venous stasis	Varicose veins	Malignant tumors
Heart failure	Aneurysms	Trauma and burns
Atrial fibrillation	Atherosclerosis	Lupus anticoagulant
		Oral contraceptives

CASE STUDIES

Case 1 A 34-YEAR-OLD MOTHER OF FOUR COMPLAINS OF EASY FATIGABILITY

Clinical history A 34-year-old woman with four children who does not work outside the home appears to be constantly tired. From time to time she feels short of breath and feels that her heart is speeding and skipping beats.[1] She appears otherwise healthy.

Physical findings She appears pale but otherwise no physical abnormalities were identified.

Laboratory findings

Hb—9 g/dL
Hematocrit—30%
RBC count—4.0 × 10^{12}/L
MCV—75 fL
MCH—22 pg
MCH concentration—30%[2]
WBC and platelet counts—normal[3]

The peripheral blood smear shows that the RBCs are pale and vary in size and shape. Numerous pencil-shaped RBCs are present.[4] These findings correlated with an RDW of 16% (normal, 11.5–14.5%).[5]

Additional hematologic studies revealed that the reticulocyte count was 1%.[6] Serum iron and ferritin concentration and transferrin saturation were moderately reduced.[7]

Follow-up The patient was given appropriate treatment and her blood count improved.[8]

Questions and topics for discussion
1. Are fatigue, shortness of breath, and palpitation diagnostic of any specific hematologic disease? Which diseases should be included in the differential diagnosis?
2. Interpret these hematologic findings.
3. What is the significance of these findings? Which disease do these findings exclude?
4. Use the appropriate technical terms for these microscopic findings. What diseases could cause these changes?
5. What is the RDW? How is it measured?
6. What is the significance of the reticulocyte count?
7. Discuss the possible causes of increased or decreased iron in the blood. What was the most likely cause of iron depletion in this patient?
8. What would be the appropriate treatment in this case?

Case 2 A 48-YEAR-OLD MAN COMPLAINING OF NIGHT SWEATS AND FEVER

Clinical history A 48-year-old man complains of bouts of low-grade fever and night sweats.[1] He also noticed that he has lost 15 pounds over the last few months.[2]

Physical findings The patient seems well nourished and has no obvious major external signs of disease. He has no fever, and his pulse rate is normal. There was slight sternal tenderness on palpation. He has no lymph node enlargement, but his spleen and liver are enlarged.[3]

Laboratory findings

Hb—14 g/dL
Hematocrit—36%
RBC count—4.2 × 10^{12}/L
WBCs—45 × 10^9/L
Platelets—850 × 10^9/L

Differential count revealed 1% promyelocytes, 7% metamyelocytes, 30% bands, 30% segmented neutrophils, 15% lymphocytes, 5% eosinophils, 4% basophils, and 1% monocytes.[4]

Diagnostic procedures Bone marrow biopsy was performed and revealed marked hypercellularity, with predominance of WBC precursors. Blasts accounted for 22% of all cells.[5] Cytogenetic studies revealed a reciprocal translocation of portions of the long arm of chromosomes 9 and 22.[6]

Follow-up The patient was treated and a complete remission of his disease was induced. After a year he was readmitted complaining of increased bruising, and bleeding from his gums.[7] He also feels tired and exhausted. He has fever and is short of breath. Radiographic examination revealed that he has pneumonia.[8]

Questions and topics for discussion
1. What is the pathogenesis of low-grade fever of unknown origin and night sweats?
2. What is the pathogenesis of involuntary weight loss?
3. What is the significance of hepatosplenomegaly in this patient?
4. Interpret the laboratory findings.
5. What is the diagnostic significance of hypercellularity of the bone marrow and the presence of blast cells?
6. Explain the molecular biologic events that occur following this chromosomal translocation. Is it pathognomonic for a specific disease or could such a translocation occur in other blood diseases as well?

7. Explain the pathogenesis of this bleeding diathesis.
8. Explain the pathogenesis of this pneumonia.

Case 3 A 60-YEAR-OLD MAN COMPLAINING OF BACK PAIN, FATIGUE, AND WEIGHT LOSS

Clinical history A 60-year-old man complains of progressively worsening back pain.[1] He feels weak and depressed and is often short of breath.[2] He has also noticed polyuria and is often constipated.

Physical findings No abnormalities were found on physical examination. The radiographic study revealed punched out lesions in the pelvic bones.[3]

Laboratory findings

Mild normochromic anemia
RBC—formed rouleaux in peripheral blood smears
WBC and platelet counts—normal
Serum calcium—elevated
Albumin, alkaline phosphatase, and alkaline phosphatase—normal.[4]

Diagnostic procedures Serum electrophoresis revealed a monoclonal spike in the globin area, which on further analysis proved to be IgG.[5] Urine protein electrophoresis revealed immunoglobulin light chain.[6]

Follow-up The patient did not respond to chemotherapy and radiation therapy. He died from renal failure 2 years later.[7]

Questions and topics for discussion
1. Is back pain a specific symptom of any hematologic disease?
2. What is the significance of these relatively nonspecific symptoms?
3. Explain the pathogenesis of these radiologic findings.
4. Explain the significance of these laboratory findings. Could hypercalcemia be related to any of the clinical and radiologic findings? What are the possible complications of hypercalcemia?
5. Is an IgG monoclonal spike diagnostic of a specific hematologic disease? Which conditions should be taken in the differential diagnosis?
6. In which conditions does immunoglobulin light chain appear in the urine? Is this patient at risk of developing amyloidosis? How is amyloidosis diagnosed?
7. Why did renal failure develop in this patient?

Case 4 A 40-YEAR-OLD WOMAN WITH DIARRHEA, FAINTING, AND PURPURA

Clinical history A 40-year-old woman, who was previous healthy and almost never visited doctors, developed profuse diarrhea, with bouts of vomiting and fever. She related the onset of symptoms to a "common cold" that she had 3 days before the onset of diarrhea. She also complained of severe headache with blurry vision. She fainted and was brought to the hospital semiconscious.[1]

Physical findings The patient was obtunded and sweating profusely. There were numerous ecchymoses on her face, chest, and extremities.[2] Her temperature was 38.5°C, the blood pressure was 110/60 mm Hg, the pulse rate was 110/min, and the respiration rate was 30/min.[3]

Laboratory findings Reduced RBC count and Hb, with RBC parameters suggesting mild normocytic anemia. There was leukocytosis and a reduced platelet count ($50 \times 10^9/L$)[3]. The peripheral smear showed many fragmented RBCs, microspherocytes, schistocytes, keratocytes, and RBCs showing polychromasia.[4] The reticulocyte count was 3% and there were occasional nucleated RBCs.[5] Serum contained increased amounts of bilirubin.[6] Special studies for the detection of unusually large von Willebrand's factor multimers (ULvWF) gave negative results.[7]

Urine contained RBCs and 3+ protein, but the total urinary output was only slightly decreased and there was no oliguria or anuria. Serum creatinine and BUN were mildly elevated.[8]

Follow-up The patient underwent plasmapheresis and plasma exchange using fresh frozen plasma.[9] She recovered within hours.

Questions and topics for discussion
1. Which diagnosis do these symptoms suggest? Which diseases should be considered in the differential diagnosis?
2. Why did the patient develop a bleeding tendency? Is the diagnosis of purpura justified in this case?
3. Define thrombocytopenia. What is the pathogenesis of thrombocytopenia? Why is it associated with a bleeding tendency?
4. Interpret these hematologic findings. What is the pathogenesis of RBC fragmentation and deformity?
5. What is the pathogenesis of reticulocytosis? Is it related to polychromasia seen in the peripheral blood smear?

6. Is this hyperbilirubinemia due to an increased concentration of direct or indirect bilirubin? Will this bilirubin cause jaundice? Will it show up in the urine?

7. Why would one look for unusually large von Willebrand's factor multimers (ULvWF)? Does this negative result change the diagnosis?

8. Do these findings suggest renal injury or renal failure?

9. What is plasmapheresis? How did this procedure correct the neurologic, renal, and hematologic signs and symptoms in this patient?

Chapter 7

THE GASTROINTESTINAL TRACT

Introduction

The gastrointestinal (GI) tract is one of the vital organ systems and a site of many human diseases. The clinical significance of GI diseases in the United States may be illustrated by the following statistics from the National Institutes of Health Web site:

- The overall prevalence of GI diseases is not exactly known, but the estimate is that approximately 70 million people are affected yearly.
- Gastrointestinal diseases account for 50 million physician office visits per year.
- Approximately 10 million people are hospitalized for GI diseases yearly, which account for 15% of all hospitalizations.

- Approximately 200,000 people die every year from GI diseases, mostly neoplasms.

Gastrointestinal diseases belong to the most common human diseases. For example close to 100 million cases of diarrhea are registered yearly in the United States. Some 30 to 50 million Americans have lactose intolerance. Approximately 10 million adults have hemorrhoids, and 4.5 million people suffer from constipation. Estimates are that 3% to 7% of all Americans have gastroesophageal reflux disease. Approximately 3.5 million physician office visits are for diagnosis, treatment, and follow-up of irritable colon disease.

Gastrointestinal disease may have many causes. The relative clinical significance of various GI diseases is presented graphically in Figure 7-1.

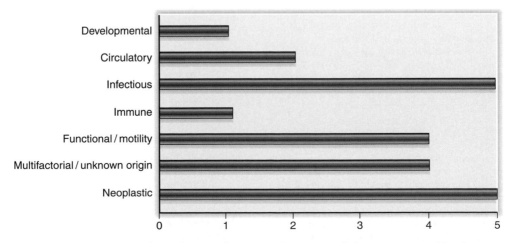

Figure 7-1 Relative clinical significance of various gastrointestinal diseases grouped by their cause.

KEY WORDS

Anatomy and Physiology

Absorption   Uptake of nutrients and fluid from the intestinal lumen into the circulation. Most of the absorption of nutrients occurs in the small intestine, but some nutrients are absorbed in the stomach and the large intestine as well.

Anus   Terminal part of the gastrointestinal tract, lined in part by columnar mucosa similar to the rest of the large intestine, and in part by squamous epithelium.

Appendix   Usual term for vermiform ("wormlike") appendix, an outpouching of the cecum.

Chyme   Semifluid mixture of partially digested food and digestive juices formed in the stomach and passed into the small intestine.

Digestion   Complex process leading to the breakdown of food into water-soluble elementary components that can be readily absorbed.

Duodenum   Part of the small intestine linking the stomach with the jejunum.

Enteroendocrine cells   Neuroendocrine cells found into the small and large intestine. They secrete various polypeptide hormones (e.g., cholecystokinin, gastrin) and can be impregnated with silver stains (thus called "argentaffin"). These cells contain membrane-bound cytoplasmic granules, which can be seen by electron microscopy. In microscopic sections they are best demonstrated by immunohistochemistry using antibodies to chromogranin or synaptophysin (staining all neuroendocrine cells) or antibodies to specific polypeptide hormones. These cells give rise to tumors known as carcinoids or neuroendocrine carcinomas.

Enterokinase   Enzyme in the brush border of enterocytes in the small intestine. It activates trypsinogen.

Esophagus   Intrathoracic tubular organ lined by squamous epithelium connecting the pharynx with the stomach.

Ingestion   Process that begins with the intake of food, followed by chewing (mastication), moistening by saliva, and swallowing (deglutition).

Large intestine (colon)   Part of the lower gastrointestinal tract connecting the ileum and the anus. It consists of several parts: cecum, ascending colon, transverse colon, descending colon, sigmoid colon, and rectum.

Mucosa-associated lymphoid tissue (MALT)   Lymphoid tissue organized into follicles that are found inside the mucosa of the gastrointestinal or respiratory system. These aggregates may be seen microscopically or macroscopically, as in the small intestine where they form Payer's patches.

Small intestine   Longest part of the gastrointestinal tract, connecting the stomach with the large intestine. It comprises the duodenum, jejunum, and ileum.

Stomach   Part of the gastrointestinal tract between the esophagus and the duodenum. It begins at the cardia and ends at the pylorus. The main part of the stomach is called the body. The upper part of the stomach is called the fundus, and the lower the pyloric antrum. The stomach contributes to digestion by secreting hydrochloric acid, pepsin, and several gastroenteric hormones such as gastrin.

Clinical and Laboratory Findings and Procedures

Achlorhydria   Secretory failure of the stomach that makes it unable to produce hydrochloric acid.

Anorexia   Loss of appetite or refusal to eat.

Constipation   Reduced defecation caused by delayed transit of intestinal contents. For practical purposes it means passing fewer than three stools per week.

Diarrhea   Increase in stool frequency or volume. In Western countries it usually means that the stool weighs more than 300 g/day and contains more water than normal. It is said that the stool takes the form of its container.

Dyspepsia   Term used for a variety of symptoms pertaining to the upper gastrointestinal tract and stomach. Such symptoms include abdominal pain, bloating, nausea, or general discomfort after feeding.

Dysphagia   Subjective feeling of difficulty while swallowing food or fluids. It can be caused by anatomic obstruction of the esophagus or functional disturbances in esophageal motility.

Encopresis   Involuntary or voluntary defecation in adults or children older than 4 years of age.

Endoscopy   Examination of the inside of a hollow organ using a flexible or rigid endoscopic instrument. Depending on the organ examined the endoscopic procedures are called esophagoscopy, rectoscopy, colonoscopy, and so on.

Flatulence   Passing of gases from the anus.

Hematemesis   Vomiting of blood.

Hematochezia   Passing of blood from the rectum.

Ileus   Failure of caudal progress of bowel contents because of defective propulsive motility of the intestines ("adynamic or paralytic ileus").

Laparoscopy   Procedure for visualizing the internal organs with an endoscopic instrument introduced into the abdominal cavity through the abdominal wall.

Melena   Passing of black stools, typically due to bleeding from the upper gastrointestinal tract. The black color results from the interaction of the hydrochloric acid with the blood in the stomach or the small intestines.

Nausea   Unpleasant subjective sensation in the throat or epigastrium usually accompanied by an urge to vomit.

Vomiting   Forceful expulsion of the upper gastrointestinal contents through the mouth. It is typically associated with nausea. It is mediated by involuntary spasmodic contractions of the abdominal and chest musculature and the relaxation of the lower esophageal sphincter. If no gastrointestinal contents are expulsed the process is called retching or dry heaves. Rumination is effortless regurgitation of the swallowed food without nausea and spasmodic contractions.

Gastrointestinal Diseases

Achalasia   Inability to relax, specifically used to describe spasms of the lower esophageal sphincter that cause dysphagia and proximal dilatation of the esophagus.

Anastomosis   Communication between two hollow organs surgically attached to one another.

Angiodysplasia   Acquired vascular abnormality most often located in the large intestine of older persons. It is an important cause of occult intestinal bleeding.

Atresia Congenital absence of a lumen of a hollow organ (e.g., esophageal or intestinal atresia) or an orifice (e.g., atresia of the anus).

Barrett's esophagus Esophageal disease characterized by intestinal metaplasia of the normal squamous epithelium.

Carcinoid Low-grade malignant tumor of neuroendocrine cells. May be found anywhere in the gastrointestinal tract and the bronchi, but most often in the small intestine.

Carcinoma of the colon and rectum Adenocarcinoma, originating in various parts of the large intestine.

Carcinoma of the esophagus Adenocarcinoma or squamous cell carcinoma, most frequently found in the lower third of the esophagus.

Carcinoma of the stomach Adenocarcinoma, originating in various parts of the stomach.

Celiac disease Also known as celiac sprue or gluten-sensitive enteropathy. An autoimmune intestinal disease characterized by malabsorption related to intolerance of certain grains (gluten, gliadin).

Colitis Inflammation of the large intestine. It may be acute or chronic, diffuse or segmental. It may be caused by infection or toxins or it may be idiopathic, as in ulcerative colitis and Crohn's disease.

Crohn's disease Inflammatory bowel disease of unknown origin. It is transmural and typically affects the terminal ileum and the right side of the colon in a discontinuous manner.

Dumping syndrome Syndrome caused by rapid passage of food from the stomach into the small intestine, most often encountered in persons who have partial gastric resection of gastrointestinal anastomoses. Clinically it is characterized by dizziness, sweating, nausea, tachycardia, and subsequent diarrhea.

Enteritis Inflammation of the small intestine that may involve the entire small intestine or only some of its parts (e.g., duodenitis, ileitis). It is often associated with colitis and thus called enterocolitis. It is typically associated with diarrhea or, if chronic, with malabsorption. It may be infectious or autoimmune (e.g., celiac disease) or idiopathic (e.g., Crohn's disease).

Familial polyposis coli Autosomal dominant syndrome characterized an occurrence of multiple colonic polyps that almost invariably undergo malignant transformation into colon cancer.

Gastritis Inflammation of the mucosa of the stomach. It may be acute or chronic, atrophic or hypertrophic, erosive or nonerosive. It may be caused by infections (e.g., *Helicobacter pylori*), chemicals and drugs (e.g., alcohol and nonsteroidal anti-inflammatory drugs), or autoimmune mechanisms.

Gastroesophageal reflux disease (GERD) Set of clinical symptoms related to the reflux of gastric acid into the esophagus due to inadequate function of the lower esophageal sphincter, diaphragmatic hernia, or increased intra-abdominal pressure compressing the stomach.

Gastrointestinal stromal tumor (GIST) Benign or malignant tumor composed of undifferentiated stromal cells. Such tumors may be found anywhere in the gastrointestinal tract from the esophagus to the anus and even in the mesentery and extraintestinal sites of the abdomen.

Gastrointestinal tumors Tumors originating in the gastrointestinal tract, including benign tumors (tubular and villous adenomas); adenocarcinomas of the esophagus, stomach, and intestines; squamous cell carcinoma of the esophagus; carcinoids and neuroendocrine carcinomas; lymphomas and various benign and malignant stromal tumors.

Hemorrhoids Dilated veins of the internal or external hemorrhoidal plexus, often harboring thrombi.

Hereditary nonpolyposis colorectal carcinoma (HNPCC) Autosomal dominant condition characterized by the appearance of adenocarcinomas of the large intestine. It is related to the mutation of the mismatch repair genes and microsatellite genetic instability.

Hernia Protrusion of abdominal contents (e.g., intestinal loops) outside of the abdominal cavity. Includes inguinal, diaphragmatic, and umbilical hernias, but also several other less common forms.

Irritable bowel syndrome Functional disturbance of unknown origin characterized by recurrent bouts of abdominal pain, bloating, and diarrhea alternating with constipation.

Ischemic bowel disease Intestinal changes related to acute or chronic ischemia, usually related to atherosclerotic narrowing of intestinal arteries or thrombi and emboli. May manifest in the form of minor functional disturbances (e.g., pain, colic, diarrhea, or constipation), hematochezia, or catastrophic extensive intestinal necrosis.

Lactase deficiency Deficiency of lactase in the intestinal mucosa, characterized by diarrhea precipitated by ingestion of milk or milk-containing food.

Malabsorption syndrome Gastrointestinal syndrome characterized by incomplete absorption of nutrients and fluids from the intestinal lumen. It may be caused by intestinal, pancreatic, biliary, or gastric diseases.

Obstruction Failure of passage or caudal progression of food in the upper alimentary tract or intestinal contents due to a mechanical barrier. May be caused by tumors; fecal impaction; foreign bodies; or intestinal adhesions, hernia, volvulus, and intussusception.

Peptic ulcer disease Multifactorial inflammatory disease, often related to *H. pylori* infection, causing a bleeding defect in the duodenal and gastric mucosa.

Peritonitis Inflammation of the peritoneal lining of the abdominal cavity, which may be caused by infection and chemicals (sterile peritonitis).

Pneumoperitoneum Accumulation of air inside the abdominal cavity, usually due to perforation of the stomach or intestines.

Pyloric stenosis Narrowing of the pyloric part of the stomach due to hyperplasia and hypertrophy of the pyloric sphincter. Most often encountered in male infants.

Ulcer Mucosal defect caused by ischemia, infection, or complex mechanisms such as occurs in peptic ulcers of the stomach and duodenum.

Ulcerative colitis Inflammatory bowel disease of unknown origin involving the colon in a diffuse manner and presenting with confluent mucosal ulcerations.

Varices Abnormally dilated veins, usually found in the esophagus, stomach, or the hemorrhoidal plexus of the rectum and anus.

Normal Structure and Function

NORMAL ANATOMY AND HISTOLOGY

The GI, or alimentary, tract includes the hollow organs stretching from the mouth to the anus, that is, the GI tract proper; and the solid organs, such as the salivary glands, the liver, and pancreas, that are attached to them (Fig. 7-2). In this chapter we deal only with the GI tract proper, whereas the liver and the pancreas are described in subsequent chapters.

The gastrointestinal tract can be divided for practical purposes into two parts: the upper and the lower GI tract.

The upper GI tract includes the mouth, pharynx, esophagus, stomach, and duodenum. These organs are involved in the ingestion and initial digestion of food. The mouth and pharynx can be inspected with the naked eye. The esophagus, stomach, and duodenum can be visualized by upper GI endoscopy using fiberoptic gastroscope. The mouth and the pharynx are located in the head and neck areas, whereas the esophagus extends from the neck through the thoracic region to the diaphragm. The stomach and duodenum are located in the abdomen.

The lower GI tract includes the small intestine (jejunum and ileum), appendix, large intestine, and anus. The small intestine is the primary site for the final stages of digestion and the place where nutrients are absorbed into the circulation. The anus can be inspected during routine physical examination. Rectoscopy and colonoscopy are used to visualize the large intestine. The terminal part of the ileum can be seen during colonoscopy as well, but the remainder of the small intestine cannot be visualized by routine endoscopy.

The wall of the gastrointestinal tract consists of several distinct histologic layers arranged in a similar manner from the pharynx to the anus.

The viscera of the GI tract have a stereotypic structure and consist of four principal layers: the mucosa, submucosa, muscularis propria, and serosa (Fig. 7-3).

- **Mucosa.** The mucosa consists of an **epithelial lining** and the connective tissue lamina propria mucosae. The mouth and esophagus are covered with squamous epithelium that provides protection against the coarse particles found in ingested food. In the stomach and the intestines the mucosa is composed of secretory or absorptive glandular cells that are important for digestion and absorption of food. The lamina propria consists of connective tissue, vessels, and scattered cells of the **mucosa-associated lymphoid tissue (MALT).**
- **Submucosa.** It is composed of loose connective tissue containing numerous blood and lymphatic vessels, cells of the MALT, and **submucosal (Meissner's) nerve plexus.** The submucosa is an important passageway for the blood and lymph entering or exiting the mucosa.
- **Muscle layer (muscularis propria).** The muscle layer of the esophagus and small and large intestines consists of an internal circular sublayer and an external layer containing smooth muscle cells arranged longitudinally.

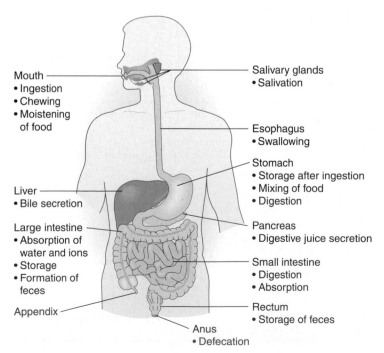

Mouth
• Ingestion
• Chewing
• Moistening
  of food

Liver
• Bile secretion

Large intestine
• Absorption of
  water and ions
• Storage
• Formation of
  feces

Appendix

Salivary glands
• Salivation

Esophagus
• Swallowing

Stomach
• Storage after ingestion
• Mixing of food
• Digestion

Pancreas
• Digestive juice secretion

Small intestine
• Digestion
• Absorption

Rectum
• Storage of feces

Anus
• Defecation

Figure 7-2 Principal components of the alimentary tract.

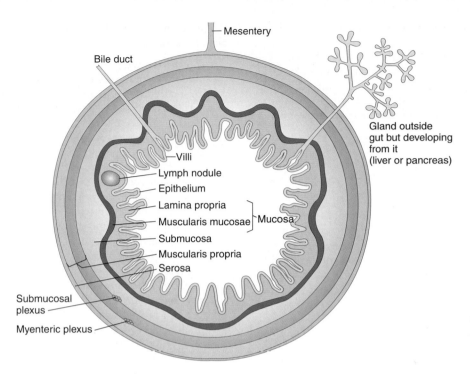

Figure 7-3 Cross section through the tubular part of the gastrointestinal tract. It is attached to the liver and the pancreas, presented here as a schematically drawn gland.

The stomach has an additional oblique middle layer of smooth muscles. The **myenteric (Auerbach's) nerve plexus** is located between the muscle sublayers of the intestines.

- **Serosa.** The external surface of the stomach and the intestines is covered with a layer of mesothelium lying on loose connective tissue that separates it from the muscle layer. The esophagus does not have a serosa and is instead enveloped by a connective tissue **adventitia.** In the abdominal cavity the serosa allows smooth movement of the intestines as they glide over each other's surface during peristalsis and contraction.

The gastrointestinal tract is subdivided into several functional units by smooth muscular sphincters that regulate the passage of contents from one part of the tract to another.

Sphincters are thickened parts of the muscle layer located in critical sites of the GI tract. Sphincters separate one part of the GI tract from another, thereby regulating the orderly forward passage of food and chyme and preventing regurgitation. The most important sphincters are as follows:

- **Upper esophageal sphincter.** It is located at the upper end of the esophagus and is composed of striated muscle. Its tone is maintained by impulses from vagal postganglionic neurons. This sphincter participates in the swallowing reflex and prevents the reflux of swallowed food from the esophagus into the pharynx.
- **Lower esophageal sphincter.** Located at the esophagogastric junction, its relaxation during peristalsis allows the passage of food from the esophagus into the stomach. It also prevents gastroesophageal reflux. It is under the control of intrinsic nervous plexus, which is influenced by the vagus nerve.
- **Pyloric sphincter.** This sphincter is located at the end of the pylorus. It represents the thickened middle layer of the gastric muscularis propria. Opening of this sphincter allows the passage of chyme from the stomach into the duodenum.
- **Ileocecal sphincter (valve).** The small intestine does not have any sphincters, and the first sphincter the chyme encounters after leaving the stomach is the ileocecal valve. It regulates the passage of chyme from the small into the large intestine. It opens on distention of the terminal ileum by chyme and closes on dilatation of the cecum.

Pearls

> The small intestine, the longest part of the GI tract, does not have any sphincters.
> The colon does not contain sphincters either. It is subdivided by smooth muscle bands into saclike segments called haustra.

■ **The internal and external anal sphincters.** These sphincters prevent involuntary passage of feces but relax during defecation, allowing the passage of stools. The external sphincter, which is composed of skeletal muscle, can be contracted or relaxed at will. If the sphincter is relaxed, defecation occurs. The internal sphincter is involved in the defecation reflex, regulating the entry of feces into the anal canal.

The mucosal lining of the stomach and the intestines contains several highly specialized cells arranged in an anatomic site-specific manner.

The mouth and esophagus on one end and the anus on the other end of the GI tract are lined by squamous epithelium. All other parts of the GI tract are lined by mucosa that contains, with some minor site-specific modifications, five cell types: (1) protective cells, (2) absorptive cells, (3) exocrine secretory cells, (4) endocrine secretory cells, and (5) stem cells considered to be the precursors of all the other more differentiated cells. Obviously some cells have more than one function and could belong to more than one of these categories. These five cells types seen in the small intestine are shown diagrammatically in Figure 7-4.

Pearl

> The histologic features of various parts of the GI tract are distinctive enough to allow the pathologist to recognize the provenance of a tissue specimen.

The main features of the epithelial cells lining the GI tract are as follows:

■ **Protective cells.** The mouth and the esophagus are lined by **squamous epithelium,** the primary function of which is the protection of the body from the adverse effects of ingested material. In the stomach and the intestine the main epithelial protective cells are the **mucus-secreting cells.** One should not forget that the GI system contains immune cells, lymphocytes, and plasma cells, forming the so-called **mucosa-associated lymphoid tissue (MALT).** These nonepithelial cells interact with the epithelial cells and contribute to their protective function.

■ **Absorptive cells.** Since most of the absorption occurs in the small intestine, it is obvious that **surface absorptive cells (enterocytes)** predominate in this part of the GI tract. Surface absorptive cells are on their luminal surface lined by **microvilli,** which increase the absorptive surface of the cell membrane. The **glycocalyx** covering the microvilli is rich in digestive enzymes such as disaccharidases and dipeptidases that facilitate the absorption of carbohydrates. The large intestine contains absorptive cells whose main function is the passive reabsorption of water, which follows the active transport of sodium from the lumen.

■ **Exocrine cells.** These cells are found in all parts of the GI system below the esophagus.

   ■ In the **stomach** the primary exocrine secretory cells are the parietal cells and the chief cells. The **parietal cells** secrete **hydrochloric acid,** the main component of the gastric digestive juice, and **intrinsic**

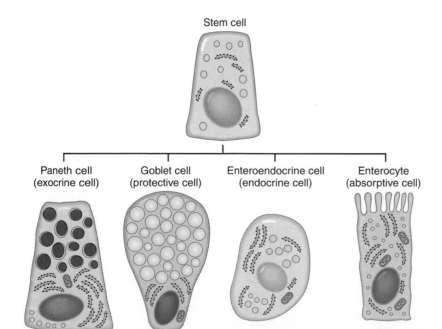

Stem cell

Paneth cell
(exocrine cell)

Goblet cell
(protective cell)

Enteroendocrine cell
(endocrine cell)

Enterocyte
(absorptive cell)

Figure 7-4 Cells of the small intestinal mucosa. This drawing shows the five cell types in the small intestine. Other parts of the intestine and stomach have slightly different cells, but they also can be classified as protective, exocrine, endocrine, absorptive, or stem cells.

factor, which is essential for the absorption of the vitamin B_{12} in the ileum. The **chief cells,** found only in the fundic glands of the gastric body, secrete **pepsin, lipase,** and several other enzymes important for the initial digestion of food. The neck of the gastric glands contains **mucus-secreting cells,** which secrete glycoproteins and glycosaminoglycans that coat the surface. This mucus is part of the **gastric mucosal barrier** that protects the gastric mucosa from autodigestion by hydrochloric acid and peptic enzymes secreted by other gastric cells.

■ In the **small intestine** the secretory cells include cells that are devoted to secretion only, such as the Paneth cells and the mucus-secreting goblet cells, and enterocytes (surface absorptive cells), which have other functions as well. The function of **Paneth cells** has not been elucidated completely. The **mucus** produced by **mucous cells** has a protective and lubricating function. The mucus also contains **bactericidal substances** including **immunoglobulin A** produced by the plasma cells residing in the intestinal mucosa. In contrast to the **enterocytes** lining the surface villi that are involved in absorption, the enterocytes in the intestinal crypts participate in **exocytosis** of fluids and minerals. These cells contribute about 3 L of fluid per day to the intestinal contents. Exocytosis includes several mechanisms, most notably: **active transport, diffusion, and facilitated diffusion.**

■ The **large intestine** contains numerous goblet cells whose main function is to produce mucus.

This mucus protects the surface of the intestines and serves as a lubricant facilitating the passage of solidified feces.

■ **Endocrine cells.** These cells are part of the diffuse enteroendocrine system and are scattered throughout the GI tract. Similar cells are found in the respiratory tract and in the islets of Langerhans. Enteroendocrine cells secrete **biogenic amines,** such as histamine and serotonin, and **polypeptide hormones** that can be classified as (1) true hormones, (2) paracrine hormones, and (3) neurocrine hormones (Table 7-1).

■ **True hormones** are released into the circulation and act on distant target organs. For example, the duodenum secretes cholecystokinin (CKK) and secretin, which enter the blood and act on the receptors in the pancreas and the biliary system.

■ **Paracrine hormones** act on cells that are adjacent to the cells that produced them. For example, somatostatin is a hormone produced by many enteroendocrine cells, and it acts by inhibiting the functions of adjacent cells.

■ **Neurocrine hormones** act on smooth muscle cells and exocrine cells by mimicking the action of sympathetic and parasympathetic nerves. For example, vasoactive intestinal polypeptide (VIP) stimulates intestinal exocytosis while relaxing circular intestinal smooth muscle cells. Enkephalins have the opposite effect. Most of the neurocrine hormones are actually synthesized by the nerve cells in the intestinal wall.

Table 7-1 Polypeptide Hormones of the Gastrointestinal Tract

HORMONE	PRIMARY SOURCE	TARGET CELL OR ORGANS	ACTION
Cholecystokinin	Duodenum and jejunum	Pancreas Gallbladder	Acinar enzyme secretion ↑ Contraction ↑
Secretin	Duodenum and jejunum	Pancreas Stomach	Ductal fluid and HCO_3^- secretion ↑
Gastrin	G cells in the antrum of stomach	Gastric parietal cells	H^+ secretion ↑
Gastrin-releasing hormone	Vagus nerve endings	G cells of antrum	Gastrin release ↑
Motilin	Small intestine	Esophageal sphincter, stomach, and duodenum	Smooth muscle contraction ↑
Somatostatin	D cells of stomach, duodenum, pancreas	Stomach Small intestine	Gastrin release ↓ Secretion ↓ Smooth muscle contraction ↑
Vasoactive intestinal polypeptide	Neurons in the GI tract	Small intestine Pancreas	Smooth muscle relaxation ↑ Exocytosis in small intestine ↑ Pancreatic secretion ↑

GI, gastrointestinal.

The innervation of the gastrointestinal tract comprises an intrinsic and an extrinsic component interacting with one another and the neuroendocrine cells.

The intrinsic innervation includes the autonomous nervous system ganglia arranged into the myenteric and submucosal plexus, and the so-called GI interstitial cells of Cajal, which act as internal pacer cells. Gastrointestinal plexuses contain both sensory and motor neurons. The sensory cells respond to the local stimuli, such as dilatation of the intestines by food, by transmitting these impulses to the motor neurons or intestinal neuroendocrine cells that regulate the autonomous contraction and relaxation of the smooth muscle cells.

The extrinsic innervation includes a sympathetic and a parasympathetic component. The sympathetic nerves release adrenalin, which inhibits the contraction of smooth muscle cells. The parasympathetic nerves are cholinergic and stimulate contraction of smooth muscle cells.

The **sympathetic** innervation stems from four ganglia: celiac, superior mesenteric, inferior mesenteric, and hypogastric. Adrenergic stimuli from these ganglia act on the nerve cells of the myenteric and submucosal plexus, or directly on the smooth muscle cells and endocrine and exocrine cells of the GI mucosa (Fig. 7-5).

The **parasympathetic** innervation is derived from the vagus nerve, which innervates the upper GI tract, and the pelvic nerve, which innervates the colon and anus. The parasympathetic system has long preganglionic fibers that extend to the ganglia in the wall of the GI tract. The intrinsic intestinal ganglion cells process the external stimuli and transmit them to the smooth muscle

cells but also to other effector cells, such as the neuroendocrine cells and exocrine mucosal cells. It is important to remember that the **vagus nerve** is composed of 75% afferent fibers and only 25% efferent fibers. It is the main conduit for pain and other sensory stimuli that reach the central nervous system from the mechanoreceptors and chemoreceptors in the GI system. It is also important for the so-called **vasovagal reflexes,** accounting for some clinically important symptoms such as nausea and vomiting and paralytic ileus.

PHYSIOLOGY

The GI tract has two main functions: to provide nutrients for the rest of the body and to eliminate the undigested food and waste products. These two main functions can be accomplished only by coordination of several basic physiologic processes, including the following:

- **Motility.** The musculature of the GI tract consists predominantly of smooth muscle cells, and thus it is not surprising that most of its movements are involuntary. These movements are under the control of the autonomic nervous system and intramural nerve plexus and are often coordinated into reflexes controlled by the autonomic centers in the medulla and the pons.
- **Secretion.** Different parts of the GI tract have different functions, and so the secretions in the stomach differ from those of the small intestine. Keep in mind that the salivary glands, the liver, and the pancreas secrete copious amounts of digestive juices that are essential for normal digestion.

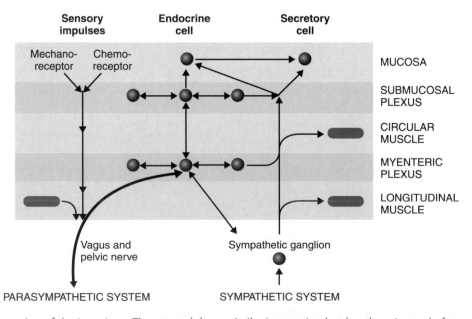

Figure 7-5 Innervation of the intestines. The stomach has a similar innervation but has three instead of two muscle layers.

■ **Intestinal fluid and electrolyte transport.** Huge amounts of fluids enter into the GI tract daily and are mostly reabsorbed, resulting in only 200 g of waste removed by defecation.

■ **Digestion.** Breakdown of foods into the basic nutrients is a prerequisite for their absorption.

■ **Absorption.** This is the final stage in the uptake of nutrients, but it is also essential for the intake of fluid, minerals, vitamins, drugs, and other exogenous substances.

■ **Defecation.** The undigested nutrients and some waste products are eliminated from the body through the anus.

The initial processing of the food begins with chewing and swallowing.

The movements of the upper GI tract participate in the processing and digestion of food. This can be broken down into several phases as follows:

■ **Ingestion.** Intake of food occurs in most instances by voluntary opening of the mouth and biting of solid food or sucking of fluids.

■ **Chewing (mastication).** Breakdown of solid food into smaller morsels is accomplished by coordinated movements of the jaws, known as chewing. It is in part based on voluntary movements and in part on a **chewing reflex** coordinated from the centers in the brainstem. It involves a coordinated action of masticatory muscles such as the masseter, medial pterygoid, and temporalis muscle.

■ **Swallowing (deglutition).** Food that has been reduced to smaller morsels is swallowed. Swallowing has three phases: an initial voluntary phase (oral phase), followed by two involuntary phases (pharyngeal and esophageal phases) (Fig. 7-6).

■ **Oral phase.** During the voluntary phase the tongue forms a bolus and pushes it into the oropharynx.

■ **Pharyngeal phase.** Once the bolus enters the oropharynx, it activates the **swallowing center** in the medulla and lower pons, which propels the food into the esophagus. At the same time the reflex leads to the closure of the glottis and vocal cords so that the food does not enter into the respiratory system.

■ **Esophageal phase.** Once the bolus has entered into the esophagus it is propelled caudally by esophageal peristalsis. Two forms of peristalsis are recognized: primary and secondary. **Primary peristalsis,** which is initiated by swallowing, is under the control of the vagus nerve, emerging from the swallowing centers in the medulla. As soon as food enters the esophagus, the upper esophageal sphincter contracts, preventing the regurgitation of the food (Fig. 7-7). The peristaltic waves of primary peristalsis are slow, and when a person is eating in an erect position the food drops faster due to gravity than to peristaltic propulsion. It should be noticed that the vagus nerve controls both the striated muscle in the upper esophagus and the smooth muscle cells. Vagotomy abolishes the primary esophageal reflex. **Secondary peristalsis,** which is initiated by the entry of food into the esophagus, is mediated by intramural mechanical stretch receptors. It is coordinated by intramural nerves, and vagotomy does not abolish it. This type peristalsis leads to the opening of the lower esophageal sphincter, and it persists until the food is passed to the stomach. Once the food has passed into the stomach the lower esophageal sphincter contracts, preventing reflux from the stomach.

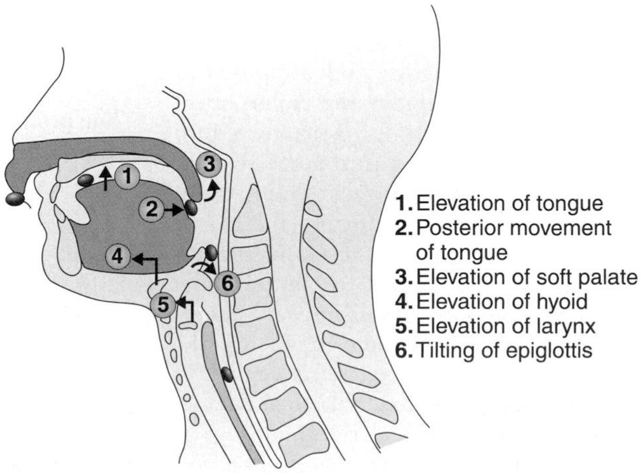

Figure 7-6 Swallowing reflex. It involves a sequential contraction and relaxation of several muscles in the mouth and throat. The sequence of events is listed numerically from 1 to 6.

1. Elevation of tongue
2. Posterior movement of tongue
3. Elevation of soft palate
4. Elevation of hyoid
5. Elevation of larynx
6. Tilting of epiglottis

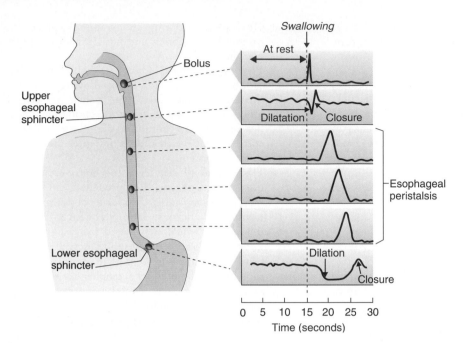

Figure 7-7 Esophageal phase of swallowing. It begins with the opening of the upper esophageal sphincter, followed by peristaltic contractions of the esophageal muscles and the opening of the lower esophageal sphincter. At the end of the passage of food the lower esophageal sphincter closes, preventing the reflux of gastric juice into the esophagus. Manometric recordings of the sequential changes of the esophageal tone are shown graphically.

In the stomach the food is transformed into chyme, which is passed into the duodenum.

Gastric processing of the food involves several processes, all of which depend on the proper motility of the muscle layers and the functioning of the mucosal cells. Several distinct processes can be recognized as follows:

- **Filling.** The swallowing of food initiates a vasovagal reflex that leads to the relaxation of the lower esophageal reflex in the proximal part of the stomach. This process is called **receptive relaxation.** The entry of food into the stomach evokes active dilatation of the fundus, known as **gastric accommodation.** This dilatation is believed to be mediated by intrinsic gastric innervation and is modulated by the vagus nerve (Fig. 7-8).
- **Mixing.** The gastric contractions needed for the mixing of food are initiated by a pacemaker that is located on the greater curvature and composed of interstitial cells of Cajal. Under the influence of hydrochloric acid the food is broken down into small morsels and transformed into a coarse mixture. This mush is propelled into the antrum, where it is churned. The food hitting the closed pyloric sphincter initiates a contraction of the antrum, which returns the food into the proximal stomach. This **propulsion, grinding,** and **retropulsion** are repeated several times, mincing the food into smaller and smaller particles until it is transformed into a semifluid material called **chyme. Expulsion of food** leads to gastric emptying, as follows.

- **Gastric emptying.** During food mixing the pyloric sphincter is closed as tightly as possible. Nevertheless small amounts of chyme escape into the duodenum. The entry of acid chyme, and especially if it contains lipids and proteins, evokes an **enterogastric reflex,** which slows down gastric emptying. The purpose of this reflex is to prevent premature emptying of the stomach and overly rapid filling of the duodenum. Nevertheless, as the mixing progresses, more and more food accumulates in the pyloric antrum, causing its gradual dilatation. The relaxation of the pyloric sphincter permits the outflow of food into the duodenum. It should be noticed that gastric emptying is also under hormonal control. Gastrin enhances the contraction of the pyloric sphincter, thereby diminishing gastric emptying. Cholecystokinin and secretin released from the duodenum filling with acid chyme also reduce the rate of gastric emptying.

The processing of food in the stomach is accomplished primarily through the action of hydrochloric acid.

Hydrochloric acid and pepsin are the main components of gastric juice. **Hydrochloric acid** (HCl) acts by dissociating and lysing cells and the extracellular matrix of animal and plant tissues. It is also essential for acidifying the luminal contents, thus providing the optimal conditions for the action of **pepsin.** Approximately 10% of the total protein is broken down completely in the stomach through the action of pepsin.

Proteins are not the only food component broken down in the stomach. Gastric **lipase** breaks down short-chain

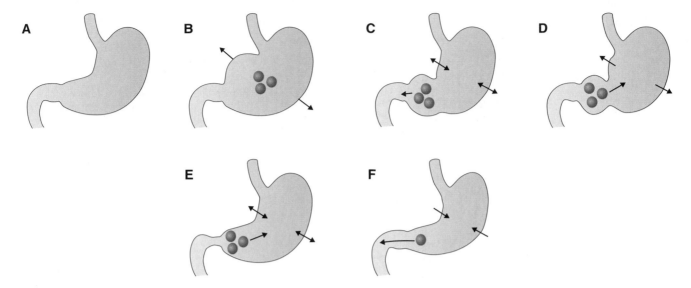

Figure 7-8 Gastric digestion. Several phases can be recognized as follows: **A,** Interval phase between feeding. **B,** Entry of food causing dilatation. **C,** Propulsion of food into the pyloric canal. **D,** Grinding. **E,** Retropulsion. **F,** Expulsion into the duodenum.

fatty acids, but in principle most lipids are not digested in the stomach. Carbohydrates continue to be digested by the salivary amylase, which is, however, soon inactivated by acid. Thus, most of the components of a food bolus are only partially digested in the stomach, and very little of these are absorbed. Most absorption involves water-soluble small molecules, which pass freely with the water into the blood.

> **Pearl**
>
> > Alcohol is water-soluble. Because water readily crosses the gastric mucosal barrier, alcohol is rapidly absorbed in the stomach.

Secretion of gastric juices is under neural and hormonal control.

Secretion of gastric juices occurs in three phases as follows:

■ **Cephalic phase.** It accounts for approximately 30% of the total gastric secretory response. The cephalic phase involves a central nervous system (CNS) reflex that can be initiated by thinking about food, or by seeing, smelling, or tasting it. The stimuli are transmitted through the vagus nerve. **Acetylcholine** (ACh) released from the nerve endings of the vagus nerve acts directly on parietal cells to secrete HCl (Fig. 7-9). Acetylcholine released from the vagus nerve also stimulates the enteroendocrine cells, indirectly evoking both stimulatory

and, to a lesser degree, inhibitory stimuli. These indirect effects on parietal cells include the action of ACh on the following cells:

■ **Enterochromaffin-like cells (ELCs).** These cells are stimulated by ACh to release histamine. **Histamine** is the strongest secretagogue and acts by binding to histamine-2 (H_2) receptors on the surface of parietal cells.

■ **G cells.** Acetylcholine also stimulates the release of gastrin from G cells. **Gastrin** binds to specific receptors on parietal cells, stimulating them to produce HCl. Gastrin also acts on ECLs, stimulating them to release histamine. Chronic stimulation of ECLs with gastrin (e.g., in Zollinger-Elllison syndrome) may even cause ECL hyperplasia.

■ **D cells.** Acetylcholine acts on D cells, which secrete **somatostatin.** Somatostatin acts on parietal cells, thus inhibiting HCl production. It also inhibits the release of gastrin from G cells.

■ **Gastric phase.** It is initiated by the mechanical stimuli created by the bolus of food as it enters the stomach. This phase accounts for most of the gastric secretory activity. The **distention** of the stomach provokes **vasovagal reflexes,** resulting in the release of ACh like in the cephalic phase. Acid pH stimulates the release of pepsin from the chief cells. Pepsin cleaves proteins to **amino acids,** some of which, notably tryptophan and phenylalanine, stimulate enteroendocrine G cells to release gastrin; this further promotes HCl production. When the acidity of gastric contents drops below

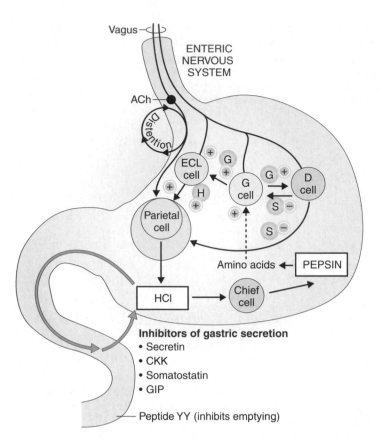

Figure 7-9 Gastric secretion is under the influence of the vagus nerve, which directly or through its connectors stimulates the parietal cells to secrete HCl. The dilatation of the stomach by food initiates the vaso-vagal reflex, which further promotes the release of acetylcholine (ACh) from the terminal branches of the vagus nerve and the parasympathetic autonomic nerves in the stomach. The vagus nerve also stimulates the enterochromaffin-like cells (ECLs) to secrete histamine (H), G cells to secrete gastrin (G), and D cells to secrete somatostatin (S). Gastrin stimulates the parietal cells. Somatostatin inhibits the secretion of gastrin and inhibits the secretion of HCl from parietal cells. HCl stimulates the chief cells to secrete pepsin. The entry of food into the duodenum leads to a release of inhibitors of gastric secretion, such as secretin, cholecystokinin (CKK), somatostatin, and gastrin inhibitory protein (GIP). The entry of chyme into the ileum leads to a release of peptide YY, which inhibits gastric emptying.

pH 3 the secretion of gastrin stops. The acidity of the contents also has an inhibitory effect on the parietal cells, and when it drops below pH 2, HCl secretion stops entirely.

■ **Intestinal phase.** This phase begins with the chyme reaching the duodenum. It accounts for only 10% of the gastric output. Initially, as long as the acidity of chyme entering the duodenum is above pH 3, the intestinal phase is characterized by prevailing stimulation of the gastric secretion. Later on, as the acidity of the chyme entering the duodenum drops below pH 3, the inhibitory effects predominate. These inhibitory stimuli include the vasovagal reflex, stimulating somatostatin release in the stomach, and inhibitory hormones, such as **secretin, CKK, somatostatin,** and **gastric inhibitory polypeptide** (**GIP**) released from the duodenum. Collectively these hormones inhibit gastric acid secretion and slow down gastric emptying. Secretin is considered to be the main inhibitor of HCl production: it acts directly on parietal cells, inhibits gastrin release, and stimulates the production of somatostatin in the duodenum and the stomach. Somatostatin released from gastric D cells is the most potent paracrine inhibitor of parietal cells. Distention of the ileum by chyme leads to the release of peptide YY, which slows down gastric emptying.

Intraluminal digestion of chyme in the small intestine requires additional mixing with digestive juices.

By the time food enters the small intestine it is semifluid. Nevertheless it must be further digested to transform all its nutrients into small water-soluble components that can be taken into the absorptive cells. To this end the food must be further mixed with pancreatic juice and bile and pushed forward through the intestinal lumen. This is accomplished by two types of intestinal contraction: segmentation and peristalsis.

■ **Segmentation** is a back-and-forth movement based on periodic 5-second contractions of small (2–3 cm long) segments of the intestine followed by relaxation. Segmentation promotes *mixing* of the food. During the contraction the chyme is propulsed backward or forward, and when the contraction relaxes it flows back into the newly dilated areas from which it was expressed by subsequent contraction (Fig. 7-10).

■ **Peristalsis** involves periodic progressive sequential contractions of the circular muscle layer that results in forward propulsion of the intestinal contents. In contrast to segmentation, which occurs at a rate of 8 to 12 contractions per minute, the peristaltic movements are slower, thus allowing enough time for the food to remain in the small intestine, which is essential for proper digestion and absorption of nutrients.

A   **B**

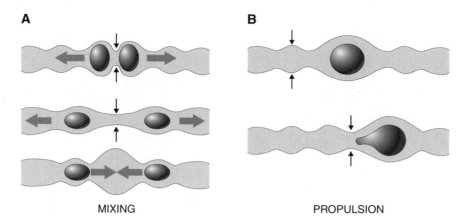

MIXING   PROPULSION

Figure 7-10 Intestinal motility. It consists of two forms of contractions: segmentation and peristalsis. **A,** Segmentation leads to mixing of food. **B,** Peristalsis leads to food propulsion.

Intestinal motility is autonomous and under the control of internal intestinal innervation. Nevertheless, external parasympathetic impulses can augment it, whereas sympathetic stimuli have an inhibitory effect. These nerves also play a role in the **intestinointestinal reflex**—the dilatation of one segment of the intestine leading to the dilatation of the rest of the small intestine. Another reflex, called the **gastroileal reflex,** is also mediated through these nerves. Increased gastric motility caused by the entry of food stimulates the contractions of the terminal ileum and the opening of the ileocecal sphincter, allowing the passage of chyme into the large intestine.

Most of the absorption of nutrients, water, and minerals occurs in the small intestine.

Food entering the small intestine is only partially digested and must be further processed. Here we briefly review the fate of the main components of food in the small intestine (Fig. 7-11).

Carbohydrates. The only dietary monosaccharides that can be properly absorbed are **glucose, galactose,** and **fructose.** Accordingly all complex carbohydrates must be broken down to these monosaccharides.

The digestion of some complex carbohydrates, such as starch, begins in the mouth through the action of salivary **α-amylase.** The bulk of carbohydrate digestion occurs in the duodenum under the influence of pancreatic digestive juice. The pancreatic juice contains large amounts of α-amylase, which acts on starch molecules reaching the duodenum. During the **intraluminal phase of digestion** the starch is hydrolyzed to maltose and several maltooligosaccharides.

The oligosaccharides generated in this process interact with the **ectoenzymes** on the brush border of enterocytes in the small intestine. These ectoenzymes include **lactase, sucrase,** and several other enzymes capable of acting on oligosaccharides. Ectoenzymes acting on oligosaccharides produce glucose, galactose, or fructose, which are taken up by the transport proteins and internalized into the cell cytoplasm. Glucose, galactose, and fructose leave the enterocyte cytoplasm on the basolateral sides through facilitated transport. From the interstitial space they diffuse into the lymphatics and blood and are carried away from the intestine.

Most carbohydrates are absorbed in the duodenum and the upper jejunum. Approximately 6% to 10% of starch that has not been digested is passed into the colon where it serves as the source of food for bacteria.

Proteins. The digestion of proteins begins in the stomach, where the mordant action of HCl disrupts cells. The acidic environment allows pepsin to hydrolyze proteins into smaller polypeptides and amino acids. Gastric pepsins reduce approximately 15% of all proteins from food to peptides and amino acids, but others must be digested in the small intestine.

Food entering the duodenum is exposed to **proteolytic enzymes from the pancreas,** including **trypsin, chymotrypsin, carboxypeptidases A** and **B,** and **elastase.** These enzymes enter the intestine from the pancreas as proenzymes (i.e., in an inactive form). In the intestine they are activated by **enteropeptidase** found on the lumina brush border of enterocytes. Approximately 50% of all proteins from food are digested and absorbed in the duodenum.

Additional protein digestion occurs on the **brush border of enterocytes,** which contain a number of peptidases. These peptidases act on longer peptides that consist of four or more amino acids.

Small peptides resulting from the action of these proteolytic enzymes are taken up and transported into the

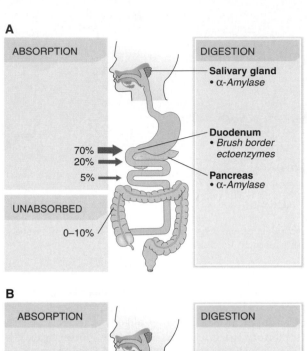

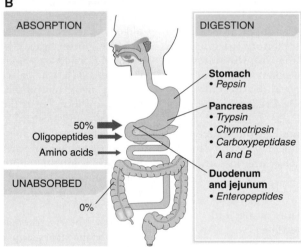

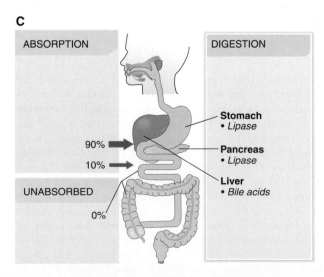

Figure 7-11 Absorption of nutrients. **A,** Absorption of carbohydrates. **B,** Absorption of proteins. **C,** Absorption of lipids.

enterocytes through specific transport mechanisms. Most dipeptides and tripeptides, accounting for most of the protein-derived nutrients, are taken up by active transport mechanisms into the cytoplasm of enterocytes of the jejunum. Inside the cytoplasm of the enterocytes the peptides are broken down to single amino acids. **Basic** and **neutral amino acids** leave the cell on its basolateral end through sodium-dependent and sodium-independent specific transport mechanisms. **Acidic amino acids** are not exported and seem to be used for internal purposes in enterocytes.

Amino acids formed by intraluminal digestion are also taken up by specific transport mechanisms. Some amino acids enter the cells by diffusion on the basolateral side. In contrast to oligopeptides, which are absorbed in the jejunum, amino acids are mostly absorbed in the ileum. In normal persons all protein in food is digested and absorbed in the small intestine. Small amounts of proteins found in feces are actually not from the food, but are derived from colonic bacteria.

Fats. Fats are absorbed in the intestines by passive diffusion. To be ready for diffusion, the fats must be degraded and made water-soluble. Even though stomach juice contains lipase, most of the digestion of fat takes place in the duodenum. **Bile acids** and lecithin emulsify fat into small globules. These globules serve as substrate for **pancreatic lipases,** which cleave the fats into fatty acids and glycerides.

Monoglycerides and **cholesterol** formed in the digestion of fats bind to bile salts to form **micelles** composed of 20 to 30 molecules of lipids and bile salts (Fig. 7-12). These micelles move along the brush border releasing the lipid on contact with the cell membrane. The lipids are internalized and then processed and packaged into **chylomicrons,** which are excreted by exocytosis. Several

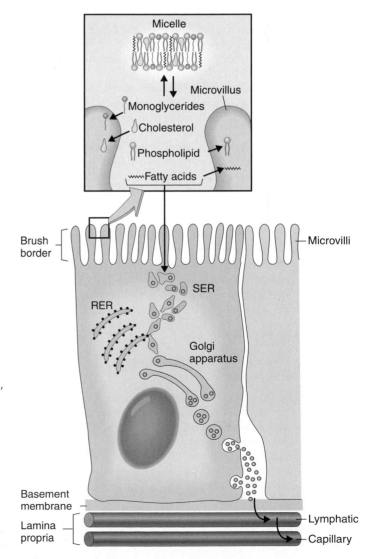

Figure 7-12 Absorption of lipids into the enterocytes. Micelles are broken down into monoglycerides, fatty acids, phospholipids, and cholesterol, each of which enters into the cytoplasm across the cell membrane on the brush border. These lipids are reconstituted in the smooth endoplasmic reticulum (SER) and linked to apoproteins synthesized in the rough endoplasmic reticulum (RER). All components are assembled into chylomicrons in the Golgi apparatus, from which they are secreted along the basolateral side of the cell. Chylomicrons enter the lymphatics for further transportation. (Modified from Sleisinger MH, Fordtran JS [eds]: Gastrointestinal Diseases, 5th ed.Philadelphia, Saunders, 1993.)

chylomicrons coalesce and enter into the lacteals and further into the lymphatic circulation. Most of the lipid is absorbed in the duodenum, and all the lipid is removed from the intestinal lumen by the time the chyme has reached the midjejunum. No lipid remains unabsorbed in the intestine in healthy persons.

Salts and water. The normal GI tract of an adult person contains approximately 7 L of fluid, which is replenished daily by 2 L of fluid in drinks and food. All 9 L of fluid is absorbed, and the feces contain only about 100 mL of water per day. Most of the GI luminal water is absorbed in the small intestine, which takes up 8.5 L per day, and the remaining 400 mL is absorbed in the colon.

Water is absorbed in the entire small intestine except in the duodenum, which actually receives more water than it absorbs. The absorption of water follows the flux of **sodium,** which is actively absorbed and transported across the cell cytoplasm into the intercellular spaces. The absorption of sodium is enhanced by glucose and neutral amino acids that cross the brush border membrane on the same carriers as Na^+. A Na^+, K^+-ATP-ase in the basolateral membranes extrudes the sodium as it enters the luminal side along a concentration gradient.

Potassium is absorbed passively together with the water in the small intestine. In the colon K^+ may be either absorbed or secreted. Secretion usually predominates.

Bicarbonate (HCO_3^-) is part of the pancreatic secretion and is secreted in large amounts into the duodenum. Most of it, however, is absorbed by the time the chyme reaches the end of the jejunum. Chloride is also absorbed in the jejunum, but not as completely. In the ileum chloride (Cl^-) is absorbed but HCO_3^- is secreted. The same happens in the colon.

Calcium (Ca^{2+}) is absorbed actively in all parts of the intestines. Intestinal absorption of Ca^{2+} depends on the solubility of the calcium salts—acidity of the gastric contents makes many of the insoluble calcium salts soluble. In the intestines the uptake of Ca^{2+} is regulated by vitamin D and parathyroid hormone, which promote Ca^{2+} absorption.

In the large intestine the intestinal contents are transformed into feces.

Most of the fluid has been removed from the chyme by the time it reaches the ileocecal valve. During the passage through the colon, an additional 400 mL of water is removed, and the contents are solidified into feces.

The intestinal contents are moved by contractions of the large intestine, which forms smooth muscle bands called haustra. Haustration is aided by peristalsis, which includes much slower movements, and periodic mass movements that occur three to four times a day and transport large amounts of fecal material into the rectum.

The waste products and residues of undigested food are eliminated from the rectum by defecation.

Under normal circumstances the rectum does not contain feces because a weak functional sphincter about 20 cm from the anus prevents the intestinal contents from filling the rectum. Also the rectum is at an angle with the sigmoid colon, which also prevents rectal filling. When the feces enter the rectum because of mass movement of the colon, the dilatation of the upper rectum initiates the **defecation reflex** (Fig. 7-13). The internal rectal sphincter is stimulated to relax, allowing fecal material to fill the anorectum. As soon as the anorectum fills over 25% of its capacity, an urge to defecate is felt. The smooth muscle in the wall of the intestine contracts, pushing the feces toward the lower anal sphincter.

The lower anal sphincter is under voluntary control and could be relaxed at will, allowing defecation to occur. Defecation can be voluntarily initiated by the relaxation of the external sphincter, at which time the rectum

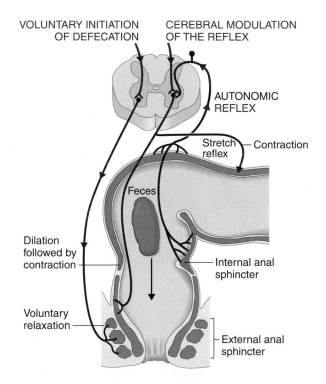

Figure 7-13 Defecation reflex. This reflex begins with the entry of the feces into the rectum. The dilatation of the rectum stimulates the sensory nerves, which transmit the impulses to the spinal cord and activate motor neurons, initially causing dilatation of the rectum and then relaxing the internal anal sphincter. After the rectum is filled the muscles in its walls contract, and the person feels the urge to defecate. Defecation occurs if the external sphincter is relaxed voluntarily. If the sphincter is not relaxed the feces remains in the rectum, but the inner anal sphincter contracts to prevent further filling.

contracts, expelling the fecal material through the anus. The pressure on the rectum can be increased by a Valsalva maneuver—closing the glottis and trying to forcefully expel the air from the lungs by mobilizing the thoracic respiratory muscles and the diaphragm. Feces can also remain in the rectum and anus, and if defecation does not occur, the upper anal sphincter will close to prevent overfilling of the anus by feces.

Clinical and Laboratory Evaluation of Gastrointestinal Diseases

FAMILY AND PERSONAL HISTORY

Family and personal history can point to some important risk factors that play a role in the pathogenesis of GI diseases. A few examples of such links and associations are given in Table 7-2.

PHYSICAL EXAMINATION

Symptoms and signs of GI diseases depend on the type of disease and on the location of the lesions, which may involve any part of the GI tract, from the mouth to the anus, and may include lesions in the head and neck area, the thoracic cage, or in the abdominal cavity. The most important signs and symptoms are as follows:

- Pain
- Dysphagia
- Dyspepsia
- Nausea and vomiting
- Anorexia and weight loss
- Constipation
- Diarrhea
- Gastrointestinal bleeding
- Ileus

Pain is a common manifestation of gastrointestinal diseases.

Gastrointestinal diseases may manifest with pain, which may be acute or chronic, mild or severe. The perception of pain varies from one patient to another, and patients tend to describe it in a number of ways. In general terms GI pain can be classified as being felt in the chest, back, or abdomen.

Chest pain. This type of pain of GI origin is usually related to esophageal diseases. It may manifest in several forms as follows:

- **Heartburn.** This substernal pain manifests as substernal burning radiating into the neck or the epigastrium. It begins after meals or after lying down and may be precipitated by efforts that increase intra-abdominal pressure, such as straining at defecation or bending. It is caused by acid reflux in GERD and may be relieved by antacids.
- **Odynophagia.** This form of chest pain during swallowing is related to esophageal disorders. It is described as a dull burning sensation, a feeling of substernal tightness, or a sharp pain that occurs on swallowing solids or liquids. A common cause of odynophagia is so-called esophageal pill ulcers, shallow mucosal defects caused by a variety of drugs, including nonsteroidal anti-inflammatory drugs and antibiotics. Odynophagia manifesting as squeezing chest pain after ingestion of cold or hot drinks that the patient has trouble swallowing is a feature of esophageal motor disorders.
- **Sharp chest pain.** This sharp pain of sudden onset, also known as "noncardiac chest pain," may be confused with coronary heart disease. The exact diagnosis may be suggested by coexistence of gastroesophageal reflux disease (GERD) or dysphagia, but often one must first exclude other diseases or perform complex esophageal testing to identify the true cause of the pain.

Table 7-2 Risk Factors for Gastrointestinal Diseases

TYPE OF RISK FACTOR	SPECIFIC DISEASES–RISK FACTOR ASSOCIATIONS
Hereditary factors	Inflammatory bowel disease
	Familial polyposis coli
	HNPCC
Social/nutritional factors	Alcoholism and gastritis
	GERD and obesity
Other GI or systemic diseases	Peptic ulcer rupture and peritonitis
Travel to tropics	Amebic colitis
	Worm infestation
Medical and surgical procedures	Dumping syndrome and gastric resection
	Short bowel syndrome and malabsorption
	Radiation therapy for cancer and stenosis
Drugs	Broad-spectrum antibiotics and pseudomembranous colitis
External mechanical factors	Trauma to the abdomen and peritonitis

GERD, gastroesophageal reflux disease; GI, gastrointestinal; HNPCC, hereditary nonpolyposis colorectal carcinoma.

Abdominal pain. Mild abdominal pain or discomfort is very common, but severe abdominal pain is usually a sign of an intra-abdominal disease. It is important to remember that not all instances of abdominal pain are caused by GI diseases. In some cases the abdominal pain is referred from extra-abdominal sites or may be a manifestation of systemic metabolic and neurologic diseases. The most important causes of abdominal pain of GI origin are listed in Table 7-3.

A complete history and physical examination will provide good guidance for further studies and even surgical intervention, which might be performed for all cases of so-called surgical abdomen. Typically the clinician must ask questions about the onset, duration, location, and spread of the pain and ask the patient to describe it or point out the most sensitive site. Laboratory and radiologic studies are usually helpful.

Dysphagia is a sign of esophageal obstruction or abnormal esophageal motility.

Dysphagia is difficulty in swallowing, which may be related to functional disorders or obstructive pathologic changes in the esophagus and oropharynx (Fig. 7-14).

Functional disorders causing dysphagia may be classified into two groups as follows:

- **Pre-esophageal dysphagia.** The cause of dysphagia lies outside of the oropharynx and esophagus. Swallowing difficulties may be related to various neurologic diseases (e.g., Parkinson's disease) or systemic muscular or autoimmune diseases (e.g., dermatomyositis, myasthenia gravis, or systemic sclerosis).
- **Esophageal motility disorders.** The most common motility disorders are esophageal spasms, which may be localized or diffuse. A less common cause of dysphagia is achalasia of the esophagus, which is caused by spasms

Table 7-3 Common Causes of Abdominal Pain Related to Gastrointestinal Disorders

ORGAN	PATHOLOGIC CONDITION
Esophagus	Perforation
	Spontaneous due to severe vomiting
	Related to diagnostic or therapeutic procedures
Stomach	Peptic ulcer
	Acute gastritis
	Gastric cancer
Duodenum	Peptic ulcer
Small intestine	Enteritis
	Obstruction or torsion or herniation
Appendix	Acute appendicitis
Large intestine	Obstruction, torsion
	Fecal impaction
	Perforation
	Inflammatory bowel disease
	Irritable bowel syndrome
	Cancer
	Diverticulitis

of the distal esophageal sphincter and dilatation of the proximal part.

Obstructive pathologic changes may be intrinsic or extrinsic.

- **Intrinsic obstructions** of the esophagus may be caused by esophageal rings and webs, chronic inflammation related to GERD or hiatal hernia, and esophageal cancer.

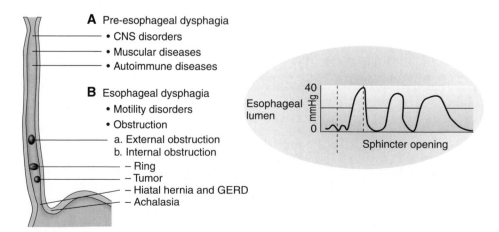

A Pre-esophageal dysphagia
- CNS disorders
- Muscular diseases
- Autoimmune diseases

B Esophageal dysphagia
- Motility disorders
- Obstruction
  - a. External obstruction
  - b. Internal obstruction
    - – Ring
    - – Tumor
    - – Hiatal hernia and GERD
    - – Achalasia

Esophageal lumen

40 mmHg 0

Sphincter opening

Figure 7-14 Dysphagia. Difficulties in swallowing may be classified as pre-esophageal or esophageal. Esophageal dysphagia may be related to functional motility disorders or external and internal obstructions. Functional motility disorders lead to a loss of normal esophageal peristalsis, which is presented graphically on the right side of the illustration. CNS, central nervous system; GERD, gastroesophageal reflux disease.

■ **Extrinsic obstruction** may be caused by mediastinal or pulmonary tumors or periesophageal fibrosis.

Obstructive dysphagia usually manifests with difficulty swallowing solid food, whereas motility disorders equally affect the swallowing of solids and liquids. Esophagoscopy is usually a reliable way of establishing diagnosis, but in some cases additional manometric measurements must be performed.

Dyspepsia is a term used to describe nonspecific upper abdominal symptoms.

Dyspepsia, a synonym for indigestion, is a noncommittal term used to describe a group of symptoms related to feeding. These include bloating, fullness, heartburn, epigastric discomfort or pain, and mild nausea. In some cases it is a manifestation of pathologic changes such as peptic ulcer, esophagitis, GERD, hiatal hernia, gastritis, or duodenitis. In many other cases the real cause of symptoms is never established, and the patient is told that he or she has **functional dyspepsia** or non-nulcear dyspepsia. These patients need only reassurance from the doctor, who also may prescribe antacids for symptomatic relief.

Dyspepsia related to *H. pylori* gastritis or peptic ulcer and other diseases must be treated medically.

Nausea and vomiting are common manifestations of gastrointestinal diseases but may have other causes as well.

Nausea, a term derived from the Greek word for seasickness, is an unpleasant feeling that one will need to vomit. Vomiting is a forceful expulsion of gastric contents via the mouth. It results from coordinated contraction of abdominal and thoracic muscles and the stomach, and relaxation of the upper esophageal sphincter coordinated by a vomiting center in the medulla oblongata (Fig. 7-15). Vomiting can be initiated by a number of stimuli, such as tickling of the back of throat. Dilatation and irritation of the stomach and duodenum are strong stimuli that can initiate vomiting. Gastrointestinal obstruction is typically associated with vomiting. Peritoneal irritation is yet another common cause. It is important to remember that nausea and vomiting are common symptoms of CNS diseases and that they also occur as a complication of medication, especially in patients being treated for cancer. The most important causes of nausea and vomiting are listed in the Table 7-4.

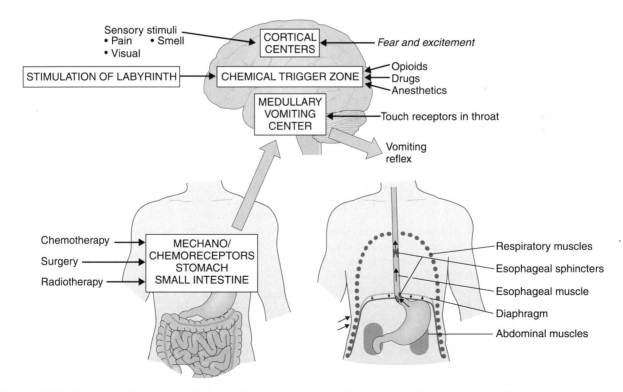

Figure 7-15 Vomiting reflex. It may be evoked by numerous stimuli as indicated in the drawing. The main anatomic/functional parts of the vomiting reflex are included in the boxes. The efferent nerve impulses stemming from the vomiting center are transmitted to the esophagus and effector muscles (respiratory muscles, diaphragm, and abdominal muscles). The contraction of these muscles combined with the relaxation of esophageal sphincters leads to the expulsion of gastric contents through the mouth.

Table 7-4 Causes of Acute Nausea and Vomiting

Gastrointestinal Inflammation
Acute chemical gastritis (e.g., alcohol abuse)
Food poisoning (bacterial toxins)
Viral gastroenteritis

Gastrointestinal Obstruction
Pyloric stenosis
Intestinal obstruction due to tumors, intussusception, volvulus
Paralytic ileus

Peritoneal Irritation
Peritonitis, localized (e.g., with appendicitis, cholecystitis)
Peritonitis, diffuse due to infection or rupture of viscera
Peritonitis, chemical (e.g., acute pancreatitis)
Mesenteric infarction

Central Nervous System and Inner Ear Diseases
Motion sickness and Ménière's disease
Migraine headaches
Meningitis and encephalitis
CNS tumors

Systemic and Metabolic Conditions and Disorders
Pregnancy
Myocardial infarction
Diabetic ketoacidosis
Renal failure

Drugs
Chemotherapy for cancer
Psychopharmaceuticals
Digoxin

Anorexia is a loss of appetite that may lead to weight loss.

Under normal circumstances body weight reflects a balance between the intake and expenditure of calories. Food intake is voluntary but is influenced by appetite, and if appetite is lost the expenditure of calories exceeds intake and the body loses weight.

Appetite and food intake are regulated by specific brain centers known as the satiety center and the hunger center. Stimulation of the satiety center decreases appetite, and the stimulation of the hunger center causes hyperphagia. Under normal circumstances these two centers are regulated by multiple neurotransmitters, which fall into two categories: **anorexigenic** substances that suppress appetite and **orexigenic** substances that stimulate feeding. The most important anorexigenic substances are corticotropin-releasing factor, glucagon-like polypeptide I, and α-melanocyte-stimulating hormone.

Many patients who have cancer of the GI tract as well as other organs develop anorexia and subsequently lose weight. The mechanism of this anorexia is not fully understood, but it is thought that peripheral stimuli either directly act on the endogenous anorexigenic factors or directly act on the CNS feeding centers. It is also possible that substances released from cancers act on the fat cells that produce **leptin,** a potent stimulator of anorexigenic factor release in the hypothalamus.

Constipation is a condition characterized by infrequent or incomplete passage of stools.

Acute constipation is reported by patients as a sudden change in bowel habits resulting in an inability to defecate. Chronic constipation is more difficult to define because it is based on the patient's perception of what is the normal pattern of defecation, and whether the feces is of normal consistency and completely evacuated during defecation. In Western countries most adults pass 3 to 12 stools per week, and thus for practical purposes it seems best to consider those who have fewer than 3 bowel movements per week as being constipated.

Acute constipation usually results from an organic cause and should be investigated until the cause is found. For example, it may result from colonic carcinoma obstructing the lumen, diverticulitis causing pericolonic fibrosis that constricts the colon, or paralytic ileus due to peritonitis.

Chronic constipation may have the same causes as acute constipation (Table 7-5). It can also develop in chronically debilitated persons, in long-lasting metabolic disorders, such as hypothyroidism, or in people who eat very little. Chronic immobility and being bedridden also cause constipation. Certain neurologic disorders, such as spinal cord injury, and some drugs, such as antidepressants

Table 7-5 Causes of Chronic Constipation

Lifestyle-related
  Sedentary lifestyle
  Immobility and lack of exercise
  Chronic hospitalization/hospice/nursing home care
Diet-related
  Low-fiber diet
  Low food intake
Chronic diseases
  Debilitating chronic diseases
  Hypothyroidism
  Diabetes mellitus
  Chronic renal failure
Neurologic and psychiatric disorders
  Spinal cord injury
  Multiple sclerosis
  Parkinson's disease
  Depression
  Dementia
Drugs
  Psychopharmaceuticals
  Calcium channel blockers
  Opiates
Obstructive lesions of colon
  Diverticulitis
  Carcinoma
  Ischemic bowel disease
Idiopathic

and anti-Parkinsonism drugs, also cause constipation. However, in most instances the cause of chronic constipation is unknown and the constipation is called idiopathic or attributed to "colonic inertia" or "pelvic floor dysfunction." Changing diet, by adding fiber to the food, or treatment with laxatives may help, but a prudent clinician always ensures that an obstructive cause of chronic constipation, such a chronic diverticulitis, has not been overlooked.

Acute diarrhea is usually caused by infection.

Diarrhea is an increased frequency of stools, usually accompanied by increased volume and decreased consistency of feces. In Western countries this means several bowel movements per day and with a weight exceeding the normal 300 g/day. The stool is softer and contains more water.

Diarrhea that lasts less than 3 to 4 weeks is called acute; if it lasts more than a month it is called chronic.

Acute diarrhea is usually caused by infection, but occasionally it is related to drugs, acute intestinal ischemia, or radiation. For practical purposes it is useful to divide acute diarrhea into two groups: noninflammatory and inflammatory.

■ **Noninflammatory acute diarrhea** manifests without fever or other signs of inflammation, and the feces do not contain leukocytes. It is most often caused by viral infection (Norwalk virus and rota virus), food poisoning with preformed enterotoxin from *Staphylococcus aureus* or *Bacillus cereus*, or enterotoxigenic *Escherichia coli* infection. *Vibrio choleae* and *Giardia intestinalis* are important causes in some parts of the world.

■ **Inflammatory diarrhea** is characterized by fever, leukocytosis, and the presence of leukocytes and even grossly visible blood in feces ("dysentery"). It is most often caused by cytotoxin-producing *E. coli* or *Clostridium difficile*, which typically causes pseudomembranous colitis. Bacteria known to invade the GI mucosa, such as *Shigella* sp., *Salmonella* sp., *Yersinia enterocolitica,* and protozoa such as *Entamoeba histolytica* are also well-known causes. Bacterial proctitis caused by *Neisseria gonorrhoeae* during genitoanal intercourse may also manifest with inflammatory diarrhea.

Pearl

> Crohn's disease (CD) and ulcerative colitis (UC) are chronic diseases. However, they usually begin as acute diarrhea and should always be included in the differential diagnosis of infectious acute inflammatory diarrheas.

Chronic diarrhea could develop due to several pathogenetic mechanisms.

Chronic diarrhea may develop from changes in the small or large intestine. Diarrhea develops if the intestines contain more fluid than can be absorbed or if the absorptive capacity of the intestines is reduced because of some intestinal disease or because the contents move too fast through the intestines (Fig. 7-16). From the pathogenetic point of view it can be subdivided into five major groups: (1) osmotic

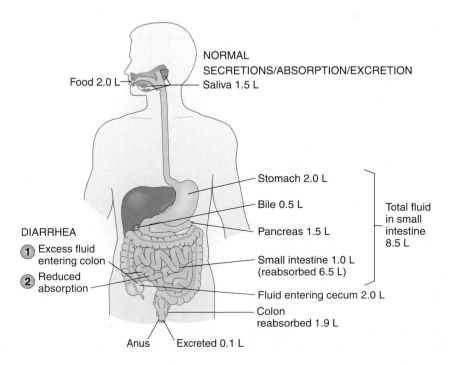

Figure 7-16 Normal intake, absorption, secretion, and excretion of water compared with usage of water in diarrhea.

NORMAL
SECRETIONS/ABSORPTION/EXCRETION

Food 2.0 L
Saliva 1.5 L

Stomach 2.0 L
Bile 0.5 L
Pancreas 1.5 L
Small intestine 1.0 L (reabsorbed 6.5 L)

Total fluid in small intestine 8.5 L

DIARRHEA
1 Excess fluid entering colon
2 Reduced absorption

Fluid entering cecum 2.0 L
Colon reabsorbed 1.9 L

Anus   Excreted 0.1 L

Table 7-6 Pathogenesis of Chronic Diarrhea

Osmotic Diarrhea
Lactose intolerance
Abuse of laxatives

Malabsorption Syndrome
Small-intestine diseases (celiac sprue, Whipple's
    disease, etc.)
Chronic pancreatitis
Bacterial overgrowth

Secretory Diarrhea
Drug-related
Polypeptide hormone tumors
Bile salt malabsorption due to ileal disease

Inflammatory Diarrhea
Inflammatory bowel disease
Radiation enteritis

Motility Disorders
Irritable bowel syndrome
Hyperthyroidism
Postvagotomy states

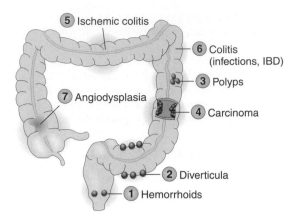

Figure 7-18 Causes of lower gastrointestinal bleeding (hematochezia) numbered in order of decreasing frequency. IBD, inflammatory bowel disease.

diarrhea, (2) diarrhea due to malabsorption syndromes, (3) secretory diarrhea, (4) inflammatory diarrhea, and (5) diarrhea due to motility disorders (Table 7-6).

Blood from gastrointestinal bleeding may be vomited, it may appear in the stool, or it may remain undetected (occult).

The signs and symptoms of GI hemorrhage depend on its location, onset (i.e., acute or chronic), duration, and amount of blood loss. Massive upper GI hemorrhage manifests with **hematemesis.** Bleeding from the rectum is called **hematochezia.** In 75% of cases it is of colonic origin.

Bleeding from the upper GI tract during which the blood is transformed by HCl to the black pigment hematein results in tarry black stools typical of **melena.** Approximately 50 to 100 mL of blood is required to cause melena. Chronic loss of small amounts of blood from bleeding peptic ulcer, cancer, or angiodysplasia of the intestines often remains undetected and manifests with **hypochromic microcytic iron deficiency anemia.** The most common causes of upper GI bleeding are shown in the Figure 7-17. The most common causes of lower GI bleeding are listed in Figure 7-18.

Ileus, a failure of propulsion of intestinal contents, may be adynamic or obstructive.

When the intestinal contents are not propelled caudally, the cause may be either a lack of bowel movement or a mechanical obstruction.

- **Adynamic ("paralytic") ileus** is most often seen in the postoperative period and is related to surgical handling of the intestines. It is of a transitory nature, and in most cases the intestines regain their normal motility within 2 or 3 days. The onset of normal bowel movements can be ascertained by auscultation: during the paralytic period the intestines do not move, and no abdominal sounds are heard. Other important causes include peritonitis and intestinal ischemia.
- Obstructive ileus can be caused by a variety of intrinsic and extrinsic factors that prevent the normal passage of the intestinal contents. The intrinsic factors include tumors, foreign bodies, impacted feces, CD, and malrotation of the intestine around its own mesentery (volvulus) or intussusception of one intestinal loop into another. External factors include compressions or strangulation of intestinal loops by the neck of a hernia sac, chronic peritonitis, postinflammatory or postsurgical connective tissue adhesions, or metastatic tumors.

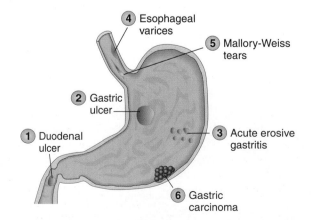

Figure 7-17 Causes of upper gastrointestinal bleeding numbered in order of descending frequency.

LABORATORY TESTS AND SPECIAL DIAGNOSTIC PROCEDURES

Most of the laboratory tests used in the diagnosis of GI disorders actually do not pertain to the GI tract itself but measure the effects of GI diseases on other organ systems. For example, chronic occult blood loss due to a bleeding peptic ulcer causes iron deficiency anemia. Malabsorption of vitamin B_{12} due to atrophic gastritis and a lack of intrinsic factor causes megaloblastic anemia, and vitamin D deficiency in malabsorption associated with steatorrhea causes osteomalacia.

Many of the previously used tests of GI function are not performed today. For example, analysis of gastric juice is rarely performed today. Certain functional tests are performed only for research purposes and in select highly specialized centers. Here we mention only a few tests that are directly relevant for the diagnosis of GI disorders.

Testing for occult blood in stool is used to screen for possible colon cancer in asymptomatic persons.

The test is based on the use guaiac-impregnated cards (e.g., "hemoccult card"). This test detects blood in stool in excess of 20 mL/day and does not react with the small amounts of blood normally present in the feces (<2mL/day). Even though it has a sensitivity of only 20% to 30% for colorectal cancer, it is widely used because no better screening tests are available.

Steatorrhea can be documented by finding fat in stool.

Fecal material is smeared on a microscope slide and stained with a fat-detecting stain such as Sudan O. The amount of fat can be also biochemically quantitated.

Microscopic examination of feces can distinguish inflammatory from noninflammatory diarrhea.

Normal feces do not contain neutrophils, and if these acute inflammatory cells are found in a patient who has diarrhea the finding is significant. The test is typically positive in colitis caused by invasive bacteria, in inflammatory bowel disease, and in pseudomembranous colitis.

Microscopic examination of the peritoneal fluid can be useful for finding the cause of peritonitis or ascites.

Microscopic examination of the peritoneal fluid may reveal leukocytes in bacterial peritonitis or malignant cells that have seeded the peritoneum and caused malignant ascites.

Gastrointestinal biopsy is a reliable and widely used test for diagnosing many gastrointestinal diseases.

Most parts of the GI tract are readily accessible to biopsy during endoscopic procedures. The only exception is the small intestine. Biopsy from the duodenum and the terminal ileum is possible, however, and specimens from these procedures are usually adequate for evaluating most small-intestine diseases.

Endoscopy and radiologic techniques are widely used to evaluate the gastrointestinal tract.

Upper GI tact endoscopy is widely used to evaluate diseases of the esophagus, stomach, and duodenum. Endoscopy has almost completely replaced radiologic techniques based on the use of barium contrast material. Likewise lower GI endoscopy, used for the evaluation of the colon and terminal ileum, is currently the most widely used method for the evaluation of this part of the GI system. Barium enema is still used for diagnosing some small-intestine diseases and for conditions like enteroenteric fistulas, which are better visualized that way than by other means. Computer tomographic imaging is widely used in clinics and has become one of the most useful techniques in gastroenterology.

Clinicopathologic Correlations

GASTROESOPHAGEAL REFLUX DISEASE

A very common disease affecting millions worldwide, gastroesophageal reflux disease (GERD) is a disease caused by increased reflux of gastric contents into the esophagus.

Gastroesophageal reflux disease is a multifactorial disorder resulting from the interaction of gastric juices and esophageal mucosa.

The exact pathogenesis of GERD is not fully understood and the condition is thought to be multifactorial. Among the many contributing factors, the following five play a critical role (Fig. 7-19):

- Abnormal tone and relaxation of the lower esophageal sphincter (LES)
- Chemical composition of the regurgitated gastric contents
- Integrity of the esophageal mucosal barrier
- Mechanical factors, such as increased intra-abdominal pressure or coexistent hiatal hernia
- Irritants in the food (e.g., pepper, hot sauces), alcohol, smoking

Under normal circumstance the LES serves as a barrier preventing the reflux of gastric contents into the esophagus. Only small amounts of the gastric contents escape back into the esophagus. In patients with GERD the LES tone is lower than normal and periodic relaxation periods last longer. The opening and closing of the sphincter are not coordinated with the contractions of the rest of the esophagus and the stomach. Certain substances in the food may cause even more relaxation and, if abused (e.g., ethanol), may contribute to LES dysfunction.

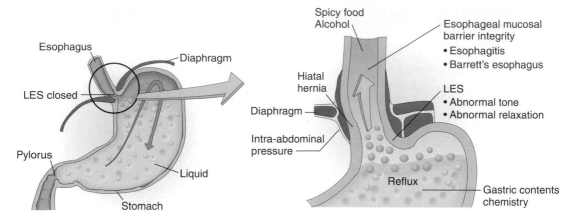

Figure 7-19 The causes of gastroesophageal reflux. The disorder is multifactorial and in many instances more than one causal factor is present. LES, lower esophageal sphincter.

The composition of the gastric juice also plays a role in the pathogenesis of GERD. As in other upper GI diseases it is the balance between the adverse effects of hydrochloric acid and pepsin and the ability of the mucosae to resist their action that determines whether pathologic changes occur, hence the importance of the integrity of the esophageal mucosa and its ability to resist peptic digestion. Certain foods or drugs may reduce this resistance or increase the mordant effect of the regurgitated gastric contents. Likewise, increased intra-abdominal pressure, caused by obesity or pregnancy, among other factors, may contribute to more pronounced reflux. Recumbent position, especially after a heavy meal, may also facilitate reflux. A hiatal hernia is present in a significant number of patients with GERD and probably plays a pathogenetic role.

Histopathologic changes in the esophagus in gastroesophageal reflux disease vary from mild to severe.

Symptomatic reflux of gastric juice may be associated with only minor histopathologic changes, but also with quite prominent chronic esophagitis. Chronic inflammation may lead to metaplasia of squamous into columnar intestinal-type epithelium, a condition known as Barrett's esophagus. Mucosae of Barrett's esophagus may become atypical and ultimately give rise to adenocarcinoma. Fibrosis caused by chronic inflammation may lead to stenosis of the esophagus.

Heartburn is the principal symptom of gastroesophageal reflux disease.

The most prominent symptom of GERD is heartburn (pyrosis), which is occasionally associated with regurgitation of the gastric contents into the mouth. The symptoms often follow heavy meals or lying down. Less commonly the gastric contents may be aspirated into the larynx causing hoarseness, and even into the lungs causing cough, asthma-like attacks, or pneumonia. In a minority of cases chronic bleeding is present and may be associated with melena or iron deficiency anemia.

The diagnosis is made on the basis of clinical data, but can be confirmed by endoscopy and esophageal biopsy. Manometric studies of esophageal motility and LES may be indicated in some patients who are resistant to therapy or those who have developed serious complications, such as long-segment Barrett's esophagus and stenosis.

PEPTIC ULCER DISEASE

Peptic ulcer is a deep defect of the mucosa related to the action of hydrochloric acid and pepsin in the gastric juice. In contrast to the superficial defects of the mucosa, ulcers extend to the muscularis mucosae or deeper into the muscularis propria of the gastric wall. Peptic ulcers are common, and it has been estimated that up to 10% of all Americans have had a peptic ulcer sometime during their life. Ulcers are most often located in the duodenum, less often in the stomach, and even less often in other sites such as the esophagus or jejunum. Most peptic ulcers are solitary lesions, but they may be multiple.

Peptic ulcers result when the mordant effects of the gastric juice surpass the protective mechanisms of the gastric mucosae.

The normal gastric mucosa is resistant to the effects of the digestive juices containing hydrochloric acid and pepsin. The mucosal barrier is maintained by normal blood flow, secretion of protective mucus, and bicarbonate that coats the surface of the mucosa. Peptic ulcers result when the mordant effect of gastric juice is increased or more often when the mucosal defense mechanisms are diminished (Fig. 7-20). The following factors play an important pathogenetic role:

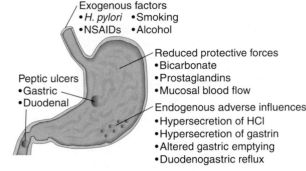

Figure 7-20 Peptic ulcer. Gastric ulcer occurs most often on the smaller curvature of the stomach. The duodenal ulcer occurs most often in the proximal duodenum. The pathogenesis of peptic ulcers is complex and includes the action of some exogenous and some endogenous adverse influences and a reduced action of protective factors. NSAIDs, nonsteroidal anti-inflammatory drugs.

- **Reduced production of bicarbonate.** The surface of the gastric mucosa has a pH close to neutral (pH 7), which is maintained by the constant buffering action of bicarbonate, which is secreted by mucosal cells. Bicarbonate is also found on the surface of the duodenal epithelium, where it protects the cells from the gastric juice permeating the chyme that enters the duodenum from the stomach. In patients with peptic ulcer bicarbonate production is reduced.
- **Reduced production of prostaglandins.** Prostaglandins have an important protective role by stimulating mucus production, maintaining the normal blood flow though the mucosa, and reducing the acid secretion. Cyclooxigenase inhibitors, such as aspirin and NSAIDs, reduce the prostaglandin production and predispose to mucosal ulceration.
- **Increased acid production.** Gastrin is a potent stimulant for gastric acid production, and excessive secretion of gastrin by neuroendocrine tumors in the Zollinger-Ellison syndrome is associated with an increased incidence of peptic ulcers. Hyperacidity of gastric contents is, however, not a prerequisite for peptic ulcer formation.
- ***Helicobacter pylori* infection.** During the last 15 years it has been conclusively shown that *H. pylori* infection plays a crucial role in the pathogenesis of peptic ulcer. *Helicobacter pylori* is found in 70% of patients with a gastric ulcer and almost 100% those with a duodenal ulcer. The bacterium is resistant to the effects of HCl and survives readily in the surface mucus of the antral mucosa. It has a complex effect on the mucosa by lowering the resistance to peptic digestion and by increasing acid production. For example, even though it does not invade the tissue it causes tissue necrosis and inflammation of the mucosa. At the same time *H. pylori*

inhibits duodenal bicarbonate secretion and stimulates gastric acid production. Nevertheless, it is not fully understood why only 10% to 20% of those infected with *H. pylori* develop peptic ulcers.

Epigastric pain is the most consistent symptom of peptic ulcer.

Duodenal ulcers, which are four times more common than gastric ulcers, typically manifest with epigastric pain that occurs 1 to 3 hours after eating. The pain is worse during the night and may even awaken the patient. It may respond to antacids in many cases. The pain related to gastric ulcer has a less characteristic pattern and may even be induced by feeding. It is also persistent. Nausea and vomiting are more common with gastric than duodenal ulcers. However, these distinctions are not consistent enough to allow clinical diagnosis with certainty. Final diagnosis is made by endoscopy. Biopsy of tissue during endoscopy is useful for demonstrating *H. pylori* and for excluding carcinoma in large gastric lesions. Treatment includes antibiotics to eradicate *H. pylori*, H₂ blockers, and proton pump inhibitors. Some ulcers recur after treatment. The most common cause for these recurrences is incomplete eradication of *H. pylori*.

Bleeding is the most common complication of peptic ulcer disease.

The most important complications of peptic ulcer disease are as follows (Fig. 7-21):

- **Bleeding.** Most peptic ulcers bleed, but most often the blood loss is relatively modest. *Chronic bleeding* may, however, cause iron deficiency anemia. In some cases *massive bleeding* occurs and results in hematemesis. Blood digested by hydrochloric acid becomes black due to the formation of hemoglobin-derived black pigment (hematein). It stains the feces black *(melena)*.

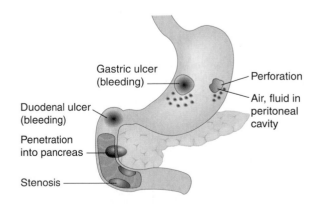

Figure 7-21 Complications of peptic ulcer. The most important complications are bleeding, perforation, stenosis, and penetration into the pancreas.

- **Perforation.** Deep ulcers may penetrate through the entire gastric wall. Gastric contents may enter into the peritoneal cavity and cause peritonitis. Air that has escaped into the peritoneal cavity may be visible radiographically as a subdiaphragmatic lucency.
- **Penetration.** Deep ulcers may penetrate through the wall into the adjacent solid organs. Most often this occurs in duodenal ulcers penetrating into the pancreas. This change is associated with pancreatic inflammation and an increased level of amylase and lipase in the blood.
- **Stenosis.** Fibrosis that develops in the wall of the pyloric channel or the duodenum may cause stenosis with considerable narrowing of the lumen. It is typically associated with gastric food retention and vomiting.

MALABSORPTION SYNDROMES

Malabsorption is a syndrome characterized by incomplete or defective absorption of nutrients, minerals, and water in the small intestine. The diseases that cause malabsorption can affect the stomach, the pancreas, the hepatobiliary system, or the small intestine (Fig. 7-22). The most important of these diseases are the following:

- Infections (e.g., tropical sprue, Whipple's disease, bacterial overgrowth)
- Autoimmune diseases (e.g., celiac disease)
- Enzyme deficiency (e.g., lactose deficiency)
- Defective function of the pancreas
- Tumors (e.g., lymphoma, neuroendocrine cell tumors, such as VIPoma)
- Surgical resection of parts of the GI tract

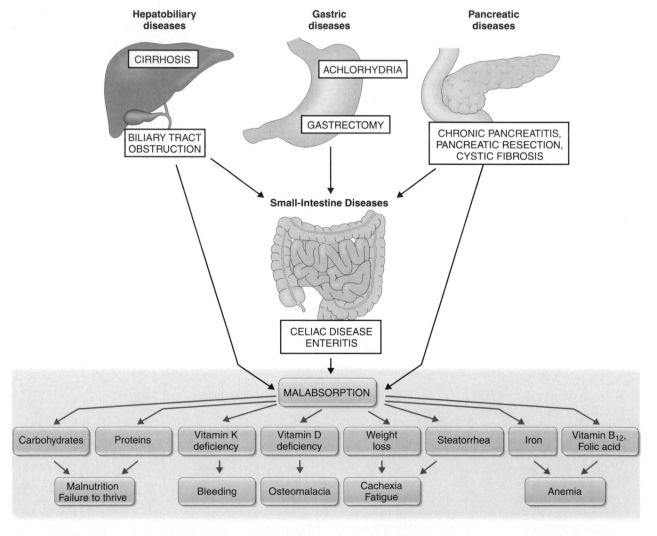

Figure 7-22 Malabsorption syndrome. It may develop due to several diseases involving the stomach, the pancreas, the hepatobiliary system, or the intestines.

Malabsorption results from defects of food digestion or absorption of nutrients and their transport into the circulation.

Digestion in the small intestine takes place inside the lumen and on the surface of enterocytes. The nutrients are then taken up into the enterocytes and transported to the interface between the enterocytes and the lymphatic or blood vessels, where they enter circulation. Defects accounting for malabsorption can thus be found in the following portions of the digestive process (Fig. 7-23):

- **Intraluminal digestion.** Since most of the enzymes filling the lumen of the intestine are derived from the pancreas, defective intraluminal digestion is most often seen in chronic pancreatic insufficiency.
- **Membrane-associated digestion on enterocytes.** This defect is seen typically in lactase deficiency. Lactase is associated with the luminal cell membrane of the enterocytes, and without it lactose cannot be absorbed.

- **Transmembrane transport.** Transport of nutrients depends on the proper functioning of the transport mechanism. Some patients demonstrate a genetic deficiency of some of these transport proteins. In abetalipoproteinemia, a genetic defect in the synthesis of beta apolipoprotein B, lipids are not properly absorbed because chylomicrons cannot be formed.
- **Obstruction of the transport from enterocytes to the circulation.** The interface between the enterocytes and the lymphatic and blood vessels may be obstructed by the imposition of abnormal proteins in amyloidosis or collagen in scleroderma.

Symptoms of malabsorption result from diarrhea and the deficiency of proteins, lipids, carbohydrates, vitamins, and minerals.

Incomplete absorption of nutrients, minerals, and water in the small intestine results in diarrhea and steatorrhea (fat-rich stools). Protein calorie deficiency causes stunted growth in childhood and weight loss in adults. Muscles may be weak and appear wasted. Hypoalbuminemia may cause

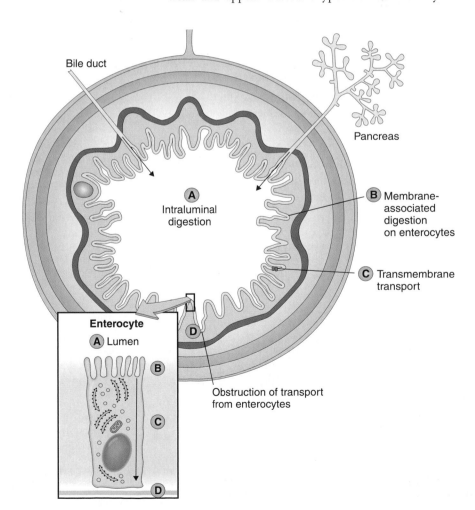

Figure 7-23 Malabsorption syndrome. Malabsorption may develop due to several defects: Deficient intraluminal digestion (A), inadequate digestion on the luminal cell membrane of the enterocytes (B), transcellular transport in the enterocytes (C), or blocked passage of nutrients from the enterocytes to the lymphatics (D).

generalized edema. Deficiency of iron and vitamin B_{12} results in anemia. Deficiency of vitamin K leads to a bleeding diathesis. Vitamin D and calcium deficiency may cause osteomalacia or rickets, as well as paresthesias and other signs of hypocalcemia.

INFLAMMATORY BOWEL DISEASE

Inflammatory bowel disease encompasses two closely related yet distinct diseases of unknown origin: Crohn's disease (CD) and ulcerative colitis (UC).

Crohn's disease and ulcerative colitis have some features in common but differ in other respects.

Although in typical cases CD and UC have characteristic features, in 10% to 15% of cases they cannot be distinguished. The common features are as follows:

- Both diseases are multifactorial and their cause is unknown.
- Both diseases are familial and may even occur in the same families.
- The peak incidence of both diseases is in the third decade.
- Both diseases have the same extraintestinal complications.
- The same drugs are used to treat both diseases.

The features that distinguish typical cases of CD pertain principally to the gross and microscopic pathology and the location of lesions.

Crohn's disease is a transmural inflammation that predominantly affects the terminal ileum and right side of the colon.

Crohn's disease typically affects the terminal ileum, and in 30% of cases the ileum is the only part of the intestine involved. If the colon is involved the disease is mostly limited to the cecum. In 15% to 20% of cases that manifest with only colonic lesions, involvement is segmental with interposed skip regions.

The disease manifests with abdominal pain, fever, and nonbloody diarrhea. Since the inflammation is transmural, it extends all the way to the serosa. Thus the intestinal wall is thickened, the lumen narrowed, and the serosa roughened. Serositis causes adhesions with other intestines, predisposing to fistula formation (Fig. 7-24). Adhesion between the intestines may form a mass that can be palpated in the right lower abdominal quadrant. On endoscopy deep ulcerations may be seen, imparting the mucosa a cobblestone appearance. Granulomas are found in biopsy specimens of about 30% of cases.

Ulcerative colitis predominantly involves the left side of the large intestine.

Ulcerative colitis involves predominantly the rectum and descending colon. In 50% of patients it is limited to the rectosigmoid colon, and in an additional 30% of cases it does not extend proximally beyond the splenic flexure (Fig. 7-25). In the remaining 20% of patients who show diffuse colitis no skip areas are evident and the entire colon is involved. The ileum is spared, although in 10% of those with diffuse colitis backwash ileitis occurs.

Inflammation in UC is limited to the mucosa. The wall is thin, and thus the intestine may dilate giving rise in some patients to toxic megacolon. Rectal bleeding may be prominent. The patients with UC are at increased risk for colon cancer.

The disease typically begins as proctitis or proctosigmoiditis and presents with urgency and frequent passing of blood-tinged mucus. As the diseases progresses, which happens in about 30% of patients, bloody diarrhea develops. It is accompanied by pain, fever, malaise, and even dehydration. Bouts of diarrhea tend to recur and may be debilitating. Extraintestinal complications develop in about 25% of patients.

The differences between UC and CD are summarized in Table 7-7.

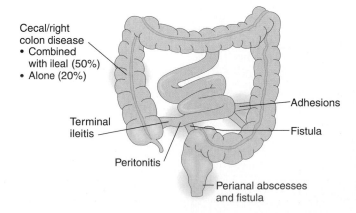

Cecal/right colon disease
- Combined with ileal (50%)
- Alone (20%)

Adhesions

Terminal ileitis

Fistula

Peritonitis

Perianal abscesses and fistula

Figure 7-24 Crohn's disease. The disease is localized in the terminal ileum and the right side of the colon. If it extends distally it skips some areas. Due to the transmural nature of the inflammation, peritonitis, with adhesions and fistula formation, is often present. The lumen is narrowed by the inflamed and thickened intestinal wall.

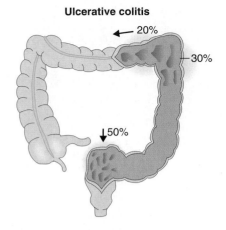

Ulcerative colitis

← 20%

—30%

↓50%

Figure 7-25 Ulcerative colitis. In approximately 50% of cases the disease is limited to the rectosigmoid areas, and in an additional 30% of cases it does not extend proximally beyond the splenic flexure. In only 20% of cases is colitis diffuse.

Ulcerative colitis and Crohn's disease have the same extraintestinal complications.

Extraintestinal complications are found in up to 25% of patients and include lesions in many organs as follows:

- Joint lesions such as arthritis of isolated large joints
- Skin lesions such as erythema nodosum and pyoderma gangrenosum
- Eye lesions such as episcleritis

- Hepatobiliary lesions such as gallstones and sclerosing cholangitis
- Thromboembolic events

These extraintestinal complications occur at different rates in UC and CD. Monoarthritis involving the large joints is the most common complication found in up to 45% patients with either UC or CD, whereas pyoderma gangrenosum is found in approximately 2% of cases.

COLORECTAL CARCINOMA

Carcinoma of the large intestine is a very common cancer; approximately 150,000 new cases occur every year in the United States, of whom 55,000 die of the disease, accounting for 10% of all cancer-related deaths in this country. Other important facts about colorectal carcinoma are as follows:

- It is the most common cancer of the GI tract.
- Its incidence increases with age.
- The peak incidence is in the 60 to 70 age group.
- Over 90% of all colorectal carcinomas occur in persons who are older than 50 years.
- Low-residue, high-fat content of the Western diet probably plays a pathogenetic role, but this still remains to be proven definitively.
- Hereditary plays an important role.
- Family history of colorectal cancer is found in 25% patients.
- Several hereditary cancer syndromes, such as familial polyposis coli, HNPCC, predispose to this type of cancer.

Table 7-7 The Differences Between Ulcerative Colitis and Crohn's Disease

FEATURE	ULCERATIVE COLITIS	CROHN'S DISEASE
Diarrhea	Bloody	Not bloody
Abdominal pain	Rare, except in severe disease	Common
Distribution	Predominantly left side of colon Diffuse	Right side of colon Patchy with skip areas
Involvement of ileum	Rare (backwash ileitis—10%)	Common (80%)
Lumen	Dilated. Megacolon a rare complication in 10%	Stenosis ("string sign")
Mucosa	Friable, surface ulceration	Deep linear ulceration Cobblestone-like
Inflammation	Limited to mucosa	Transmural
Granulomas	No	Yes (in 30%)
Serosa	Smooth, unaffected	Inflamed
Adhesions	No	Yes
Intestinal fistulas	No	Yes
Perianal abscess and fistula	No	Yes (50%)

Most colorectal carcinomas are initially asymptomatic.

Most colorectal carcinomas develop as small-intestine lesions or inside intestinal polyps and are thus asymptomatic for long periods of time. Retrospective studies show that some signs or symptoms may be present 6 to 18 months prior to the final diagnosis.

The mortality rate associated with early colorectal cancer is 20% and that of advanced cancer over 60%. Early detection is the only currently available method for reducing the mortality from this cancer. It is based on two approaches:

- **Testing of patients for occult blood in the feces.** This test is guaiac-based and can detect blood in about 70% of cancer patients and 40% of patients with polyps of the large intestine. It should be noted that it is negative in a significant number of patients with cancer and in the majority of patients with polyps.
- **Colonoscopy.** Endoscopy with flexible colonoscope is a reliable method for detecting polyps and colon carcinoma. It is especially useful in persons at increased risk for colorectal cancer, including from hereditary cancer syndromes (e.g., UC lasting more than 7–10 years).

Colorectal carcinoma may originate in polyps, and thus all neoplastic polyps should be removed preventively.

Colorectal polyps are classified as tubular adenoms, villous adenomas, or tubulovillous adenomas. Approximately 4% of all tubular adenomas undergo malignant transformation. Approximately 40% of villous adenomas give rise to cancer. The larger the polyp, the higher the risk. Likewise the number of polyps also correlates with cancer risk. In familial adenomatous polyposis coli, a condition characterized by the appearance of thousands of polyps, some of which may be quite large, the incidence of cancer is 100%.

Symptoms of colorectal cancer depend on the location of the tumor.

Carcinoma of the rectosigmoid area. Most colorectal cancers occur in the rectosigmoid area (Fig. 7-26). Such tumors may manifest with hematochezia or cause changes

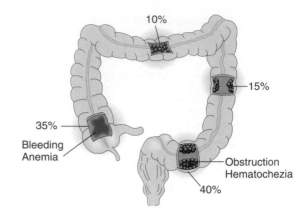

Figure 7-26 Distribution of colorectal carcinomas. Most cancers develop in the proximal or the distal large intestine.

in bowel habits. Tumors tend to narrow the lumen of the colon, obstructing the passage of feces. Pencil-like stools, constipation, and colic are encountered in some patients.

Carcinoma of the cecum and ascending colon. These tumors do not cause obstruction, mostly because the intestine is much wider there than in the rectosigmoid area. Tumors have crater-like or polypoid features and show superficial defects that tend to bleed. Loss of blood may cause iron deficiency anemia. Occult blood may be detected in the feces.

Colorectal carcinomas produce carcinoembryonic antigen, but this tumor marker cannot be used for screening purposes.

Carcinoembryonic antigen (CEA) is found in elevated concentration in the blood of approximately 70% of patients with colorectal cancer. However, it is also elevated in the blood of patients who have other carcinomas, patients with active UC, and even in chronic smokers. Hence the test for CEA is not used for screening purposes.

Carcinoembryonic antigen is measured at the time of resection of colorectal carcinoma. If the resection is complete, CEA levels in blood will normalize. Persistently elevated serum CEA is typically associated with residual cancer and is indicative of a poor prognosis. Recurrence of cancer is also associated with an elevation of CEA.

CASE STUDIES

Case 1 HEARTBURN UNRESPONSIVE TO ANTACIDS IN AN OBESE MAN

Clinical history   A 50-year-old bus driver complained of long-standing heartburn occasionally associated with regurgitation of the food into the mouth.[1] He smokes two packs of cigarettes a day, likes to eat spicy food, and on weekends drinks a case of beer. He was given antacids and was told to lose weight, stop smoking, and change his drinking and eating habits.[2] For the last 3 months he has had difficulties swallowing solid food.[3] Since the heartburn did not respond to antacids he was scheduled for an upper gastrointestinal (UGI) endoscopy.[4]

Physical findings   The patient is obese, but otherwise in relatively good health.

Laboratory findings   No abnormalities were detected.

Diagnostic procedures   A UGI endoscopy revealed that the normal esophageal mucosa has been replaced by velvety red patches and streaks extending 5 cm above the gastroesophageal junction. A biopsy was performed on this part of the esophagus, and the diagnosis of Barrett's esophagus without signs of epithelial atypia or dysplasia was made.[5]

Questions and topics for discussion
1. What is the most likely cause of heartburn in this patient? Explain the pathogenesis of heartburn in general.
2. How is obesity related to heartburn? What other risk factors for heartburn can you identify in his history?
3. Does this patient have dysphagia or odynophagia? How does the difficulty swallowing hard food differ from difficulty in swallowing liquids?
4. What could one expect to find by endoscopy in this patient?
5. Describe the histopathologic findings in Barrett's esophagus. Why is it important to know whether epithelial dysplasia is present in a case of Barrett's esophagus?

Case 2 UPPER ABDOMINAL PAIN IN A 40-YEAR-OLD SURGEON

Clinical history   A 40-year-old surgeon complained of periodic upper abdominal pain that typically begins 2 to 3 hours after meals and often recurs during the night, waking him up.[1] He was taking antacids and H₂ blockers whenever his symptoms flared up. Since the pain intensified recently he was scheduled for an upper gastrointestinal (UGI) endoscopy.[2]

Physical findings   No abnormalities were detected.

Laboratory findings   Mild hypochromic microcytic anemia was noticed.[3]

Diagnostic procedures   UGI endoscopy revealed a bleeding ulcer in the duodenum.[4] The stomach showed erythema and the biopsy chronic gastritis. *Helicobacter pylori* was identified in the mucus covering the antral mucosa.[5]

Follow-up   The *H. pylori* infection was treated, and the patient was given proton pump inhibitors.[6] His symptoms disappeared.

Questions and topics for discussion
1. Is it important to note that the patient is a surgeon? What are the most common causes of upper abdominal pain?
2. What diseases should be considered in the differential diagnosis at this point? Make lists of diseases that cause pain in other parts of the abdomen and those that cause diffuse abdominal pain.
3. What could be the cause of anemia in this patient?
4. Do all peptic ulcers bleed? What are the other possible complications of peptic ulcers?
5. How is *H. pylori* related to the patient's symptoms? Could it be the cause of both gastritis and duodenal ulcer?
6. Explain the effect of proton pump inhibitors.

Case 3 FAILURE TO THRIVE AND FOUL-SMELLING BULKY STOOLS IN A 4-YEAR-OLD BOY

Clinical history   Mother noticed that the child is restless and cranky and complains often of abdominal distention and pain in his legs and arms. He has had two to three bulky, foul-smelling stools per day for the last year.[1]

Physical findings   The child has a potbelly and thin arms and legs. He is short for his age and is in the 15th percentile on the growth curve for his age group.[2] Petechial hemorrhages are seen on both legs.[3] The bones of the extremities are sensitive to palpation. Mild generalized edema is present.[4]

Laboratory findings   Hypochromic microcytic anemia,[5] hypoalbuminemia, and hypocalcemia are evident. The stools contained fat.

Diagnostic procedures   Duodenal biopsy revealed blunting of the villi and elongation of crypts. T lymphocytes were found infiltrating the intestinal epithelium.[6] Antiendomysial antibodies were present in the serum.[7]

Follow-up   A gluten-free diet was prescribed, and the patient improved remarkably.[8]

Questions and topics for discussion

1. Does this patient have diarrhea or steatorrhea or both?
2. What are the possible causes of failure to thrive (FTT) in general? What is the cause of FTT in this case?
3. What bleeding conditions of childhood cause skin petechiae? Which laboratory finding could explain the bleeding tendency in this child?
4. Which laboratory finding could explain edema in this child?
5. Is this anemia related to iron or vitamin deficiency or both?
6. Are these microscopic findings diagnostic of any specific disease? Could similar findings be seen in the intestinal biopsy specimens of asymptomatic relatives of this patient?
7. What is the significance of antiendomysial antibodies?
8. What would a repeat biopsy of the duodenum show in a patient who responded favorably to a gluten-free diet?

Case 4 BLOODY DIARRHEA IN A 22-YEAR-OLD COLLEGE STUDENT

Clinical history   The patient noticed blood in stools, which he passed three to four times per day for the last 4 weeks.[1] Initially the stools were hard, but during the last few days they became softer and he had up to 10 bowel movements per day.[2] Passing of stools was associated with cramps and urgency. He noticed weight loss, had a mild fever, and was constantly thirsty.[3]

Physical findings   Diffuse abdominal tenderness could be elicited by palpation, but no masses were palpable. The patients appeared dehydrated and exhausted.

Laboratory findings
- Anemia; low hematocrit and RBC count[4]
- Leukocytosis
- ESR elevated[5]
- Examination of feces revealed blood and neutrophils.[6]

Diagnostic procedures   Colonoscopy revealed diffuse ulceration of the friable mucosa of the rectum, sigmoid, and descending colon. No skip lesions were noticed. Biopsy of the colon revealed cryptitis and crypt abscesses.[7]

Follow-up   Aminosalicylates were prescribed, and the patients' condition improved.[8]

Questions and topics for discussion

1. Does this patient have acute or chronic diarrhea? Is this diarrhea caused by small-intestine or large-intestine disease?
2. What is the significance of the changing clinical picture?
3. Explain the pathogenesis of weight loss, thirst, and fever in this patient.
4. What is the cause of anemia?
5. Why does this patient have leukocytosis and an elevated ESR?
6. List several diseases associated with the finding of neutrophils in the feces.
7. Are these pathologic changes diagnostic of any specific disease, or should they be interpreted in the context of other clinical findings?
8. What is the effect of aminosalicylates?

Case 5 CONSTIPATION AND BLOOD IN STOOLS IN A 60-YEAR-OLD MAN

Clinical history   This 60-year-old man, who had suffered from constipation for many years, complained of a sense of abdominal fullness and difficulties in passing stools.[1] He did not have bowel movements for 3 to 4 days, and when he went to the toilet he had to strain to pass the stools. The stools came out thin like a pencil.[2] There was also blood on the stools. He also felt tired and noticed he had lost weight.

Physical findings   Distended descending colon could be palpated on the left side of the lower abdomen.

Laboratory findings
- Anemia
- Elevated ESR
- Guaiac test—positive

Diagnostic procedures   Colonoscopy revealed a mass lesion partially obstructing the rectum. A biopsy of the lesion proved the mass to be an adenocarcinoma.[3] The serum level of CEA was elevated.

Treatment and follow-up   Additional radiologic studies were performed, but no masses were identified outside the colon.[4] The patient underwent partial colectomy. The tumor was sent to the pathology department for further examination. The report indicated that the tumor had penetrated through the muscle layer and invaded the subserosal fat tissue. Two of 15 mesenteric lymph nodes examined histopathologically were involved by metastatic carcinoma.[5] On the first follow-up examination, 1 month after surgery, CEA in blood was within normal limits.[6]

Questions and topics for discussion

1. Define constipation. How could you prove that somebody has constipation?
2. What is the significance of pencil-like stools?
3. Does this mean that the patient has a primary colonic tumor?
4. Why were these studies performed?
5. Stage this tumor according to the TNM system. What is the prognosis for a 5-year survival in this patient?
6. Interpret the significance of the CEA test in this case.

Chapter 8

THE LIVER AND BILIARY SYSTEM

Introduction

The liver is the largest internal organ in the body and accounts for 3% to 5% of total body weight. Although it is anatomically part of the gastrointestinal tract, physiologically it belongs to the entire body. It participates in almost all aspects of intermediary metabolism and is the main site of turnover of carbohydrates, lipids, proteins, hormones, nutrients, drugs, and toxins. The liver has many remarkably complex secretory functions and is the main source of most plasma proteins, lipoproteins, and carbohydrates released from its own stores. It also excretes bile, which is a major pathway for metabolizing some lipids (e.g., cholesterol), oligominerals, some minerals (e.g., copper), and drugs. Because of it size, it is a common site for tumors, either primary or metastatic.

Hepatic diseases are an important cause of human morbidity and mortality. Their clinical significance may be illustrated by the following facts:

- Liver diseases account for more than 40,000 deaths annually in the United States alone.

- Approximately 4 to 5 million Americans are infected with viral hepatitis C, but the real number of infected persons is unknown.
- Symptoms of liver disease are often not obvious: approximately 40% of patients who have end-stage liver disease have no significant symptoms.
- Abnormal liver function tests are found in at least 20% of hospitalized persons, and in an even higher number of those who are severely ill, have just undergone surgery, or have experienced trauma.
- Adverse drug reactions involve the liver in a significant number of cases.
- Enlarged livers are found in most patients with congestive heart failure and in many other common diseases and afflictions such as diabetes, obesity, and alcoholism.

Liver diseases may have many causes. The relative clinical significance of various liver diseases is presented graphically in Figure 8-1.

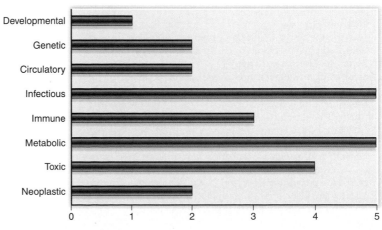

Figure 8-1 Relative clinical significance of various liver diseases.

KEY WORDS

Anatomy and Physiology

Bilirubin   Yellow pigment derived from the heme portion of hemoglobin. Oxidation of heme gives rise to biliverdin, which is converted to bilirubin. Biochemically it is composed of four pyrrole rings ("open tetrapyrrole"). This unconjugated bilirubin is water-insoluble. It is bound to albumin and thereby transported to the liver. In the liver it is conjugated by UDP-glucuronyltransferase and thus made water-soluble. Through bile it is excreted into the intestine, where it is transformed by bacteria into urobilinogen and partially recirculated through the blood back to the liver. Conjugated bilirubin is referred to as direct and unconjugated as indirect. Bilirubin accounts for the yellow discoloration of the skin and mucosae in jaundice.

Common bile duct   Main extrahepatic bile duct. It is a continuation of the common hepatic duct from the point where that duct is joined by the cystic duct to the orifice of the common bile duct in the duodenum at the papilla of Vater. It serves as a conduit for bile.

Gallbladder   Hollow organ attached by the cystic duct to the main extrahepatic biliary ducts. It serves as a storage reservoir for bile.

Glisson's capsule   Peritoneum with underlying fibrous tissue enveloping the liver. Fibrous strands extend from the capsule into the liver parenchyma along the biliary ducts and blood vessels. Glisson's capsule contains sensory nerves.

Hepatic artery   Artery originating from the celiac trunk and providing most of the arterial blood to the liver.

Hepatic lobule   Term for the hypothetical anatomic unit of the liver composed of a centrally located central vein surrounded by hepatocytes. Portal tracts containing the smallest branches of hepatic artery, portal vein, and bile ducts are located on the periphery of the lobule.

Hepatic vein   Vein that drains venous blood from the liver into the inferior vena cava.

Hepatocyte   Also known as the liver cell, it represents the principal metabolic cell in the liver.

Kupffer cell   Fixed macrophage of the liver found in the hepatic sinusoids.

Papilla of Vater   Small duodenal mucosal elevation at the site of entry of the common bile duct and pancreatic duct into the intestine.

Porta hepatis   Also known as the hepatic hilum, it is the part of the visceral (inferior) surface of the liver through which the major blood vessels and extrahepatic bile duct enter the liver parenchyma.

Portal tract   Triangular fibrous area at the periphery of the hepatic lobule that contains the terminal branches of the portal vein and hepatic artery, as well as the small biliary ducts. The limiting plate represents the sharp line separating the portal tract from the hepatocytes in the lobule (acinus).

Portal vein   Vein formed through the confluence of the splenic and pancreatic superior and inferior mesenteric veins. It drains the venous splanchnic blood into the liver.

Sinusoids   Small hepatic blood vessels, corresponding to capillaries. They differ from capillaries in that they are lined by a discontinuous ("fenestrated") endothelial layer.

Space of Disse   Narrow space between the apical surface of hepatocytes and the endothelial cells lining the sinusoids.

Sphincter of Oddi   Smooth muscle bands encircling the terminal part of the common bile duct, common pancreatic duct, and ampulla of Vater. Cholecystokinin and neural stimuli cause relaxation or constriction of the sphincter, thus regulating the flow of bile into the intestine.

Stellate cells of Ito   Stromal cells scattered at random in the spaces of Disse. They accumulate fat and vitamin A and may transform into collagen-producing myofibroblasts in cirrhosis.

Terminal hepatic venule   Also know as the central vein of the lobule, it represents the beginning of the hepatic venous system inside the lobule (acinus). It is located at the center of the lobule. It receives the blood from hepatic sinusoids and drains that blood toward the hepatic vein and the inferior vena cava.

Pathophysiology and Laboratory Medicine

Ascites   Accumulation of serous fluid in the abdominal cavity. Usually it is a sign of cirrhosis, but it may be also be a consequence of generalized hypoalbuminemia or chronic heart failure.

Cholecystitis   Inflammation of the gallbladder. It is often associated with gallstones or bacterial infection.

Cholelithiasis   Formation of gallstones in the hepatobiliary system, most often in the gallbladder.

Cholestasis   Stagnation of bile inside the biliary tree usually due to biliary obstruction. Canalicular cholestasis may be a consequence of liver cell injury and is one of the well-known hepatic signs of injury. Cholestasis is associated with conjugated hyperbilirubinemia and bilirubinuria and may be accompanied by clay-colored (acholic) stools.

Fatty liver   Also known as steatosis, it is a consequence of fat accumulation inside the hepatocytes. Fat begins to accumulate in the form of small droplets (microvesicular steatosis), which become confluent and eventually fill the entire liver cell with triglycerides (macrovesicular steatosis). The most common causes of fatty liver are obesity, diabetes, and alcohol abuse. Viral hepatitis C and some drugs (e.g., tetracycline) may also cause hepatic steatosis. Steatosis is a reversible cell change, but in some cases it may be accompanied by inflammation (steatohepatitis).

Gynecomastia   Enlargement of male breast. In patients with cirrhosis it is usually caused by hyperestrinemia, resulting from incomplete hepatic inactivation of endogenous estrogens.

Hepatic encephalopathy   Brain disturbance caused by liver disease. Symptoms include asterixis (coarse tremor and flapping of hands), loss of coordination, and progressive coma. Coma is graded on a scale from I to IV and may be lethal.

Hepatomegaly   Enlargement of the liver. It may a consequence of various metabolic disturbances leading to accumulation of fat (e.g., obesity or diabetes), hemosiderin (e.g., hemochromatosis), or congestion of the liver in heart failure. Tumors may also cause hepatomegaly.

Hepatorenal syndrome   Oliguric renal failure seen in patients with end-stage liver disease (cirrhosis) accompanied by ascites.

Jaundice (Latin, *icterus*) Yellow discoloration of the skin and mucosae that develops due to hyperbilirubinemia. It reflects the deposition of bilirubin in tissues. Jaundice becomes evident when the blood concentration of bilirubin exceeds 2 mg/dL.

Kernicterus Cerebral dysfunction caused by the deposition of bilirubin in basal ganglia. Typically it is caused by hemolytic anemia in infants due to maternofetal blood group incompatibility or severe prolonged hyperbilirubinemia, as in Crigler-Najjar syndrome type I.

Liver function tests (LFTs) Laboratory tests performed on blood to estimate the extent of liver cell injury and synthetic and excretory functions of the liver. They include measurements of serum transaminases (AST and ALT), alkaline phosphatase, bilirubin, albumin, and coagulation parameters (most often prothrombin time—PT).

Portal hypertension Elevation of blood pressure over 12 mm Hg in the portal system. The main consequences of portal hypertension are ascites, esophageal varices, and splenomegaly.

Splenomegaly Enlargement of the spleen. In cirrhotic patients it is usually related to chronic passive congestion that develops due to portal hypertension. It may be associated with signs of hypersplenism, including anemia and thrombocytopenia.

Vascular spider Also known as spider telangiectasia it represents a dilatation of small dermal blood vessels. It has a red central dotlike bulge with small branches radiating from it in all directions. Because of its resemblance to spiders it is also called spider nevus. It usually develops on the skin of the upper chest and, like palmar erythema, is a complication of hyperestrinism often found in cirrhosis.

Xanthoma Yellow skin papule, plaque, or nodule caused by hyperlipidemia. It is a feature of primary biliary cirrhosis and is associated with hypercholesterolemia. It may be found in primary disorders of lipid metabolism. If found on the palpebrae it is called xanthelasma.

Liver Diseases

Abscess of the liver Localized purulent inflammation of the liver caused by bacteria. The infection may reach the liver through the bile ducts (cholangitic abscess) or the branches of the portal vein (pylephlebitic abscess).

Acute hepatitis Inflammation of the liver, characterized by sudden-onset jaundice or other symptoms of relatively short duration.

Alcoholic liver disease Spectrum of diseases related to alcohol abuse, including fatty change, alcoholic steatohepatitis, and alcoholic cirrhosis. Fatty liver is almost always found in patients after excessive drinking of alcohol. Alcoholic hepatitis and cirrhosis develop in a minority of chronic alcohol abusers.

α_1-Antitrypsin deficiency Genetic disease characterized by liver and pulmonary diseases. The affected liver may show signs of chronic hepatitis or cirrhosis. Symptoms may appear in any age group. This genetic defect is the most common cause of neonatal hepatitis.

Autoimmune hepatitis Autoimmune disease predominantly affecting young women. Associated with antismooth muscle antibodies (ASM), antinuclear antibodies (ANAs), and other autoimmune diseases. It responds to corticosteroid treatment but may also persist and progress to cirrhosis.

Budd-Chiari syndrome Syndrome caused by thrombosis of the hepatic vein and massive enlargement of the liver due to congestion. Most often it is a complication of such hematologic diseases as polycythemia, leukemia, and thrombophilia.

Cholangitis Inflammation of intrahepatic or extrahepatic bile ducts. It may be suppurative owing to bacterial infection, or nonsuppurative as in various autoimmune diseases (e.g., primary biliary cirrhosis).

Chronic hepatitis Chronic inflammation of the liver, most often caused by viral hepatitis C. It may persist and be relatively asymptomatic or it may progress to cirrhosis. Similar changes can be seen in various immune diseases of the liver and drug-related liver diseases.

Cirrhosis Chronic liver disease causing liver failure. The liver is of abnormal size and shape and subdivided into small nodules by abundant collagenous connective tissue. Cirrhosis may have many causes, the most important of which are chronic alcohol abuse and chronic viral hepatitis C infection. The cause of cirrhosis cannot be established in 15% to 20% of patients, and in such cases it is called cryptogenic.

Crigler-Najjar syndrome Hereditary unconjugated hyperbilirubinemia caused by absolute or relative deficiency of glucuronosyltransferase in liver cells.

Dubin-Johnson syndrome Hereditary conjugated hyperbilirubinemia, presenting as mild jaundice. It is caused by a blockage in bilirubin excretion from hepatocytes owing to the defect in the function of the ATP-binding cassette (ABC) of the canalicular multispecific organic anion transporter protein.

Gilbert syndrome Genetic disorder characterized by recurrent bouts of jaundice caused by unconjugated hyperbilirubinemia. It is related to mutation of the gene encoding uridine glucuronosyltransferase.

Hereditary hemochromatosis Genetic disease related to mutations of the *HFE* gene encoding the regulator of iron absorption in the small intestine. It is characterized by excessive absorption of iron from food. Excess iron is stored in the body, damaging multiple tissues. The most common complications of iron storage are cirrhosis, diabetes, hyperpigmentation of the skin, arthropathy, and cardiomyopathy.

Liver tumors Tumors of the liver can be classified as benign or malignant. The most common benign tumor is hemangioma. Other benign tumors are hepatocellular adenoma and focal nodular hyperplasia. Malignant tumors may be primary or metastatic. Primary tumors of the liver are hepatocellular carcinoma, cholangiocarcinoma, and angiosarcoma. Metastases to the liver can occur from any other primary site. Metastases are the most common malignant tumors of the liver.

Nonalcoholic steatohepatitis Chronic liver disease of unknown origin characterized by fatty change of hepatocytes, intralobular fibrosis, and focal infiltrates of inflammatory cells. It may cause portal hypertension and progress to cirrhosis.

Primary biliary cirrhosis Autoimmune liver disease primarily affecting women. It is a nonsuppurative cholangitis leading to destruction of bile ducts and progressive jaundice and cirrhosis. Other symptoms include pruritus, xanthelasma, and steatorrhea. Antibodies to mitochondria are a clue to the diagnosis.

Primary sclerosing cholangitis Disease of unknown origin but considered to be immune in nature. In 60% to 70% of cases it is associated with ulcerative colitis. The diagnosis is made by cholangiography, which shows typical "sausage-like" narrowing and dilatation of intrahepatic and extrahepatic bile ducts. Liver biopsy shows concentric fibrosis around large- and medium-sized bile ducts. The disease has a tendency to progress to cirrhosis.

Wilson's disease   Rare autosomal recessive genetic disorder characterized by accumulation of copper in the liver and other tissues. Cirrhosis develops together with degeneration of basal ganglia of the brain, resulting in Parkinsonism. A brownish green ring (Keyser-Fleischer ring) can be seen by slit lamp examination on the limbus of the cornea.

Normal Structure and Function

ANATOMY

The most important aspects of the macroscopic anatomy of the liver are its (1) location, (2) size and shape, (3) anatomic links with the other abdominal organs, and (4) blood supply.

The liver is located in the right upper abdominal quadrant underneath the diaphragm and mostly behind the rib cage.

The liver is located in the right upper quadrant of the abdomen behind the lower part of the rib cage (Fig. 8-2). Cranially its superior surface is in contact with the diaphragm. From the clinical point of view these anatomic facts are important for the following reasons:

- The liver can be localized by percussion through the chest wall. In contrast to the resonant sound of the percussed lung, over the liver the percussion produces a dull sound. The distance between the upper and lower border of this dullness is used to estimate the size of the liver.
- During each inspiration the liver is pushed caudally by the expanded lung, and the anterior edge can be palpated underneath the right costal margin while the patient is taking a deep breath.
- Percutaneous liver biopsy is performed through the intercostal space.

The size and the shape of the liver are relatively constant but may change under pathologic conditions.

The liver is roughly conical in shape. It consists of a larger right lobe that forms the base of the pyramid and a smaller left lobe that forms the apex of the pyramid. The falciform ligament on the diaphragmatic surface of the liver forms the border between these two lobes. Each major lobe can be subdivided into smaller segments, each of which has a separate blood supply. This subdivision is not important functionally, but it is of paramount importance to surgeons engaged in partial hepatectomy.

The size of the liver depends on body size. On average, top to bottom it has a span of less than 13 cm when measured in the midcostal line. The size of the liver can be estimated by percussion, or by combining percussion and auscultation. Unfortunately these techniques lack precision and reproducibility. More accurate measurements can be made by ultrasonography or radiologic imaging. Ultrasonography may be also used to determine whether the liver has a normal shape and smooth surface, is irregularly

A   **B**

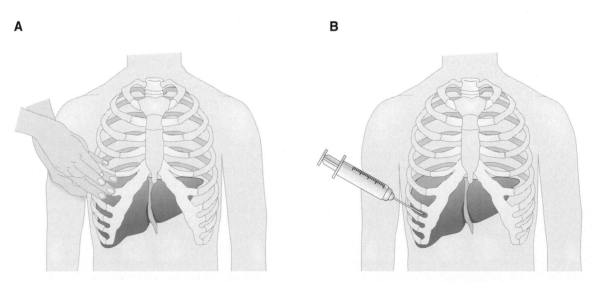

Figure 8-2 The location of the liver. The liver is located in the right upper quadrant of the abdomen and is mostly covered by the rib cage. **A,** Its size can be determined by percussion or even better by ultrasound. **B,** The biopsy needle is usually introduced through the intercostal spaces.

shaped, or contains irregular masses. These abnormalities are visible in computed tomography (CT) scans as well.

Pathologically altered livers can be of normal size, enlarged, or reduced in size.

- **Liver of normal size.** In the course of most diseases, the size of the liver does not change significantly.
- **Hepatomegaly.** The enlargement of the liver may have numerous causes. The most common is *congestive hepatomegaly* caused by right heart failure and consequent stagnation of the blood inside the liver. *Inflammatory hepatomegaly* may be encountered in acute viral hepatitis. *Metabolic hepatomegaly* may be seen in diabetes, which is characterized by an accumulation of lipids and glycogen in hepatocytes. Inborn errors of metabolism, such as glycogenosis type I (von Gierke's disease) or galactosemia, may cause hepatomegaly in infants and children. Chronic alcohol abuse causes accumulation of fat in the liver cells and enlargement of the liver. *Neoplastic hepatomegaly* can be caused by primary liver tumors or metastases to the liver.
- **Small livers.** Shrunken livers are typical of end-stage liver failure. The liver can decrease to half of its normal size during *acute massive hepatic necrosis*. At the time of surgery such livers appear small and soft and have a shrunken capsule. *Cirrhotic livers* are also small. In contrast to acute hepatic necrosis, small cirrhotic livers are firm and nodular.

Pearls

> More than one half of patients found to have enlarged liver by palpation have no signs of liver disease.
> If during palpation you discover that the liver has a very hard lower edge or contains distinct nodules think of cancer rather than cirrhosis.

The liver has relatively limited mobility and is linked through the bile ducts with the intestine.

The liver is enclosed by folds of the peritoneum, which together with the falciform ligament keep it fixated in the subdiaphragmatic position. The peritoneum covering the liver is known as *Glisson's capsule.* On the visceral side of the liver the peritoneum covers the hilar structures (i.e., the gallbladder) and forms the lesser omentum surrounding the portal vein, hepatic artery, and the extrahepatic biliary ducts (Fig. 8-3).

Pearls

> Glisson's capsule contains sensory nerves.
> Venous congestion of the liver causes expansion of the capsule and is accompanied by pain.
> Do not forget to anesthetize the capsule prior to liver biopsy.

The extrahepatic biliary ducts begin as the main hepatic ducts, which fuse into a common hepatic duct. The common bile duct joins the cystic duct, and from that point downward it is called the *common bile duct,* or *ductus choledochus.* It passes through the head of the pancreas, at which point it usually joins with the main pancreatic duct to terminate in the duodenum at the ampulla of Vater.

The bile flow from the liver into the duodenum depends on a balance between the production and the need for bile. The flow is primarily regulated by the sphincter of Oddi, which forms smooth muscle layers around the choledochus, pancreatic duct, and the ampulla of Vater. The sphincter of Oddi has sympathetic and parasympathetic innervation, the former causing its relaxation and the latter its contraction. Cholecystokinin, a polypeptide hormone produced by intestinal cells, promotes bile flow into the duodenum by causing relaxation of the sphincter of Oddi simultaneously with the contraction of the gallbladder.

The *sphincter of Oddi* has three functions: (1) regulation of the flow of bile and pancreatic juices into the duodenum, (2) prevention of reflux of duodenal contents into the bile duct and pancreas, and (3) promotion of filling of the gallbladder with hepatic bile.

During feeding the sphincter of Oddi is relaxed, allowing the diluted hepatic bile to enter into the duodenum. Between the meals the sphincter of Oddi is contracted and the bile from the common hepatic bile duct cannot enter into the duodenum; instead it is redirected into the gallbladder where it is concentrated and stored. The gallbladder is not essential for the excretion of bile as evidenced by the fact that it can be removed surgically without significant consequences.

Pearls

> Prolonged or irregular contractions of the sphincter of Oddi may lead to reflux of bile into the pancreas and cause pancreatitis.
> Inadequate contraction of the sphincter of Oddi may facilitate the entry of bacteria into the common bile duct. Such bacteria may cause ascending cholangitis.

The liver has a dual blood supply.

The liver is full of blood, and under normal circumstances the blood accounts for 30% of the total weight of the liver. The liver could be considered as a blood reservoir because normally it contains approximately 15% of the total circulating blood. This reservoir may expand under certain conditions: in circulatory shock or chronic heart failure the blood content of the liver can increase dramatically.

The liver has a dual blood supply. The *hepatic artery,* a branch of the hepaticoduodenal artery originating from the celiac axis, provides the arterial blood, which accounts for 25% to 30% of the total hepatic blood supply. The *portal*

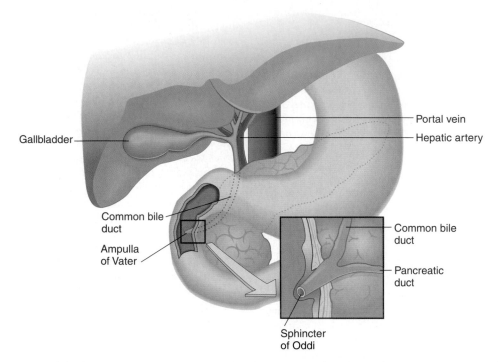

Figure 8-3 Anatomy of the liver. The liver is covered by the Glisson's capsule, a layer of peritoneum that also forms the lesser omentum. In the hilum of the liver the most important structures are the hepatic artery, portal vein, and the extrahepatic bile duct, which connects the liver to the duodenum. The confluence of the common bile duct and the pancreatic duct results in the formation of the ampulla of Vater, which is enveloped by the smooth muscles of the sphincter of Oddi.

vein, a large valveless vein draining the venous blood from the intestines, stomach, pancreas, and spleen, brings in the remaining 70% to 75% of the blood. The venous blood leaves the liver through the hepatic veins, which drain into the inferior vena cava.

On entering the liver at the porta hepatis the portal vein and the hepatic artery divide into progressively smaller and smaller branches until they reach the portal tracts in the hepatic lobule, or acinus. From the portal tract the blood enters into the sinusoids and is finally collected into the terminal hepatic venule. From terminal hepatic venules the blood flows into the larger veins, which finally form the main hepatic vein. The hepatic vein is connected to the lower vena cava, through which the hepatic venous blood reaches the right atrium.

The *portal vein* and its branches are a low-pressure blood flow system. Blood pressure varies from 3 to 10 mm Hg, depending on several factors including posture and respiratory phase. Coughing, Valsalva maneuver, or compression of the abdomen may also temporarily increase the portal pressure. These physiologic and short-term elevations of portal blood pressure must be distinguished, however, from *portal hypertension*, which is defined as persistent elevation of portal blood pressure over 12 mm Hg.

In most instances **portal hypertension** is a consequence of liver disease. If the blood cannot be drained from the portal system through the liver and the portal blood pressure exceeds 20 mm Hg, anastomoses, or *collaterals*, develop between the portal and systemic venous system. These anastomoses develop through the dilatation and reopening of small veins that normally connect the portal and systemic venous systems. Under normal circumstances these small veins contain very little blood, but in portal hypertension they transform into congested, tortuous, widely opened venous channels that can be visualized by angiography. These anastomotic collaterals most often develop in the area of the *lower esophagus and gastric fundus, internal hemorrhoidal veins and retroperitoneum, and the periumbilical veins* (Fig. 8-4). The dilatation of periumbilical veins is traditionally called *caput Medusae*, in reference to the Gorgon from Greek mythology whose hair was made of snakes.

HISTOLOGY

The liver is composed of hepatocytes, bile ductular cells, vascular cells, and connective tissue cells. Hepatocytes account for 70% of all cells in the liver. Because of their large size they account for 95% of the liver's volume.

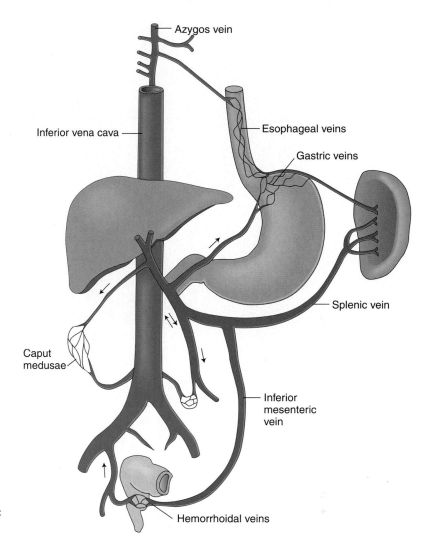

Azygos vein

Inferior vena cava

Esophageal veins

Gastric veins

Splenic vein

Caput medusae

Inferior mesenteric vein

Hemorrhoidal veins

Figure 8-4 Portal hypertension. Portal vein obstruction leads to the formation of collaterals between the portal and systemic venous system.

Hepatocytes perform most complex liver functions.

Hepatocytes, or *liver cells,* are polarized cells interconnected along their apical sides with intercellular junctions. Tight junctions are important for the maintenance of liver cell polarity; they also ensure the structural stability of liver cell cords. In the midportion of the apical surface two adjacent liver cells form intercellular canaliculi, which are filled with bile secreted by the hepatocytes. The cell surface that does not have tight junctions is called the basolateral side. It delimits the space of Disse, which on the other side is separated from the lumen of the sinusoids by endothelial and Kupffer cells (Fig. 8-5).

Hepatocytes have numerous functions, and it has been estimated that each moment some 70 metabolic functions are performed simultaneously in every liver cell. These functions can be classified into several categories as follows:

■ Bilirubin metabolism and the formation and excretion of bile

■ Intermediary metabolism of carbohydrates, lipids, proteins, and minerals
■ Synthesis of plasma proteins
■ Detoxification; inactivation; or metabolic conversion of hormones, drugs, and toxins

Sinusoids are essential for the normal exchange of metabolites between the blood and liver cells.

The **vascular system** of the liver consists of branches of the hepatic artery, hepatic vein, and portal vein. These three systems all communicate with one another through the *sinusoids,* which receive the blood from the hepatic artery and portal vein and drain into the hepatic vein. All these arteries and veins are lined by a continuous layer of endothelial cells, in contrast to the sinusoids, which have a discontinuous endothelial layer. Such fenestration of sinusoids facilitates the passage of metabolites and other substance from the liver cells into the blood and vice versa.

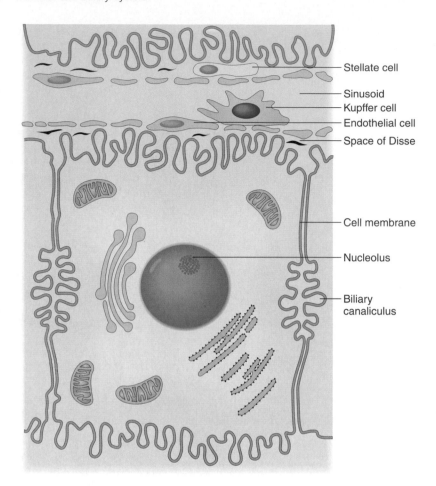

Stellate cell

Sinusoid
Kupffer cell
Endothelial cell
Space of Disse

Cell membrane

Nucleolus

Biliary canaliculus

Figure 8-5 Liver cell. The liver cell is polarized and has an apical side, containing the biliary canaliculus, and a basolateral domain, which abuts the sinusoids. The sinusoids are lined by fenestrated endothelial cells and phagocytic Kupffer cells. Between the liver cells and endothelial cells of the sinusoids is the narrow space of Disse.

In addition to the endothelial cells, the sinusoids contain scattered *Kupffer cells,* which act as fixed macrophages. These cells have major scavenger functions and participate in the removal of particulate material, bacteria, and immune complexes from the circulation. Inside the spaces of Disse are scattered the *stellate cells of Ito,* which have a capacity to store lipids and, if properly stimulated, also synthesize collagenous extracellular matrix. These cells play a major role in the formation of fibrous tissue in liver cirrhosis.

Pearl

> Deposition of collagen in the walls of sinusoids in cirrhosis is accompanied by capillarization of the sinusoids with a *loss of fenestration*. Continuous basement membranes encasing the vascular spaces of the liver acini impair exchange between the liver cells and the blood, thus contributing to liver failure.

The liver produces large amounts of lymph.

Hepatic lymph is formed as plasma passes into the extravascular *spaces of Disse*. In contrast to capillaries, which in other organs allow the passage of only 0.01% of the plasma volume into the lymphatic channels, in the sinusoids 0.3% of the total hepatic blood is transformed into the lymph. From the spaces of Disse this lymph is drained into the main *lymphatic channels* running parallel to the branches of the portal vein toward the hilum. From the porta hepatis the lymph enters *cysterna chyli,* mixing with the lymph from the intestines and the lower extremities. Cirrhosis with intrahepatic scarring or a surgical procedure in the hepatic hilum may interfere with the outflow of the lymph from the liver. These changes block and thus redirect the flow of the lymph, which seeps into the peritoneum, thus contributing to the formation of ascites.

The biliary ducts and the gallbladder are lined by cuboidal to cylindrical cells specializing in the excretion of bile.

The **biliary excretory system** begins with *intercellular bile canaliculi* on the apical (intercellular) surface of the hepatocytes (Fig. 8-6). From these canaliculi the bile flows into minor *bile ducts* in the portal tracts as well as medium-sized and larger (septal) bile ducts draining the bile toward the hepatic bile ducts in the porta hepatis. All bile ducts are lined by cuboidal to cylindrical cells lying in a polarized manner on a basement membrane. Similar polarized cells line the major *extrahepatic bile ducts* all the way to the papilla of Vater. These cells produce some components of the bile and are also important for the maintenance of bile outflow from the liver. The cells lining the *gallbladder* resemble those in the bile ducts. However, gallbladder cells are unique in that they can actively absorb sodium and chloride from the bile. The resorption of sodium chloride is followed by a passive outflow of water and concentration of bile.

Connective tissue extends along the bile ducts and blood vessels all the way to the portal tracts in the center of hepatic acini.

Connective tissue forms the liver capsule, and from the surface it extends into the parenchyma along the blood vessels and bile ducts. The ultimate part of this connective tissue

skeleton is the strands of collagen in the portal tracts. The acinus itself does not contain banded collagenous stroma beyond the limits of the portal tract. This boundary is called the *limiting plate.* The skeleton of acini consists of the delicate matrix produced by the endothelial and interstitial cells.

> **Pearl**
>
> > As inflammatory cells invade the acinus from the portal tract, the limiting plate becomes irregular. This histologic finding, called *piecemeal necrosis,* or *interface hepatitis,* is a sign of active hepatitis that may progress to cirrhosis.

Liver cells are arranged into functional units called lobules or acini.

All hepatocytes are interchangeable among themselves and thus all of them can perform all hepatic functions. Under normal circumstances the function of each hepatocyte nevertheless depends on it location in the hexagonal microscopic unit called the lobule or acinus (Fig. 8-7).

According to 19th century histologic teaching, the concept of **lobule** is based on the idea that hepatocytes are arranged around a small central hepatic vein. Sinusoids and liver cell plates radiate from the central veins, forming a hexagonal unit demarcated on its periphery with portal tracts. Portal tracts containing the bile ducts and the terminal branches of the hepatic artery and portal vein are surrounded by fibrous tissue. The blood flows into the portal tracts through the lobular sinusoids, toward the central vein, and from there into the larger branches of the hepatic vein out of the liver. The bile flows in the opposite direction from the center of the lobule toward its periphery.

The concept of **acinus** points out some of the misconceptions related to the concept of the lobule. For example, the so-called central hepatic vein has a very thin wall and is actually a venule. From a hemodynamic point of view it is not located centrally but rather at the periphery of the functional unit and is more appropriately called the terminal hepatic venule (THV).

According to the concept of acinus, which is a reverse image of the lobule, the blood enters the functional unit through the centrally located portal tract and flows through the sinusoids toward several peripherally located THVs. Pressure gradients are formed as the blood flows from the center to the periphery, and bile flows from the periphery to the center.

The hepatocytes located along these pressure gradients have different functions, probably determined by the oxygen supply (which is higher around the portal tracts than around the THV) and the concentration of nutrients and metabolites. The acinus can be thus divided into three functional zones: (1) *periportal zone 1,* (2) *perivenular zone 3,* and

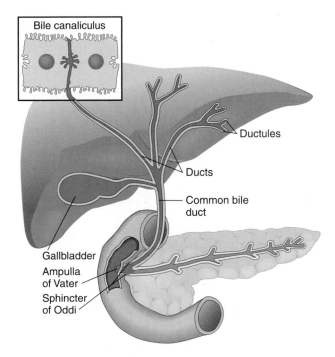

Bile canaliculus

Ductules

Ducts

Common bile duct

Gallbladder

Ampulla of Vater

Sphincter of Oddi

Figure 8-6 Biliary system. Liver cells secrete bile into the canaliculi, from which it flows into progressively larger and larger ducts.

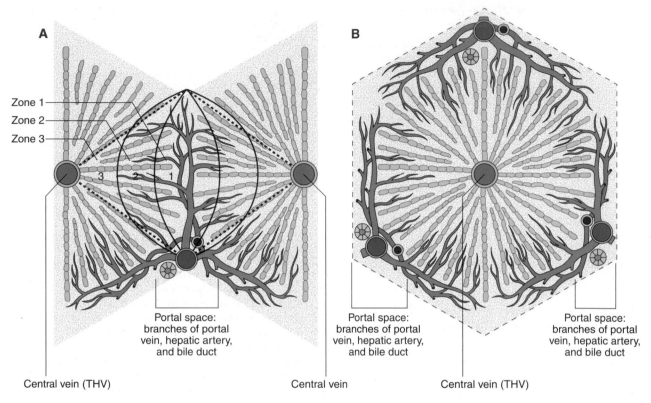

Figure 8-7 Comparison of the acinar (**A**) and the lobular (**B**) concept of hepatic microarchitecture. THV, terminal hepatic venule. (From Underwood JCE, [ed]: General and Systemic Pathology, 4th ed. Edinburgh, Churchill Livingstone, 2004, p. 402.)

(3) *zone 2 in between zones 1 and 3.* Furthermore it was shown that the falling blood pressure from the center of the acinus toward its periphery is accompanied by a decreasing concentration of oxygen in hepatic blood and a decreased concentration of various metabolites and toxins. For example, ammonia is mostly extracted from portal blood as soon as it enters into the acinus (zone 1) so that very small amounts of this substance reach the perivenular periphery of the acinus. The hepatocytes of zone 1 are more active in oxidative phosphorylation and gluconeogenesis than those in zone 3. Perivenular hepatocytes, adapted to relative hypoxia, tend to engage more in anaerobic glycolysis and lipogenesis.

The concept of the acinus explains several clinicopathologic findings, some of which can be appreciated by liver biopsy and deserve to be mentioned here:

- Most direct hepatotoxins are taken up by hepatocytes in zone 1. This principle explains periportal zone 1 liver cell necrosis, which is caused by phosphorus.
- Substances that become toxic only after being metabolized, such as carbon tetrachloride (CCl_4), mostly damage hepatocytes in zone 3. CCl_4 is taken

up by hepatocytes of zone 1, activated, and then released into the sinusoids. It is carried downstream and taken up in its active form by perivenular hepatocytes of zone 3, lethally damaging these cells.

- Zone 3 hepatocytes are more susceptible to ischemia and are the first to undergo necrosis in systemic hypoxia and vascular hypoperfusion during shock.
- Signs of bile flow obstruction first become evident in zone 3, the part of the bile canalicular system that is most distant from the major bile ducts in the hepatic hilum. Bile ultimately kills these perivenular cells and causes the formation of *bile lakes*. These changes are important for diagnosing biliary obstruction in liver biopsy specimens.

Pathophysiology

When attempting to understand the pathophysiology of the liver we must ask ourselves: *What could go wrong?*

Since almost all functions of the liver cells are performed simultaneously and are thus interconnected, the answer might not be so simple. For didactic purposes we, nevertheless, discuss each of the major functions separately and outline the most important consequences of liver cell dysfunction, including the following processes:

- Intermediate metabolism of carbohydrates, lipids, and proteins
- Hepatic synthetic functions
- Detoxification of endogenous and exogenous substances
- Bilirubin metabolism and excretion
- Bile circulation

DISTURBANCES OF INTERMEDIATE METABOLISM

The liver plays a crucial role in the metabolism of carbohydrates, lipids, and proteins. The intermediate metabolism of each of these main components of all living cells is closely interrelated. For practical purposes it is thus best to concentrate on end-point metabolites in blood or liver cells. Let us consider some examples.

Glycogen accumulates in the liver of infants who lack glucose-6-phosphatase.

The glucose taken up from blood is stored in the liver in the form of glycogen. Glycogen stores (70–80 g) are sufficient to meet the body's demand during 24 hours of fasting, after which gluconeogenesis from amino acids becomes the primary source of glucose. In children who have **von Gierke's disease,** or **glycogenosis type I,** the hepatocytes lack glucose-6-phosphatase and therefore cannot form glucose to be exported into the blood (Fig. 8-8). Such children suffer from hypoglycemia. At the same time glucose-1-phosphate accumulates, promoting glycogen accumulation in liver cells and resulting in hepatomegaly. Compensatory metabolic changes lead to hyperlipidemia and lactic acidosis.

Lipids can accumulate in liver cells due to increased supply and influx, increased endogenous lipogenesis, lowered utilization, or decreased excretion.

Lipids are transported by blood to the liver from food absorbed in the intestines or from fat stores and other tissues (Fig. 8-9). The fat absorbed from food in the intestines is packaged into chylomicrons, which enter the intestinal lymph and from there enter the blood. During the passage of such blood through the small blood vessels of the skeletal muscle and fat tissue, the endothelial lipoprotein lipase acts on the chylomicrons, resulting in the formation of glycerol, free fatty acids, and cholesterol-enriched chylomicron remnants. Most of the glycerol and fatty acids thus formed are absorbed by muscle cells and fat cells, whereas the chylomicron remnants reach the liver and are taken up through the low-density lipoprotein (LDL) and LDL-related receptors.

Free fatty acids liberated from chylomicrons but not taken up by other tissues also end up in the liver. In addition to these exogenous lipids the lipid pool inside the hepatocytes also contains endogenously formed cholesterol and lipids that have arrived into the liver through the endogenous LDL receptor-mediated uptake. These lipids may be further metabolized as follows:

- Oxidized and used for production of energy.
- Used for the synthesis of acetoacetate, which accounts for most of the ketone bodies released from the liver into the blood. Ketone bodies are a major source of energy in the skeletal muscles, brain, and kidneys.
- Esterified into phospholipids, which can be coupled with apoproteins and secreted into the blood as lipoproteins, or used for the synthesis of structural proteins that are found in all cell membranes.
- Used for synthesis of cholesterol, which may be further used for endogenous purposes, excreted in bile, metabolized to bile acids and excreted in bile, or

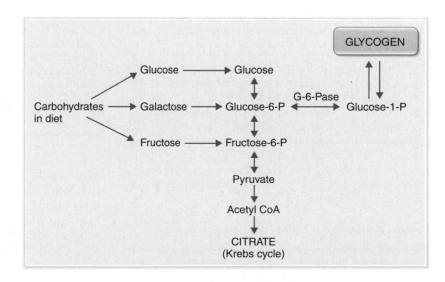

Figure 8-8 Glycogen accumulation in glycogenosis type I. Deficiency of glucose-6-phosphatase (glucose-6-P) leads to the accumulation of glucose-1-phosphate (glucose-1-P), promoting deposition of unused carbohydrates in the form of glycogen.

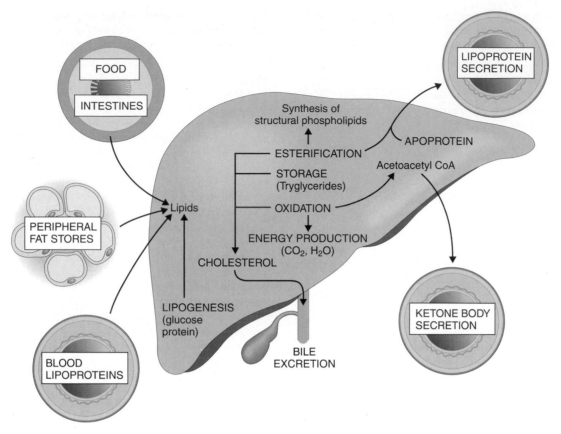

Figure 8-9 Lipid metabolism in the liver. Free fatty acids (FFAs) and chylomicron remnants derived from the fat absorbed in the intestine from food, the FFAs derived from the endogenous peripheral fat stores, and the lipid contained in circulating lipoproteins enter into the liver. In the liver FFAs can be esterified, used up through oxidation, stored in the form of triglycerides, or used for the formation of structural phospholipids. Lipids can be secreted as lipoproteins or as ketone bodies or excreted in bile. Lipids can be also formed in the liver from carbohydrates and proteins.

packaged into very low density lipoproteins (VLDLs) and secreted into the blood.

■ Stored in the hepatocytes in the form of triglycerides.

Fatty liver (**steatosis**) can be induced by increasing the supply of lipids by overeating. Obesity, diabetes, and alcoholism are also associated with overabundance of lipid influx into the liver. Alcohol mobilizes free fatty acids from peripheral fat tissue stores, but it also promotes the esterification of intrahepatic fatty acids into triglycerides, and it inhibits the synthesis of the apoproteins essential for synthesis and export of VLDLs. Starvation and protein-deficient malnutrition may cause fatty liver due to inadequate synthesis and export of lipoproteins. The most important causes of fatty liver are listed in Table 8-1.

Protein synthesis is a major function of liver cells.

Liver cells synthesize proteins for endogenous purposes but also for export. Proteins for exogenous purposes are synthe-

Table 8-1 Common Causes of Fatty Liver

Obesity	Drugs
Diabetes	Tetracycline
Alcohol abuse	Zidovudine
Chronic viral hepatitis C	Corticosteroids
Inborn errors of metabolism	Tamoxifen
(e.g., Wilson's disease,	Cisplatin
glycogenesis I, Wollman's	Methotrexate
disease)	Amiodarone

sized in the cisterns of the rough endoplasmic reticulum, glycosylated or folded, and actively secreted into the blood. Most of the plasma proteins are synthesized in the liver. Liver disease results in marked reduction of plasma protein synthesis, which is usually associated with significant pathophysiologic changes. For example, **hypoalbuminemia** occurs in chronic liver disease, resulting in diminished oncotic pressure of the plasma and predisposing to edema formation.

Abnormal synthesis of some proteins may also cause structural changes in hepatocytes, which are visible by light and electron microscopy. The best example is **α₁-antitrypsin (AAT) deficiency,** an autosomal recessive disorder characterized by the inability of liver cells to excrete AAT. The defect lies in the abnormal folding of the AAT in the cisterns of the rough endoplasmic reticulum of hepatocytes, which cannot then complete the synthesis of the protein and retains the abnormal intermediate product inside the cytoplasm in the form of round globules (Fig. 8-10). Deficiency of AAT predisposes the affected person to cirrhosis but also to pulmonary emphysema.

Amino acids are metabolized to urea and ammonia, which may be toxic.

Amino acids absorbed from the intestines in surplus to the needs of the body as well those that are released after normal cell turnover are used for the production of energy, for the synthesis of new proteins, or for ketogenesis or glucogenesis, or are metabolized further into urea (Fig. 8-11). Urea is excreted in urine and feces. Urea that is excreted in kidneys leaves the body, but the urea excreted into the intestine is again cleaved by urease-containing bacteria, and the newly formed ammonia is absorbed into the portal circulation and sent back to the liver. Approximately 10 to 20 g of nitrogen are produced every 24 hours in an average adult and excreted.

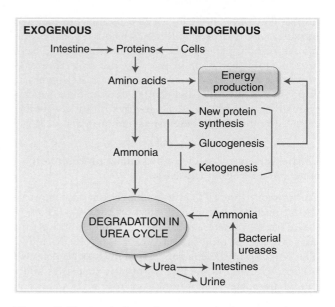

Figure 8-11 Metabolism of amino acids. Amino acids entering the liver cell are used for energy production, new protein synthesis, glucogenesis, or ketogenesis. Unused amino acids are degraded through the urea cycle. Urea is excreted in the urine or into the intestines. In the intestines urease-rich bacteria metabolize urea into ammonia, which is recirculated to the liver.

DISTURBANCES OF HEPATIC SYNTHETIC FUNCTIONS

Chronic liver disease leads to decreased synthesis of serum albumin and hypoalbuminemia.

Albumin is the most abundant serum protein, but it occurs also in interstitial fluids. In an adult the total body pool of albumin is approximately 300 g, of which 40% is inside the circulating blood and 60% in the extravascular pool. Its normal blood concentration is 3.5 to 5 g/dL, and the liver must produce about 12 g of albumin a day to keep it in that range.

Since the liver is the only source of albumin, chronic destructive liver disease and especially cirrhosis manifest with hypoalbuminemia. **Hypoalbuminemia** is therefore one of the best indicators of reduced hepatic synthetic capacity. Not every patient with chronic liver disease, and even many with cirrhosis, demonstrates hypoalbuminemia. The half-life of albumin in the plasma is 21 days, and thus even if production ceases it takes some time before the concentration in the serum drops below the normal range. Furthermore, the loss of liver synthetic function is usually in part compensated for by adaptive reduction in the degradation of albumin. However, demonstrable hypoalbuminemia is a reliable sign of chronic liver insufficiency.

Hypoalbuminemia may be aggravated in patients with portal hypertension by excessive leakage of albumin from the blood into the ascites fluid or the lymph away from its

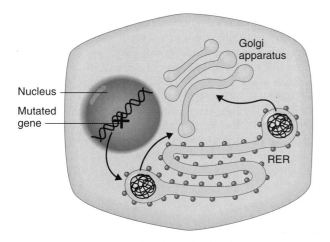

Figure 8-10 α₁-Antitrypsin (AAT) deficiency. Genetic mutation interferes with the folding of the AAT in the cisterns of rough endoplasmic reticulum (RER), inhibiting the transfer of proteins from the rough endoplasmic reticulum to the Golgi apparatus. The abnormal AAT accumulates in the form of round aggregates inside the RER.

normal flow through the liver. Hypoalbuminemia may also be partly related to poor nutrition, which is especially common in cirrhotic patients who are chronic alcoholics. Finally, bear in mind that albumin is a *"negative acute-phase reactant";* that is, the liver reduces the synthesis of albumin in response to many acute and chronic diseases. Since patients with advanced cirrhosis usually feel sick, this is yet another reason why they might have hypoalbuminemia.

Cirrhosis is associated with prolonged prothrombin time and a bleeding tendency.

Prothrombin time (PT) is a functional test that measures the intrinsic and common coagulation pathways. The normal PT is 12 minutes, and it depends on a normal plasma concentration of prothrombin and factors VII, IX, and X. The synthesis of these factors is vitamin K-dependent and occurs exclusively in the liver. In massive acute liver injury caused by acute viral infection or toxins, as well as in chronic liver diseases such as cirrhosis, PT is prolonged. Impaired absorption of fat due to defective bile synthesis and excretion may affect the absorption of fat-soluble vitamins, such as vitamin K, thus contributing to the reduced production of coagulation factors.

Serum levels of ceruloplasmin are reduced in Wilson's disease.

Ceruloplasmin is a serum protein involved in the transport of copper. Like most other serum proteins it is synthesized by the liver. In Wilson's disease, an inborn error of copper metabolism, serum levels of ceruloplasmin are markedly reduced. Although the reasons for this phenomenon are unknown, low ceruloplasmin concentration is a reliable sign of Wilson's disease, especially if associated with a high concentration of copper in liver biopsy specimens or urine.

Acute and chronic diseases stimulate the liver to secrete acute-phase reactants.

Various inflammatory diseases, as well as chronic debilitating diseases such as cancer, may stimulate the liver to synthesize a variety of proteins known as acute-phase reactants. This group of proteins includes the C-reactive protein; a number of serum transport proteins, such as transferrin and ceruloplasmin; some coagulation factors, such as fibrinogen; and enzyme inhibitors, such as antichymotrypsin. Interleukins produced by the inflammatory cells are the mediators of this liver response, but its purpose remains unknown.

C-reactive proteins (CRPs) can be estimated indirectly by a widely used test—the *erythrocyte sedimentation rate* (ESR). In this test, a calibrated tube is filled with venous blood and allowed to settle for 1 and 2 hours. The extent of separation of the red blood cells from the plasma is measured in millimeters and expressed as the observed ESR value.

C-reactive protein, the main acute-phase reactant, is routinely measured in clinical practice and provides the same information as ESR, meaning that it indicates whether the patient has some systemic disease or demonstrates a focus of inflammation in the body. C-reactive protein is a elevated in patients who have myocardial infarction, but its serum concentration falls during recovery. Persistently high values for serum CRP or their rise after normalization is a good predictor for the recurrence of myocardial ischemia following an infarction.

Among acute-phase reactants produced by the liver, the **serum amyloid A precursor** is also worth mentioning. This protein, if produced in large quantities, may be deposited in the kidneys, liver, adrenals, spleen, and other organs in the form of amyloid, thereby causing systemic amyloidosis. This disease may have a protean manifestation, but overall it has a poor prognosis and cannot be cured with our present means.

DISTURBANCES OF DETOXIFICATION

The liver is involved in the detoxification and degradation of numerous endogenous and exogenous potentially toxic substances, drugs, and metabolites. It also plays a role in degradation and inactivation of hormones.

The liver detoxifies drugs and toxins.

The liver is the major site of drug metabolism and detoxification of toxins. Some drugs are ingested in an inactive form and become active only after conversion into an active form in the liver. Lipid-soluble drugs are made water-soluble by the **cytochome P$_{450}$** family of enzymes. During this process P$_{450}$ unmasks or introduces into the drugs polar groups such as —OH or —NH$_2$. Thereafter many of these drugs can be excreted by the kidneys, whereas others need to be further conjugated to make them less lipophilic. This conjugation includes binding to glucuronic, sulfuric, or acetic acid. **Glucuronidation** is the most common form of drug conjugation in the liver. Glucuronidation of drugs is inefficient in neonates; many drugs cannot therefore be inactivated and are potentially toxic during the neonatal period. Detoxification of drugs is defective in patients who have cirrhosis; thus the blood concentration of many antibiotics, psychopharmaceuticals, and hypoglycemics may remain high for prolonged periods in such patients.

The liver degrades and neutralizes ammonia, thus disabling its toxicity.

Cirrhosis and massive liver necrosis may reduce the capacity of the liver to remove ammonia formed from the degraded amino acids. In cirrhotic patients with portal hypertension the blood bypasses the liver through the portal-systemic anastomoses, further contributing to body's inability to remove ammonia. If the portal hypertension-related esophageal varices rupture and the patient has a massive bleed, the swallowed blood becomes yet another source of ammonia. Blood is a protein-rich fluid, and when it arrives into the intestines, the proteins are degraded into amino acids and further into ammonia. Hyperammonemia resulting from any of these complications of cirrhosis has a potentially toxic effect on the brain and is considered to play an important pathogenetic role in hepatic encephalopathy (Fig. 8-12).

The liver inactivates and degrades hormones.

Many hormones act on the liver. For example, glucagon and insulin regulate the uptake and metabolism of glucose in the liver. Many hormones are inactivated or degraded by the liver. All steroid hormones, such as corticosteroids, aldosterone, and sex hormones, are inactivated and degraded in the liver. The liver is involved in the metabolism of parathyroid and thyroid hormone, insulin, and many others.

> **Pearl**
>
> > Inadequate degradation of estrogen in cirrhotic livers leads to hyperestrinemia, which may cause gynecomastia, spider telangiectasias, and palmar erythema.

DISTURBANCES OF BILIRUBIN METABOLISM AND EXCRETION

Bilirubin derived from the heme component of the hemoglobin is bound to albumin and carried to the liver.

Approximately 4 mg/kg of bilirubin is formed daily, mostly from the heme component of hemoglobin released from effete red blood cells (Fig. 8-13). A smaller part of the newly formed bilirubin (15% to 20%) is derived from ineffective

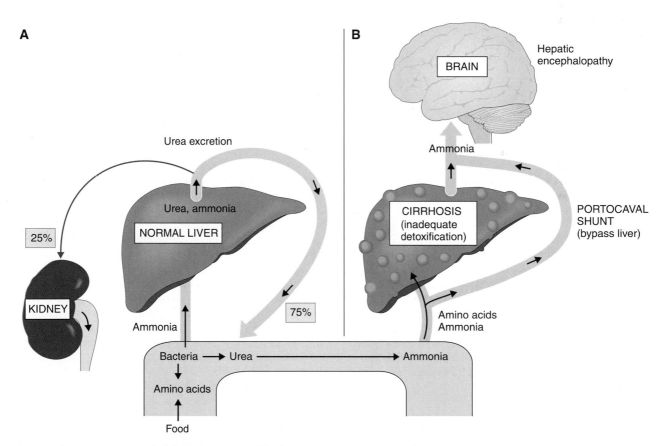

Figure 8-12 Hepatic encephalopathy. **A,** Normal liver. Amino acids absorbed from the intestines are metabolized by the liver, and the potentially toxic ammonia is converted into urea and excreted into the intestines or urine. Ammonia formed in the intestines through the action of bacteria is neutralized by the liver as well. **B,** Cirrhosis. The liver cannot degrade the ammonia entering the portal vein system from the intestines. Furthermore, the portocaval anastomoses provide venues for the ammonia-containing portal blood to bypass the liver. Thus, the systemic circulation is flooded with extra ammonia, which is toxic and can induce hepatic encephalopathy.

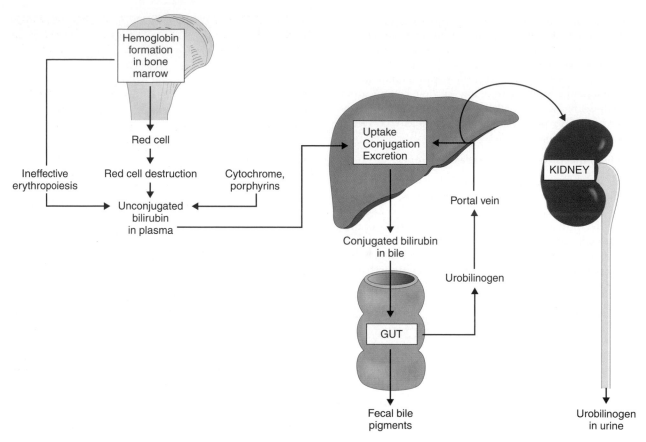

Figure 8-13 Bilirubin formation and excretion.

hematopoiesis and heme-containing enzymes such as P_{450} oxidoreductases or other porphyrins.

Biliribin formed from heme is water-insoluble. It must attach to albumin to be transported to the liver for further processing and excretion in the bile. Since it has not been conjugated in the liver it is also known as **unconjugated bilirubin.** Owing to the links to albumin it cannot enter into the urine and it does not cross the normal blood–brain barrier.

Unconjugated bilirubin is elevated in the serum in conditions that lead to increased hemolysis, such as autoimmune hemolytic anemia, hereditary spherocytosis, or sickle cell anemia. Ineffective hematopoiesis, as in megaloblastic anemia caused by vitamin B_{12} or folic acid deficiency, may also cause unconjugated hyperbilirubinemia (i.e., prehepatic jaundice).

Bilirubin taken up by hepatocytes is conjugated to glucuronide.

The bilirubin–albumin complex binds to the basolateral side of hepatocytes. It dissociates from albumin and is actively transported across the plasma membrane into the cytoplasm of liver cells. At least three distinct mechanisms participate in this process. In the cytoplasm bilirubin is

transferred into the endoplasmic reticulum, most likely by direct membrane-to-membrane transfer. In the endoplasmic reticulum bilirubin is then conjugated through the action of uridine disphosphate (UDP) and uridine glucuronyltransferase (UGT) into monoglucuronides and diglucuronides and readied for excretion (Fig. 8-14).

UGT is a large family of enzymes that are active in many organs. In the liver UGT1A1 performs most of the glucuronidation of bilirubin. Hence it is to no surprise that mutations of the gene encoding UGT1A1 account for most hereditary unconjugated hyperbilirubinemias. The most important among these diseases are the Gilbert and Crigler-Najjar syndromes.

- **Gilbert syndrome** is an common periodic unconjugated hyperbilirubinemia that is related to mutations in the promoter region of the *UGT1A1* gene or a missense mutation of the *UGT1A1* gene itself.
- **Crigler-Najjar syndrome** is an unconjugated hyperbilirubinemia that occurs in two forms. Type I of the syndrome is characterized by severe congenital hyperbilirubinemia that has a high mortality rate in infancy. It is also related to the mutation of the *UGT1A1* gene, resulting in the complete lack of the enzyme in liver

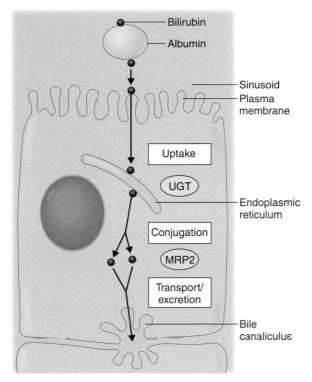

Figure 8-14 Intrahepatic processing of bilirubin. The unconjugated bilirubin bound to albumin is delivered in the blood to the liver, where it binds to the cell surface thus dissociating from albumin. Bilirubin enters into the liver cells and is transferred to the endoplasmic reticulum. Inside the endoplasmic reticulum bilirubin is bound to glucuronic acid through the action of uridine glucuronosyltransferases (UGTs). Water-soluble bilirubin monoglucuronides and diglucuronides, which account for 80% of the total conjugated bilirubin, are transported into the bile canaliculi by enzymes such as multidrug resistance protein 2 (MRP2).

cells. In Crigler-Najjar syndrome type II, the activity of UGT1A1 is markedly reduced, but it still can form monoglucuronides.

Uptake and conjugation of bilirubin in hepatocytes may be affected by many forms of **hepatocellar injury** and **various drugs.** Functional immaturity of hepatocytes combined with increased hemolysis of fetal red blood cells in the early postnatal period accounts for **neonatal physiologic jaundice.**

Bilirubin is excreted into the bile canaliculi in a water-soluble form.

Bilirubin monoglucuronides and diglucuronides are water-soluble and are readily excreted into the bile. Conjugated bilirubin is transported across the plasma membrane by canalicular organic anion transporter multidrug resistance protein 2 (MRP2). Mutation of the gene for the ATP-binding

cassette (ABC) of the canalicular organic anion transporter protein MRP2 results in **Dubin-Johnson syndrome,** which is characterized by conjugated hyperbilirubinemia and mild jaundice but no other major problems.

Bilirubin reaches the intestine through the bile ducts.

Bilirubin in bile has an average concentration of 0.2%, yet it gives the bile its typical yellow-brown color. Bile flows from the intercellular canaliculi into the bile ducts in the portal tracts and from there through larger bile ducts to the hilum of the liver and into the common bile duct. Obstruction of bile ducts causes regurgitation of bilirubin into the blood and *conjugated hyperbilirubinemia.* Clinically it manifests as **obstructive jaundice.** The most important causes of obstructive jaundice are illustrated in Figure 8-15.

Bilirubin is transformed in the intestines by bacteria into urobilinogen.

Bacteria in the intestines hydrolyze the conjugated bilirubin into free bilirubin, which is further reduced into several pyrroles known as urobilinogen. Most of the urobilinogen is excreted in feces, but approximately 20% is reabsorbed and through the enterohepatic recirculation returns to the liver. Part of reabsorbed urobilinogen is excreted in the urine, accounting for its yellowish color.

DISTURBANCES OF BILE CIRCULATION

The liver cells produce bile and excrete it into the bile ductules.

Bile is a complex bicarbonate-rich fluid produced by the liver cells and excreted through the biliary ducts into the intestines. Approximately 450 mL of canalicular bile is

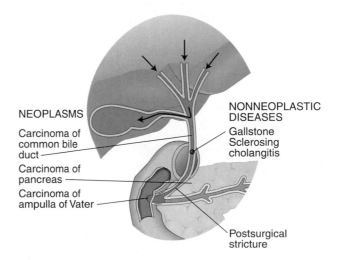

Figure 8-15 Extrahepatic obstructive jaundice. The diseases causing jaundice are classified as neoplastic or nonneoplastic.

produced daily, which is supplemented with about 150 mL of ductular secretion to account for a total of 600 mL.

The bile is a complex fluid that consists principally of water (97%) and the following solutes:

- Bile acids
- Phospholipids (lecithin)
- Cholesterol
- Proteins
- Bilirubin
- Minerals

The concentration of various solutes in the bile varies enormously. Primary biliary acids, cholic and chenodeoxycholic acids, account for 10% to 50% of organic solutes of bile, whereas phospholipids account for 10% to 20%, cholesterol for 3% to 10%. The relationship between these three components determines whether cholesterol remains in a soluble form or precipitates. Proteins account for 3% to 5%, and bilirubin for 0.3% to 2% of organic solutes.

Primary bile acids are produced in the hepatocytes from cholesterol and conjugated to glycine or taurine (Fig. 8-16). Once excreted from the liver cells, bile acids combine with cholesterol and phospholipids to form *micelles*, which are important for the emulsification and subsequent absorption of fat in the small intestine. Bile ductular cells secrete mucus, composed of proteins and carbohydrates, as well as water and minerals.

Primary bile acids are almost completely reabsorbed together with some urobilinogen in the terminal ileum and recirculated back to the liver (*"enterohepatic circulation of biliary acids"*). Small amounts of primary bile acids that reach the colon are transformed by bacteria into *secondary bile acids*, deoxycholic acid and lithocholic acid. Secondary bile acids are mostly lost in the feces, but some are reabsorbed and recirculated to the liver. At any point in time 85% of the total bile acid pool is either in the intestines or in the gallbladder. Thus the liver must replace only a small portion of the total bile acid pool, which is good because the liver has a limited capacity for bile acid production.

A large portion of this hepatic bile is extruded into the duodenum during the meals (Fig. 8-17). Between meals the sphincter of Oddi contracts and redirects the bile flow into the gallbladder, where it is concentrated by a removal of water and stored until needed.

Bile acid concentration can be measured in the serum, and although it changes in various liver diseases, the methods for measuring bile acid concentration in the serum are rather cumbersome. Accordingly, this biochemical test is not widely used in practice.

The liver diseases affect the excretion of bile.

The bile produced by pathologically altered livers differs from normal bile, which might affect the absorption of fats from the intestine. Long-term changes in the composition of bile are associated with steatorrhea and deficiencies in fat-soluble vitamins A, D, E, and K.

Vitamin K deficiency contributes to the prolongation of PT and may account in part for the bleeding tendency of patients who have cirrhosis.

Changes in the composition of bile may predispose to formation of gallstones.

The solutes found in bile remain in a soluble form as long as the relative concentration of cholesterol, bile salt, and lecithin remains in the normal range (Fig. 8-18). Changes in the composition of bile and the presence of substances that promote "nucleation of bile" (e.g., bacteria) may lead to the formation of gallstones.

The conditions that most often predispose to **gallstone** formation include:

- **Hypersaturation of bile with cholesterol.** The excretion of cholesterol is increased in persons who are obese and consume excessive amounts of fat-rich foods. Cholesterol excretion may be increased by blood cholesterol-lowering drugs ("statins"). Because

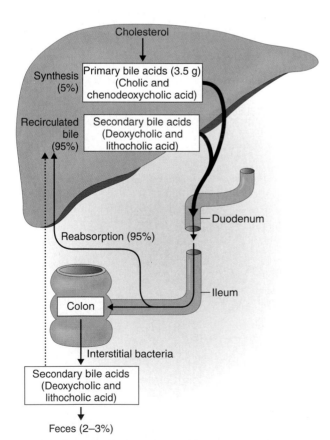

Figure 8-16 Recirculation of bile.

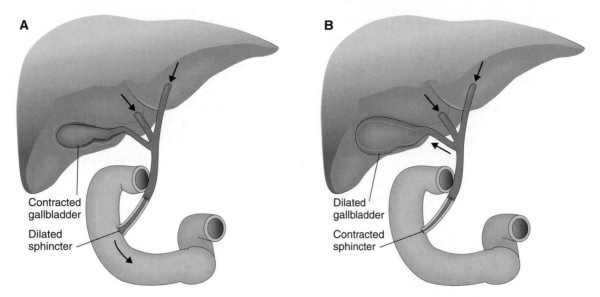

Figure 8-17 Bile flow during feeding and fasting. **A,** During feeding the sphincter of Oddi is relaxed and bile flows into the intestine. The gallbladder contacts, adding the concentrated bile to the newly synthesized bile flowing out of the liver. **B,** During fasting the sphincter of Oddi is contracted and the flow of bile in the common bile duct is redirected into the gallbladder, where it is stored and concentrated.

cholesterol is insoluble in water it must be kept in solution by bile acids and phospholipids, primarily lecithin. If the concentration of cholesterol exceeds the capacity of bile acids and lecithin to keep cholesterol in solution, it begins forming aggregates. However, hypersaturation of bile with cholesterol is not enough for the production of gallstones. Apparently, cholesterol does not always "nucleate" unless other factors are present that promote this process. Thus, the pathogenesis of gallstones is considered to be

mutifactorial and cannot be explained only in terms of hypersaturation of bile with cholesterol.

■ **Obstruction of bile flow.** These changes influence the absorptive properties of the gallbladder's mucosa, favoring the absorption of water and concentration of bile. Grossly visible sludge that is formed from cholesterol crystals in hypersaturated bile is normally expelled by the vigorous gallbladder contractions. Such contractions cannot occur if the gallbladder is infected or if the biliary ducts are obstructed. Pregnancy also

Figure 8-18 Phase diagram for plotting different mixtures of bile salt, lecithin, and cholesterol. Mixtures containing 4% to 10% of solids (e.g., point A in the curved area) are nonlithogenic. Any mixture that is out of that zone (e.g., point B) is potentially lithogenic. (From Andreoli TE, Carpenter CCJ, Griggs RC, Loscalzo J: Cecil Essentials of Medicine, 6th ed. Philadelphia, Saunders, 2004, p. 425.)

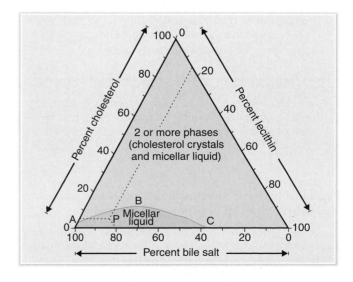

promotes lithogenesis by causing relaxation of smooth muscle cells in the gallbladder and thus reducing its contractility. Mucus, which accumulates in biliary obstruction, also promotes nucleation, and any irritation that stimulates mucus production promotes gallstone formation. Reduced concentration of substances that inhibit gallstone formation, like apolipoprotein A-I, also promotes nucleation.

■ **Infection.** Bacteria alter the function of the gallbladder's mucosa in a way that is similar to the effects of obstruction. Bacteria may serve as "nucleation centers" and also change the composition of bile, thus promoting gallstone formation. In many pigmented stones bacteria can be found. Furthermore, bacteria damage the mucosal cells, and the cell debris may serve as nucleation particles that begin the formation of gallstones.

■ **Excess bilirubin.** Bilirubin produced in excess in chronic hemolytic anemias, such as sickle cell disease, may predispose to the formation of another type of stones—bilirubin stones. Intestinal diseases that promote bacterial deconjugation of bilirubin into less-soluble compounds also promote formation of bilirubin stones.

Gallstones occur in two forms: as cholesterol stones or pigment stones.

Gallstones are classified as cholesterol stones or pigment stones.

■ **Cholesterol stones** (75%) are composed predominantly of cholesterol crystals. Cholesterol accounts for the yellow color of these stones. They may be solitary, ovoid, and large, or multiple and multifaceted. Pure cholesterol stones are not visible on plain radiographs. They are asymptomatic in more than 80% of cases.

■ **Pigment stones** (25%) are either brown or black. They are composed predominantly of calcium bilirubinate and other calcium salts. Due to their calcium content they are visible in plain radiographs. They are often small, multiple, and friable. Thus they may more easily obstruct the cystic duct and cause biliary colic than the larger cholesterol stones.

Pearl

> Since most gallstones do not contain calcium and are not visible radiographically; ultrasound is the best way to detect gallstones.

Intestinal bacterial overgrowth causes deconjugation and dehydroxylation of primary biliary acids.

Surgically generated intestinal pouches and anastomoses may produce so-called *blind loop syndrome*, in which a part of the intestinal loop is overgrown by bacteria. These bacteria may transform primary biliary salts into less efficient secondary biliary salts. Secondary salts are not only less efficient emulsifiers, but they are also more readily lost in the feces. Malabsorption with steatorrhea develops in such cases. Chronic intestinal infections also predispose to gallstone formation by promoting the deconjugation of bilirubin into less-soluble derivatives, which tend to form precipitates in the gallbladder more often than the soluble derivatives do.

Interruption of the enterohepatic circulation of bile acids causes diarrhea.

Most of the bile acids are absorbed in the terminal part of the small intestine. Diseases that affect the terminal ileum, such as Crohn's disease, or surgical resection of the terminal ileum may interrupt the enterohepatic circulation of the bile acids. This may affect the intestinal digestion in two ways and produce either a choleretic secretory diarrhea or steatorrhea.

■ **Choleretic diarrhea** results from an excess of bile salts entering the colon. These salts stimulate the colonic cells to secrete water, and a watery diarrhea develops. Bile acid binders, such as cholestyramine, can reduce the flux of bile acids into the colon and reduce the watery diarrhea.

■ **Steatorrhea** develops once the loss of bile acids has depleted the bile acid pool, and the liver synthesis cannot compensate for the loss of bile acids in the stools. Lack of bile acids in the bile reaching the small intestine results in impaired absorption of lipids from food.

Clinical and Laboratory Evaluation of Liver Diseases

Initial evaluation of patients suspected of having liver disease includes a complete history and physical examination and standard laboratory testing. If indicated, additional testing with ultrasound, CT scanning, and invasive techniques such as liver biopsy may be recommended.

FAMILY AND PERSONAL HISTORY

Family and personal history may be important because such data may identify potential risk factors and point to the cause of liver disease. Furthermore one may determine whether the liver disease is limited to that organ or is part of a multisystemic disease, whether it is acute or chronic, and what the nature of the disease is. Risk factors for liver diseases that can be noticed in family and personal history are listed in Table 8-2.

Constitutional symptoms are common in most liver diseases. These nonspecific symptoms include fatigue, loss of appetite (anorexia), easy fatigability, malaise, and weight loss.

Fever is associated with many forms of hepatic infection, such as viral hepatitis or bacterial and parasitic liver and biliary tract infections. Systemic infections and sepsis may also affect the liver.

Table 8-2 Risk Factors for Various Liver Diseases

RISK FACTORS	LIVER DISEASE
Family history of liver disease	Hemochromatosis Wilson's disease α_1-Antitrypsin deficiency
History of blood transfusion, professional exposure to blood, unsafe sex practice	Viral hepatitis B, C
Travel to tropical countries	Viral hepatitis A, amebic abscess
Alcohol consumption	Alcoholic hepatitis, cirrhosis
Medications	Drug-induced acute or chronic hepatitis
Autoimmune diseases, such as SLE, Hashimoto's thyroiditis, atrophic gastritis	Autoimmune hepatitis, primary biliary cirrhosis
Ulcerative colitis	Primary sclerosing cholangitis
Pulmonary emphysema	α_1-Antitrypsin deficiency
Diabetes mellitus	Steatohepatitis or fatty liver
"Four F's" (female, fertile, over forty, and fat)	Gallstones

SLE, systemic lupus erythematosus.

PHYSICAL EXAMINATION

Symptoms and signs of liver disease are not limited to the liver itself and may be seen in many other parts of the body. The most important symptoms and signs suggesting liver diseases or their major complications are as follows:

- Jaundice
- Abdominal swelling due to ascites and splenomegaly
- Hemorrhagic diathesis and bleeding into the skin
- Gastrointestinal bleeding
- Vascular spiders and palmar erythema
- Gynecomastia and loss of libido (in men)
- Hepatomegaly and sensitivity of the liver to palpation
- Pruritus and xanthomas
- Shortness of breath
- Oliguria and renal insufficiency
- Neurologic disturbances (e.g., asterxis), somnolence or coma

Jaundice results from hyperbilirubinemia and the deposition of bilirubin in tissues.

Jaundice (Latin, *icterus*) is characterized by yellow discoloration of skin and mucosae. It is associated with hyperbilirubinemia, an elevation of blood bilirubin concentration over the normal value of 1 mg/dL (17 μmol/L). Jaundice usually becomes clinically apparent when the concentration of bilirubin in blood exceeds 2 mg/dL (34 μmol/L).

Under normal circumstances the serum contains less than 1 mg/dL bilirubin. All this bilirubin is an **unconjugated form.** Since it cannot be measured directly by adding the reagent (diazotized sulfanilic acid) to the serum it is called indirect bilirubin. **Conjugated** bilirubin, which is present only in jaundiced patients, can be measured directly and is thus called direct bilirubin. Although no conjugated bilirubin is present in the blood of healthy persons, up to 30% of the unconjugated bilirubin reacts in a direct manner. Thus, using routine laboratory tests it is not possible to estimate the "true" value of conjugated bilirubin in normal blood and even in low-grade hyperbilirubinemia under 4 mg/dL.

Hyperbilirubinemia that accompanies jaundice can be classified as predominantly unconjugated or conjugated. The causes of predominantly **unconjugated hyperbilirubinemia** (direct bilirubin < 20% of elevated level of total bilirubin) are, in practice, limited to hematologic conditions characterized by hemolysis and inefficient hematopoiesis, or hereditary diseases involving conjugation of bilirubin (Gilbert and Crigler-Najjar syndromes). Conjugated hyperbilirubinemia may be caused by hereditary liver diseases (e.g., Dubin-Johnson and Rotor's syndrome), acute and chronic liver diseases (e.g., viral hepatitis or cirrhosis), or intrahepatic and extrahepatic biliary obstruction. Major causes of predominantly unconjugated or conjugated jaundice are listed in Table 8-3.

Ascites and splenomegaly are signs of portal hypertension.

Ascites is a form of localized edema in which serous fluid accumulates in the abdominal cavity. Splenomegaly is defined as enlargement of the spleen that can be clinically detected. When found together, ascites and splenomegaly are almost invariably caused by portal hypertension. Remember, however, that both ascites and splenomegaly may occur independently and may have many causes.

Table 8-3 Causes of Jaundice (Hyperbilirubinemia)

PREDOMINANTLY UNCONJUGATED HYPERBILIRUBINEMIA	PREDOMINANTLY CONJUGATED HYPERBILIRUBINEMIA
Hemolysis Blood transfusion reaction Autoimmune hemolytic anemia, hemoglobinopathies (sickle cell anemia, thalassemia, etc.) **Inefficient Hematopoiesis** Vitamin B$_{12}$ deficiency Folic acid deficiency **Defective Uptake and Conjugation** Neonatal jaundice Gilbert syndrome Crigler-Najjar syndrome Hepatocellular injury Drugs (e.g., rifampin, chloramphenicol) Radiographic contrast agents	**Defective Excretion from Liver Cells** Dubin-Johnson syndrome Rotor syndrome **Liver Cell Injury** Viral hepatitis Drugs and toxins Shock and sepsis Chronic hepatitis of various origins **Bile Duct Obstruction** Gallstones Tumors of the head of pancreas, common bile duct, ampulla of Vater Biliary strictures—congenital (stenosis or atresia) or acquired (postsurgical fibrosis)

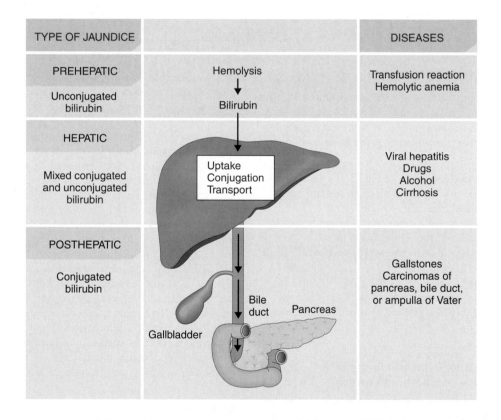

In clinical practice it is important to determine the cause of ascites. Accordingly, it is advisable to take a sample of ascites fluid and analyze it. Cytologic examination determines whether malignant cells are present. The presence of neutrophils and positive bacteriologic findings point to an infectious cause. The presence of amylase and lipase are evidence of pancreatic disease.

One of the most important tests performed on ascites fluid is the measurement of protein content and, most importantly, albumin. Albumin content of ascites is expressed as a ratio of albumin in serum and ascites. *High serum–ascites albumin ratio* (>1.1 g/dL) is typical of portal hypertension, but may be found is some other conditions as well, most notably in congestive heart failure. *Low serum–ascites albumin ratio* (< 1.1 g/dL) is found in ascites caused by malignant peritoneal tumors, infection, or pancreatitis (Table 8-4).

Pearls

> Ascites caused by cirrhosis and ascites causedcongestive heart failure are both characterized by a high S/A ratio. Protein concentration in the ascites fluid helps to distinguish these two conditions: In cirrhosis the protein content is less than 2.5 g/dL; in heart failure protein content is greater than 2.5 g/dL.
> Sudden onset of ascites is a sign of Budd-Chiari syndrome, which may be caused by thrombi, hematologic disease, or liver tumors obstructing the hepatic vein.

Other factors besides portal hypertension may contribute to the pathogenesis of ascites.

All patients with cirrhosis who develop ascites have portal hypertension, but not all of those who have cirrhosis have ascites. Obviously, something else besides portal hypertension is at work. Three major theories have been proposed to explain why fluid accumulates in the abdominal cavity and how ascites is related to renal handling of water and minerals: the (1) underfilling theory, (2) overflow theory, and (3) theory of increased sympathetic activity.

The underfilling theory postulates that the process is initiated by portal hypertension, which leads to transudation of fluid into the abdominal cavity. The water drained from the blood vessels generates a sense of underfilling, triggering a baroreceptor response. It stimulates the renin–angiotensin–aldosterone system to reduce sodium and water excretion in the kidneys, resulting in water retention. According to the *overflow theory*, the initial event is the renal retention of sodium and water with a subsequent overflow of this water into the peritoneal cavity. The third theory postulates that *increased sympathetic activity* and subsequent peripheral arterial dilatation are the primary events. According to this theory hyperactivity of the sympathetic system leads to dilatation of the peripheral vasculature, causing a sense of underfilling. At the same time the dilatation of the splanchnic vasculature leads to portal hypertension and stimulates the transudation of fluid into the peritoneal cavity.

Irrespective of the arguments about the initial events, the pathogenesis of ascites could be related to three major disturbances (Fig. 8-19). These pathogenetic factors are:

- Mechanical obstruction of the blood flow through the liver
- Reduced synthetic activity of the liver
- Hormonal and sympathetic regulation of blood flow

Mechanical obstruction of the blood and lymph flow through the cirrhotic liver is a consequence of fibrosis, formation of regeneratory nodules, and a loss of normal hepatic architecture. Obstruction of the blood flow leads to *portal hypertension* and *transudation of fluid* from the congested splanchnic veins. Obstruction of the lymph flow leads to the pouring of *lymph fluid* into the abdominal cavity.

Reduced synthetic activity of the liver accounts for the *hypoalbuminemia.* Since albumin concentration of blood determines its osmotic potential, hypoalbuminemia is associated with the inability of plasma to keep the water inside the blood vessels resulting in hypo-osmotic edema.

Increased sympathetic activity is found in most cases of cirrhosis with ascites. Sympathomimetic stimuli lead to dilatation of splanchnic vessels and increased blood influx into the portal system, contributing to portal hypertension. At the same time arterioles in the systemic vasculature dilate, leading to a disproportion between the arteriolar space and the amount of fluid to fill it. The heart must work harder and pump more blood, again promoting transudation in the peripheral vessels.

Dilatation of arterioles generates the "underfilling effect," which triggers the baroreceptors to activate the renin–angiotensin–aldosterone system. Retention of sodium and water ensues in the kidney, resulting in oliguria and "overflow" of fluid into the ascites. Severe form of water retention results in oliguric renal failure, a phenomenon called hepatorenal syndrome.

Portal hypertension can be classified as hepatic, prehepatic, or posthepatic.

Portal hypertension is most often caused by cirrhosis, but it can have other causes as well. Accordingly, portal hypertension can be classified as (1) sinusoidal, (2) presinusoidal, and (3) postsinusoidal (Fig. 8-20).

Table 8-4 Causes of Ascites

LOW ALBUMIN CONTENT (S/A albumin > 1.1 g/dL)	HIGH ALBUMIN CONTENT (S/A albumin < 1.1 g/dL)
Cirrhosis*	Peritoneal carcinomatosis*
Congestive heart failure*	Pancreatitis
Constrictive pericarditis	Cholecystitis
Budd-Chiari syndrome	Peritonitis
Liver tumors	Hematoperitoneum
Nephrotic syndrome	Nephrotic syndrome
Hypothyroidism	

*Most important causes of ascites.
S/A albumin, serum/ascites ratio of albumin.

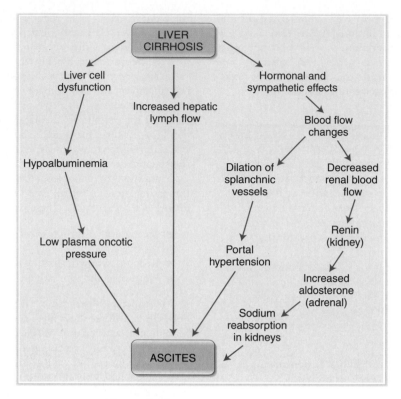

Figure 8-19 Pathogenesis of ascites.

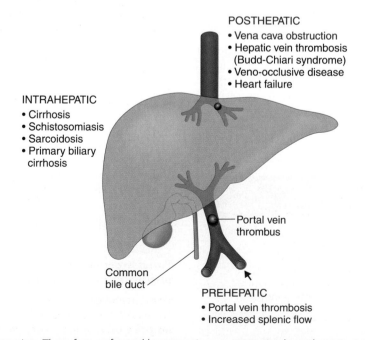

Figure 8-20 Portal hypertension. Three forms of portal hypertension are recognized: posthepatic, intrahepatic, and prehepatic.

Sinusoidal portal hypertension occurs in various liver diseases but is in most instances caused by cirrhosis. Alcoholic hepatitis, congenital hepatic fibrosis, and primary or secondary tumors may also cause this type of portal hypertension.

Presinusoidal portal hypertension may involve the portal vein or the hilus of the liver and the intrahepatic branches of the portal vein all the way to the portal tracts. Accordingly it may be subdivided into two forms: prehepatic and intrahepatic. Portal vein thrombosis or tumors may obstruct the portal veins. Hepatocellular carcinomas have a tendency to invade the veins inside the liver. Portal tract and hilar fibrosis may also be a cause.

Postsinusoidal portal hypertension may be intrahepatic or extrahepatic. Intrahepatic postsinusoidal portal hypertension is most often caused by Budd-Chiari syndrome; that is, obstruction of the hepatic vein with thrombi, hyperviscous blood, or tumors. Constrictive pericarditis, cor pulmonale, and pulmonary hypertension are posthepatic causes of portal hypertension.

Ascites can become infected by bacteria.

Approximately 10% to 20% of patients with long-standing ascites develop signs of bacterial peritonitis. Such infection could originate from the following:

- Inadvertent *iatrogenic infection* (e.g., following tapping of the ascites or surgical interventions)
- *Intra-abdominal infections* spreading to the peritoneal fluid from an infectious focus such as appendicitis or cholecystitis
- No obvious predisposing conditions. This **spontaneous bacterial peritonitis** (SBP) is defined as bacterial infection of ascites without any obvious causes of intra-abdominal infection. SBP occurs most often in patients who have large-volume ascites and a low protein content (<1.5 g/dL).

Spontaneous bacterial peritonitis is the most common cause of infected ascites. Typical symptoms of SBP include fever, abdominal pain, and abdominal tenderness. However, many patients are asymptomatic. Suspected infection can be documented by finding neutrophils in freshly prepared smears or by counting the cell content in ascites fluid. Typically infection is present if the neutrophil count is more than 250 neutrophils/μL. Bacteriologic cultures become positive, especially if the ascites fluid is drained into the bacteriologic tube at the bedside.

The pathogenesis of SBP is unknown, but several factors may contribute as follows:

- *Increased permeability of the intestinal wall* caused by ascites fluid and portal hypertension. Since the intestine normally contains saprophytic bacteria, it is easy to envision these bacteria crossing the intestinal wall and infecting the ascites fluid.
- *Rupture of small branches of the portal vein.* In portal hypertension the venous blood in the intestines may

contain bacteria that have entered the slow-flowing blood in dilated enteric veins.
- Collaterals between portal and systemic veins allow the portal blood to bypass the liver and its system for elimination of bacteria (i.e., sinusoidal Kupffer cells).

In typical SBP ascites usually contains a single bacterium. Most often such cultures yield enterogenic bacteria, such as *Escherichia coli* and enterococci (group D streptococci). In contrast to SBP, infections due to iatrogenic causes or foci of infection are multimicrobial.

Pearl

> Polymicrobial outgrowth from cultured ascites fluid should prompt a search for a focus of intra-abdominal infection.

Hemorrhagic diathesis is a consequence of reduced synthesis and inactivation of coagulation factors by the liver.

Cirrhotic patients have a hemorrhagic diathesis evidenced by a tendency to bleed spontaneously into the skin and mucosae after surgical procedures or trauma. Both the *prothrombin time* (PT) and the *activated partial thromboplastin time* (aPTT) are prolonged, indicating that neither the intrinsic nor the extrinsic coagulation pathway is functioning normally.

The primary reason for the prolonged PT and aPTT is the reduced synthesis of coagulation factors in the damaged liver. The second reason lies in the defective scavenger function of the liver. Under normal circumstances the liver regulates the coagulation cascade by removing the activated coagulation factors from circulation. If these activated factors are not removed, a state of smoldering intravascular coagulation persists and depletes coagulation factors from the blood.

Splenomegaly may cause thrombocytopenia, anemia, and leukopenia.

Some cirrhotic patients have *thrombocytopenia, anemia,* and *leukopenia.* These hematologic abnormalities are consequences of splenomegaly and are part of a hematologic syndrome called **hypersplenism.** Primarily it is a consequence of increased sequestration of blood cells in the enlarged spleen. Thrombocytopenia may contribute to the hemorrhagic diathesis in patients with cirrhosis.

Gastrointestinal bleeding is a complication of portal hypertension and hemorrhagic diathesis.

Gastrointestinal mucosal bleeding occurs in two forms: (1) capillary mucosal bleeding that occurs due to splanchnic congestion and portal hypertension; and (2) major bleeding from ruptured esophageal varices.

Massive bleeding from esophageal varices has the following symptoms and complications:

- **Hematemesis.** Massive bleeding and vomiting of blood may cause significant hypotension. Ensuing hypovolemic shock due to blood loss may be lethal. The mortality rate is still high, ranging from 30% to 60%.
- **Melena.** Black discoloration of stools results from hematin, the black pigment formed from hemoglobin exposed to hydrochloric acid in the stomach.
- **Hepatic encephalopathy.** It is mostly related to an influx of ammonia formed from the digested amino acids in the protein-rich blood that was digested in the intestines.
- **Hepatorenal syndrome.** It is most likely precipitated by hypotension caused by massive blood loss and ensuing circulatory disturbances.

Relative hyperestrinemia may cause several symptoms that can be discovered on physical examination.

Hyperestrinemia in patients with cirrhosis has two causes: (1) estrogen that is not inactivated in the pathologically altered liver remains in an active form in circulation, (2) testosterone that is not inactivated in the liver undergoes peripheral conversion in the fat tissue, generating additional estrogen.

Estrogens may produce *palmar erythema* and *vascular spiders* (telangiectasiae) on the skin of the chest. In men estrogen may induce *gynecomastia*. It may have inhibitory effects on the pituitary testicular axis, reducing *libido* and ultimately causing *testicular atrophy*.

Hepatomegaly may be a sign of liver cell cancer but can also occur in non-neoplastic liver diseases.

Rapidly growing tumors may cause enlargement of the liver. However, many other non-neoplastic inflammatory and metabolic diseases, such as acute viral hepatitis or fatty liver of alcoholism, may cause liver enlargement. Other causes of hepatomegaly are listed in Table 8-5.

Chronic biliary obstruction is accompanied by itching and formation of xanthomas.

Liver diseases (e.g., primary biliary cirrhosis) that cause long-standing obstructive jaundice are associated with increased blood concentrations of cholesterol and bile acids—substances that cannot be excreted in the bile. Excess *cholesterol* is deposited in the skin and taken up by macrophages that form small yellow skin nodules called xanthomas. Similar yellow nodules and plaques on the eyelids are called xanthelasma. An excess of *bile acids* in circulating blood acts on sensory nerves in the skin causing itching (Latin, *pruritus*).

Table 8-5 Causes of Hepatomegaly

Inflammatory Liver Diseases
Acute viral hepatitis
Alcoholic hepatitis
Septic hepatomegaly
Bacterial cholangitis or abscesses
Parasitic infections (e.g., echinococcosis, schistosomiasis)

Chronic Liver Diseases
Chronic hepatitis
Cirrhosis
Autoimmune diseases, systemic or limited to the liver (e.g., autoimmune hepatitis, primary biliary cirrhosis)

Metabolic Diseases
Fatty liver (e.g., due to obesity, alcoholism, diabetes)
Genetic metabolic/storage diseases
Amyloidosis
Hepatic porphyria

Biliary Diseases
Biliary obstruction
Drug-induced cholestasis
Congenital polycystic liver disease

Circulatory Liver Diseases
Acute or chronic congestive hepatomegaly due to heart disease
Shock
Budd-Chiari syndrome

Neoplasms
Primary liver tumors
Metastases
Leukemia and lymphoma

Shortness of breath may be a sign of the hepatopulmonary syndrome.

Shortness of breath and even dyspnea at rest are found in 10% to 15% patients with cirrhosis. These symptoms are related to functional changes in pulmonary blood flow called the **hepatopulmonary syndrome.** Functional changes are not accompanied by any detectable pathologic changes in the lung parenchyma. The changes include precapillary vascular dilatation and arteriovenous right-to-left shunting of blood. Accordingly, the venous blood does not reach the alveolar capillaries and remains unoxygenated. Because of hypoxemia the patients experience dyspnea. At present there is no known treatment for this complication of cirrhosis.

Oliguria and renal failure are signs of the hepatorenal syndrome.

Cirrhosis accompanied by ascites may lead to renal failure and oliguria without any pathologic changes in the kidneys. This functional renal failure, considered to be a consequence of renal hypoperfusion brought about by severe intrarenal cortical vasoconstriction, is called the **hepatorenal syndrome.** The diagnosis is based on the following findings:

- Progressive oliguria (<500 mL/day)
- Declining glomerular filtration rate evidenced by serum creatinine above 1.5 mg/dL and 24-hour creatinine clearance below 40 mL/min
- Azotemia that shows a high BUN to creatinine ratio
- Low urine sodium content (<10 mEq/L)
- Absence of granular casts and cellular detritus in the urinary sediment and lack of proteinuria (<500 mg/24 hour)
- Absence of any urinary obstruction or primary kidney disease
- Unresponsiveness to treatment with plasma volume expanders. These findings help in distinguishing this phenomenon from tubular necrosis.

The hepatorenal syndrome is found in less than 5% of all patients with decompensated cirrhosis. Most often it is precipitated by (1) sepsis, (2) attempts to remove ascites by paracentesis, and (3) intensive diuretic treatment. It has a mortality rate of 95%. The kidneys are structurally normal, and if the patient dies they can be used for transplantation.

The hepatorenal syndrome must be distinguished from prerenal azotemia typically found in cardiac failure or acute renal failure due to tubular necrosis. In most instances the clinical data indicate the most likely cause of oliguria, but if that does not help, the sodium concentration in serum, urinary osmolality, and the urine-to-plasma creatinine ratio may be used (Table 8-6).

Hepatic encephalopathy may be acute and severe or chronic and progressive.

Hepatic encephalopathy develops due to a loss of hepatic metabolic functions and the inability of the liver to detoxify ammonia and other potentially toxic substances (e.g., mercaptans or γ-aminobutyric acid [GABA]) absorbed from the intestines. Portal–systemic shunts allow the portal blood to bypass the liver and thus contribute to raising the concentration of neurotoxins in the systemic circulation.

Acute hepatic encephalopathy is dominated by cerebral edema that typically develops after acute massive or subtotal liver necrosis. **Chronic hepatic encephalopathy** develops in patients who have cirrhosis, portal hypertension, and esophageal varices. It is characterized by a progressive evolution of neurologic symptoms, which may be initially quite subtle, but soon become obvious and ultimately end in coma and death.

The early neurologic symptoms may include nothing more than forgetfulness or sleep disturbances, such as sleeping during the day and being awake at night. Mild motor disturbances, evidenced as poor handwriting or an inability to reproduce simple designs (e.g., cannot draw a star or connect numbered dots), are noticed. These patients emit a special s,. As the encephalopathy deepens, the symptoms and signs become more pronounced, and loss of mental capacity (*dementia*), loss of motor coordination, and an inability to perform simple tasks (*apraxia*) ensue. Typical findings include a sweet musty odor called *fetor hepaticus*, considered to be caused by mercaptans, and a flapping tremor of extended hands called *asterixis*. *Coma* is progressive, and although most patients in chronic liver failure respond to treatment it often has a lethal outcome. In stage 4 coma the survival rate is only 20%. The clinical features of the four stages of hepatic encephalopathy are given in Table 8-7.

Hepatic encephalopathy may be a sign of progressive hepatic decompensation, but it may also be precipitated by several events as listed in Table 8-8.

Treatment usually includes restricted intake of animal proteins and reduction of bacterial flora in the intestines using broad-spectrum antibiotics. Lactulose given by mouth remains in the intestinal lumen, where it is fermented into lactic acid. This acid lowers the pH of the intestinal contents, thus trapping ammonia and preventing it from entering the circulation.

LABORATORY FINDINGS

Laboratory tests are important indicators of liver function and are classified into several groups as follows:

- **Markers of liver cell injury.** Serum transaminases are the most sensitive indicators of liver cell injury.

Table 8-6 Laboratory Data Useful for Distinguishing Hepatorenal Syndrome from Prerenal Renal Failure and Renal Failure Due to Renal Tubular Necrosis

LABORATORY FINDINGS	HEPATORENAL SYNDROME	PRERENAL RENAL FAILURE	RENAL TUBULAR NECROSIS
Na+ in urine	<10 mEq/L	<10 mEq/L	>30 mEq/L
Cr urine/plasma ratio	>30	>30	<20
Urine/plasma osmolality	Urinary 100 mOsm > plasma	Urinary 100 mOsm > plasma	Urinary osmolality = plasma osmolality
Urinary sediment	Normal	Normal	Granular casts, debris

Data from Zakim D, Boyer TD: Hepatology: A Textbook of Liver Diseases, 2nd ed. Philadelphia, Saunders, 1990.

Table 8-7 Clinical Stages of Hepatic Encephalopathy

STAGE OF ENCEPHALOPATHY	LEVEL OF CONSCIOUSNESS	NEUROLOGIC ABNORMALITIES
Stage 1	Mild confusion, depression, or irritability Inverted sleep pattern (day–night reversal)	Slight tremor Incoordination Poor handwriting Asterixis
Stage 2	Drowsiness, disorientation Personality changes	Asterixis Muscle rigidity Abnormal reflexes
Stage 3	Stupor—asleep but can be roused When awake, sounds confused and unable to perform higher mental tasks Incoherent speech	Asterixis Hyperactive reflexes Extensor plantar responses
Stage 4	Coma—unarousable	Decerebrate posture Response only to painful stimuli Pupillary reflexes preserved

Bilirubin also leaks into the blood from injured liver cells. Its concentration in blood correlates positively with the extent of liver injury.

- **Measures of synthetic function of liver cells.** The best indicators of synthetic function of liver cells are serum albumin and coagulation factors, usually estimated by measuring PT.
- **Markers of biliary obstruction.** The best indicators of biliary obstruction are serum levels of bilirubin and alkaline phosphatase.
- **Evidence of immunologic disorders.** Elevated total serum immunoglobulin concentration is the best sign of autoimmune hepatitis. Additional antibodies, such as antimitochondrial antibodies, are useful for diagnosing specific immune-mediated diseases.
- **Virologic markers.** These markers are essential for the diagnosis of viral hepatitis.
- **Markers of genetic diseases.** These can include specific proteins, such as α_1-antitrypsin isoforms, or genetic markers for specific diseases.
- **Tumor markers.**

Serum levels of transaminases are raised more in acute than in chronic liver diseases.

Two clinically important transaminases, serum **aspartate aminotransferase (AST)** and **alanine aminotransferase (ALT)**, are the best indicators of liver cell injury. Normal serum contains less than 8 to 20 IU/L of ALT, and 10 to 30 IU/L of AST, but values of up to 60 IU/L may be found in healthy persons. ALT is found almost exclusively in the liver, but AST is nearly ubiquitous, and besides in the liver it also occurs in most major organs, such as the kidneys, skeletal muscle, and brain. Elevation of serum AST may be a conse-

Table 8-8 Causes of Hepatic Encephalopathy

Massive gastroesophageal bleeding from ruptured varices
Infection, especially sepsis
Intensive diuretic treatment
Renal or prerenal azotemia, electrolyte and acid–base disturbances
Surgery, trauma, shock
Excess dietary proteins (especially animal proteins!)
Psychotropic drugs, such as benzodiazepines and opiates

quence of heart or muscle injury, but if combined with an abnormal ALT, it is a reliable sign of liver cell injury.

Marked elevation of AST and ALT, more than 15 times the normal (i.e., over 500 U/L), is indicative of acute liver cell injury. Such laboratory findings are typical of acute viral or drug-induced hepatitis, necrosis induced by shock due to sepsis, or cardiac failure and trauma. These changes are usually associated with **conjugated hyperbilirubinemia,** which may manifest as jaundice.

In chronic liver disease that does not cause massive liver cell necrosis, such as in chronic viral hepatitis C or cirrhosis, AST and ALT are elevated in serum two to five times above normal. Similar mild elevation of transaminases may be found in obstructive jaundice as well.

Prothrombin time and serum albumin are the best measures of the synthetic functions of liver cells.

Prothrombin time (PT) is a measure of intrinsic and common coagulation pathway factors. Normally it is 9 to 13 seconds, but it can also be expressed as a ratio of measured-to-control PT, called the international normalized ratio (INR).

Since the half-life of these coagulation factors is short, from a few hours to a few days, the PT becomes abnormal soon after the onset of acute liver failure. Even a short prolongation of PT, for example from 13 seconds (upper limit of normal) to 18 seconds, is a reliable sign of severe acute liver failure. PT is also prolonged in decompensated cirrhosis, but it is relatively insensitive for detecting minor reduction of the synthetic liver cell function.

Albumin is found in serum in a concentration from 3.5 to 5 g/dL. It is produced by the liver at a rate of 10 to 15 g/day. However, since its half-life in circulation is 21 days, the serum albumin pool does not become depleted in acute liver injury. Low levels of serum albumin are typically found in decompensated cirrhosis. Alcohol inhibits protein synthesis, and malnutrition typically encountered in chronic alcoholics contributes further to hypoalbuminemia. Note that hypoalbuminemia may be encountered in many chronic diseases and cachexia. Protein loss in malabsorption syndromes, protein-losing enteropathy, nephrotic syndrome, or skin burns may also cause hypoalbuminemia.

Bilirubin and alkaline phosphatase are the best markers of biliary obstruction.

Bilirubin is present in serum in a range from 0.2 to 1.2 mg/dL (3.4–17.1 μmol/L). It occurs exclusively in an unconjugated form, but 15% may react in a direct manner with the van den Bergh colorimetric reaction, thus giving the impression that the serum contains some conjugated (direct) bilirubin as well. Because of this technical problem fractionation into conjugated and unconjugated bilirubin should not be performed if hyperbilirubinemia is less than 4 mg/dL. In medical practice, fractionation is rarely performed, and only if hyperbilirubinemia is present without an elevation of other liver function tests (LFTs), and in neonatal jaundice.

Hyperbilirubinemia may be caused by unconjugated or conjugated bilirubin. Unconjugated hyperbilirubinemia is related to hemolysis or inefficient hematopoiesis. Hyperbilirubinemia of hepatic origin may be caused by congenital errors of bilirubin metabolism, liver cell injury, or obstruction of bile flow. Except in Gilbert and Crigler-Najjar syndromes, two types of unconjugated hyperbilirubinemia, it is always caused by an increased amount of conjugated bilirubin.

Hyperbilirubinemia is best interpreted in the context of other LFTs. In the presence of high serum AST and ALT levels it is a sign of liver cell injury, for instance that caused by hepatitis virus or drugs. Hyperbilirubinemia associated with an elevation of alkaline phosphatase suggests obstruction of the bile ducts.

Alkaline phosphatase in the serum has a normal concentration of 42 to 98 IU/L in females and 53 to 128 IU/L in males. Most of the enzyme is derived from the liver and the bones, but during pregnancy it may be also of placental origin. High levels are found in the blood of growing children and adolescents. In the elderly, isolated elevation of alkaline phosphatase in serum is most likely related to Paget's disease of bones.

Alkaline phosphatase is located in the intercellular bile canalicular portion of the liver cell plasma membrane. As such it is excreted in the bile, and any biliary obstruction causes a reflux of alkaline phosphatase into the blood. Alkaline phosphatase is typically elevated in the serum of patients who have obstructive jaundice or diseases (e.g., primary biliary cirrhosis or graft-versus-host reaction) that destroy the bile ducts. These diseases cause hyperbilirubinemia. Isolated elevation of alkaline phosphatase in serum without hyperbilirubinemia may be seen in patients who have localized liver disease, such as an abscess, hepatic tumors, or partial biliary obstruction.

γ-Glutamyl transpeptidase (GGT) is a microsomal enzyme that leaks out of damaged liver cells. It is elevated in biliary obstruction but also in other hepatic diseases. In practice it is used primarily for two purposes: to determine whether the elevated alkaline phosphatase is of hepatic or bone origin, and as a marker of alcoholic liver diseases. In contrast to alkaline phosphatase, which is found both in the liver and bones, GGT is found only in the liver. Elevated serum levels of alkaline phosphatase and GGT thus indicate liver disease, whereas alkaline phosphatase elevated in the presence of normal GGT suggests bone disease. GGT is considered a sensitive but, unfortunately, insufficiently specific marker of alcoholic liver injury.

Immunologic markers are important for the diagnosis of primary biliary cirrhosis and autoimmune hepatitis.

Three liver diseases are considered to have an immune pathogenesis:

- primary biliary cirrhosis
- autoimmune hepatitis
- primary sclerosing cholangitis

The first two diseases are often associated with other autoimmune diseases, such as Hashimoto's thyroiditis and autoimmune atrophic gastritis. Primary sclerosing cholangitis is associated in 60% to 70% cases with ulcerative colitis, a disease of unknown origin and frequently associated with immune system abnormalities.

Although one might expect that serum immunoglobulins would be a good marker of immunologic liver disease, this is unfortunately not so. Total immunoglobulins may be elevated in the serum of patients with any type of chronic hepatitis or cirrhosis. Electrophoresis usually reveals **polyclonal hypergammaglobulinemia.** Nevertheless, significant elevation of immunoglobulins, usually two times normal (from 2.7 g/dL to over 5 g/dL), and the reversal of the normal albumin:globulin ratio from 2:1 to 1:1.5 may be indicative of autoimmune hepatitis.

More specific antibodies are found in primary biliary cirrhosis and autoimmune hepatitis. Primary biliary cirrhosis is associated in 90% of cases with **antimitochondrial antibodies.** Autoimmune hepatitis is associated with **anti-smooth muscle antibodies.** A good response to corticosteroid treatment is yet further evidence that this disease may be of immune origin. In primary sclerosing cholangitis it is not uncommon to find ANA or antibodies to neutrophil cytoplasmic antigens (ANCA), but these antibodies are not specific for that particular liver disease.

Serology is essential for diagnosis of viral hepatitis.

All patients who have laboratory evidence of acute or chronic liver disease must be tested to rule out a viral cause of their disease. These tests include antibodies to viral markers of hepatotropic viruses A, B, C, D, and E. If the test is positive, the final diagnosis of viral infection is documented by measuring the number of viral particles in the blood. This is usually accomplished with molecular biology techniques. Such techniques are also used to determine genetically the strain of hepatitis C virus (HCV).

Genetic testing is used for the final diagnosis of hereditary diseases.

Many liver diseases are genetic. These diseases can be suspected from the standard laboratory data. For example in Wilson's disease, an inborn error of *copper* metabolism, the serum contains *ceruloplasmin*, the copper transport protein, in abnormally low concentration. In hereditary hemochromatosis the serum and the liver and many other organs contain increased amounts of *iron*.

The final diagnosis is currently made by genetic testing. The search for specific gene mutations is useful for documenting **hereditary hemochromatosis, Wilson's disease, AAT deficiency,** and **congenital glucogenesis,** but also many others.

Liver cell carcinoma secretes α-fetoprotein, a protein that is not found in the serum of adults.

α-Fetoprotein (AFP) is the most abundant serum protein in the fetal blood. It is produced by the fetal liver, but its production ceases soon after birth. Normal adult serum contains less than 10 ng/mL of AFP. The reappearance of AFP in the serum of an adult is a rather reliable sign of liver cell neoplasia.

The explanation of this finding relates to the dedifferentiation of liver carcinoma cells, which assume some of the properties of fetal liver cells. This reversion to a fetal phenotype may be associated with the activation of genes that are active only during fetal life and are not expressed in the adult liver. *AFP* is apparently one of these fetal genes that is reactivated in malignant liver cell tumors.

SPECIAL TECHNIQUES FOR EVALUATING THE LIVER

The discussion of special techniques currently used in clinical practice is beyond the scope of this textbook. Suffice to say that many modern techniques can be used for the following purposes:

- **Ultrasound** is used to measure the size of the liver, determine its shape, and detect masses inside the liver. Ultrasound is also the method of choice for studying the biliary tract and detecting gallstones. Doppler ultrasound is the method of choice for detecting intrahepatic thrombi.
- **Computed tomography (CT)** is very useful for studying tumors in the liver, but it can also provide information about the cirrhotic liver, the extent of splenomegaly, and the presence of ascites. Computed tomography can detect a fatty liver and accumulation of iron inside the liver.
- **Endoscopic retrograde cholangiopancreatography (ERCP)** is useful for demonstrating obstructions of the biliary system (Fig. 8-21). It is the method of choice for diagnosing primary sclerosing cholangitis. This disease shows a typical beading pattern due to multiple fibrous rings, causing segmental stenosis of the extrahepatic and intrahepatic bile ducts.
- **Angiography** is useful for demonstrating the vasculature of the liver. For example vascular tumors as well as the abnormal blood vessels formed around primary liver tumors can be nicely demonstrated with this technique.
- **Liver biopsy** is used to obtain information about the histologic changes in the liver in various diseases. It can provide information about the nature of the disease, its activity, and the extent of liver injury or repair. The most important indications for liver biopsy are given in Table 8-9.

Clinicopathologic Correlations

In this section we briefly discuss several prototypical liver diseases, most notably (1) acute hepatitis, (2) chronic liver diseases, (3) cirrhosis, (4) biliary diseases, and (5) liver tumors.

ACUTE HEPATITIS

Acute hepatitis is an inflammation of the liver, but the term has different meanings for clinicians and pathologists.

Acute hepatitis is an inflammation of the liver. *Clinicians* use this term to denote a liver disease of sudden onset and short duration. Most often it is accompanied by jaundice (**icteric acute hepatitis**), but it may also manifest in an **anicteric form** as a nonspecific gastrointestinal disease. In the severe form, it is called **fulminant acute hepatitis.**

A

B

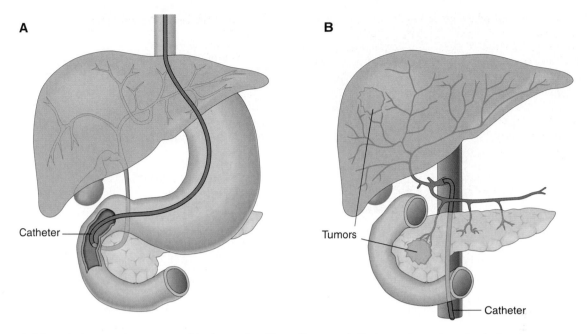

Catheter

Tumors

Catheter

Figure 8-21 Radiologic techniques used in the study of liver diseases. **A,** Endoscopic retrograde cholangiopancreatography is performed by injecting the radiographic contrast material into the common bile duct cannulated through the ampulla of Vater. **B,** Angiography is performed by injecting radiographic contrast material into the hepatic artery.

Pathologists use the term to describe widespread liver cell injury and the body's reaction to it (Fig. 8-22). The key histologic features are as follows:

- Liver cell injury—manifesting as vacuolar swelling ("*ballooning degeneration*") of hepatocytes and *apoptosis* in the form of "acidophilic bodies"
- Cholestasis—evidenced by "feathery degeneration" of hepatocytes and intercellular canaliculi bile plugs
- Immune response—evidenced by infiltrates of lymphocytes in the portal tracts and inside the acini
- Scavenger cell reaction—evidenced by an increased number of Kupffer cells and macrophages

Table 8-9 Indications for Liver Biopsy

Acute hepatitis of nonviral origin
Massive liver necrosis
Suspected drug reaction or hepatitis
Abnormal laboratory findings suggesting chronic hepatitis
Positive serologic test for viral hepatitis C
Intrahepatic cholestasis
Cirrhosis
Space-occupying lesions suggestive of malignancy
Post-transplantation monitoring of transplant rejection or recurrence of the original disease that caused cirrhosis

Note that the inflamed liver does not contain neutrophils, as is typically seen in acute bacterial inflammation, but rather lymphocytes. These immune cells infiltrate the liver in response to viral antigens or autoantigens expressed on damaged liver cells.

Fulminant acute hepatitis is characterized by massive necrosis of hepatocytes (Fig. 8-23). In the most severe form almost all hepatocytes except for a few cells around the portal tracts are lost, a condition called **subtotal hepatic necrosis.**

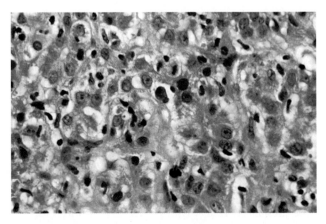

Figure 8-22 Viral hepatitis (photomicrograph). Liver biopsy specimen shows swelling of liver cells, scattered acidophilic (apoptotic) hepatocytes, and an increased number of macrophages (hematoxylin and eosin stain).

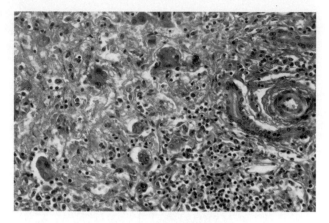

Figure 8-23 Massive hepatic necrosis (photomicrograph). Hepatocytes are lost (*left*) but the bile ducts (*right*) are still preserved (hematoxylin and eosin stain).

Pearl

> Liver biopsy is useful for confirming the diagnosis of acute hepatitis, but the final diagnosis is always made by correlating the pathologic findings with clinical and laboratory data.

Acute hepatitis has many causes.

Acute viral hepatitis may have many causes, which can be broadly classified as infectious or noninfectious (Table 8-10).

All forms of acute hepatitis may be icteric, meaning that they are associated with jaundice, or are subclinical and unrecognized. Typical features of clinical findings related to acute liver injury are shown in Figure 8-24.

Table 8-10 Causes of Acute Hepatitis

Viral hepatitis
   Hepatotropic viruses (HAV,* HBV, HCV,* HDV, HEV)
   Herpesviruses (herpes simplex virus 1 and 2, CMV, Epstein-Barr virus)
   Yellow fever virus
Toxins and drugs
   Alcohol†
   Acetaminophen poisoning‡
   Isoniazid
   Chlorpromazine
   Herbs and plant products
Genetic diseases
   Wilson's disease
   α_1-Antitrypsin deficiency
Immunologic diseases
   Autoimmune hepatitis
Idiopathic

*Indicates the most common causes in the United States.
†Acute alcoholic hepatitis is a relatively rare disease, especially when taking into account the prevalence of alcohol abuse in the United States.
‡A common cause of massive subtotal hepatic necrosis.
CMV, cytomegalovirus; HAV, HBV, HCV, HDV, HEV, viral hepatitis A, B, C, D, and E, respectively.

Hepatitis A virus is directly cytopathic, whereas the hepatitis B and C viruses evoke a cytotoxic immune response.

Hepatitis A virus (HAV) invades liver cells. It replicates inside the hepatocytes, causing their apoptosis (Fig. 8-25). On the other hand, hepatitis B virus (HBV) and hepatitis C virus (HCV) are not directly cytotoxic. On entry into the hepatocytes these viruses are incorporated into the cell's genome, where they replicate and at the same time produce viral antigens. The appearance of viral antigens on the cell

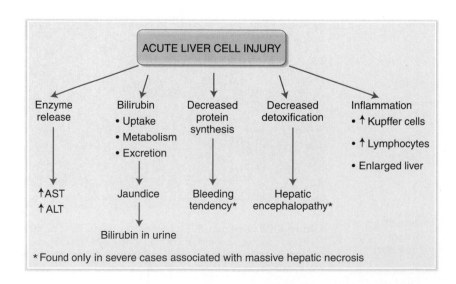

Figure 8-24 Clinical findings in acute hepatitis. Coagulopathy and encephalopathy are found only in severe forms of acute hepatitis associated with massive hepatic necrosis.

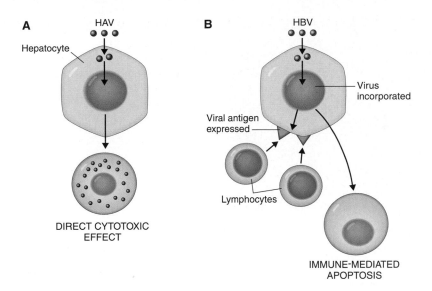

Figure 8-25 Liver cell death in viral hepatitis. **A,** Hepatitis A virus (HAV) is directly cytotoxic to hepatocytes. **B,** Hepatitis B virus (HBV) is incorporated into the liver cells.

surface elicits an immune response, which causes apoptosis of infected hepatocytes.

Hepatitis A virus causes a short-lived acute disease.

Hepatitis A virus is a common human pathogen infecting millions of persons in all parts of the world every year. Serologic evidence indicates that approximately 50% of all Americans have been infected by the age of 50 years, but in some underdeveloped countries the prevalence of anti-HAV antibodies is over 90%. The most important facts about HAV infection are as follows:

- Fecal–oral transmission: "dirty hands," contaminated water and food
- Short incubation (15–45 days)
- Infectivity for 2 to 3 weeks around the appearance of jaundice
- May be sporadic or epidemic
- Clinically mild with full recovery
- No carrier state or chronicity
- Vaccine available

Figure 8-26A shows the short incubation period, the period of infectivity due to the appearance of HAV in stools, a short period of jaundice and elevated serum ALT, and the appearance of antibodies. IgM antibodies are a sign of acute infection, whereas IgG antibodies indicate immunity due to past disease or immunization.

Hepatitis B may cause acute or chronic hepatitis.

Hepatitis B virus infection may cause acute or chronic hepatitis and a spectrum of immunologically mediated reactions, such as a serum-sickness likeness-like skin rash or cryoglobulinemia. Chronic HBV-related hepatitis may progress to cirrhosis and liver cell carcinoma. The most important facts about HBV infection are as follows:

- Transmission by blood and body fluids
- Transfusion, blood-contaminated needles or instruments
- Sexual contact
- Perinatal infant infection
- Long incubation period (4 weeks to 6 months)
- Infection may persist long term
- Carrier state, chronic hepatitis, cirrhosis, or liver cancer
- Infectivity may persist
- Complex antibody response—important for diagnosis
- Vaccine available

Figure 8-26B illustrates the long incubation period, the appearance of diagnostic viral antigens (HBeAg and HBsAg) and antibodies (anti-HBc, anti-HBs, anti-HBe), the persistence of elevated ALT after the disappearance of jaundice, and the transition to chronic hepatitis. Typical serologic findings in HBV infections are shown in Table 8-11.

Hepatitis C virus is clinically the most common infectious hepatitis in the United States.

Approximately 4 million Americans have antibodies to HCV and 70% contain viral particles in the blood, indicating that they have a chronic persistent infection. Every year some 40,000 men and women are infected with HCV in the United States, 85% of whom will develop a chronic persistent infection. A significant number of these develop cirrhosis, which may ultimately give rise to liver cancer. The most important facts about HCV infection are as follows:

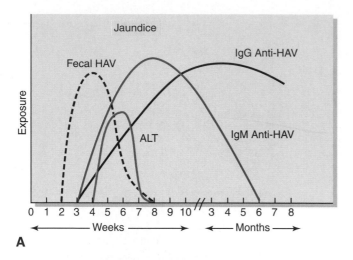

A

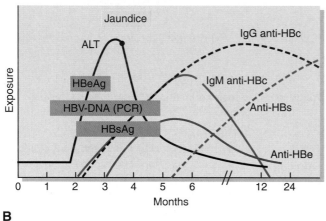

B

Figure 8-26 Sequence of clinical and laboratory findings in acute viral hepatitis A (HAV) (**A**) and viral hepatitis B (HBV) (**B**). ALT, alanine aminotransferase; PCR, polymerase chain reaction. (From Andreoli TE, Carpenter CCJ, Griggs RC, Benjamin I: Andreoli and Carpenter's Cecil Essentials of Medicine, 7th ed. Philadelphia, Saunders, 2007, p. 443.)

- Transmission by blood or blood-contaminated needles and instruments
- Transfusions are safe, but 2 per million are still associated with post-transfusion hepatitis caused by inadvertently transfused HCV.
- In more than 50% the mode of infection cannot be determined.

- Incubation is variable, 2 to 26 weeks (average, 5–10 weeks)
- Often asymptomatic, even though the biopsy shows portal inflammation
- May progress to chronic hepatitis and cirrhosis
- Diagnosis made by demonstrating antibodies to HCV

Table 8-11 Serologic Findings in Hepatitis B Virus Infection

HBsAg	Anti-HBs	Anti-HBc	HBeAg	Anti-HBe	INTERPRETATION
+	−	+ (IgM only)	+	−	Acute infection, high infectivity
+	−	+ IgG (may also have IgM)	+	−	Chronic infection, high infectivity
+	−	+ IgG	−	+	Chronic infection, low infectivity
−	−	+ IgM	+ or −	+ or −	Acute infection
−	+	+ IgG	−	+ or −	Recovery from acute infection, developing immunity
−	+	−	−	−	Vaccinated (immune)
−	−	+ IgG	−	−	False-positive. Repeat!

+, positive; −, negative.

- Quantitation of viral particles in blood to determine viral load
- Extent of disease and transition to cirrhosis established by biopsy
- No vaccines available

The Figure 8-27 illustrates the value of the virologic test for early diagnosis of HCV infection and the tendency of HCV infection to persist and periodically cause elevation of serum transaminases.

Pearls

> Acute HCV infection can be diagnosed only by periodic serologic testing performed after a documented exposure to HCV-positive blood.
> HCV hepatitis invariably recurs in all liver allotransplants.

Drugs can induce changes that are indistinguishable from those in acute or chronic hepatitis.

Many drugs can induce liver injury. In liver biopsy specimens such injury may manifest as ballooning degeneration or apoptosis and necrosis of hepatocytes, cholestasis, fatty change, fibrosis, and so on. In most instances these changes can be classified as drug-induced hepatitis, which is indistinguishable from viral hepatitis.

Drug-induced hepatitis may be acute or chronic and can be classified as predictable or unpredictable.

Predictable. This reaction is dose-dependent and can be anticipated. Usually it is possible to document an overdose or long-term cumulative effect of a drug. Sometimes exposure to a combination of drugs can be documented, each of which is not toxic, but if given together may cause hepatotoxicity. For example, acetaminophen is innocuous if taken as an analgesic, but taking 50 tablets causes acute submassive necrosis of the liver. Acetaminophen taken with alcohol is even more toxic.

Unpredictable. Such reactions cannot be foreseen and are also called *idiosyncratic*. In some cases drugs act as haptens and evoke an immune reaction to hepatocytes, whereas in others the affected person is apparently "too sensitive" and responds inappropriately to small doses of a drug that is tolerated well by most other people.

To diagnose drug-induced hepatitis the following facts must be established:

- Document exposure to a drug.
- Provide data from the literature that this particular drug may be a cause of liver diseases.
- Exclude serologic viral diseases.
- Exclude autoimmune viral diseases.
- Exclude genetic liver diseases.

Even though the diagnosis of drug-induced hepatitis is mostly made by exclusion, its significance cannot be overstated.

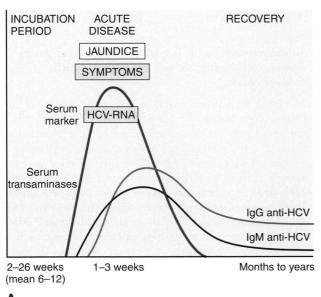

A

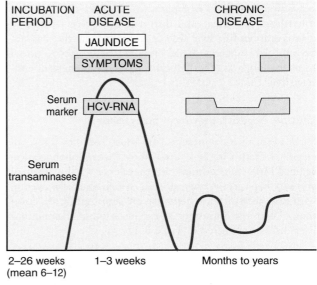

B

Figure 8-27 Sequence of clinical and laboratory findings in viral hepatitis C (HCV). **A,** Acute infection. **B,** Chronic disease following acute infection. (From Kumar V, Abbas AK, Fausto N [eds]: Robbins Pathologic Basis of Disease, 7th ed. Philadelphia, Elsevier, 2004, p. 895.)

Rough estimates are that 2% of all persons taking drugs have some laboratory evidence of liver cell injury, such as mild elevation of AST and ALT. Approximately 10% of all clinically recorded drug reactions involve the liver.

> **Pearls**
>
> > Histologic features of drug-induced hepatitis cannot be distinguished from those of viral hepatitis.
> > Most drug reactions are mild and temporary, meaning that they disappear after withdrawal of the drug.

Exacerbation of chronic liver diseases may clinically manifest as acute hepatitis.

Some chronic genetic liver diseases, such as Wilson's disease or AAT deficiency, or immunologic diseases, such as autoimmune hepatitis, may be diagnosed during an exacerbation, which may erroneously lead to diagnosis of acute hepatitis. Liver biopsy usually helps by providing evidence of chronicity and pointing to some diagnostic findings, such as elevated AAT cytoplasmic globules, or the presence of numerous plasma cells in autoimmune hepatitis.

CHRONIC LIVER DISEASES

Chronic diseases are defined clinically as inflammation of the liver that lasts more than 6 months. Persistent liver disease can be documented clinically, by means of laboratory tests and liver biopsy. Chronic inflammatory liver diseases may persist for many years or progress to cirrhosis. The transition to cirrhosis is gradual, and thus it is not always possible to distinguish chronic liver disease from cirrhosis that has not become decompensated and complicated by ascites, portal hypertension, and other typical sings and symptoms of end-stage liver failure.

Chronic hepatitis may have many causes.

Viral hepatitis C represents the most common cause of chronic hepatitis in the United States. Active immunization against HBV has reduced the prevalence of this form of chronic hepatitis. Other causes, which partially overlap with the cause of acute hepatitis, are significantly less common. The most important causes of chronic inflammatory liver diseases are listed in Table 8-12.

Chronic viral hepatitis caused by HBV and HCV are diagnosed serologically and documented by liver biopsy.

Persistence of HBV is best documented serologically by demonstrating HBV-related antigens in blood (HBsAg and HBeAg) and quantitating the viral particles in blood. Per-

Table 8-12 Causes of Chronic Hepatitis

Chronic viral hepatitis
　Hepatotropic viruses (HBV, HCV,* HDV, HEV)
Toxins and drugs
　Alcohol abuse*
　Isoniazid
　Chlorpromazine
　Herbs and plant products
Genetic diseases
　Hereditary hemochromatosis
　Wilson's disease
　α_1-Antitrypsin deficiency
Immunologic diseases
　Autoimmune hepatitis
　Primary biliary cirrhosis
Diseases of the biliary system
　Primary sclerosing cholangitis
　Cholelithiasis and biliary obstruction
Idiopathic chronic hepatitis

*The most common causes in the United States.
HBV, HCV, HDV, HEV, viral hepatitis B, C, D, and E, respectively.

sistence of HCV infection is documented by quantitating HCV particles in the blood.

Liver biopsy is important for determining the activity of inflammation and the extent of fibrosis. A grading system classifies the disease as mild, moderate, or severe. Mild inflammation and fibrosis limited to portal tracts are hallmarks of stable nonprogressive hepatitis (Fig. 8-28). Severe interface hepatitis and spilling of inflammatory cells into the lobules and bridging fibrosis are signs of aggressive disease that may progress to cirrhosis.

Autoimmune hepatitis is typically a disease of young women and it responds well to treatment with corticosteroids.

Autoimmune hepatitis (AIH) is a chronic disease of unknown origin mediated by an abnormal immunologic reaction in the portal tracts and extending into the lobules. The diagnosis is based on clinical, serologic, and biopsy findings.

The serologic findings are of diagnostic value and are useful for classifying AIH into two major groups: In **type 1** AIH, which accounts for most of the cases in the United States, autoantibodies to smooth muscle antigen (SMA) and antinuclear antibodies (ANAs) are present. In **type 2** AIH, which is the most common form of the disease in children, antibodies to liver/kidney microsomes residing in cytochrome P_{450} enzyme system are present. Two thirds of type 2 patients have also antibodies to HCV, which probably plays a role in the pathogenesis of this disease.

Approximately 20% of AIH patients have a form of disease that shows an overlap with primary biliary cirrhosis. These patients have antimitochondrial antibodies and show destructive cholangitis in liver biopsy specimens.

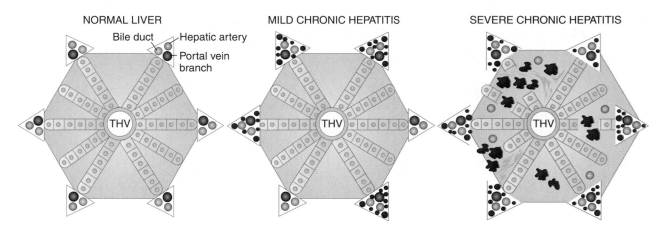

Figure 8-28 Chronic hepatitis. In mild chronic hepatitis, the portal tract is expanded by infiltrates of lymphocytes, but the inflammation does not extend into the acinus. In severe chronic hepatitis, infiltration of chronic inflammatory cells extends into the acinus and the inflammation is accompanied by progressive fibrosis, which may lead to cirrhosis. THV, terminal hepatic venule.

The most important aspects of AIH are as follows:

- Females are more often affected than males, in a ratio of 4:1.
- Most patients are younger than 30 years of age at the time of diagnosis, and some of them are even prepubertal children.
- The disease has an insidious onset, but in 40% symptoms appear suddenly and resemble acute hepatitis.
- Serum contains increased amounts of IgG, in excess of 1.5 times the normal and autoantibodies to smooth muscle cells, nuclear antigens, or liver/kidney microsomes.
- Concurrent autoimmune diseases involving other organs (e.g., thyroiditis or gastritis) are found in 30% of patients.
- Liver biopsy specimens shows aggressive chronic hepatitis with extensive interface hepatitis and infiltrates of plasma cells in portal tracts extending into the lobules.
- All patients respond favorably to corticosteroid treatment. Without steroid treatment 40% of patients die within 6 months. Even with a good response to steroids, 45% of type 1 and over 80% of type 2 patients ultimately develop cirrhosis.

Primary biliary cirrhosis is an autoimmune cholangitis that leads to progressive jaundice and biliary cirrhosis.

Primary biliary cirrhosis (PBC) is a disease of unknown origin that presents as a nonsuppurative cholangitis (Fig. 8-29). The destruction of bile ducts leads to progressive jaundice and portal to portal fibrosis, progressing to cirrhosis. The diagnosis is based on clinical, serologic, and liver biopsy findings.

The most important aspects of PBC are as follows:

- Females are more often affected than males in a ratio of 6:1.

- The disease may begin any time between 20 and 80 years of age, but the peak incidence is between 40 and 50 years.
- The onset of the disease is insidious and includes fatigue, loss of appetite, and pruritus, often followed by jaundice. Biliary obstruction causes steatorrhea and malabsorption of fats, hypercholesterolemia, and formation of dermal xanthomas.
- Diagnostic antimitochondrial antibodies are present in over 90% of all patients. These antibodies react with the E2 subunit of the pyruvate dehydrogenase complex, dihydrolipoamide acetyltransferase.
- Liver biopsy specimens show destructive nonsuppurative cholangitis progressing to ductopenia and fibrosis. Ultimately cirrhosis develops in almost all patients 10 to 15 years after the onset of initial diagnosis of PBC.

Primary sclerosing cholangitis is a chronic disease characterized by periductal fibrosis and obliteration of bile ducts.

Primary sclerosing cholangitis (PSC) is a disease of presumptive immune origin, characterized by progressive fibrosis around the intrahepatic and extrahepatic bile ducts (Fig. 8-30). It is thought that this fibrosis occurs as a fibroblastic response to cytokines secreted by activated T lymphocytes. It is possible, however, that the fibrosis results from nonimmune stimuli and even from ischemia or chemicals. The events initiating this progressive fibrosis are not fully understood, but it is worth noting that 70% of PSC patients have ulcerative colitis.

The most important aspects of PSC are as follows:

- The disease is more common in males than females in a ratio of 2:1.

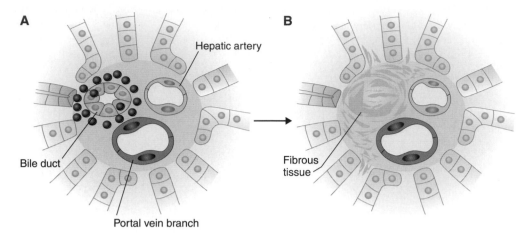

Figure 8-29 Primary biliary cirrhosis. **A,** In early stages of the disease the portal tact is infiltrated with lymphocytes, some of which invade and destroy the bile duct. **B,** In later stages of the disease ductopenia occurs; that is, the ducts have been destroyed and replaced with fibrous tissue that extends into the acinus.

- The median age of patients at the time of diagnosis is 45 years.
- The onset of symptoms is insidious and includes fatigue, itching, and jaundice. With time bile duct obstruction develops with consequent fat malabsorption and steatorrhea.
- Biliary obstruction is associated with elevations of serum alkaline phosphatase.
- Autoantibodies are not found, and serology is used only to exclude other diseases. In 10% of patients antibodies, such as ANA or ANCA, are present, but they are nonspecific and of no diagnostic significance.
- No association with autoimmune diseases is evident in other organs, but 70% of patients have ulcerative colitis.
- Endoscopic retrograde cholangiopancreatography is used in diagnosis and shows typical beading of the bile ducts.
- Liver biopsy specimens show concentric fibrosis around medium-sized and larger bile ducts. Ultimately fibrosis progresses to cirrhosis.
- These patients are at increased risk for cholangiocarcinoma.

> **Pearl**
>
> > In chronic cholestatic diseases such as PBC and PSC, serum levels of alkaline phosphatase are more elevated than transaminases, whereas in chronic hepatitis caused by viruses and drugs, AST and ALT are more elevated than alkaline phosphatase levels.

Hereditary hemochromatosis is characterized by deposition of iron in the liver and several other organs.

Hereditary hemochromatosis (HHC) is a common autosomal recessive disease characterized by iron overload due to the mutation of the *HFE* gene. Homozygosity of the mutated gene is found in 1 of 220 persons, but only 20% of these develop clinical disease.

The *HFE* gene encodes intestinal protein that regulates the uptake of dietary iron in the duodenum. The most common mutation, *C282Y,* involving replacement of tyrosine by cysteine on position 282, accounts for 90% of cases, whereas mutation

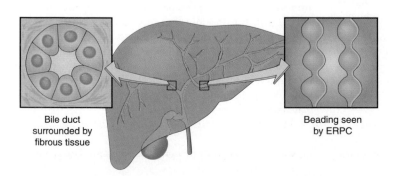

Bile duct surrounded by fibrous tissue

Beading seen by ERPC

Figure 8-30 Primary sclerosing cholangitis. Endoscopic retrograde cholangiopancreatography (ERCP) shows typical beading of the intrahepatic and extrahepatic bile ducts.

H63D is found in 10% cases. Both mutations can be detected by molecular biology techniques, and these tests are used for providing the final diagnosis of HHC in clinical settings.

Abnormal gene product results in an inability to limit the absorption of iron in the intestine, which leads to iron overload throughout the body and the deposition of iron in the form of hemosiderin in the liver, skin, and many other tissues. Normally the body contains approximately 4 g of iron. In HHC this upper limit of normal is exceeded by the time an affected person reaches 10 years of age. Symptoms begin in midlife when the total body iron reaches 25 to 30 g. Cirrhosis develops after iron stores exceed 40 g (i.e., 10 times higher than normal). Coincidental alcohol abuse or viral hepatitis C infection accelerates the development of cirrhosis.

Liver disease is a common manifestation of HHC. Liver injury is accompanied by fibrosis progressing to cirrhosis.

Cirrhosis is associated with hyperpigmentation of the skin and diabetes mellitus ("bronze diabetics"). Other symptoms include various endocrine disturbances, such as hypothyroidism or infertility, arthropathy, and cardiomyopathy. For unknown reasons hand joints are most often affected (Fig. 8-31).

Diagnostic tests include (1) saturation of transferrin in serum, (2) serum ferritin, (3) genetic testing, and (4) liver biopsy. For more details, see Chapter 3.

Pearl

> Hereditary hemochromatosis must be distinguished from secondary hemochromatosis seen in chronic hemolytic anemias, following repeated transfusions, or in chronic viral hepatitis C.

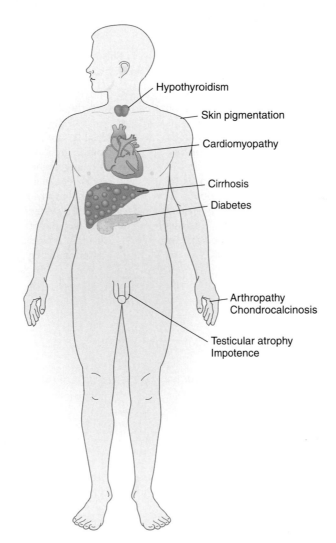

Hypothyroidism
Skin pigmentation
Cardiomyopathy
Cirrhosis
Diabetes
Arthropathy
Chondrocalcinosis
Testicular atrophy
Impotence

Figure 8-31 Hemochromatosis. Clinical findings are evident in several major organs, including the liver, pancreas, heart, and endocrine glands.

Wilson's disease is characterized by the deposition of copper in the liver, basal ganglia of the cerebrum, and the limbus of the eye.

Wilson's disease is an autosomal recessive disorder related to the mutation of the *ATP7B* gene encoding a transmembrane copper-transporting ATPase. Due to this defect, copper cannot be excreted in the bile and accumulates in the liver, basal ganglia of the cerebrum, and the limbus of the eye. Urinary excretion of ceruloplasmin is increased (Fig. 8-32). Typical features include the following:

- *Liver failure* of acute onset or slowly evolving chronic liver disease. The disease can begin at any age, but is uncommon in children younger than 6 years of age.
- *Psychiatric and neurologic (Parkinsonian)* symptoms may be the first manifestations.
- Deposits of copper in the limbus of the eye form the so called *Keyser-Fleischer* ring visible as a brownish green rim by slit-lamp examination.
- Increased amounts of *copper* can be found in *urine*. Under normal circumstances the urine contains less than 50 µg/24 hours. In Wilson's disease the urine contains more than 100 µg/24 hours.
- Serum *ceruloplasmin* levels are typically low. Normally, serum contains 20 to 40 mg/dL, but in Wilson's disease it is less than 20 mg/dL.
- Liver biopsy findings are highly variable and include steatosis, accumulation of glycogen in the nuclei, and chronic hepatitis or cirrhosis.
- Copper can be demonstrated in the hepatocytes by histochemical techniques. The excess of copper in liver biopsy specimens can be quantitated by special biochemical methods. Normally the liver contains less than 50 µg/g dry weight, but in Wilson's disease it contains greater than 250 µg/g dry weight.

Alcohol is a very common cause of liver disease.

Alcohol abuse is the most common cause of liver disease in the western world. Pathologically the injury manifests in several forms (Fig. 8-33):

- **Fatty liver.** It occurs in essentially all alcoholics and even after a binge of drinking or a single intake of more than 200 mL of pure alcohol (3 six-packs of beer, 3 L of wine, or 15–20 mixed drinks). Fatty liver rarely causes clinical symptoms and is reversible.
- **Acute alcoholic hepatitis.** This condition develops in chronic alcoholics, unpredictably or after a major "binge." It is characterized by fever, leukocytosis, pain around the liver, and possibly jaundice and ascites. Still, even this condition may be reversible, but if the alcohol intake is not curtailed it may progress to cirrhosis.
- **Alcoholic cirrhosis.** It develops in 15% to 20% of all chronic alcoholics and clinically is no different from other forms of cirrhosis.

The following aspects of alcohol-induced liver disease are worth remembering:

- The risk of liver disease increases proportionately with the duration and the amount of alcohol intake.
- The risk of liver disease varies because of individually variable sensitivity to alcohol. For unknown reasons women are more sensitive to alcohol than men.
- The progression from fatty liver to alcoholic hepatitis or cirrhosis is unpredictable.
- Alcohol has an adverse effect on the course of liver disease induced by viruses (HBV or HCV) or hemochromatosis.
- The liver is not the only organ affected by alcohol. Alcohol has adverse effects on the brain, heart, pancreas, skeletal muscles, gastrointestinal system, hematologic

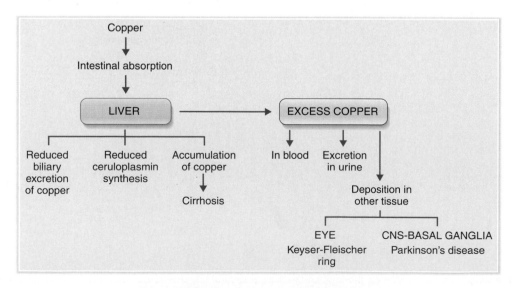

Figure 8-32 Clinical findings in Wilson disease.

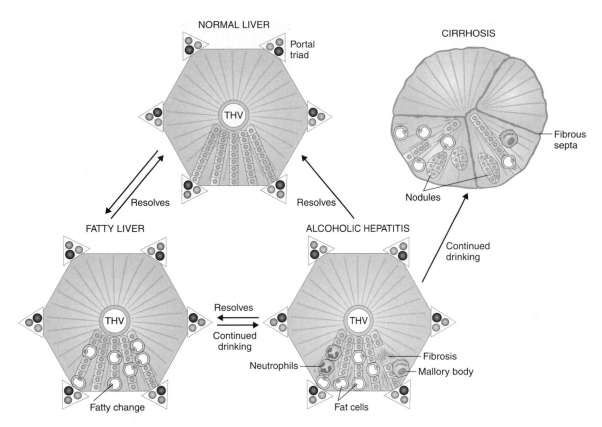

Figure 8-33 Alcoholic liver disease. Almost all alcoholics have a fatty liver, which in some progresses to alcoholic hepatitis or cirrhosis. Alcoholic hepatitis is still reversible; cirrhosis is irreversible. THV, terminal hepatic venule.

system, and endocrine organs (i.e., it affects the entire body in one way or another).

There are no definitive diagnoses of alcoholic liver disease. The most common abnormalities found are listed in Table 8-13.

CIRRHOSIS

Cirrhosis is essentially a pathologic diagnosis. Clinically it denotes irreversible end-stage liver disease. Pathologically it is characterized by a loss of normal liver architecture,

which is replaced by strands of fibrosis and nodules composed of regenerating hepatocytes. For the clinician, to quote the famous Yale gastroenterologist Howard Spiro, "Cirrhosis is a disorder of protean manifestations, plenteous pitfalls, and infinite opportunity for frustration and befuddlement."

Cirrhosis has many causes.

Cirrhosis is the end stage of many liver diseases and is most often preceded by chronic hepatitis. Thus, it is no wonder that the list of causes of cirrhosis shows considerable overlap

Table 8-13 Laboratory Findings in Alcoholic Liver Disease

MARKER	ABNORMAL IN PERSONS > 60 g ALCOHOL/DAY	COMMENT
GGT	75%	Sensitive (90%) but nonspecific
AST:ALT ratio >1	90%	Highly suggestive of alcohol abuse
MCV > 100 μL	80%	Due to folic acid or vitamin B_{12} deficiency
Transferrin > 400 mg/dL	80%	Abnormal only in alcoholics who have normal AST
Alcohol in blood	75%	Take blood at random!

ALT, alanine aminotransferase; AST, aspartate aminotransferase; GGT, γ-glutamyltranspeptidase; MCV, mean corpuscular volume.

with the list of causes of chronic hepatitis. The causes of cirrhosis are listed in Table 8-14.

Liver biopsy is important for the diagnosis of cirrhosis, but the correlation between pathology and clinical findings is poor.

A cirrhotic liver is composed of hepatocellular nodules surrounded by fibrous septa (Fig. 8-34). Pathologists subdivide cirrhosis into the following types:

- Macronodular versus micronodular, depending on the size of the nodule
- Regular versus irregular (also known as "postnecrotic"), depending on the size and shape of nodules and the distribution of scars
- Portal versus biliary, depending on the pathogenesis of cirrhosis and the type of fibrosis in early stages of the disease

Table 8-14 Causes of Cirrhosis

Chronic viral
  HCV*
  HBV
Excessive intake of alcohol*
Nonalcoholic fatty liver disease (also called nonalcoholic steatohepatitis [NASH])
Autoimmune hepatitis
Biliary diseases
  Primary biliary cirrhosis
  Primary sclerosing cholangitis
  Biliary atresia in children
Genetic diseases
  AAT deficiency
  Hemochromatosis
  Wilson's disease
  Glycogen or lipid storage diseases
Prolonged exposure to some drugs and toxins
Heart failure of venous outflow obstruction
Idiopathic* (20%)

*The three most common causes are marked by asterisks.
AAT, α₁-antitrypsin; HBV, hepatitis B virus infection; HCV, hepatitis C virus infection.

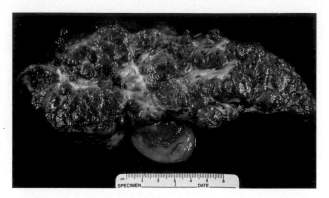

Figure 8-34 Cirrhosis. The normal liver architecture has been replaced by nodules surrounded by fibrous strands.

These pathologic designations have very little if any clinical significance. In some cases the liver biopsy specimen reveals cirrhosis, but the patient is essentially asymptomatic. In that case we say that the cirrhosis is *compensated*. Ultimately cirrhosis becomes *decompensated*, and symptoms of portal hypertension and hepatocellular dysfunction appear.

Clinical manifestations of cirrhosis are consequences of portal hypertension and liver cell dysfunction.

Most of the clinical signs and symptoms of cirrhosis represent the consequences of portal hypertension or liver cell dysfunction (Fig. 8-35). In many instances both portal hypertension and liver cell dysfunction play an equal pathogenetic role.

The most common physical findings in patients with cirrhosis are listed in Table 8-15.

The consequences of cirrhosis are noticed in many other organs.

It cannot be overemphasized that cirrhosis, the end stage liver disease, has profound effects on other organs systems. The most important effects are as follows:

Circulatory system. The heart is overburdened by an increased amount of fluid in the circulation. Plasma volume is increased by one third over normal. It is irregularly distributed, and tends to pool in the splanchnic circulation. Increased sympathomimetic functions cause peripheral arteriolar dilatation and strain the heart directly and indirectly.

Pulmonary system. Circulatory disturbances and the presence of right-to-left shunts reduce the oxygenation of the blood and cause hepatopulmonary syndrome.

Gastrointestinal system. Nausea and vomiting and bouts of diarrhea may lead to depletion of potassium and nutrients.

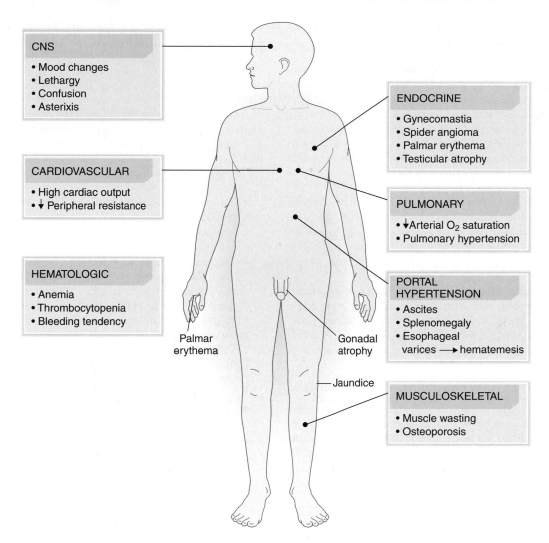

Figure 8-35 Clinical features of cirrhosis.

Table 8-15 Physical Findings in Cirrhosis

PHYSICAL FINDINGS	INCIDENCE (%)
Palpable liver	96
Jaundice	68
Ascites	6
Spider angiomas	49
Dilated abdominal wall veins	47
Splenomegaly	46
Testicular atrophy	45
Palmar erythema	37
Fever (noninfectious)	22
Hepatic coma	18
Gynecomastia	15
Dupuytren's contracture	5

Data from Powell W, Klatskin G: Duration of survival in patients with Laennec's cirrhosis. Am J Med 44:406–414, 1968.

The metabolism of bile, bilirubin, and digestion in general may be affected.

Renal system. Blood flow through the kidneys is shunted from the cortex to the medulla, possibly resulting in tubular acidosis. Ultimately the pronounced vasospasm of cortical blood vessels may lead to hepatorenal syndrome and renal failure.

Endocrine system. Many hormones that are processed in the liver are not inactivated, and like estrogens may cause profound body changes. The liver is the major source of hormone-binding and transport proteins, and cirrhosis therefore affects the metabolism of many hormones such as thyroxin and insulin.

Hematopoietic system. Cirrhosis is associated with anemia, which may be macrocytic due to folic acid and vitamin

B_{12} deficiency or hypochromic microcytic due to iron deficiency. A profound bleeding tendency also occurs.

Immune system. Some liver diseases are immune-mediated, but even those that are not affect the immune system. For example IgA is cleared through the liver, and in patients who have cirrhosis IgA circulates in high concentrations in the blood. This IgA may be deposited in the glomeruli and cause mesangial proliferative IgA nephritis. Most patients with cirrhosis are more susceptible to infections, indicating that their immune system does not function properly.

Skin. Best known changes on the skin include vascular spider, palmar erythema, and petechial hemorrhages. Itching caused by an excess of bile acids in the blood, or xanthomas due to hypercholesterolemia, is typical of chronic cholestasis.

Central nervous system. The inability of the liver to eliminate endogenous and exogenous toxins and neurotropic substances has profound effects on the brain and ultimately causes hepatic encephalopathy. These changes are reversible and the symptoms disappear after liver transplantation.

Transplantation is the only definitive cure for cirrhosis.

Cirrhosis was previously an incurable disease, but today most patients can be treated by liver allotransplantation. Both whole livers harvested postmortem and parts of the liver obtained from living donors can be used. The survival rate at 1 year post-transplantation if over 90%, but transplant failure occurs in about 10% to 25% of patients, who will then receive a second transplant.

Liver transplantation is a major operation and only patients with advanced liver disease should be treated in this way. Transplantation is performed on patients who have either acute liver failure due to massive hepatic necrosis or end-stage cirrhosis. The patients in the latter groups are evaluated according to the Child criteria, a point-by-point semiquantitative system (Child-Pugh system) used to determine hepatic functional reserve. These criteria are listed in Table 8-16.

Liver transplantation has dramatically changed the treatment of cirrhosis, a previously incurable disease. More than 85% of all patients resume normal activities and more than 90% have no major health problems.

The reasons for transplant failure may be as follows:

- **Surgery-related complications.** These complications include graft failure due to dehiscence of sutures or postoperative stenosis of bile ducts, or vascular thrombosis or infection.
- **Immune transplant rejection.** In most instances transplant rejection can be suppressed with modern immunosuppressant drugs. *Ductopenic rejection* marked by a loss of bile ducts and portal fibrosis is a late complication that cannot be treated effectively.
- **Recurrence of the original hepatic disease.** Essentially all patients infected with viral hepatitis C infect their new liver, and the disease may progress to cirrhosis. Autoimmune diseases such as primary biliary cirrhosis also may recur in transplants.
- **Infections related to immunosuppression.** Most common in this group of complications is cytomegalovirus (CMV) infection, which occurs in 15% to 25% of cases. It can be controlled by antiviral drugs. Ascending bacterial infection may be caused by normal intestinal saprophytes. Fungal infection may be found in patients severely immunosuppressed and treated with antibiotics.
- **Functional complications.** In about 20% to 30% of patients functional disturbances occur involving the

Table 8-16 Child-Pugh Criteria for Estimating Hepatic Functional Reserve

PARAMETERS/LABORATORY FINDINGS	MINIMAL (1 POINT)	MODERATE (2 POINTS)	ADVANCED (3 POINTS)
Serum bilirubin (mg/dL)	<2.0	2.0–3.0	>3.0
Serum albumin (g/dL)	>3.5	2.8–3.5	<2.8
Ascites	None	Moderate, easily controlled	Tense, poorly controlled
Prothrombin time (PT) (seconds prolonged)	1–3	4-6	>6
INR*	<1.7	1.7–2.3	>2.3
Encephalopathy	No evidence	Minimal, stage 1–2	Severe, stage 3–4

Total points:
  5-6: Child-Pugh class A
  7-9: Child-Pugh class B
  10-15: Child-Pugh class C
*International normalized ratio (INR) is a standardized prothrombin time, corrected by the sensitivity of the reactive to anticoagulants.
Data from Pugh RNH, Murray-Lyon IM, Dawson JL, et al: Transection of the oesophagus for bleeding oesophageal varices. Br J Surg 60:649, 1973.

kidney, lungs, or the central nervous system. These complications are usually encountered during the first few months after transplantation.

BILIARY DISEASES

Biliary diseases are an important cause of morbidity. Among these diseases the most important are (1) cholelithiasis, (2) infections of the biliary tree, and (3) tumors.

Gallstones have many causes and are very prevalent.

Cholelithiasis is one of the most common hepatobiliary diseases. The most important risk factors for gallstone formation are as follows:

Female sex. The incidence of gallstones is three times higher in women than in men. Estrogens inhibit enzymatic conversion of cholesterol to bile acids and thus increase the concentration of cholesterol in bile. Progesterones inhibit contraction of the gallbladder and delay its emptying, thus allowing slush to accumulate in the lumen. Pregnancy-related increase of estrogen and progesterone has an additive effect.

Age. The incidence of gallstones increases with age in both females and males. The ratio of females to males is 3:1 before menopause, but males "catch up," and the ratio drops to 2:1 after menopause.

Obesity. Hyperlipidemia leads to increased excretion of cholesterol in the bile.

Hereditary hypercholesterolemia and hyperlipidemia. Genetic factors play an important role and probably account for some of the ethnic differences seen in the prevalence of gallstones. Gallstones have the highest incidence among Pima Indians, but all Native Americans have a very high predisposition to gallstones. It seems that diet and life-style have a dominant role. For example, the introduction of western diet has increased the prevalence of gallstones in Japan, a country that had previously a low prevalence.

Hepatic diseases. Change in the metabolism of bile acids, cholesterol, and phospholipids that occurs in cirrhosis is associated with an increased incidence of gallstones.

Gastrointestinal disease. Many intestinal diseases, such as blind intestinal loop with bacterial overgrowth, motility disorders, and regional enteritis (Crohn's disease), alter the excretion and enterohepatic recirculation of bile and contribute to the formation of gallstones.

Hemolytic anemia. Excessive generation of bilirubin from hemolysis of red blood cells in hereditary spherocytosis, sickle cell anemia, and other chronic hemolytic anemias may promote the formation of pigmentary stones.

Biliary tract infections. Bacteria promote nucleation of biliary micelles and are an important cause of gallstone formation. In tropical countries liver flukes (e.g., *Opistorchis sinensis*) are an important cause of biliary diseases and contribute to the formation of gallstones.

Gallstones cause acute symptoms by entering into the extrahepatic biliary ducts.

Despite their prevalence, gallstones are most often clinically silent. Most gallstones are composed predominantly of cholesterol. These stones tend to be solitary and rapidly attain a size precluding their entry into the cystic duct. Thus they do not interfere with bile flow and do not cause pain that would result from smaller stones becoming impacted in the cystic or common bile duct.

Acute symptoms and complications of gallstone disease depend on the location of the gallstones (Fig. 8-36) but in general include the following: (1) biliary pain, (2) acute cholecystitis, and (3) bile duct obstruction.

Biliary pain. The pain results from impaction of gallstones in the cystic or common bile duct. The pain usually begins

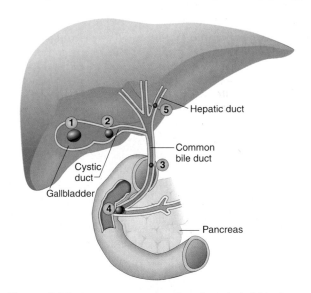

Figure 8-36 Acute symptoms related to cholelithiasis. Symptoms vary depending on the location of the gallstones. 1, Gallstones in the gallbladder may be asymptomatic. 2, Impaction of the cystic duct causes acute cholecystitis and biliary colic. 3, Obstruction of the common bile duct causes biliary colic and jaundice. 4, Obstruction of the ampulla of Vater or the ampullary part of the common bile duct may cause jaundice and signs of pancreatitis. 5, Obstruction of the hepatic duct may be asymptomatic or it may cause jaundice and signs of inflammation of the bile duct and the liver.

15 minutes to 1 to 2 hours after a fatty meal. The pain often wakes up the patient in bed. In some instances it occurs even after a nonfatty meal, and it may be sometimes completely unrelated to food intake. Although it is known as 'biliary colic," the pain does not have a crampy quality, but is rather dull and slowly evolving. It usually lasts a few hours and may be accompanied by nausea and vomiting.

Acute cholecystitis. Gallbladder inflammation is a complication of cystic duct obstruction. It is chemically mediated, but in most instances a secondary bacterial infection supervenes a few hours after the onset of symptoms. The inflammatory mediators, such as prostaglandins and cytokines, are formed due to the interaction of the stagnant bile and the gallbladder cells. Circulatory disturbances caused by increased intravesical pressure may cause ischemic necrosis, bleeding, and exudation of neutrophils. The entire wall of the distended gallbladder becomes inflamed and sensitive to palpation. **Murphy's sign,** right subcostal pain provoked by deep inspiration typically so intense that it stops the patient from breathing, is typically evident. Leukocytosis confirms the presence of acute inflammation, but the liver function tests and amylase remain within normal limits or are only minimally elevated. Hyperbilirubinemia and elevation of alkaline phosphatase indicate common bile duct obstruction or ascending cholangitis. Elevation of amylase points to pancreatitis. Bacterial superinfection occurs almost invariably. Broad-spectrum antibiotic treatment is usually followed by cholecystectomy.

Bile duct obstruction. Small gallstones may pass from the gallbladder through the cystic duct and enter into the common bile duct. In some patients the stones form in the common bile duct. This is typically the case in patients who had previous cholecystectomy. Intracholedochal stones obstruct the bile flow. Clinically common bile duct obstruction is accompanied by pain that is similar to the pain caused by the obstruction of the cystic duct, except that the former is typically followed by hyperbilirubinemia and jaundice. Liver function tests become abnormal, and most prominently serum alkaline phosphatase is significantly elevated. In prolonged obstruction AST and ALT levels drop to normal levels, but the elevation of alkaline phosphatase may persist. Obstruction at the level of the ampulla of Vater may cause reflux of bile into the pancreatic duct and acute pancreatitis.

Pearls

> Ultrasound is the method of choice for detecting gallstones (sensitivity > 95%).
> Endoscopic retrograde cholangiopancreatography is an excellent method for diagnosing and also for removing bile stones from the common bile duct.
> Hepatobiliary scintigraphy with radioactive imidodiacetic acid derivatives (IDA) is an excellent technique for diagnosing cystic duct obstruction—an almost universal feature of acute cholecystitis.

Chronic cholelithiasis is usually asymptomatic and rarely causes complications that would require surgery.

Sixty percent to 80% of all patients who have gallstones have no symptoms, and only 3% to 5% of them ultimately require cholecystectomy. Some of the possible complications of chronic cholecystitis are illustrated algorithmically in Figure 8-37.

Gallstones may cause mechanical irritation of the gallbladder, which is usually accompanied by mild inflammation. Symptoms of chronic cholecystitis are usually vague and nonspecific. Chronic inflammation may cause adhesions with the adjacent intestines and ultimately lead to the formation of a cholecystointestinal fistula. Gallstones passing through the fistula into the intestine may cause obstructive ileus.

Occasionally chronic inflammation is associated with extensive fibrosis and calcification known as porcelain gallbladder. Obstruction of the cystic duct and inflammation may cause symptoms of acute cholecystitis. Rupture of the infected gallbladder may result in peritonitis. Furthermore, infection from the gallbladder can spread into the hepatic bile ducts and cause ascending cholangitis and liver abscesses.

Obstruction of the common bile duct may result in jaundice, pancreatitis, and even malabsorption.

Cholecystitis associated with certain diseases tends to be clinically more severe. Accordingly prophylactic cholecystectomy is recommended for patients who in addition to gallstones have the following diseases:

- **Diabetes mellitus.** These patients are prone to infections and may develop acute bacterial cholecystitis more readily than others. The removal of infected gallbladders is associated in these patients with a mortality rate of 10%, and therefore a prophylactic cholecystectomy is warranted.
- **Sickle cell anemia.** Pigmentary stones that form in these patients often cause attacks of cholecystitis, which may be difficult to distinguish from hepatic crisis.
- **Porcelain gallbladder.** This form of chronic cholecystitis, in which the gallbladder is distended rigid, and calcified, is a well-known risk factor for carcinoma of the gallbladder.

LIVER TUMORS

Liver tumors can be benign or malignant. The most common benign liver tumor is the **hemangioma,** which is found in 7% of normal persons. Usually such tumors are recognized by CT scanning and are not treated.

Benign **liver cell adenomas** are relatively uncommon. They occur more often in women than men. They must be distinguished from focal nodular hyperplasia (FNH), a tumor-like proliferation of liver cells usually around a fibrous scar. Liver cell adenomas may progress to liver cell cancer and are usually resected, whereas FNH is not associated with progression to malignancy and is not resected unless of considerable size.

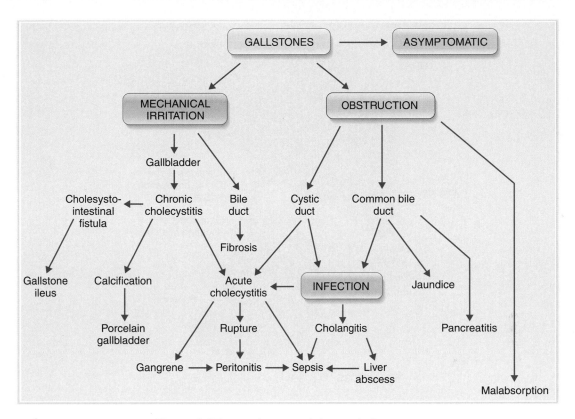

Figure 8-37 Complications of chronic cholecystitis.

Malignant liver tumors can be primary or secondary (metastatic). In the United States, metastatic tumors are more common than primary liver tumors. Primary malignant tumors may be classified as (1) **hepatocellular carcinomas (HCCs),** (2) **cholangiocellular carcinoma,** and (3) **sarcomas originating from Kupffer cells** or other stromal cells of the liver (Fig. 8-38). Tumors originating from the gallbladder and extrahepatic bile ducts have the same histologic features as cholangiocarcinoma. We limit our discussion here to hepatocellular carcinomas.

Hepatocellular carcinoma usually develops in the context of cirrhosis.

Cirrhosis is the major risk factor for HCC. Patients who have cirrhosis caused by viral hepatitis B and C and hemochromatosis are at a higher risk than those who have cirrhosis caused by alcohol or primary biliary cirrhosis.

However, for practical reasons all cirrhotic patients should be considered to be at risk for liver cell cancer. For unknown reasons HCC is more common in males than females, and the M:F ratio is 4:1. Patients with primary sclerosing cholangitis are at risk for cholangiocarcinoma. Note that approximately 25% to 30% of HCCs develop in livers that are not affected by cirrhosis.

Hepatocellular carcinoma differs from other nodules in a cirrhotic liver.

The only hope for curing HCC lies in the early detection of the malignant tumor. Such early cancers can be diagnosed by proper monitoring with ultrasound, CT, or magnetic resonance imaging (MRI), and serologic testing for AFP, followed by targeted biopsy of the suspicious nodules. The malignant nodules differ from surrounding regenerating nodules, and such differences can be noticed as follows:

■ **Ultrasound.** Most liver cancers are hypoechogenic, but any mass that has a variable echogenicity and differs from adjacent parenchyma should be suspect.
■ **Computed tomography.** Since the liver cancers promote angiogenesis the flow through the tumor is more rapid. Computed tomography combined with an intravascular contrast medium reveals quick enhancement

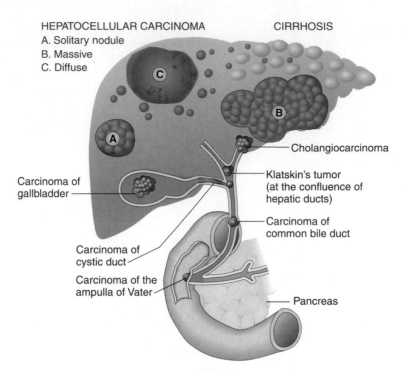

HEPATOCELLULAR CARCINOMA
A. Solitary nodule
B. Massive
C. Diffuse

CIRRHOSIS

Cholangiocarcinoma

Klatskin's tumor
(at the confluence of
hepatic ducts)

Carcinoma of
common bile duct

Carcinoma of
gallbladder

Carcinoma of
cystic duct

Carcinoma of the
ampulla of Vater

Pancreas

Figure 8-38 Hepatobiliary malignant tumors.

during the arterial phase and rapid de-enhancement in the venous phase.

■ **Magnetic resonance imaging.** Tumors are hypointense in T1-weighted images and hyperintense in T2-weighted images. Administration of gadolinium enhances the tumor's image.

■ **α_1-Fetoprotein.** Hepatocellular carcinomas secrete AFP, which is a relatively good marker for liver cancer. Even small hepatocellular carcinomas raise the level of AFP to 10 times more than normal (normal < 40 ng/dL). Values of serum AFP in the range of 2000 to 5000 ng/dL are common.

Hepatocellular carcinoma causes liver enlargement.

Pathologically, hepatocellular carcinoma can present in one of the following three forms:

■ Solitary nodule
■ Large localized mass
■ Diffusely infiltrating/multifocal tumor

Only the localized solitary nodule or a few small nodules limited to a portion of the liver are curable by hepatectomy followed by liver transplantation. Even so, many of them are surrounded by satellite nodules, indicative of progressive infiltrative growth of the tumor. Such localized small tumors usually produce no obvious clinical signs or symptoms. Unfortunately in 60% to 70%

of cases HCC manifests as massive lesions or diffusely infiltrating multifocal tumors. Such tumors cause progressive enlargement of the liver, which can be readily palpated and is accompanied by subcostal right upper quadrant pain.

> **Pearls**
>
> > Not all liver masses are malignant. Keep that in mind, especially if the patient does not have cirrhosis.
> > The differential diagnosis should include inflammatory conditions (e.g., liver abscess, ameboma, echinococcus cyst), congenital developmental cysts (e.g., polycystic liver disease), or benign tumors, which may be large (e.g., liver cell adenoma or focal nodular hyperplasia, FNH).

Hepatocellular carcinoma destroys the liver and invades into blood vessels.

Hepatocellular carcinoma destroys the surrounding liver, causing elevation of LFTs and jaundice. The tumor has a propensity to invade the veins and thus cause sudden elevation of portal pressure. Invasizzon of veins is accompanied by thrombosis. Due to vascular obstruction the amount of ascites may increase in size and it may become hemorrhagic. The entry of tumor cells into the hepatic veins is accompanied by metastases in the lungs.

Hepatocellular carcinoma may cause paraneoplastic syndromes and metabolic disturbances.

An HCC is composed of liver-like cells that are metabolically active. For example hypoglycemia has been seen in 30% of patients with HCC. In part it is due to increased sequestration of glucose from blood and increased glucose consumption. It has been shown that some HCCs secrete the insulin-like growth factors (IGF-2), which further contributes to hypoglycemia. Some tumors secrete cholesterol that cannot be eliminated in bile and causes hypercholesterolemia. Erythropoietin secretion may cause erythrocytosis. Parathyroid-hormone-like activity causes hypercalcemia, and hyperthyroidism is caused by an excess of thyroid-stimulating hormone. The most common disturbances are listed in Table 8-17.

The pathogenesis of the most important clinical findings is illustrated in Figure 8-39.

Pearl

> Metastases to the liver are times more common than primary malignant tumors (in the United States). Any malignant tumor can metastasize to the liver, but the most common ones originate from five organs, which can be remembered with the mnemonic **LIMPS** (**l**ung, **i**ntestinal, **m**ammary, **p**ancreas, and **s**tomach).

Table 8-17 Possible Metabolic and Hormonal Effects of Hepatocellular Carcinoma

Erythrocytosis
Hypoglycemia
Hypercalcemia
Hypercholesterolemia
Hyperthyroidism
Gynecomastia
Pseudoporphyria

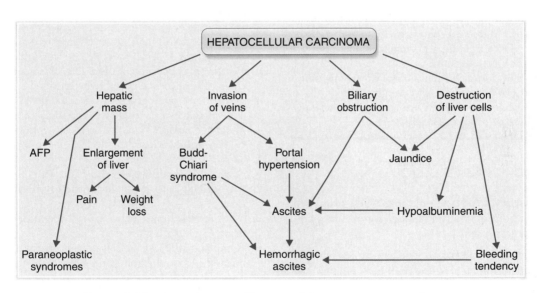

Figure 8-39 Clinical features of hepatocellular carcinoma. AFP, a-fetoprotein.

CASE STUDIES

Case 1 JAUNDICE OF SUDDEN ONSET

Clinical history A 30-year-old, previously healthy woman returned from vacation in Central America. Two weeks later she developed mild fever and noticed fatigue and loss of appetite. A few days later her friend noticed that she was jaundiced,[1] and the woman noticed that her urine was brown and foamy.[2]

Laboratory findings Bilirirubin[3] was elevated in the blood. The bilirubin was mostly of the direct type.[4]

Serologic findings Antibody to viral hepatitis A was present in a high titer. The antibody was of the IgM type.[5]

Outcome She recovered completely after a few weeks.[6]

Questions and topics for discussion
1. What is jaundice? How do you diagnose jaundice?
2. Why is the urine brown and foamy? Does the urine change color in every form of jaundice?
3. What is bilirubin? How is it formed?
4. What is the difference between direct and indirect bilirubin? Does the blood normally contain both direct and indirect bilirubin?
5. Why is it important to determine whether the antibodies to HAV are of the IgM or IgG type?
6. What is the outcome of HAV infection? Are there any significant late complications?

Case 2 VOMITING OF BLOOD

Clinical history A 50-year-old man who was in good health had a bout of vomiting blood[1] and was hospitalized in hypotensive shock.

Family and passt history The patient used intravenous drugs as a student. He does not drink and has had no previous surgery and received no blood transfusions.[2]

Clinical finding Mild ascites, pedal edema, and splenomegaly[3] were found. Endoscopy revealed esophageal varices,[4] which were ligated and cauterized. Ultrasound disclosed a small liver.[5]

Laboratory findings
- Low serum albumin[6]
- Slight elevation of AST,[6] ALT,[6] and alkaline phosphatase[6]
- Bilirubin slightly elevated in blood[6]
- Prothrombin time prolonged[6]
- RBC[6] and hemoglobin low[6]
- MCV normal[6]
- Antibodies to hepatitis C virus positive[7]

Liver biopsy A transjugular liver biopsy[8] revealed irregular fibrosis surrounding small nodules. Prominent infiltrates of lymphocytes were evident in the fibrous strands. The liver cells showed focal fatty change.[9]

Outcome The patient was listed for possible liver transplantation.[10]

Questions for discussion
1. Is vomiting of blood the same as hematemesis? What are the most common causes of hematemesis?
2. What is the significance of these historical data? Which other questions would you ask to determine the possible cause of portal hypertension?
3. Explain the pathogenesis of ascites, pedal edema, and splenomegaly. Are they interrelated?
4. What are varices? What is the most common cause of esophageal varices?
5. Why is the liver small?
6. What is the significance of these laboratory findings?
7. Are antibodies to HCV diagnostic of this viral disease?
8. Why was the biopsy performed through the jugular vein?
9. Are these pathologic findings diagnostic of any liver disease? Do these findings provide a clue about the causes of the liver disease in this case?
10. Why should this patient consider liver transplantation? Will the disease recur in the liver transplant?

Case 3 PROLONGED JAUNDICE AND ITCHING IN AN ADULT WOMAN

Clinical history A 50-year-old woman complained mild jaundice and persistent itching.[1]

Family and past history Family history is unremarkable. She has a history of hypothyroidism[2] for which she has been treated for 5 years.

Clinical findings Jaundice and scratch marks on the arms, legs, and the back. There is xanthelasma[3] around both eyes.

Laboratory findings Hyperbilirubinemia and hyperlipidemia were found.[4] Bilirubin was found in the urine as well. Other findings were within normal limits.

Serologic findings for viral antigens were negative. Antimitochondrial antibodies[5] were present in high titer. Antinuclear antibodies (ANAs) and antismooth muscle (ASM) antibodies[6] were negative.

Liver biopsy Percutaneous liver biopsy revealed prominent periportal infiltrates of lymphocytes and macrophages with destruction of bile ducts.[7] Portal tract fibrosis extended into the lobules. Intralobular cholestasis was evident.[8]

Outcome The patient was treated with cholestyramine, with follow up every 6 months.

Questions for discussion

1. Is pruritus just a fancy name for itching? What could cause itching? What is the pathogenesis of itching in a jaundiced person?
2. How could hypothyroidism be linked to liver problems in this woman?
3. What are xanthelasmas? Do they differ from xanthomas?
4. Could hyperbilirubinemia and hyperlipidemia have the same pathogenesis?
5. What is the significance of antimitochondrial antibodies?
6. What is the significance of ANA and ASM?
7. Do the liver biopsy results explain the pathogenesis of jaundice? Is this hyperbilirubinemia caused by conjugated or unconjugated bilirubin?
8. Could this portal fibrosis progress to cirrhosis? How often does this happen in this liver disease?

Case 4 ENLARGING PAINFUL LIVER

Clinical history A 60-year-old man known to have cirrhosis[1] noticed pronounced swelling of the abdomen, which became painful.[2] He also complained of pain under the right costal margin.

Family and past history Family history is unremarkable. He had no blood transfusions, never used illicit drugs, and had no contact with blood products. He is monogamous and never had any sexual contacts with any other person. He does not drink alcohol, he has no diabetes, and he is not obese.

Clinical findings The patient has ascites and an enlarged liver.[3] The anterior edge of the liver is palpable and hard. The spleen is markedly enlarged. Endoscopy revealed esophageal varices and internal hemorrhoids.

Dynamic CT scan revealed a mass[4] in the cirrhotic liver that has prominent blood filling.

Laboratory findings

- Hypoalbuminemia, INR 2.0
- AST, ALT, and alkaline phosphate all slightly elevated
- All viral and immunologic markers negative
- α-Fetoprotein in blood 10 times normal

Liver biopsy A malignant tumor was identified by ultrasound-guided transjugular biopsy.[5] It was composed of atypical polygonal cells resembling liver cells.[6]

Outcome The patient developed hepatic vein thrombosis complicated with pulmonary emboli and died.[7,8]

Questions for discussion

1. Cirrhosis that develops after viral infection is called "posthepatic." Do you know any other forms of cirrhosis? What is the name for the cirrhosis that has no obvious cause?
2. What is the cause of progressive abdominal swelling in a patient with cirrhosis? Could similar symptoms occur in a person who does not have cirrhosis? Make a list of conditions that could cause "abdominal swelling."
3. What are the possible causes of liver enlargement? Why would a cirrhotic liver enlarge?
4. What is the liver mass discovered by CT?
5. Why was the biopsy ultrasound-guided and transjugular?
6. Interpret the liver biopsy findings. What are the diagnosis and differential diagnosis of these findings?
7. Why did this patient develop hepatic vein thrombosis?
8. Does this patient have Budd-Chiari syndrome?

Case 5 PAIN OF SUDDEN ONSET UNDER THE RIGHT COSTAL MARGIN

Clinical history A 40-year-old woman who is 30-weeks pregnant experienced excruciating pain under the right costal margin, accompanied by nausea and vomiting.[1] The pain began after the Thanksgiving dinner and as it did not subside she was hospitalized.

Family and past history Family history is unremarkable. She had three previous pregnancies, which were all unremarkable. She is obese but cannot lose weight.[2]

Clinical findings The patient is in distress and restless. She has mild fever and is sweating. She has a positive Murphy's sign. The right upper abdominal quadrant is sensitive to palpation. Ultrasound examination revealed gallstones.[3]

Laboratory findings
- Leukocytosis
- All other tests, including the liver function tests, were normal.[4]

Outcome A cholecystectomy was performed with complete recovery.[5]

Questions for discussion
1. What caused these symptoms?
2. Which risk factors for gallstones does this woman have?
3. Does this woman have cholelithiasis or cholecystitis or both?
4. If she had hyperbilirubinemia, what would be the significance of that finding?
5. How is a cholecystectomy performed? Can a person live without the gallbladder?

Chapter 9

THE EXOCRINE PANCREAS

Introduction

The pancreas is a mixed exocrine-endocrine gland attached to the duodenum. The exocrine pancreas produces digestive enzymes that are excreted into the lumen of the intestine. The hormones produced by the endocrine cells enter into the bloodstream and are distributed throughout the body. Hence, the diseases of the exocrine pancreas are in the domain of the gastroenterologist, whereas diabetes and other endocrine diseases are traditionally treated by endocrinologists.

The relative clinical significance of various pancreatic diseases is presented in Figure 9-1. Diseases of the exocrine pancreas are not as common as other gastrointestinal diseases, but are nevertheless a significant clinical problem. Carcinoma of the pancreas is the sixth most common human cancer, and its incidence is increasing.

Normal and Structure and Function

ANATOMY AND HISTOLOGY

To understand the clinical manifestations of pancreatic diseases a brief review of the development and macroscopic and microscopic anatomy of the pancreas is in order.

The pancreas is a solid retroperitoneal organ that has three main parts: head, body, and tail.

The normal pancreas measures approximately 15 cm and extends from the duodenum to the spleen. It is located in the retroperitoneum anterior to the aorta of the epigastrium and is fixed by fibrous tissue to the posterior abdominal wall. It is best visualized by computed tomography (CT, Fig. 9-2).

The connective tissue of the retroperitoneum contains numerous nerve endings and Pacinian corpuscles, which accounts for the pain that often accompanies pancreatic disease.

The exocrine pancreas drains into the duodenum.

The pancreas is a mixed exocrine-endocrine gland that has three parts: head, body, and tail (Fig. 9-3). The digestive juices produced by the exocrine part of the pancreas drain into the duodenum through a system of ducts. Minor interlobular ducts originating from the intercalated ducts at the center of the acini fuse and ultimately form a **major pancreatic duct** *(duct of Wirsung)*. Prior to entering into the duodenum, the duct of Wirsung fuses with the common bile duct forming an ampulla of Vater in 60% of cases. In the

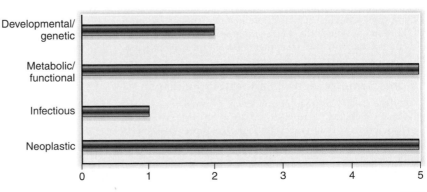

Figure 9-1 Relative importance of the most common pancreatic diseases.

KEY WORDS

Anatomy and Physiology

Acinus   Secretory unit of the exocrine pancreas. It is composed of several serous cells surrounding a lumen into which these cells secrete various digestive proenzymes.

Cholecystokinin   Polypeptide stimulating the secretion of enzyme from the pancreatic acinar cells. It is produced, like secretin, by the endocrine cells of the duodenum.

Ductal cells   Cuboidal cells lining the ducts of the pancreas. Serous cells secrete bicarbonates, whereas the mucous cells secrete mucus into the pancreatic juice.

Endopeptidases   Group of pancreatic hydrolytic enzymes comprising trypsin, chymotrypsin, and elastase. These enzymes cleave polypeptides into smaller units (oligopeptides) composed of two to six amino acids. Approximately 70% of proteins in food are broken down by endopeptidases.

Intercalated duct   Small duct that drains the acinar cell secretions into the larger pancreatic ducts.

Pancreas   Major exocrine gland that also contains endocrine elements in the form of the islets of Langerhans. It is located retroperitoneally and extends from the duodenum to the spleen.

Pancreatic ducts   The main pancreatic duct (duct of Wirsung) extends from the tail to the head of the pancreas. It joins the common bile duct prior to entering into the duodenum at the greater duodenal papilla (papilla of Vater). The accessory pancreatic duct (duct of Santorini) may be found in some people, bifurcating from the main duct and entering the duodenum at the lesser duodenal papilla.

Pancreatic enzymes   Several digestive enzymes produced by the acinar cells of the pancreas. These enzymes act on lipids (lipase and phospholipase), proteins (trypsin, chymotrypsin, carboxypeptidase), carbohydrates (amylase), nucleic acids (deoxyribonuclease, ribonuclease), and elastic tissue (elastase), just to mention the most important ones.

Secretin   Polypeptide hormone that stimulates pancreatic secretion of fluid rich in bicarbonate. It is produced by the endocrine cells in the duodenum.

Trypsin   Pancreatic endopeptidase that cleaves proteins into oligopeptides composed of several amino acids. It is secreted by pancreatic acinar cells as trypsinogen, an inactive proenzyme that is activated in the intestine into trypsin through the action of enterokinases located in the intestinal brush border.

Zymogen granules   Cytoplasmic granules containing proenzymes in acinar cells. These enzymes are excreted into the intercalated ducts and from there through the main pancreatic duct into the intestine.

Signs, Symptoms, and Laboratory Findings

Amylase test   Normal serum levels of amylase are less than 140 IU/dL. Serum amylase is a sensitive marker of pancreatic diseases, especially if amylase is present in high concentration (>700 IU/dL). However, amylase is also produced by salivary glands and may be elevated in the serum in a number of other diseases, such as liver and intestinal diseases or renal failure. Amylase is excreted in the urine and may be detected in the urine in patients who have elevated serum amylase.

Cholecystokinin test   Test used to detect chronic pancreatitis. Intravenous administration of cholecystokinin and secretin increases the volume of pancreatic secretion, which may be assessed by measuring the volume of juice in the duodenum and the concentration of bicarbonate and amylase. The test is technically difficult to perform. A peak bicarbonate concentration of less than 80 mEq/L is highly specific and suggestive of pancreatic insufficiency.

Endoscopic retrograde cholangiopancreatography (ERCP)   Noninvasive radiologic technique based on the injection of contrast medium into the pancreatic and biliary ducts through a catheter introduced into the duodenal papilla of Vater. It is used to visualize the ductal abnormalities of the pancreas, including ductal fibrosis, obstruction, pancreatic stones, and tumors. The catheter introduced into the pancreatic duct may be used to obtain cytologic samples for microscopic diagnosis of cancer. Approximately 5% of all patients develop acute pancreatitis after this procedure.

Fecal fat content   Test is based on collection of fecal material over 72 hours. Steatorrhea is defined as fecal fat content in excess of 7 g per 24 hours. The test is insensitive and becomes positive only if more than 90% of pancreatic acini are lost.

Lipase test   Normal serum contains less than 130 IU/L lipase. Serum lipase is a sensitive marker of pancreatic disease. It is more sensitive and more specific for acute pancreatitis than amylase, especially after the first day of the onset of disease.

Magnetic resonance cholangiopancreatography   Noninvasive radiologic technique used to visualize the pancreas and bile ducts, similar to ERCP.

Sweat test   Test is based on measuring the concentration of sodium (Na^+) and chloride (Cl^-) in sweat. The test is used to diagnose cystic fibrosis. On injection of pilocarpine the sweat of homozygous patients contains an increased concentration of Na^+ and Cl^- (>60 mEq/L). Sweat Cl^- is a more sensitive test for cystic fibrosis than sweat Na^+.

Trypsin test   Normal serum contains 20 to 80 μg/L of trypsin. Serum trypsin elevation is a very sensitive test of pancreatic disease. It has, however, low specificity since trypsin may be elevated in serum in hepatobiliary, intestinal, and renal diseases. The serum trypsin is measured by a radioimmune assay, which makes it impractical for routine usage.

Pancreatic Diseases

Acute pancreatitis   Acute inflammation of the pancreas related to intrapancreatic activation of pancreatic enzymes. It is characterized by autodigestion of the pancreas and adjacent tissues. The entry of activated pancreatic enzymes into the systemic circulation is typically associated with signs of shock.

Carcinoma of the pancreas   Malignant tumor most often originating from the pancreatic ducts.

Chronic pancreatitis   Chronic inflammation of the pancreas characterized by progressive fibrosis and calcification. Loss of pancreatic acini is accompanied by pancreatic insufficiency and malabsorption, whereas fibrosis usually causes persistent back pain.

Cystic fibrosis   Autosomal recessive genetic disease related to the mutation of the gene encoding the cystic fibrosis transmembrane conductance regulator (CFTR). The disease is characterized by abnormal secretion of pancreatic juices, as well as abnormal Cl^- secretion in the mucus in the bronchi, hepatobiliary tract, and sweat. These patients are prone to infection and usually die in early adulthood due to repeated respiratory infections.

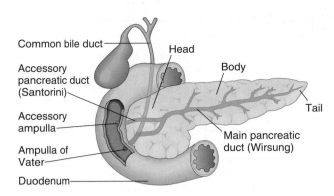

Figure 9-3 Diagram of the main anatomic components of the pancreas.

remaining 40% such a fusion does not occur, and many anatomic variants are present instead. Most people also have a separate **accessory duct** (the *duct of Santorini*), which branches from the main duct, entering the duodenum separately at its own ampulla. In many people such an ampulla does not exist, and the accessory duct ends blindly.

Pancreatic ducts are best visualized by **endoscopic retrograde cholangiopancreatography (ERCP).** This noninvasive radiologic technique is based on the injection of contrast medium into the pancreatic and biliary ducts through a catheter introduced into the duodenal papilla of the ampulla of Vater or the variant forms of the common bile duct and pancreatic ducts.

The pancreas develops from two primordia that fuse during fetal development.

The pancreas develops from a dorsal and a ventral bud of cells in the fetal duodenum. These two primordia fuse: the ventral giving rise to the head of the pancreas, and the dorsal forming the body and the tail. The main and the accessory pancreatic ducts are also formed in this process. Abnormal morphogenesis occurs in about 5% of persons, resulting in developmental anomalies, such as pancreas divisum, annular pancreas, or aberrant heterotropic pancreas in the wall of the stomach or intestine or in the liver.

Pearls

> Developmental anomalies are important for the radiologist performing ERCP, but in most instances they cause no clinical symptoms.
> Incomplete fusion of the ductal system may predispose to retention of pancreatic juices in parts of the pancreas, which may predispose to chronic pancreatitis.

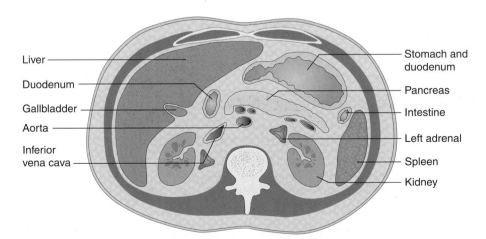

Figure 9-2 Pancreas as seen radiologically by computed tomography. It is located retroperitoneally between the spleen and the liver.

Histologically the exocrine pancreas consists of acini and ducts.

The secretory unit of the exocrine pancreas consists of acinar cells and excretory ducts (Fig. 9-4). The acinar cells are specialized protein-secreting cells arranged coronally around a centrally located intercalated duct. They are cuboidal and have abundant cytoplasm filled with zymogen granules. Zymogen granules contain proenzymes (zymogens) that are excreted into the ducts. The ductal cells are polarized and specialized for fluid and electron transport. These cells contribute bicarbonates, minerals, and water to the pancreatic juices. The ducts also contain scattered mucus-producing cells.

PHYSIOLOGY

The pancreas produces approximately 1500 mL of digestive juices per day. This pancreatic juice consists of (1) water, (2) minerals, (3) enzymes, (4) nonenzymatic proteins, and (5) mucus.

The pancreatic secretion has three main functions: (1) to provide digestive enzymes, (2) to protect the tissues from autodigestion by its own enzyme, and (3) to neutralize the acidity of the chyme arriving in the duodenum from the stomach.

Digestive enzymes are produced by the acinar cells.

Pancreatic acinar cells produce some 20 enzymes, which represent the primary digestive components of the pancreatic juice. These enzymes are proteins synthesized on the rough endoplasmic reticulum and packaged into membrane-bounded cytoplasmic granules. The contents of these granules are extruded into the intercalated ducts. Functionally these enzymes can be classified into several groups, most important of which are proteolytic, lipolytic, and amylolytic enzymes, and nucleases (Table 9-1).

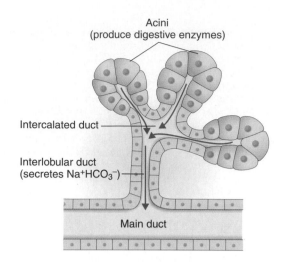

Figure 9-4 Diagram of the exocrine pancreatic acini and ducts.

All proteolytic enzymes are secreted in an inactive form, meaning as proenzymes that require additional activation to become functionally active. Other enzymes are secreted in an active form.

Nonenzymatic proteins secreted by acinar cells have regulatory functions but may also play a role in pancreatic diseases.

In addition to the enzyme, acinar cells secrete several proteins, the function of which is not fully understood. Nevertheless, it appears that these proteins play some regulatory roles. Some of these nonenzymatic secretory products are listed as follows:

- **Trypsin inhibitor.** It inactivates the prematurely activated trypsinogen. It is copackaged into granules together with trypsinogen, thus serving as an internal

Table 9-1 Pancreatic Enzymes

ENZYME CLASS	FUNCTION	TYPICAL ENZYMES
Proteolytic enzymes	Split peptide bonds of proteins forming oligopeptides and free amino acids	Trypsinogen Chymotrypsinogen Proelastase Procarboxypeptidase A and B
Lipolytic enzymes	Hydrolyze the bonds between fatty acids and glycerol or cholesterol esters	Lipase Phospholipase A_2 Carboxylesterlipase Colipase
Amylolytic enzymes	Breakdown of starch	Amylase
Nucleases	Breakdown of DNA and RNA	RNase DNase

blocker of this proteolytic enzyme. Note that the activation of trypsinogen into trypsin occurs only in the small intestine under the influence of intestinal *enterokinase.*

- **Protein GP2.** It is linked to the inner surface of zymogen granules and is thought to prevent reflux of the extruded enzymes from the intercalated duct into the acinar cells.
- **Lithostathine.** The function of this protein is unknown, but it is thought that it may prevent the formation of pancreatic stones. However, both protein GP2 and lithostathine may form intraductal plugs in dehydrated persons and those with cystic fibrosis and chronic pancreatitis.
- **Pancreatitis-associated protein.** This protein is found in low concentration under normal conditions, but it is present in high concentration in pancreatitis. It has been suggested that it has a bacteriostatic role, preventing infection and the formation of pancreatic abscesses.

Pancreatic juice contains salts and bicarbonates.

Pancreatic juice contains several ions in large concentration. These ions include Na^+, K^+, Ca^{2+}, Cl^-, and bicarbonate (HCO_3^-). Calcium is secreted by the acinar cells, whereas HCO_3^- and other ions are secreted by the ductal cells. The concentration of Na^+ and K^+ does not change, but the concentration of HCO_3^- and Cl^- does. The entry of Cl^- into the lumen of ducts depends on the proper function of the **cystic fibrosis transmembrane conductance regulator (CFTR).** Ductal cells have receptors for secretin, and on stimulation with secretin they secrete HCO_3^-. In that process Cl^- is exchanged for HCO_3^-, and accordingly the juices flowing from a stimulated pancreas are rich in HCO_3^-. Bicarbonate renders the pancreatic juice alkaline, and its pH rises over 8.0. The alkalinity of pancreatic juices discharged into the intestine neutralizes the acidity of the gastric juices as they enter the duodenum, and thus allows normal functioning of the pancreatic enzymes in the intestinal chyme.

Pancreatic secretion is low during the fasting phase but increases 10-fold during the digestive phase.

The secretory activity of the pancreas is under complex neurohumoral control. Two secretory phases are recognized: the fasting state and the digestive phase.

In the **fasting state** (*interdigestive period*) the basal secretory rate of the pancreas is relatively low. It is predominantly under parasympathetic control. Acetylcholine released from the terminal branches of the vagus nerve maintains a low level of constitutional secretory activity, which is inhibited by adrenergic stimuli.

Basal pancreatic secretion oscillates depending on intestinal motility. However, even with heightened stimulation during intestinal contraction, pancreatic secretion reaches only 10% to 20% of the maximum achieved during the digestive phase.

In the **digestive phase,** when the food enters the gastrointestinal tract, pancreatic secretion increases approximately 10 times over the basal rate. This increase is a consequence of stimulation by the intestinal hormones cholecystokinin and secretin.

- **Cholecystokinin (CCK)** is released from the duodenal neuroendocrine cells 10 to 30 minutes after ingestion of the food. The most potent stimulants for the release of CCK are lipids, but small peptones and amino acids in the food also stimulate these cells. The neuroendocrine cells of the duodenum that produce CCK-releasing factors may have a paracrine effect and also stimulate CCK release. Cholecystokinin stimulates the acinar cells to secrete pancreatic enzymes.
- **Secretin** is released from the neuroendocrine cells in the small intestine mostly in response to intestinal acidification by the gastric contents admixed with the food. Bile acids and lipids also stimulate secretin release. Secretin stimulates release of bicarbonates in the pancreas. It appears that CCK and secretin act in concert because injection of pure secretin never has the same effect as a combined CCK-secretin stimulation or, for that matter, as food itself.

The digestive phase pancreatic secretion has three interval phases: cephalic, gastric, and intestinal.

Like other parts of the gastrointestinal tract the pancreatic digestive phase stimulated by food has three interval phases called cephalic, gastric, and intestinal (Fig. 9-5).

- **Cephalic phase.** Mere exposure to food triggers the so-called cephalic phase, which is a reflex and most likely mediated by acetylcholine (ACh) released from the vagus nerve. It account for about 25% of the pancreatic secretion.
- **Gastric phase.** Entry of food into the stomach starts the second phase. The pancreas is stimulated by polypeptide hormones released from the gastric neuroendocrine cells, vagal stimulation, and the changes in the pH in the contents that reach the duodenum. This phase accounts for 10% to 20% of the pancreatic secretion.
- **Intestinal phase.** The third phase of stimulated pancreatic secretion begins with the entry of food into the duodenum. It provides 50% to 80% of the pancreatic secretion and is mediated mostly by CCK and secretin.

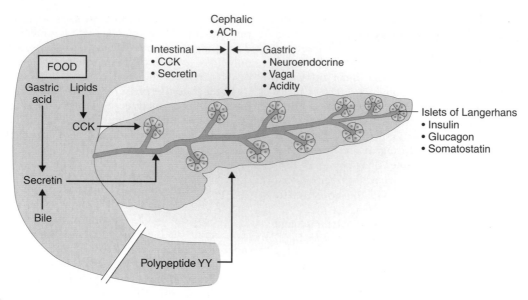

Figure 9-5 Neurohumoral control of pancreatic function. The stimulatory and inhibitory factors stem from the vagus and sympathetic nerves and the gastrointestinal hormones. Cholecystokinin (CCK) and secretin play the pivotal role in stimulating pancreatic secretion. ACh, acetylcholine.

> **Pearl**
>
> > The pancreas has a huge reserve capacity and is capable of producing much larger amounts of enzyme than needed. Hence, pancreatic insufficiency becomes clinically apparent only after a loss of 80% to 90% of all acini.

Stimuli from the distal small intestine inhibit digestive phase pancreatic secretion.

The exact mechanisms that reduce digestive phase pancreatic secretion are not fully understood. It is, however, well known that lipid in the distal small intestine has a negative feedback effect and is a potent stimulus for the reduction of pancreatic secretion. Polypeptide YY is the most significant inhibitor substance. Somatostatin and glucagon also contribute to the inhibition of pancreatic secretion.

Clinical and Laboratory Evaluation of Pancreatic Diseases

The evaluation of suspected acute or chronic pancreatic disease includes taking a complete history and performing a physical examination, as well as conducting standard laboratory tests and specialized tests aimed at detecting pancreatic disease. Additional testing includes sampling of the ascites fluid, if present, CT and ultrasound examination, or ERCP.

FAMILY AND PERSONAL HISTORY

Family and person history may provide some clues about the nature of pancreatic diseases. Here we concentrate on acute pancreatitis as the prototype of pancreatic diseases. Later we will see that acute pancreatitis can progress to chronic pancreatitis. The risk factors for acute pancreatitis that may be discovered by careful history taken from the patient are listed in Table 9-2.

PHYSICAL EXAMINATION

Symptoms and signs of pancreatic disease are most pronounced in the epigastrium but may also be seen in other parts of the body. The most important signs and symptoms are as follows:

- Pain
- Nausea and vomiting
- Abdominal tenderness
- Ascites
- Ileus
- Jaundice
- Shock, disseminated intravascular coagulopathy, and multiorgan failure
- Weight loss with or without steatorrhea
- Palpable epigastric mass

These symptoms may be present in both acute and chronic diseases of the pancreas, albeit in varying proportions (Table 9-3).

Table 9-2 Risk Factors for Acute Pancreatitis

TYPE OF RISK FACTOR	SPECIFIC DISEASE/ ASSOCIATION
Hereditary and metabolic diseases	Cystic fibrosis Hyperlipidemia Hyperparathyroidism Hemochromatosis End-stage renal disease Diabetic ketoacidosis
Social/nutritional factors	Alcoholism Severe malnutrition
Hepatobiliary diseases	Biliary stones Biliary/ampullary tumors
Infections	Viral infections: mumps, coxsackie B, HIV Worm infestation
Medical and surgical procedures	Post-ERCP Surgery of the biliary/ duodenal/pancreatic lesions Postrenal transplant
Drugs	Thiazides, furosemide, valproic acid, azathioprine, corticosteroids, oral contraceptives, sulfonamides
External factors	Trauma to the abdomen Hypothermia Scorpion bites Organophosphate poisoning

ERCP, endoscopic retrograde cholangiopancreatography; HIV, human immunodeficiency virus.

Epigastric pain is a feature of both acute and chronic pancreatitis and pancreatic cancer.

The pancreas has a rich innervation and contains numerous afferent nerve fibers that end in the celiac ganglia and the superior mesenteric ganglion (Fig. 9-6). Thus, many pancreatic diseases are accompanied by pain. However, the intensity, duration, and nature of the pain vary.

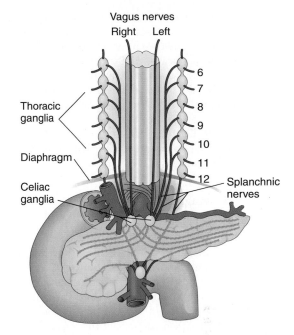

Figure 9-6 Diagram of the pancreatic innervation. The vagus nerves provide the predominant cholinergic stimuli, whereas the sympathetic inhibitory signals arise from the sympathetic ganglia. Sensory nerve fibers converge into the celiac ganglia and the superior mesenteric ganglion.

■ *Acute pancreatitis* is associated with pain in 80% to 90% of instances. It is intense, epigastric, and deep ("visceral") and tends to radiate into the back. Often it is associated with "*acute abdomen*," a term used if the patient is incapacitated by severe widespread abdominal pain, accompanied by nausea and vomiting, fever, and generalized tenderness to palpation. Such diffuse pain is a consequence of peritoneal irritation.

■ *Chronic pancreatitis* is accompanied by persistent nagging epigastric pain radiating into the back. Pain is often the most prominent symptom of disease, but its pattern, intensity, and frequency vary considerably. It

Table 9-3 Incidence of Common Symptoms and Signs in Acute and Chronic Pancreatic Diseases

FINDINGS	ACUTE PANCREATITIS	CHRONIC PANCREATITIS	CARCINOMA OF THE PANCREAS
Pain	Intense, 90–100%, lasts a few days	Dull, 80–90%, tends to diminish over time	Dull, 30–60%, tends to become more severe over time
Nausea and vomiting	50–90%	—	30–40%
Abdominal tenderness, ileus, and ascites	50–80%	—	—
Jaundice	20–30%	0–20%	60–90% (head), 15% (tail)
Shock	30–60%	—	—
Weight loss	—	15–30%	60–90%

may be mild or severe and intolerable. Sometimes it may be persistent, or it may last a few days, then stop for a day or two and then recur. The pain may be alleviated by bending forward and is aggravated by standing up. It may be worsened by intake of alcohol or food.

■ *Pancreatic cancer* is accompanied by pain in 60% to 80% of patients. It begins gradually and usually becomes more pronounced as the tumor spreads and invades the celiac plexus. Tumors of the tail and body are more likely to produce pain than tumors of the head of the pancreas.

Nausea and vomiting are common symptoms of acute pancreatitis but occur also in some patients with chronic disease.

Nausea, that is, an unpleasant sensation in the throat and epigastrium, often accompanied by vomiting, is a common symptom of acute pancreatitis. Both the nausea and the vomiting result from the sensory impulses emanating from the inflamed pancreas.

Vomiting is a reflex mediated by the vomiting center in the lateral reticular formation close to the nucleus of the vagus nerve. In acute pancreatitis the initial stimuli from the inflamed pancreas reach the vomiting center through the afferent vagal and sympathetic nerves. Any food or fluids taken by mouth are rapidly vomited. To prevent this from occurring it a standard practice to introduce a nasojejunal tube and thus try to rehydrate and nourish the patient.

Approximately 20% to 30% patients with carcinoma of the head of the pancreas have an urge to vomit. This may be due to the compression or obstruction of the duodenum, in which case the tumor prevents the passage of food, which triggers the vomiting reflex.

Pain in acute pancreatitis may be a consequence of chemical peritonitis.

Leakage of enzymes and chemical mediators of inflammation from the acutely inflamed or necrotic pancreas may cause **"chemical" peritonitis.** This inflammation is typically associated with formation of protein-rich *ascites.* The fluid aspirated from the abdominal cavity contains pancreatic enzymes (e.g., amylase and lipase). In contrast to bacterial peritonitis, the fluid is sterile, and the bacteriologic studies give negative results.

Acute peritonitis is accompanied by *fever, diffuse abdominal pain,* and *tenderness of the anterior abdominal wall to palpation.* In about 60% of cases it is associated with *paralytic ileus,* and in such cases no bowel movements are heard on auscultation. Persistent ileus makes the intestinal walls permeable and allows the bacteria to cross into the peritoneal cavity. This is marked by the transition of chemical peritonitis into an infectious bacterial peritonitis that has a high accompanying mortality rate.

Pancreatic jaundice results from obstruction of the common bile duct.

Both acute and chronic pancreatic disease may cause jaundice. Jaundice is typically caused by an obstruction of the terminal part of the common bile duct as it passes through the head of the pancreas. Biochemically it is characterized by an elevation of conjugated bilirubin and alkaline phosphatase.

Acute pancreatitis may be accompanied by biliary obstruction, which is caused by the swelling and inflammation of the head of the pancreas. Such jaundice is of sudden onset, mild, and transient. As the inflammation subsides and inflammatory edema disappears, the bile flow resumes and the jaundice disappears.

Pancreatic carcinoma often manifests with jaundice. The accompanying jaundice is usually described as "painless," although about 30% patients complain of some pain. Jaundice occurs in most patients with carcinoma of the head of the pancreas, but it is not an early symptom in those who have carcinoma of the tail. As the tumors grow, all tumors of the pancreas can produce jaundice. The jaundice is typically progressive, associated with pruritus, and may require palliative surgery. Mild chronic jaundice can be seen in some patients with chronic pancreatitis.

Acute pancreatitis may result in shock, accompanied by disseminated intravascular coagulation and multiorgan failure.

Acute pancreatitis may be accompanied by an entry of pancreatic enzymes into the systemic circulation. In the most severe form of acute pancreatitis these enzymes trigger **disseminated intravascular coagulation (DIC)** and cause **shock** with multiorgan failure. Loss of fluids due to vomiting and leakage of albumin-rich fluid into the peritoneal cavity aggravate the clinical condition by causing hypovolemia and hypotension and by reducing the oncotic pressure of the plasma.

Respiratory failure characterized by profound hypoxemia is a hallmark of severe acute pancreatitis. The exact mechanism of this complication is unknown, but it is thought that DIC and the entry of various enzymes and cytokines into the circulation contribute to the circulatory disturbances that occur in the lungs. Intrapulmonary shunting of blood may reach 30%, and since one third of the total blood passing through the lungs never reaches the alveoli, and thus is never oxygenated, dyspnea and pulmonary insufficiency develop.

Cardiovascular failure results in hypotension and hypoperfusion of vital organs. This aspect of shock is most likely caused by the pooling of blood in the splanchnic area and transudation of fluid into the peritoneal cavity and the formation of ascites. Dilatation of peripheral blood vessels mediated by inflammatory cytokines is yet another important pathogenetic mechanism. Fluid replacement by intravenous infusion is thus important, but if that does not help, adrenaline infusion should be considered.

Renal failure results from hypoperfusion of the kidneys due to hypotension and hypovolemic shock. Fluid replacement therapy is the treatment of choice, but it may be supplemented with adrenergic drugs.

A *bleeding tendency* is a common complication of acute pancreatitis. In most severe cases the pancreas shows massive necrosis and hemorrhage *(acute hemorrhagic necrosis of the pancreas)*. This bleeding results from the action of pancreatic proteolytic enzymes such as trypsin and elastase acting on the blood vessels of the pancreas and adjacent tissues. Disseminated intravascular coagulation leads to consumption of coagulation factors and platelets and the widespread appearance of dermal ecchymoses. Internal bleeding is especially common in the gastrointestinal tract.

Pearls

> *Cullen's sign*, referring to the periumbilical bruise, may be found in 3% to 5% of patients with acute pancreatitis. It is not specific and is seen in other conditions, such as extrauterine pregnancy.
> *Grey Turner's sign* is similar to the bruising seen on the flanks in acute pancreatitis.

Weight loss is a common symptom of chronic pancreatitis and pancreatic carcinoma.

Weight loss is one of the cardinal symptoms of *chronic pancreatitis*. It is a consequence of malabsorption due to a lack of pancreatic enzymes. Typically it is associated with steatorrhea, which develops after the total output of pancreatic digestive enzymes has been reduced by 85% to 90%. Malabsorption of fats may cause deficiency of fat-soluble vitamins A, D, E, and K.

Cachexia and weight loss are found in almost all (>90%) patients with *carcinoma* of the pancreas. The reasons for weight loss are complex and include, among others, the increased energy expenditure to meet the requirements of the growing tumor cells and the digestive problems caused by the occlusion of the pancreatic and biliary duct and destruction of pancreatic acini.

A palpable epigastric mass in the area of the pancreas may be a malignant tumor, a cystic benign tumor, or a pseudocyst.

Malignant tumors of the pancreas are rarely palpable in the early stages of the disease. A palpable mass found during the initial examination has been reported only in 15% of all patients. More often pancreatic tumors cause enlargement of the liver (found in 80% of patients), which is often a consequence of hepatic metastases or distention of the gallbladder (30%). Enlargement of the spleen may be caused by the obstruction of the splenic vein or the spleen.

Benign tumors of the pancreas are rare, accounting for only 5% of all pancreatic tumors. Due to their slow growth such tumors often attain a considerable size and, in relative terms, are more often palpable than malignant tumors. Benign tumors are also cystic, and the mucus or serous fluid filling the cavities of the tumor tends to contribute to the mass effect.

Pseudocysts developing after a bout of acute pancreatic necrosis may manifest as distinct masses that are palpable in approximately one half of all cases. The diminishing size of a mass is usually a sign that the fluid in a pseudocyst is being absorbed or drained.

LABORATORY FINDINGS

The most important laboratory tests used for diagnosing pancreatic disease are as follows:

- **Markers of pancreatic acinar cell injury.** These tests typically measure the serum or urine concentration of amylase, lipase, or trypsin.
- **Markers of overall tissue injury.** The most widely used test is serum lactate dehydrogenase, a ubiquitous enzyme released from many damaged organs and even hemolyzed red blood cells.
- **Study of pancreatic functional reserve or loss of parenchyma.** These tests include cholecystokinin-secretin test, measurement of fecal fat, and various ultrasonic and radiologic techniques.
- **Tests of pancreatic and biliary duct obstruction.** These tests include measurements of serum bilirubin and alkaline phosphatase, ERCP, and radiographic techniques.
- **Tumor markers.** These include carbohydrate antigen 19-9 (CA 19-9) and carcinoembryonic antigen (CEA).

Amylase is a good marker of pancreatic acinar cell injury.

Amylase, also known as α-1,4-glucosidase, is the most important pancreatic enzyme involved in the digestion of carbohydrates. It hydrolyzes the terminal α-1,4-glucosidic bonds of starch. Amylase is normally present in serum in low concentration (i.e., <200 U/L). It is also present in urine, and its activity is in the range from 0 to 300 U/L.

The pancreas and the salivary glands are the major sources of serum amylase, but small amounts are derived from the fallopian tubes, the liver, kidneys, and some other internal organs. In healthy persons most of the serum amylase is derived from the salivary glands. Amylase has no known function in the blood.

Amylase occurs in the serum in two isoforms: *P-amylase* is derived almost exclusively from the pancreas, and *S-amylase* is derived from other organs. These two isoamylase forms can be separated from one another by electrophoresis. Both forms of amylase have a short half-life of approximately 2 hours. P-amylase is excreted through the kidneys in urine, whereas S-amylase is taken up by the fixed macrophages of the spleen and liver. Kidney diseases and a reduced glomerular filtration rate could cause elevation of serum P-amylase.

Serum amylase is a good marker of acute pancreatitis. However, since an elevation of serum amylase may be caused by salivary gland disease (e.g., bacterial sialadenitis, mumps, Sjögren syndrome, irradiation of the neck), biliary tract disease, or renal insufficiency (reduced GFR) it is important to interpret the laboratory findings in the context of other clinical data.

In a patient who has the typical features of acute pancreatitis, the serum amylase concentration increases two to three times or higher over the normal within 2 to 12 hours after the onset of symptoms (Fig. 9-7). Serum amylase remains elevated for 3 to 5 days. A persistently elevated serum amylase level after the symptoms of acute pancreatitis have subsided is a sign of such complications as pancreatic pseudocysts or pancreatic ascites.

In 1% to 2% of adults who have neither pancreatic nor salivary gland disease, serum amylase is elevated due to so-called *macroamylasemia*. In this condition, amylase is bound to another plasma protein, such as immunoglobulin, and cannot be excreted in the urine.

The most important causes of hyperamylasemia are listed in Table 9-4.

Amylase activity in the urine is elevated in patients with acute pancreatitis. The urinary amylase appears with a lag of several hours and remains elevated longer than in the serum. Elevated urinary amylase is seen in patients with pseudocysts of the pancreas and in 10% of patients with chronic pancreatitis.

Normally the ratio of amylase clearance to creatinine clearance is between 1% and 4%; an elevation over 5% is a usually typical of pancreatic disease. In macroamylasemia

Table 9-4 Causes of Elevation of Serum Amylase

DISEASE	PATHOGENESIS OF HYPERAMYLASEMIA

Pancreatic diseases
  Acute pancreatitis
  Pancreatic pseudocyst
  Pancreatic carcinoma
  ERCP
  Pancreatic surgery
	Release of amylase from damaged pancreatic acinar cells

Gastrointestinal disease
  Peptic ulcer penetrating into the pancreas
  Small-bowel obstruction
  Peritonitis
	Release of amylase from damaged pancreatic acinar cells

Salivary gland disease
  Mumps
  Sialoadenitis
  Sialolithiasis
	Release of salivary gland amylase

Ectopic (tubal) pregnancy	Release of amylase from fallopian tube
Renal insufficiency	Reduced renal clearance of amylase
Opiates	Reflux of amylase due to the spasm of the sphincter of Oddi
Macroamylasemia	Binding of amylase to plasma proteins
Tumors (acinic cell carcinoma of pancreas, carcinoma of lung, carcinoma of ovary)	Paraneoplastic production of amylase by tumor cells

ERCP, endoscopic retrograde cholangiopancreatography.
Modified from Marshall WJ, Bangert SK: Clinical Biochemistry. Metabolic and Clinical Aspects. New York, Churchill Livingstone, 1995.

and in chronic renal diseases the concentration of amylase in the urine is within normal limits, and hyperamylasemia is not accompanied by increased amylase activity in the urine.

The activity of serum lipase and trypsin also rise during acute pancreatitis.

Lipase, a hydrolytic enzyme that cleaves the fatty acids from glycerol, is an important component of pancreatic juice. The pancreas is the only source of this enzyme. The serum activity of lipase is normally under 280 IU/L. In acute pancreatitis serum levels of lipase rise in parallel with the activity of amylase, reaching a maximum of more than five times the normal within 24 to 30 hours (see Fig. 9-7). Serum lipase activity remains high longer than that of amylase, falling to normal levels 8 to 12 days after the onset of the attack. Lipase may be found in the urine, but urinary measurement is rarely performed in clinical practice.

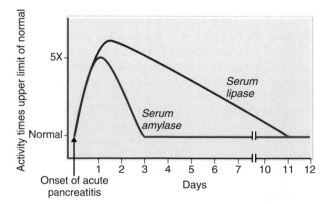

Figure 9-7 Serum amylase and lipase in the course of acute pancreatitis. Amylase and lipase rise in serum at the same rate. The amylase remains detectable in the urine longer than in serum.

By ordering serum amylase and lipase tests at the same time one may increase the sensitivity and specificity of laboratory diagnosis of pancreatitis and exclude nonpancreatic causes of amylasemia or macroamylasemia.

Trypsin circulates in serum as an inactive proenzyme (trypsinogen) or bound to protease inhibitors α_1-antitrypsin and α_2-macroglobulin. Trypsin activity increases in acute pancreatitis, but the test is difficult to perform and is rarely used in clinical practice.

Lactate dehydrogenase is used as a marker of tissue necrosis and an indicator of the severity of acute pancreatitis.

Lactate dehydrogenase (LDH) is a ubiquitous enzyme and it is present in the blood in concentrations of 100 to 270 IU/L in males and 122 to 220 IU/L in females. Serum LDH is derived from various organs and also from aging and destroyed red and white blood cells. Lactate dehydrogenase is elevated in serum in various diseases, such as myocardial infarction or liver necrosis, and is thus also elevated in the blood of patients who have acute pancreatic necrosis. Overall, the concentration of LDH in serum reflects the severity of tissue necrosis and the size of hematoma formed at the site of acute pancreatitis. LDH levels over 400 IU/L are one of the signs of severe pancreatic injury. Protracted elevation of LDH in blood after an attack of acute pancreatitis is usually a sign of remaining complications, such as pancreatic pseudocysts.

The cholecystokinin-secretin test is used to measure pancreatic secretory reserve.

The **cholecystokinin-secretin test** is a functional test designed to measure the capacity of the pancreas to produce enzymes and bicarbonates. It is performed by measuring the basal pancreatic secretion of amylase and bicarbonate content in the duodenum and by comparing it with changes seen 30 minutes after intravenous injection of CCK and 60 minutes after injection of secretin. The CCK-secretin test gives low values in chronic pancreatitis, but only after more than 85% to 90% of the total pancreatic parenchyma has been lost.

Newer tests have been introduced to replace the rather laborious older CCK-secretin tests. In these tests, the labeled substrates for pancreatic enzymes are administered orally, and the products of enzymatic digestion are measured in the urine or breath. For example in the *bentiromide test*, *N*-benzoyl-L-tyrosine-*p*-aminobenzoic acid is given orally, and *p*-aminobenzoic acid, the product of proteolytic cleavage, is measured in the urine.

Pancreatic insufficiency causes steatorrhea, which can be documented by measuring the fat content of feces.

Steatorrhea is characterized by bulky, foul-smelling, greasy stools. The diagnosis can be made by inspecting the feces or by measuring its fat content. This is usually done by collecting feces over a 3-day period. In steatorrhea feces contain more than 7 g of fat per 24 hours. A rough estimate can be made by microscopically examining feces for **fat particles** that were stained by special stains such as Sudan III or Oil red O. Note that steatorrhea can be not only of pancreatic but also of intestinal or biliary origin.

Carcinoma of the head of the pancreas causes biliary obstruction.

Signs of biliary obstruction are often the first evidence of carcinoma of the head of the pancreas. Typically, biliary obstruction results in jaundice and is accompanied by an elevation of serum *conjugated bilirubin* and *alkaline phosphatase*. Biliary obstruction and jaundice are found also in 25% of patients with acute pancreatitis and 10% of those with chronic pancreatitis.

Carbohydrate antigen 19-9 is a tumor marker found in the serum of most pancreatic cancer patients, but this test has low sensitivity and specificity.

The search for specific serologic markers of pancreatic adenocarcinoma has been disappointing so far. The most widely used marker is **CA 19-9,** a sialosyl-fucosyl-lactotetrose found in cell membrane glycolipids and glycoproteins of the mucus secreted by pancreatic carcinomas. This tumor marker is found in increased concentration in the serum of 75% of patients with pancreatic carcinoma. Unfortunately the test has a sensitivity of only 60%, and it cannot be used for screening purposes. Furthermore CA 19-9 may be found in the serum of patients who have cancer of other organs besides those of the pancreas.

SPECIAL TECHNIQUES FOR EVALUATING PANCREATIC DISEASES

Due to its location the pancreas is inaccessible to palpation during physical examination. Nevertheless, it can be visualized by ultrasound and radiologic techniques. Ultrasound, CT, and ERCP are widely used for diagnosing pancreatic diseases as follows:

- **Ultrasound** is the method of choice for demonstrating acute swelling of the pancreas in acute pancreatitis. It is also good for detecting pancreatic cysts, pseudocysts, and tumors. It is also used in the initial stages of evaluating suspected chronic pancreatitis. Ultrasonographic examination may be difficult and also unreliable because of the superimposition of gas-containing intestinal loops overlying the pancreas.
- **Computed tomography** is widely used for evaluating chronic pancreatic disease. In chronic pancreatitis CT can demonstrate a loss of parenchyma, irregularity of the pancreatic outline, and cystic dilatation of ducts. Calcification inside an atrophic pancreas can be seen in approximately one third of all patients with chronic pancreatitis.

■ **Endoscopic retrograde cholangiopancreatography** is the most complex but also the most reliable test currently used to diagnose chronic pancreatitis and pancreatic tumors. Its specificity for diagnosing chronic pancreatitis is over 90%. It is often combined with cytologic examination of ductal contents and is thus the most reliable way to distinguish chronic pancreatitis from pancreatic carcinoma.

> ### Pearl
>
> > Radiologic techniques have supplanted functional tests in the diagnosis of chronic pancreatitis and pancreatic insufficiency.

Clinicopathologic Correlations

CYSTIC FIBROSIS OF THE PANCREAS

Cystic fibrosis (CF) is a systemic genetic disease caused by mutation of the *CF* gene, located on chromosome 7. Cystic fibrosis is the most common lethal genetic disease in the United States, affecting 1:3,000 whites, 1:13,000 blacks, and 1:62,000 East Asians.

The *CF* gene encodes the protein known as the cystic fibrosis transmembrane conductance regulator (CFTR), which acts as a transmembrane chloride channel and a regulator of chloride and sodium flux across the membrane of epithelial cells of many organs. As mentioned earlier CFTR plays an important role in regulating the influx of chloride ions into the lumen of ducts and the formation of the pancreatic juice. Disturbances of CFTR result in the formation of viscous pancreatic secretions that tend to plug the ducts. Obstruction of the ducts leads to backpressure and atrophy of the acini. Loss of exocrine pancreatic tissue is accompanied by pancreatic insufficiency and malabsorption.

Viscous mucus is formed not only in the pancreas but in other organs as well.

Abnormal CFTR function results in the formation of viscous mucus, causing functional problems in several organs as follows (Fig. 9-8):

■ **Intestinal obstruction.** Viscous meconium causes obstruction of the intestines in neonates (meconium ileus). Obstructed intestines may rupture and cause meconium peritonitis. In older children CF may cause distal intestinal obstruction syndrome and fibrosing colonopathy with frequent rectal prolapse.
■ **Pancreatic obstruction.** Inspissated mucus may cause obstruction of the major pancreatic duct and thus prevent the entry of pancreatic digestive enzyme into the intestine. Lack of pancreatic enzymes causes steatorrhea and malabsorption. At the same time the retrograde pressure caused by the ductal plugs leads to atrophy of the pancreatic acini, and a pathologic picture indistinguishable from chronic pancreatitis develops. In one third of these patients loss of acini is accompanied by a loss of islets of Langerhans and clinical signs of diabetes mellitus.

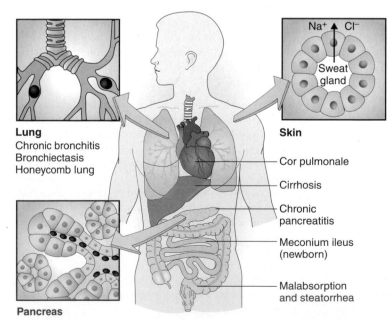

Lung
Chronic bronchitis
Bronchiectasis
Honeycomb lung

Skin

Cor pulmonale

Cirrhosis

Chronic pancreatitis

Meconium ileus (newborn)

Malabsorption and steatorrhea

Pancreas

Figure 9-8 Cystic fibrosis. The disease affects predominantly the lungs and the gastrointestinal tract, including the liver and the pancreas. The sweat test is important for the diagnosis of cystic fibrosis in infants and children.

■ **Bronchial obstruction.** Mucus in the bronchi predisposes to chronic infection and formation of bronchiectasis. Recurrent pneumonias are the most common cause of death in these patients. Death usually occurs by the third decade.

■ **Biliary obstruction.** Mucous plugs in the biliary ducts may cause obstructive jaundice, cholelithiasis, and secondary biliary cirrhosis.

> ### Pearl
>
> > The old name for cystic fibrosis is mucoviscidosis! It is still the best way to describe the main feature of this disease (viscid mucus) in one word.

Cystic fibrosis causes changes in the excretion of sodium and chloride in sweat.

Abnormal function of the CFTR results in abnormal loss of Na^+ and Cl^- in sweat. In extreme cases this loss of mineral ions may lead to hypochloremic and hyponatremic metabolic alkalosis, predisposing such children to heat stroke.

Excessive Cl^- in sweat can be stimulated by pilocarpine. In this **pilocarpine sweat test** a sweat concentration of Cl^- over 60 mmol/L is diagnostic of CF in children. In adults a value of over 70 mmol/L is consistent with CF, and a genetic test is recommended to confirm the diagnosis.

Genetic tests are used to confirm the diagnosis of cystic fibrosis.

Although more than 1000 distinct mutations of the *CF* gene have been identified, more than 70% of all cases are caused by the **mutation Δ*F508*.** Most testing laboratories provide testing for the 87 most common mutations, but in some cases additional testing might be required in specialized reference centers. Family members should also be offered the same type of testing to detect asymptomatic carriers. In the general population in the United States 1 in 28 white persons carries the mutated gene.

ACUTE PANCREATITIS

Acute pancreatitis is an acute inflammation caused by an injury of pancreatic acinar cells during which pancreatic digestive enzymes leak into the tissue of the pancreas and adjacent organs. Autodigestion of the pancreas is accompanied by an acute inflammation and vascular changes. Massive necrosis may be found in 10% to 20% of cases. Systemic multiorgan failure that follows is associated with significant mortality and, in patients who survive, significant complications such as pancreatic pseudocysts and chronic pancreatitis.

Table 9-5 The Most Important Causes of Acute Pancreatitis

Common causes
  Biliary disease (gallstones)
  Alcohol abuse
Uncommon causes
  Drugs (e.g., diuretics, ACE inhibitors, azathioprine, methyldopa)
  Infections (e.g., mumps, *Ascaris*, coxsackievirus, *Mycobacterium avium intracellulare* complex)
  ERCP
  Surgery of pancreas and upper abdomen
  Abdominal trauma
  Genetic diseases (e.g., hypertryglyceridemia, cystic fibrosis)
  Gastroduodenal diseases (e.g., peptic ulcer)
Idiopathic (15%)

ACE, angiotensin-converting enzyme; ERCP, endoscopic retrograde cholangiopancreatography.

Acute pancreatitis is in most instances a complication of biliary tract disease or alcohol abuse.

Acute pancreatitis has an incidence of 5 to 20 cases per 100,000 per year. As shown in Table 9-5 acute pancreatitis may have many causes. However, in practical terms, biliary obstruction and alcohol abuse account for 75% to 80% of all cases (Fig. 9-9).

Biliary stones are the most common identifiable cause of acute pancreatitis. Obstruction of the ampullary part of the common bile duct and pancreatic duct may have two principal consequences:

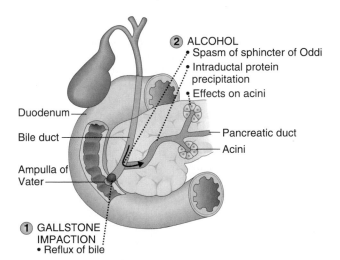

Figure 9-9 Acute pancreatitis. Biliary obstruction causing reflux of bile into the main pancreatic duct and chronic alcoholism are the main causes of acute pancreatitis. Alcohol causes spasms of the sphincter of Oddi but also affects the pancreatic cells directly.

■ Increased intraductal pancreatic pressure
■ Reflux of bile into the pancreatic duct

Increased intraductal pressure may be transmitted into the acini and thus ultimately cause the rupture of acinar cell membranes. Reflux of bile may cause premature intrapancreatic activation of proenzymes such as trypsinogen. Enzyme leakage from the disrupted cells is associated with fat necrosis, proteolysis of other parenchymal cells, and formation of chemotactic factors, which attract neutrophils and initiate acute inflammation. The entry of pancreatic enzyme into the blood vessels causes thrombosis, and the subsequent ischemia contributes even further to pancreatic necrosis.

Alcohol, the most common cause of acute pancreatitis in the United States, has a more complex role in the pathogenesis of acute pancreatitis. Alcohol could have multiple effects, some of which are listed here:

■ **Spasm of the sphincter of Oddi.** The contracture of the sphincter is accompanied by a reflux of bile into the pancreatic duct.
■ **Precipitation of intraductal proteins.** These changes are accompanied by the formation of plugs and pancreatic ductal stones.
■ **Secretin release.** Alcohol stimulates acid secretion in the stomach, which triggers a release of secretin. Secretin promotes secretion of pancreatic juices, thus further contributing to intrapancreatic pressure.
■ **Acinar cell injury.** Alcohol acts on acinar cells by causing increased cell membrane permeability and disruption of cytoskeletal fibers. It also changes blood flow through the pancreas. These events make cells more vulnerable to autodigestion by enzymes released from damaged acinar cells.
■ **Inhibition of lithostatin secretion.** Lithostatins are nonenzymatic proteins secreted by acinar cells. Their function is to prevent the aggregation of calcium carbonate crystals and the formation of intraductal plugs and concretions. In the absence of lithostatins, plugs form and tend to calcify into intraductal calculi, which obstruct the flow of the pancreatic juices.

Although there is ample evidence that alcohol has adverse effects on the pancreas, acute pancreatitis develops only in a minority of people who abuse alcohol. Obviously other genetic, nutritional, and environmental factors probably contribute to the onset of disease.

Acute pancreatitis is a "chemical inflammation," and the tissue injury results from the action of pancreatic digestive enzymes.

Acute pancreatitis begins with an inappropriate activation of pancreatic enzymes (Fig. 9-10). As mentioned earlier, essentially all proteolytic enzymes, such as trypsin and chymotrypsin, are excreted from pancreatic acinar cells in an inactive form (i.e., as proenzymes). These enzymes remain inactive in the pancreatic ducts and are activated by enterokinase on entry into the small intestine. Premature activation of trypsin, as seen in acute pancreatitis, has devastating effects on the pancreas and is considered today to be the primary event that initiates the destruction of tissue in this disease.

The cause of acute pancreatitis remains unknown in about 15% of cases.

In patients who do not have biliary disease and do not abuse alcohol, acute pancreatitis may be related to some other factors. The most important among those are various *drugs*. Numerous drugs have been implicated as a possible cause of pancreatitis. A small number of cases are related to *viral* or *bacterial infections*, and in some instances there is a history of trauma. Even so, at least 15% of cases are considered to be *idiopathic* and unrelated to any identifiable exogenous cause.

Acute pancreatitis has a sudden onset and manifests with local and systemic symptoms.

The clinical presentation of acute pancreatitis varies greatly and may range from mild to severe. In typical cases it usually manifests with sudden pain in the epigastrium. In many cases it occurs 12 to 24 hours after a large meal or episode of binge drinking. Pain radiates into the back and is usually associated with nausea, vomiting, and abdominal wall guarding. Fever and sweating and signs of severe distress are common. The most common signs and symptoms in uncomplicated acute pancreatitis are listed in Table 9-6.

In severe cases there are systemic signs of shock, such as tachycardia, hypotension, and oliguria due to renal failure. Respirations are rapid and shallow, and hypoxia develops due to acute respiratory distress syndrome (ARDS). Disseminated intravascular coagulation develops and is accompanied by a bleeding tendency. Enzyme spilling through the abdominal cavity may cause peritonitis, which is sterile and chemically mediated. Ileus may also be present, which may facilitate the passage of bacteria through the intestinal wall and contribute to the formation of bacterial peritonitis or pancreatic abscesses. In most severe cases bacteremia and sepsis are also evident. The most important features of complicated acute pancreatitis are listed in Table 9-7.

Laboratory findings are essential for the diagnosis of acute pancreatitis.

Acute pancreatitis is associated with the usual signs of pancreatic tissue destruction, acute inflammation, dehydration, shock, and multiple organ failure. The most important laboratory findings are as follows:

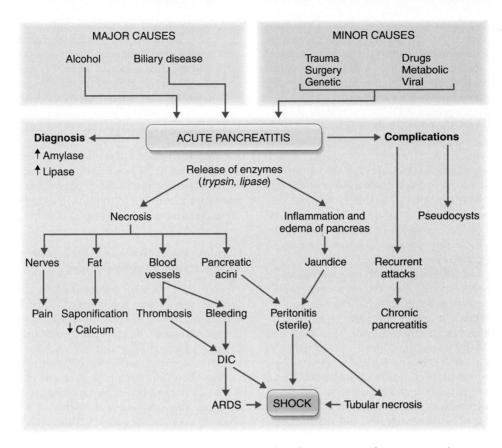

Figure 9-10 Acute pancreatitis. All clinical findings can be related to the activation of enzymes, such as trypsinogen, amylase, lipase, elastase, and others. Trypsinogen activation is considered to be the key event and it leads to activation of other enzymes. ARDS, acute respiratory distress syndrome; DIC, disseminated intravascular coagulation.

- **Leukocytosis.** It is a sign of acute inflammation of the pancreas. Leukocytosis over $16 \times 10^9/L$ in nonalcoholic cases, and over $18 \times 10^9/L$ in alcoholics, is a bad prognostic sign.
- **Hemoconcentration.** Hematocrit is elevated due to dehydration. A hematocrit decrease of more than 10 points within 48 hours is a bad prognostic sign.

Table 9-6 Signs and Symptoms of Uncomplicated Acute Pancreatitis

SIGNS AND SYMPTOMS	FREQUENCY (%)
Abdominal pain	85–95
Sensitivity to palpation of abdomen	70–90
Nausea and vomiting	50–80
Fever	50–60
Dehydration	30–50
Generalized distress	40–60
Paralytic ileus	40–60

Table 9-7 Signs and Symptoms of Severe Acute Pancreatitis

Peritonitis
   Ascites
   Ileus
Shock
   Hypotension
   Tachycardia
   Renal failure
   ARDS with dyspnea and tachypnea
   Disseminated intravascular coagulation
Bleeding tendency
   Ecchymoses
   Gastrointestinal bleeding
   Cullen's sign (periumbilical bruise)
   Grey Turner's sign (flank bruise)
Infection
   Pancreatic abscess
   Bacterial peritonitis
   Sepsis

ARDS, acute respiratory distress syndrome.

- **Amylase and lipase elevation in blood.** These pancreatic enzymes leak from the damaged pancreas into the blood. Amylase can be detected in the urine as well as in the ascites fluid. LDH, which is not restricted to the pancreas, is also used to gauge the extent of tissue injury in pancreatitis.
- **Lactate dehydrogenase (LDH).** Serum levels of LDH increase proportionately with the extent of pancreatic injury. Lactate dehydrogenase over 400 IU/L is a bad prognostic sign.
- **Hypocalcemia.** It develops during the second or third day after onset of pancreatic inflammation. It is caused by the formation of calcium soaps at the sites of fat necrosis in the pancreas and the fat tissue of the abdominal cavity. Formation of fat soaps leads to depletion of circulating calcium. Calcium levels below 8 mg/dL are a bad prognostic sign.
- **Bilirubin and alkaline phosphatase elevation in serum.** These changes reflect the obstruction of bile ducts that occurs in about 20% of cases.
- **Hyperglycemia.** Injury to the islets of Langerhans causes a relative deficiency of insulin. This "acute diabetes" is usually reversible. Glucose concentration in the blood of over 200 mg/dL is a bad prognostic sign.
- **Creatinine and BUN elevation in the blood.** Azotemia occurs in patients who have renal insufficiency.
- **Thrombocytopenia and coagulation disorders** (e.g., prolonged bleeding time, PT, and aPTT). These changes are found in patients who develop DIC.
- **Respiratory alkalosis.** It develops in patients who are hyperventilating and are also hypoxemic. These patients also have low Pao_2.
- **Metabolic alkalosis.** It develops due to the release of minerals and other cations from destroyed tissues.
- **Metabolic acidosis.** It develops due to prolonged renal failure.
- **Respiratory acidosis.** It is usually found in severe cases with ARDS and pulmonary hyaline membrane formation. Pao_2 of less than 60 mm Hg after 48 hours of onset of the attack of pancreatitis is a bad prognostic sign.

Severe acute pancreatitis may have serious complications.

Severe acute pancreatitis still has a mortality rate of close to 10%. Those patients that survive may develop serious complications, the most important of which are as follows:

- **Pancreatic abscess.** It results from invasion of bacteria into the necrotic pancreatic tissue. Such infections may be resistant to treatment.
- **Pancreatic pseudocyst.** These cavitary lesions develop at the site of massive tissue necrosis in the pancreatic parenchyma. The cavity contains enzymes and tissue debris. Because some enzymes leak into the blood, pseudocysts may be associated with elevated blood concentration of amylase, lipase, and LDH. Such pseudocysts may be resistant to treatment and require special surgical drainage and resection.
- **Chronic pancreatitis.** It usually develops from incompletely healed acute pancreatitis or recurrent bouts of acute inflammation.

CHRONIC PANCREATITIS

Chronic pancreatitis is a relatively rare disease characterized by destruction of the pancreatic parenchyma and the replacement of acini by fibrous tissue. Most often it is preceded by acute pancreatitis, but in some cases it develops without any obvious predisposing conditions.

Chronic pancreatitis is in most instances a complication of alcohol abuse.

Alcohol abuse can be documented in about 70% of all patients with chronic pancreatitis. The pathogenesis of this disease is, however, not fully understood—only 10% of all chronic alcoholics develop pancreatic insufficiency. Other causes of chronic pancreatitis, such as biliary disease, are less common. Approximately 15% cases are idiopathic.

Even though the exact pathogenesis of chronic pancreatitis is not fully understood, it is thought that the disease is, in most instances, related to repeated injuries of acinar cells or the obstruction of ducts (Fig. 9-11). Thus, it is thought that it has the same pathogenesis as acute pancreatitis. In many patients recurrent attacks of acute pancreatitis can be documented.

Chronic pancreatitis manifests with pain and malabsorption.

Chronic pancreatitis most often manifests with dull pain in the epigastrium radiating to the back. The clinical findings are relatively nonspecific until pancreatic insufficiency supervenes, causing steatorrhea and malabsorption. The signs of malabsorption include malnutrition, anemia, hypoalbuminemia, and deficiency of fat-soluble vitamins A, D, E, and K.

Radiologic techniques are used for diagnosing chronic pancreatitis.

Loss of pancreatic acinar cells results in atrophy of the pancreas, which can be best visualized by CT. Calcifications are also evident, and the pancreatic ducts are typically dilated (Table 9-8). Endoscopic retrograde cholangiopancreatography is usually performed to demonstrate loss of parenchyma but also to obtain cytologic smears and thus exclude pancreatic carcinoma. Carcinoma occurs at an increased rate in the context of chronic pancreatitis.

Laboratory findings are not of much use in the diagnosis of chronic pancreatitis. Some patients show signs of biliary obstruction. Others show signs of persistent acinar cell injury evidenced by elevation of serum amylase and lipase.

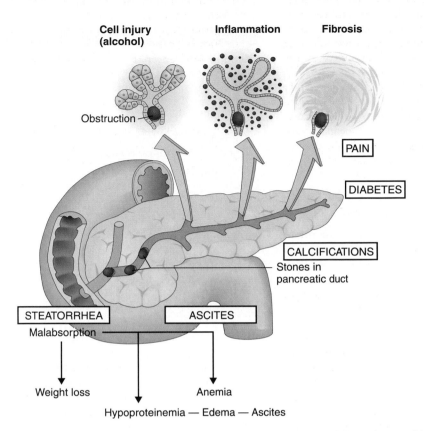

Figure 9-11 Chronic pancreatitis. The pathogenesis of the disease is not fully understood but most likely it includes direct pancreatic cell injury (e.g., by alcohol) or obstruction of the ducts and atrophy and destruction of acinar cells due to back-pressure. The symptoms are related to the destruction of acini and consequent pancreatic insufficiency. Destruction of the islets of Langerhans may cause secondary diabetes mellitus. Pain results from nerve trapping in the fibrous tissue. Calcifications and intraductal stones may be seen radiographically.

CARCINOMA OF THE PANCREAS

Carcinoma of the pancreas is a very common cancer, and since it has a very bad prognosis it represents a major health problem. The most important facts about carcinoma of pancreas are as follows:

Table 9-8 Signs and Symptoms of Chronic Pancreatitis

Pain in the epigastrium radiating to the back
Radiologic signs of chronic pancreatic disease—
   calcification, atrophy, duct dilatation
Steatorrhea and malabsorption of nutrients
   Hypoproteinemia
   Edema
   Ascites
   Anemia
   Weakness
   Weight loss

- It is the fourth most common cause of cancer death in the United States.
- It is the second most common cancer of the gastrointestinal tract in the United States.
- The risk increases with age.
- Genetic predisposition is the most important risk factor.
- The mortality rate is over 90%.

Carcinoma of the pancreas is most often an adenocarcinoma originating from the ducts.

Over 90% of all tumors of pancreas are histologically classified as adenocarcinomas originating from the ducts. The remaining tumors are rare acinic cell carcinomas, serous and mucinous adenomas and adenocarcinomas, and islet cell tumors.

Most of the tumors, approximately 60%, originate from the head of the pancreas. Approximately 10% of tumors are limited to the tail, whereas the remaining 30% of tumors involve the entire organ.

Histologically, most pancreatic carcinomas are composed of nondescript neoplastic glands and tubules surrounded by abundant fibrous tissue. Histologically it is impossible to distinguish pancreatic adenocarcinomas from adenocarcinomas of the hepatobiliary system or desmoplastic adenocarcinomas in other sites. Occasionally, the tumors are less desmoplastic, and more produce mucin or form cystic spaces.

Metastases are found in most cases at the time of diagnosis. The most common sites for metastases are the peripancreatic lymph nodes and the liver, but distant metastases also develop quite often.

Weight loss, jaundice, and epigastric pain are the most common symptoms of pancreatic carcinoma.

Most pancreatic carcinomas are diagnosed after the tumor has reached a rather large size or has already metastasized. Thus, *weight loss* and *weakness* are the most common clinical findings. Remember that tumors act as a "parasite" and drain energy from the body, using the essential metabolites for their own growth.

Most carcinomas originate in the head of the pancreas, and thus it is not surprising that these tumors often manifest with *jaundice*. This jaundice, in many textbooks, is still described as "usually painless," but it is in most cases in fact accompanied by dull epigastric pain. The appearance of jaundice depends on the location of carcinoma: tumors of the head of the pancreas tend to produce

jaundice earlier than those of the body and the tail. Tumors of the tail tend to cause more pain than those of the head. The most common symptoms of pancreatic carcinoma are listed in Table 9-9 and Figure 9-12.

Table 9-9 Signs and Symptoms of Pancreatic Carcinoma

SIGNS AND SYMPTOMS	INCIDENCE (%)
Head of the Pancreas	
Weight loss	90
Jaundice	80
Pain	60
Enlargement of the liver	50
Nausea and vomiting	40
Diarrhea	20
Migratory thrombophlebitis	2
Body and Tail of the Pancreas	
Weight loss	90
Epigastric/back pain	80
Enlargement of the liver	40
Nausea and vomiting	40
Constipation	20
Jaundice (usually a late symptom)	20
Migratory thrombophlebitis	2

Data from several studies. The numbers are rounded up and represent approximations.

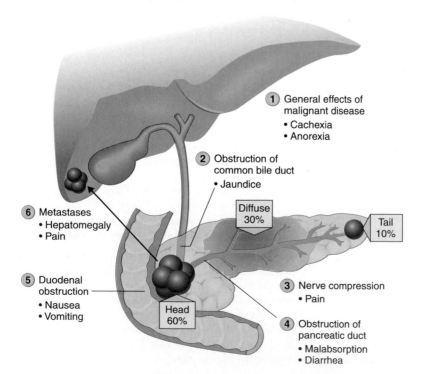

Figure 9-12 Carcinoma of pancreas. Signs and symptoms result from six major pathophysiologic and/or pathologic changes.

Pearls

> *Courvoisier's sign*—a painlessly distended gallbladder that can be palpated in some jaundiced patients with carcinoma of the head of the pancreas.
> *Trousseau's syndrome*—migratory thrombophlebitis occasionally found in patients with pancreatic carcinoma. Thrombi form because of the entry of tumor-derived thromboplastin into the circulation.

Radiologic techniques are the gold standard for diagnosing pancreatic carcinoma.

Due to the location of the pancreas, pancreatic tumors rarely manifest in the form of palpable masses. Most of the palpable tumors are actually cystic and have a better prognosis than the "garden-variety" invasive adenocarcinoma, which represents most of the malignant tumors of the pancreas. Thus, the diagnosis depends mostly on visualizing the tumors by ultrasonic and radiologic techniques, which are widely used in clinical practice.

Many tumors are visible by CT, but smaller tumors require the use of more sensitive techniques. Endoscopic retrograde cholangiopancreatography is the method of choice for the diagnosis of small ampullary, intraductal, and periductal carcinomas. Endoscopic ultrasound, a technique in which the ultrasound probe is introduced into the lumen of the intestine, combined with needle biopsy can be used to detect tumors as small as 2 cm in diameter.

Biochemical tests are not useful for the diagnosis of carcinoma of the pancreas.

The carbohydrate antigen 19-9 test, performed on the serum, is positive in 70% of patients with pancreatic carcinoma. Unfortunately the test has low sensitivity and specificity and cannot be used for early diagnosis or screening purposes.

Carcinoembryonic antigen (CEA) is found in the blood of more than 70% of patients with pancreatic carcinoma. This test is also not suitable for early diagnosis or screening purposes. Neither one of these two serologic tests can distinguish adenocarcinomas of the pancreas from carcinoma of the hepatobiliary tract, stomach, or the intestines, or, for that matter, in the bronchi or even the ovaries.

CASE STUDIES

Case 1 RECURRENT PULMONARY INFECTIONS IN A MALNOURISHED BOY

Clinical history   A 4-year-old boy was hospitalized for recurrent respiratory infections.[1] At the time of admission he had a high fever, he was short of breath, and he was expectorating large amounts of mucopurulent material.[2] He was also found to have frequent smelly and greasy stools.[3]

Physical findings   The child is malnourished and shorter than expected for his age.[4] Auscultation and radiography disclosed patchy consolidation of both lungs and chronic pulmonary changes consistent with bronchiectasis.

Laboratory findings   Leukocytosis and anemia were evident.[5] *Pseudomonas aeruginosa* was cultured from the sputum. Fat globules were found in the feces. A sweat test showed increased concentration of Na^+ and Cl^-.[6] Molecular biology tests were performed to confirm the diagnosis.[7]

Outcome   He was treated with antibiotics and released.

Questions for discussion
1. Which childhood diseases are associated with recurrent respiratory infections?
2. In this case what was the cause of mucopurulent expectoration? Which other pathogens could cause purulent expectoration? How is mucopurulent expectoration related to the formation of bronchiectasis?
3. Which diseases cause greasy smelly diarrhea? Why do feces contain fat?
4. What are the possible causes of slower than normal growth in children? Is fat in feces related to this child's stunted growth?
5. Why does the child have leukocytosis and anemia?
6. How is the sweat test performed? What are the indications for performing the sweat test? What does one look for in a sweat test?
7. What is the final diagnosis in this case? What is the prognosis? Would you offer the genetic test to the relatives of this patient?

Case 2 SEVERE ABDOMINAL PAIN IN A MIDDLE-AGED ALCOHOLIC

Clinical history   A 50-year-old alcoholic was admitted complaining of severe abdominal pain.[1] The pain was localized in the epigastrium and radiated to the back. It was associated with nausea and vomiting.[2]

Physical findings   He is in extreme pain and sweating profusely. He feels thirsty and has dry lips.[3] The abdomen is bulging and sensitive to palpation. There are no bowels sounds.[4] He has fever, tachycardia, tachypnea, and hypotension.[5]

Laboratory findings   Leukocytosis, elevated serum amylase and lipase.[6] During the second day of hospitalization he developed hypocalcemia.

Outcome   The acute attack subsided, but the patient continued to have upper abdominal pain. Using CT a cystic mass was found in the body of the pancreas, and his serum amylase remained slightly elevated.[7]

Questions for discussion
1. What are the possible causes of abdominal pain? Is your differential diagnosis narrowed when you learn that the pain is predominantly epigastric and that it radiates to the back?
2. What could cause nausea and vomiting?
3. What are the signs of dehydration? Why did dehydration develop in this patient?
4. What is the significance of this finding?
5. What is the significance of these findings? Explain their pathogenesis.
6. What are the possible causes of elevated serum amylase and lipase?
7. What is the significance of these findings?

Case 3   WEIGHT LOSS, JAUNDICE, AND EPIGASTRIC PAIN IN AN ELDERLY MAN

Clinical history   A 72-year-old man noticed a slowly evolving jaundice of his sclerae, skin, and oral mucosa. His urine was dark brown and foamy.[1] He also complained of a nagging pain in the epigastrium and reported a weight loss of 20 pounds over a period of 4 months.[2]

Physical findings   The patient appears emaciated and weak. Computed tomography revealed a mass in the head of the pancreas.[3] Endoscopic retrograde cholangiopancreatography revealed an obstruction of the ampullary region of the common bile duct and the main pancreatic duct.[4] Cytologic examination of pancreatic juice aspirated during the procedure revealed malignant cells.[5]

Laboratory findings   High erythrocyte sedimentation rate and anemia are evident. Serum levels of bilirubin and alkaline phosphatase were elevated.[6] Carbohydrate antigen 19-9 was elevated in the serum.[7]

Outcome   The patient discussed various treatment options but refused them all and decided to have only palliative treatment.[8]

Questions for discussion
1. Is this jaundice related to conjugated or unconjugated hyperbilirubinemia?
2. What is the significance of these findings in a jaundiced patient?
3. What is the significance of this radiologic finding? What would you do next?
4. What is ERCP? How is ERCP performed?
5. Are these findings sufficient for the final diagnosis or do you have to obtain solid tissue by pancreatic biopsy?
6. Why is alkaline phosphatase elevated in the serum?
7. Is elevation of CA 19-9 a definitive proof of pancreatic malignancy?
8. What is the final diagnosis? What are the treatment options? What is the prognosis?

Chapter 10

THE ENDOCRINE PANCREAS

Introduction

The endocrine pancreas consists of the islets of Langerhans, which are scattered between the acini and ducts of the exocrine part of the gland. The clinical syndromes related to the pathology of the islets of Langerhans result from either underproduction or overproduction of hormones normally produced by the cells forming the islets. The most important disease resulting from the underproduction of insular hormones is diabetes mellitus (DM). The syndromes related to overproduction of insular hormones are typically caused by tumors, which are also discussed here (Fig. 10-1). These tumors are relatively rare, accounting for 1% to 3% of all pancreatic neoplasms.

Normal Structure and Function

ANATOMY AND HISTOLOGY

The islets of Langerhans consist of several cell types (Fig. 10-2):

- Alpha (α) cells, which secrete glucagon
- Beta (β) cells, which secrete insulin, proinsulin, C peptide, and amylin
- Delta (δ) cells, which secrete somatostatin
- F cells (PP cells), which secrete pancreatic polypeptide but only in some islets

In most islets beta cells account for approximately 70%; alpha cells account for 20%; and delta cells, F cells, and nonfunctioning cells account for the remaining 10% of cells.

PHYSIOLOGY

Hormones produced by the islets of Langerhans are the key regulators of the intermediary metabolism of carbohydrates, lipids, and proteins.

Insulin is a polypeptide formed from inactive precursors.

Insulin is a short polypeptide composed of 51 amino acids arranged into two chains linked together by two disulfide bonds (Fig. 10-3). Insulin synthesis occurs in several steps:

- **Preproinsulin.** The original gene product, called preproinsulin, is a polypeptide that contains the A and B chains of insulin linked together with a long C polypeptide and a signal sequence on the N-terminal.
- **Proinsulin.** It is formed in the cisterns of the rough endoplasmic reticulum through the cleavage of the signal sequence and the formation of the interchain and intrachain disulfide.

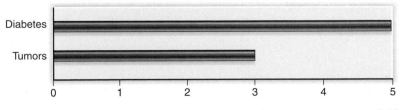

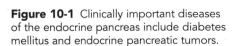

Figure 10-1 Clinically important diseases of the endocrine pancreas include diabetes mellitus and endocrine pancreatic tumors.

Anatomy and Physiology

Glucagon   Polypeptide hormone produced by insular alpha cells that regulates the metabolism of carbohydrates. It promotes glycogenolysis in the liver, thus causing hyperglycemia. It may be produced by some pancreatic endocrine tumors (glucagonomas).

Glucose   Key component of carbohydrate metabolism, present in free form in the blood or complexed into oligo- and polysaccharides in tissues. The normal concentration of glucose in serum or plasma is 70 to 110 mg/dL (3.9–6.1 mmol/L).

Insulin   Polypeptide hormone produced by insular beta cells that is involved in regulating the metabolism of carbohydrates, lipids, and proteins. It has many functions, the most important of which is the promotion of glycogenesis in the liver and the uptake and utilization of glucose in muscle, fat cells, and several other tissues, thus lowering the blood concentration of glucose. It may be produced by some pancreatic endocrine tumors (insulinomas).

Insulin receptor   Tyrosine kinase-linked cell membrane receptor that binds circulating insulin. Its activation leads to metabolic changes, the most important of which is increased influx and utilization of glucose. Defective function of insulin receptors leads to diabetes mellitus type 2.

Islets of Langerhans   Endocrine part of the pancreas. Each islet is composed of several cell types: alpha cells that secrete glucagon, beta cells that secrete insulin, delta cells that secrete somatostatin, and F cells that secrete pancreatic polypeptide.

Pancreatic polypeptide   Polypeptide secreted by endocrine and exocrine pancreatic cells and intestinal cells. It inhibits the secretion of pancreatic enzymes and the contraction of the gallbladder.

Somatostatin   Polypeptide hormone produced by insular delta cells and intestinal endocrine cells. It inhibits the release of several other hormones, such as growth hormone, glucagons, insulin, and gastrin. It may be produced by some pancreatic or intestinal endocrine tumors (somatostatinomas).

Vasoactive intestinal polypeptide   Polypeptide hormone widely distributed in the body, but most prominently found in the central nervous system and intestines. It leads to intestinal vasodilatation and hypermotility, as well as gastrointestinal water and electrolyte secretion. It may be produced by some pancreatic endocrine tumors (VIPomas).

Diseases of Endocrine Pancreas

Diabetes mellitus   Metabolic syndrome characterized by hyperglycemia related to absolute or relative insulin deficiency or tissue resistance to insulin.

Gastrinoma syndrome   Metabolic syndrome also known as Zollinger-Ellison syndrome, caused by gastrin-secreting tumors, most often located in the head of the pancreas. It is characterized by hypergastrinemia, gastric acid hypersecretion, and peptic ulcers that are often multiple and found in atypical locations. It is also sometimes characterized by a resistance to conventional antiulcer therapy.

Glucagonoma syndrome   Metabolic syndrome caused by glucagonoma (i.e., a glucagon-secreting islet cell tumor composed of alpha cells). The syndrome includes mild diabetes, migratory erythematous skin necrosis, anemia, thrombosis, and a predisposition to bacterial infections.

Hyperglycemia   Increased concentration of glucose in serum (>120 mg/dL), typically seen in diabetes mellitus as well as in a variety of endocrine diseases (e.g., Cushing's syndrome, hyperthyroidism) and acute pancreatitis. Any type of shock increases serum glucose levels. It may be also drug-induced (e.g., by thiazide diuretics, phenytoin, and epinephrine).

Hypoglycemia   Decreased concentration of glucose in serum (<40 mg/dL). Reactive hypoglycemia may occur after feeding (postprandial hypoglycemia). Fasting hypoglycemia is typically found in association with insulinoma, insulin abuse, or insulin overdose (in diabetic patients), but may be also found in association with some glycogen-storing or -consuming tumors and in severe systemic diseases.

Insulinoma syndrome   Syndrome caused by insulinoma (i.e., an insulin-secreting islet cell tumor composed of beta cells). It is characterized by hypoglycemia, sweating, nervousness, lethargy, or fainting that may occasionally progress to hypoglycemic coma.

Islet cell tumors   Group of endocrine tumors originating from the islets of Langerhans. These tumors may be benign or malignant, solitary or multiple, hormonally active or inactive. On the basis of the type of cells that form these tumors they are classified as insulinomas (most common), glucagonomas, gastrinomas, somatostatinomas, vasoactive intestinal polypeptide-secreting tumors (VIPomas), or pancreatic polypeptide-secreting tumors (PPomas). Histologically they resemble carcinoid tumors of the gastrointestinal and respiratory tract. By electron microscopy they contain dense membrane-bounded granules. Highly malignant tumors may resemble small-cell (oat cell) carcinomas of the lung.

Somatostatinoma syndrome   Metabolic syndrome caused by somatostatinomas (i.e., somatostatin-secreting islet cell tumors). It is characterized by mild diabetes, steatorrhea, gastric hypochlorhydria, and gallstones.

VIPoma   Metabolic syndrome, also known as Verner-Morrison syndrome, caused by VIPomas (i.e., pancreatic islet tumors composed of vasoactive polypeptide [VIP]-secreting cells). It is characterized by watery diarrhea, hypokalemia, and gastric hypochorhydria or even achlorhydria.

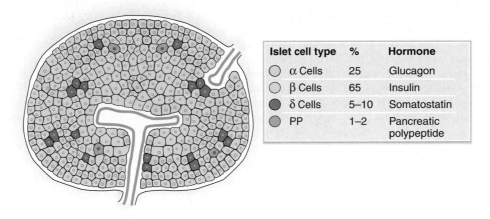

Islet cell type	%	Hormone
α Cells	25	Glucagon
β Cells	65	Insulin
δ Cells	5–10	Somatostatin
PP	1–2	Pancreatic polypeptide

Figure 10-2 Islets of Langerhans. Insulin-secreting beta (ß) cells account for two thirds of all cells in the islets of Langerhans.

■ **Insulin.** It is formed from proinsulin through the cleavage of the C peptide in the Golgi apparatus, from which it is transferred to the storage granules in the cytoplasm. From these granules insulin is released into the circulation by endocytosis. The circulating insulin has a short half-life (6 minutes), during which period it has the opportunity to bind to insulin receptors, predominantly in the liver, muscle, and fat cells. It is degraded by hepatic insulinase.

Secretion of insulin and glucagon is regulated by blood glucose, other metabolites, and some hormones.

Insulin and glucagon have diametrically opposite effects on the intermediary metabolism, and thus it is logical that the regulation of the synthesis and release of these two hormones is closely interlinked.

Factors that regulate the secretion of insulin can be classified as stimulatory and inhibitory.

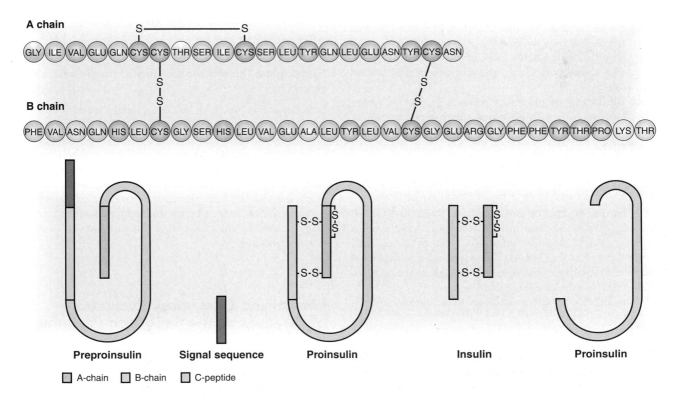

Figure 10-3 Simplified structure of insulin and its precursor molecules.

- **Stimulation of insulin release.** High **blood glucose** directly stimulates beta cells, and it is thus the most important stimulus for insulin production and release. Other food constituents and metabolites, such as **amino acids** and **fatty acids,** may stimulate insulin release directly, but most often their effect is indirect, since these metabolites affect the utilization or release of glucose into the bloodstream. Intestinal **secretin,** released on feeding, stimulates insulin release. **Cortisol** and **growth hormone** induce peripheral insulin resistance and increase blood glucose concentration, thus stimulating the release of insulin.
- **Inhibition of insulin release.** Insulin secretion is reduced physiologically during starvation and decreased **food intake.** Acute inhibition of insulin secretion during stress or trauma is mediated by **epinephrine,** which stimulates release of glucose from the liver and fatty acids from fat tissues, but also acts on pancreatic beta cells to decrease their sensitivity to glucose. **Somatostatin** has a paracrine inhibitory effect on insulin secretion.

Glucagon secretion is regulated by the same factors that regulate insulin secretions, but in a reverse manner.

- **Stimulation of glucagon release.** The most potent stimulus for glucagon release is **low blood glucose** concentration, as occurs in hunger. **Epinephrine** release during stress or trauma also promotes glucagon release. It also overrides the effects of excess glucose release from the liver, which acts directly on the insular cells. **Amino acids** also stimulate glucagon release, thus counteracting their stimulatory effect on insulin release.
- **Inhibition of glucagon release.** The most important inhibitor is **high blood glucose** concentration. **Ketone bodies** and **free fatty acids** have the same effect.

Insulin and glucagon regulate the intermediary metabolism of carbohydrates, lipids, and proteins.

The actions of insulin and glucagons are closely interlinked. Insulin has predominantly anabolic effects and is "anticatabolic," whereas glucagon has predominantly catabolic effects (Fig. 10-4). This is reflected in the blood **insulin-to-glucagon ratio,** which is high in the fed condition and low in a fasting state.

Insulin acts predominantly on liver, muscle, and fat tissue.

- **Liver.** In the liver it promotes storage of **glucose** in the form of glycogen by promoting glycogen formation and its lysis into glucose. The net outflow of glucose from the liver is reduced. Excess glucose is used for the synthesis of lipids, which are stored in

liver cells in the form of triglycerides (TGs). Insulin also affects lipid metabolism by inhibiting ketogenesis and promoting synthesis of very low density lipoproteins (VLDLs). When VLDLs are released into the bloodstream they are taken up by muscle cells or fat cells and stored or used for energy production. Insulin stimulates the uptake of amino acids into liver cells.
- **Muscle.** In the muscles insulin promotes the uptake of glucose from the blood and glycogen synthesis. It also inhibits glycogen phosphorylase and slows down glycogenolysis. Insulin stimulates the entry of amino acids into muscle cells and protein synthesis.
- **Fat tissue.** Insulin stimulates glucose uptake and promotes TG storage by promoting the uptake of fat and fatty acid esterification and by inhibiting lipolysis of TGs.

Glucagon acts predominantly on the **liver,** and it counteracts the hypoglycemic effects of insulin. In the liver it stimulates glycogenolysis by promoting the breakdown of glycogen into glucose. It stimulates gluconeogenesis (i.e., the formation of glucose from lactate or amino acids). Both effects lead to an increased concentration of glucose in the blood. Glucagon promotes the oxidation of fatty acids, which results in the formation of ketone bodies from acetyl CoA. It also stimulates the uptake of amino acids in the liver.

The main effects of insulin and glucagon are listed in Table 10-1.

Somatostatin inhibits the secretion of insulin and glucagon.

Somatostatin is produced by the delta cells. It acts locally in a paracrine manner on alpha and beta cells; in an autocrine manner by inhibiting its own release from δ cells; and in an endocrine manner on absorptive, secretory, and contractile cells of the gastrointestinal system. Somatostatin release is stimulated by high levels of blood glucose, some amino acids, and also in a local paracrine manner by glucagon. Its paracrine effects are inhibitory, and it suppresses the release of both insulin and glucagon. It also inhibits pancreatic exocrine secretion.

Clinical and Laboratory Evaluation of Diseases of the Endocrine Pancreas

FAMILY AND PERSONAL HISTORY

Except for **diabetes mellitus (DM),** which affects millions of people worldwide, other diseases of the endocrine pancreas are relative rare. Hence, in this chapter the major

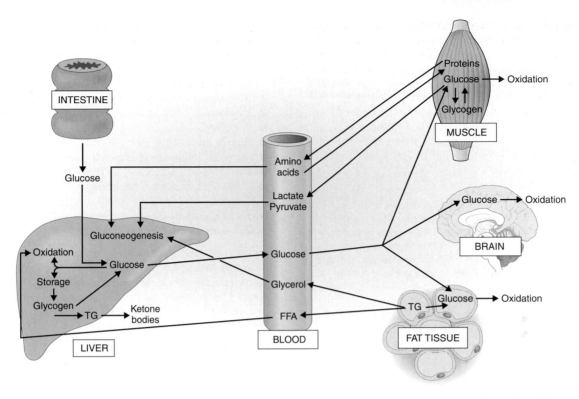

Figure 10-4 Effects of insulin and glucagons on intermediary metabolism in the liver, muscles, and peripheral fat tissue. FFA, free fatty acid; TG, triglyceride.

emphasis is on DM and its complications. The risk factors for DM and other less common pancreatic endocrine disorders can be discovered by careful taking of the patient's history and are listed in Table 10-2.

The American Diabetes Association (ADA) recommends screening for type 2 diabetes in all adults older than 45 years who have one or more risk factors. Screening should be repeated every 3 years thereafter. Fasting glucose testing of plasma is the preferred test, but one may use random plasma or serum glucose measurements also. If a random plasma glucose is 160 mg/dL or more, a fasting plasma glucose should be measured.

Table 10-1 Metabolic Effects of Insulin and Glucagon

ORGAN	FUNCTION/FINDING	INSULIN	GLUCAGON
Liver	Glycogen formation/storage	↑	↓
	Glycogen breakdown	↓	↑
	Lipid synthesis (TGs, VLDLs)	↑	↓
	Fatty acid oxidation	↓	↑
	Amino acid uptake	↑	↑
Muscle	Glucose uptake	↑	—
	Glycogen formation/storage	↑	—
	Amino acid uptake	↑	—
Fat tissue	Lipid uptake	↑	—
	Fatty acid esterification to TGs	↑	—
	Triglyceride lysis	↓	—
Blood	Glucose concentration	↓	↑
	VLDL concentration	↑	↓
	Ketone bodies concentration	↓	↑

TG, triglycerides; VLDL, very low density lipoproteins; ↑, increased activity or concentration; ↓, decreased activity or concentration.

Table 10-2 Risk Factors for Diabetes Mellitus (DM) and Other Less Common Pancreatic Endocrine Disorders

TYPE OF RISK FACTOR	SPECIFIC DISEASES–RISK FACTOR ASSOCIATIONS
Hereditary factors	Type 1 and type 2 DM Multiple endocrine neoplasia syndromes
Social/nutritional factors	Obesity-related type 2 DM
Other diseases of the pancreas	Acute and chronic pancreatitis and secondary DM
Other endocrine diseases	Hyperglycemia due to Cushing's syndrome, or acromegaly
Medical and surgical procedures	DM after resection of the pancreas for tumors
Drugs	Drug-induced hyperglycemia or DM
External mechanical factors	Pancreatic necrosis due to seat belt trauma and secondary DM

Increased incidence of type 2 diabetes in children and adolescents has prompted the ADA to recommend screening of children at age 10 years if the child has the following risk factors:

- Overweight (BMI >85th percentile or weight 120% of ideal)
- Family history of diabetes
- High risk race/ethnicity (e.g., Native Americans, Hispanic Americans)
- Signs of insulin resistance (e.g., dyslipidemia, acanthosis nigricans, hypertension, or polycystic ovary syndrome)

PHYSICAL EXAMINATION AND HISTORY OF PRESENT DISEASE

The most important clinical findings pointing to DM or other endocrine pancreatic disorders are:

- Polyuria
- Polydypsia
- Polyphagia
- Weight loss
- Increased incidence of bacterial infections
- Sensory disturbances
- Coma with Kussmaul breathing

Polyuria and polydipsia are common manifesting signs of diabetes mellitus.

Polyuria is defined as an excessive volume of urine, typically over 3 L/day. In DM it is typically combined with excessive excretion of glucose and thus it is best classified as osmotic. Loss of water elicits dehydration, which in turn causes thirst. Typically polyuria is thus accompanied by **polydipsia** (increased intake of water).

It is important to note that polyuria may be related to excessive intake of water, as in people who have an urge to drink **("psychogenic polydipsia"),** and other **endocrine disorders** (e.g., hyperparathyroidism and other forms of hypercalcemia). Many intracranial lesions interfering with the secretion of the antidiuretic hormone (ADH) may cause **"cranial" diabetes insipidus.** Several renal diseases and drugs and toxins that affect the kidneys may manifest as **"nephrogenic diabetes insipidus"** (Table 10-3).

Polyuria is a complication of hyperglycemia, which leads to glucosuria. Glucose in the urine "draws out" the water and thus leads to an **osmotic polyuria.** It is associated with a loss of fluid, minerals, and glucose in the urine. **Dehydration** may cause clinical symptoms such as dry skin and mucosal surfaces and reduced skin turgor. A hyperglycemia-related **hyperosmolar state** may cause blurry vision because of exposure of the lens and retina to hyperosmolar plasma.

Table 10-3 Causes of Polyuria

CLINICAL CONDITION	MECHANISM	FINDINGS
Psychogenic polydipsia	Water intake ↑	Plasma sodium → or ↓
Diabetes mellitus	Osmotic water loss	Plasma osmolality ↓
Hyperparathyroidism	Osmotic water loss	Plasma/urine glucose ↑
Cranial diabetes insipidus (reduced renal water reabsorption)	Lack of ADH	Plasma/urine calcium ↑
Renal diseases	Inability to concentrate urine	Urine osmolality ↓ (<600 mOsm/kg)
Drugs (e.g., lithium)	Renal effects	Plasma osmolality ↑ (>300 mOsm/kg)
Heavy-metal toxicity	Renal effects	Other signs of kidney disease

ADH, antidiuretic hormone; →, normal; ↓, reduced; ↑, increased.

Reduced plasma volume (**hypovolemia**) may cause hypotension, syncope, and dizziness.

Polyphagia results from increased metabolic demands.

Many patients who develop type 1 DM have increased appetite and consume large amounts of food (polyphagia). Even though these patients eat a lot they tend to lose weight. Subcutaneous fat may appear depleted.

The reasons for polyphagia are not quite obvious but are directly or indirectly related to disturbances of the feeling of hunger. The eating behavior of each person is a function of hypothalamic centers known as the satiety and hunger centers (Fig. 10-5). These centers receive numerous impulses, which can be classified as **anorexigenic** (i.e., suppressing appetite) or **orexigenic** (promoting appetite). The secretion of orexins that act on the hunger center is stimulated by low glucose concentration in the blood. This correlates with the well-known fact that hypoglycemia, induced by exogenous insulin or insulin-producing tumors, manifests with hunger. Patients who have type 1 DM apparently lose the function of **"glucose-sensitive neurons"** and persistently secrete orexins. Another stimulus for overeating in type 1 DM might be a lack of **glucagon** or **cholecystokinin (CCK),** a pancreaticointestinal polypeptide that under normal circumstances inhibits hunger. The effects of CCK are seen only in the presence of an intact **vagus nerve,** which may be affected by diabetic neuropathy or the hyperosmotic state caused by hyperglycemia. **Catecholamines,** and especially norepinephrine, which are elevated in type 1 DM due to stress and poor glycemic control, also act by stimulating eating.

Longer lasting effects on the hunger center are most likely coming from the fat cells. Under normal circumstances fat cells secrete an appetite-suppressing substance called **leptin.** A lack of insulin leads to a loss of peripheral fat, causing a reduced secretion of leptin. Polyphagia and **obesity** typically found in type 2 DM are multifactorial and usually precede the development of clinical symptoms of DM.

Weight loss results from loss of glucose and lack of insulin.

Weight loss is a common feature of type 1 DM. In part it is related to a **loss of glucose** in the urine that leads to a negative caloric balance, and in part it is caused by a **lack of anabolic stimulation** by insulin. In advanced and poorly controlled DM weight loss may be due to complex **metabolic disturbances,** ketoacidosis, and the adverse effects of repeated infections.

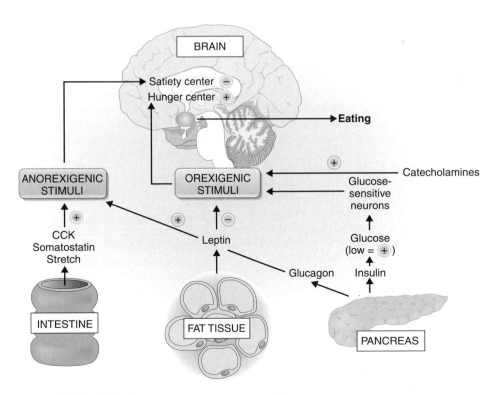

Figure 10-5 Control of eating behavior. CCK, cholecystokinin.

Increased incidence of infection is related to reduced resistance caused by hyperglycemia.

Hyperglycemia is frequently associated with infections. In part this is related to the increased availability of glucose in tissues promoting bacterial and fungal growth. It is well known that carbohydrates promote the growth of many pathogens—bacteria and fungi are like children, they like sweets. Hyperglycemia and especially ketoacidosis in poorly controlled DM adversely affect the function of leukocytes, reducing their response to infections. Most often the infections are caused by bacteria and involve the skin and the urinary tract. *Candida albicans* infection of the vulva is a common complication of DM.

> ### Pearl
>
> > Recurrent vaginal candidiasis may be an early presenting sign of DM.

Neurologic disturbances are very common in diabetes mellitus.

Hyperosmolality of the plasma due to hyperglycemia affects the peripheral and central nerve cells and is an important cause of sensory and motor disturbances seen in DM patients. Additional metabolic disturbances, such as acidosis, the presence of ketone bodies, reduced potassium stores, and dehydration found in uncontrolled DM, contribute even more to neural dysfunction. **Microangiopathy** (i.e., changes in the basement membrane of small blood vessels providing blood to the nerves) contributes to chronic changes, which manifest as combined **sensory and motor neuropathy.**

Ketoacidosis may cause clouding of the consciousness and **coma.** Typically it is associated with **Kussmaul breathing—** rapid deep respiratory excursions typical of metabolic acidosis. The breath may have a sweet acetone odor.

Visual disturbances are a common complication of DM. Hyperglycemia and hyperosmolar states lead to the swelling of the lens and retina and cause blurry vision. Long-term retinal changes known as diabetic retinopathy are a major cause of blindness. The incidence of cataracts increases probably because of the deposition of sorbitol and other by-products of carbohydrate metabolism.

LABORATORY TESTS AND SPECIAL DIAGNOSTIC PROCEDURES

Physical examination and a detailed medical history are important for the initial evaluation of suspected DM or other pancreatic endocrine disorders. However, the final diagnosis is ultimately made, as in many other metabolic and endocrine disorders, on the basis of laboratory data. The most important findings are

- Hyperglycemia
- Hypoglycemia
- Hyperketonemia

Hyperglycemia results most often from inadequate insulin regulation of metabolism.

The fasting whole blood glucose fluctuates in healthy persons in the **reference range** from 60 to 100 mg/dL (3.3–5.6 mmol/L). When measured in serum or plasma the glucose concentration is slightly higher, in the range from 70 to 110 mg/dL (3.9–6.1 mmol/L).

Hyperglycemia is empirically defined as fasting blood glucose concentration exceeding the upper limits of the normal range. If the glucose concentration is in the range of 110 to 125 mg/dL (5.6–6.9 mmol/L), it is considered to be in the **prediabetic range.** Fasting blood glucose above 126 mg/dL (7.0 mmol/L) obtained on at least two occasions is a sign of DM.

> ### Pearl
>
> > High blood sugar is most often a consequence of inappropriate blood sampling from patients who have not fasted prior to the test. Thus every abnormal glucose test should be repeated at least once and the blood should be drawn after 8 hours of fasting.

Since insulin is the principal regulator of intermediary carbohydrate metabolism, a lack of insulin or a lack of an appropriate response of peripheral tissue to insulin, is the most common cause of hyperglycemia. Other causes of hyperglycemia are listed in Table 10-4.

Hyperglycemia due to insulin deficiency is caused by increased hepatic formation of glucose (**gluconeogenesis**) from amino acids, and lipids, and increased **glycogenolysis** (i.e., lysis of glycogen into glucose), which is released

Table 10-4 Causes of Hyperglycemia

Diabetes mellitus
Endocrine hyperfunction syndromes
   Glucagonoma
   Cushing's syndrome
   Growth hormone hypersecretion
   Thyrotoxicosis
   Pheochromocytoma
Acute pancreatitis
Drugs
   Thiazide diuretics
   Phenytoin
   Hormones (e.g., cortisone, thyroxin)

into the blood in excessive amounts (Fig.10-6). The reduced uptake of glucose into the peripheral tissues contributes to hyperglycemia. An excess of glucose leads to **glucosuria** and osmotic **polyuria.**

Symptoms of hyperglycemia vary but are most often related to hyperosmolar effects of glucose and consequent polyuria and depletion of water and minerals from the body (Table 10-5).

Hypoglycemia is typically caused by an excess of insulin.

Hypoglycemia results when the utilization and removal of glucose from blood exceed its production. For clinical purposes it is defined as fasting glucose levels below 50 mg/dL. Insulin, which promotes glucose uptake in the liver and inhibits its release into the circulation from the liver, is the main cause of hypoglycemia. Typically this phenomenon occurs during treatment of DM when too much insulin is administered or the use of sulfonylurea-type drugs has overstimulated the islets to produce excess of insulin. Islet cell tumors secreting insulin are rare but important causes of hypoglycemia. There are many other causes of hypoglycemia, the most important of which are listed in Table 10-6.

The clinical signs and symptoms of hypoglycemia can be attributed to the direct effects of insulin or the activation of the adrenergic system by low glucose concentration in the blood.

- **Neuroglycopenic symptoms.** These are related to the lowering of glucose concentration in the blood and include headache, confusion, slurred speech, seizures, and even coma and death.

Table 10-5 Signs and Symptoms of Hyperglycemia

Glucose increased in blood, urine, and body fluids
Polyuria—nocturia
Dehydration—dry mouth, skin, and mucosae
Polydipsia and increased thirst
Polyphagia and feeling of hunger
Weight loss/gain
Fatigue, nausea
Blurry vision and headaches
Pruritus vulvae or balanitis due to *Candida albicans*
Mood change, irritability, apathy

- **Adrenergic symptoms.** These clinical findings occur only when glucose levels drop rapidly and include feeling of distress, sweating, flushing of the face, and tremor.

> **Pearl**
>
> > More than 100 years ago, Whipple described the classic features of hypoglycemias, which are still known as **Whipple's triad** and include: (1) hypoglycemia, (2) central nervous system and vasomotor symptoms such as fainting and sweating, and (3) prompt relief of symptoms by administering glucose.

Low blood glucose stimulates the **hypothalamic regulatory centers,** which send signals into the periphery to counteract the adverse effects of hypoglycemia. In the short term the most important response is the release of epinephrine and norepinephrine from the autonomic nervous system and

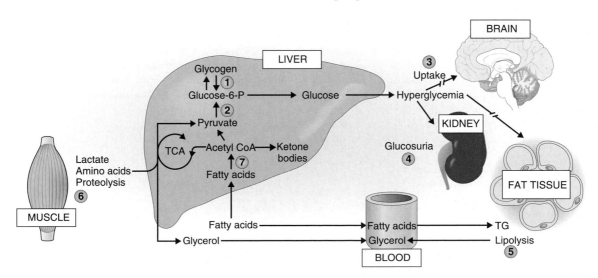

Figure 10-6 Pathogenesis of hyperglycemia. 1, Glycogenolysis. 2, Gluconeogenesis. 3, Reduced uptake of glucose-contributing hyperglycemia. 4, Glucosuria. 5, Lipolysis. 6, Proteolysis. 7, Fatty acid metabolism. Acetyl CoA, acetyl coenzyme A; glucose-6-P, glucose-6-phosphate; TCA, tricarboxylic acid; TG, triglycerides.

Table 10-6 Causes of Hypoglycemia

Diabetes therapy related
    Insulin
    Sulfonylurea
Tumors secreting insulin or IGF
    Insulinoma
    Sarcomas
    Carcinoma of liver, kidneys, adrenal glands
Drugs
    Pentamidine
    Sulfonamides
    Salicylates
Major organ failure
    Liver failure
    Kidney failure
    Heart failure
Systemic diseases
    Multiple organ failure
    Sepsis
    Malnutrition
    Alcoholism
Childhood inborn errors of metabolism
    Glycogenesis
    Galactosemia
    Mitochondria-linked enzyme deficiencies
Postgastrectomy syndrome

IGF, insulin-like growth factor.

adrenal medullary cells. **Catecholamines** counteract the adverse effects of hypoglycemia and also act on the liver to stimulate glycogenolysis and inhibit gluconeogenesis, thus contributing to the normalization of glucose concentration in the blood. Low glucose concentration in the blood stimulates the release of **glucagon,** which also contributes to raising the glucose concentration in the blood.

In the work-up of patients who have hypoglycemia it is important to determine whether it is caused by insulin or some other mechanisms (Fig. 10-7). If it is caused by an excess of insulin, then it is critical to determine whether it is due to endogenous insulin or exogenous insulin that was injected into the body. The analysis of

these problems can be achieved by measuring the blood concentration of insulin and C peptide. As mentioned before C peptide is a part of proinsulin, which is cleaved from the insulin molecule and stored in the secretory granules of beta cells. Both C peptide and insulin are secreted into the blood, and thus, if hyperinsulinemia is of endogenous origin, both the insulin and C peptide concentrations will be elevated in the blood. Exogenous insulin increases the total insulin content of the blood, but the C peptide concentration is low.

Ketone body overproduction may lead to ketoacidosis, a common complication of poorly controlled diabetes mellitus.

Ketone bodies, including acetoacetate, 3-hydroxybutirate, and acetone, are normally formed in the liver as the by-product of catabolism of carbohydrates, lipids, or amino acids (Fig. 10-8). The first step in this shunting process is the formation of acetyl coenzyme A (CoA), which through several steps gives rise to acetoacetate. Acetoacetate can be exported into the blood or transformed into acetone for storage, or it can be transformed into 3-hydroxybutyrate for export. Ketone bodies in the blood are taken up by the brain, muscle, and peripheral fat cells, where they serve as a source of energy.

Normal liver produces ketone bodies in limited amounts. It is important to note that the liver cannot convert aceto-acetate to fuel and must export it as such or convert it to 3-hydroxybutyrate. Ketone body production is increased during **starvation** when, after the depletion of glucose, ketone bodies become the main source of energy for the brain. Skeletal muscles also take up ketone bodies in the early stages of starvation, but after some time they stop utilizing the ketone bodies and rely exclusively on the endogenous lipids stored inside the muscle cells.

Insulin deficiency promotes the formation of ketone bodies, which can be detected in the blood in increased concentration **(ketonemia)** and spill over into the urine **(ketonuria).** Ultimately this leads to **ketoacidosis.** Although ketone bodies can be formed from several metabolic

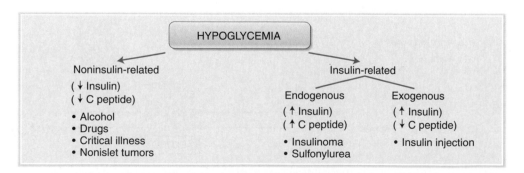

Figure 10-7 Differential diagnosis of hypoglycemia. (Modified from Boon NA, Colledge NR, Walker BR, Hunter JAA [eds]: Davidson's Principles and Practice of Medicine, 20th ed. Edinburgh, Churchill Livingstone, 2006, p. 790.)

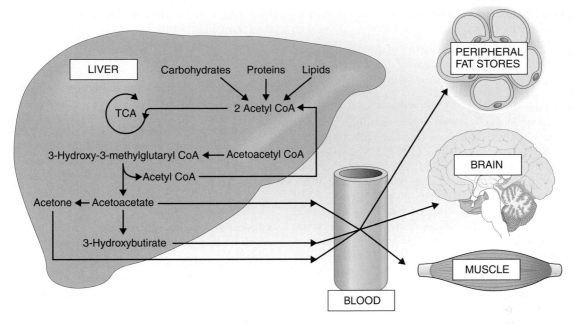

Figure 10-8 Production and metabolic utilization of ketone bodies. Ketone bodies are produced in the liver and taken up and metabolized by the cells of the peripheral fat tissue, brain, and muscle. TCA, tricarboxylic acid.

precursors, the increased influx of fatty acids into the liver is the most common cause of increased ketone body production in DM. Ketoacidosis is accelerated by the effects of catecholamines and other stress hormones, resulting in increased lipolysis and increased influx of free fatty acids into the liver.

Pearl

> **Ketonuria** is not diagnostic of DM and can occur in normal persons especially during fasting, after eating fatty food, after engaging in strenuous exercise, or even after prolonged vomiting.

Clinicopathologic Correlations

DIABETES MELLITUS

Diabetes mellitus is a name for a group of systemic diseases characterized by hyperglycemia and related to abnormal insulin secretion, insulin action, or both. Diabetes mellitus affects more than 16 million Americans, more than 50,000 of whom die every year from complications of the disease. The costs of DM treatment exceed billions of dollars annually. Hence, by all standards, DM is a major health problem.

Most cases of diabetes mellitus can be classified as type 2 or type 1 diabetes—other forms of diabetes are rare.

In most instances DM can be classified as type 1 or type 2. Type 1, also known as insulin-dependent diabetes mellitus (IDDM), accounts for 10% of cases. Type 2, also known as noninsulin-dependent diabetes mellitus (NIDDM), is the most common form of DM and accounts for more than 90% of all cases. Other forms of DM are less common (Table 10-7).

Table 10-7 Classification of Diabetes Mellitus (DM)

Type 1 DM (absolute insulin deficiency due to beta cell destruction)
Type 2 DM (insulin resistance and relative insulin deficiency)
Other types of DM
    Genetic defects involving islet cells, insulin receptors, etc.
    Genetic and chromosomal syndromes (e.g., Down, Turner's, and Klinefelter's)
    Pancreatic diseases and pancreatectomy
    Systemic diseases (e.g., hemochromatosis, autoimmune endocrine insufficiency)
    Excess of insulin antagonizing hormones (e.g., glucagons, corticosteroids, growth hormone, thyroid hormones)
Drug-induced DM (e.g., thiazide diuretics)

The clinical presentation of diabetes depends in part on the pathogenesis of the disease.

Type 1 DM develops as a consequence of the destruction of insulin-producing cells in the islets of Langerhans. These patients produce no insulin and require insulin injections to survive. Type 2 DM results from a resistance to the action of insulin or a relative insulin deficiency owing to the dysfunction of islet cells. Other important differences between type 1 and type 2 DM are listed in Table 10-8.

The exact pathogenesis of either form of DM is unknown, although it is obvious that several endogenous and exogenous factors play an important role. These include the following:

- **Genetic factors.** The strongest evidence for a genetic basis of diabetes was obtained from the study of **twins**. If one of the identical twins has type 1 DM, there is approximately a 50% chance that the second twin will develop diabetes. In type 2 DM the concordance in identical twins is up to 90% (see Table 10-8). The increased incidence of type 2 DM in some **ethnic/racial** groups, such as Native Americans, is yet another evidence of genetic predisposition. **Mutations of the genes** encoding insulin or insulin receptors and transcription factors account for a small but significant number of cases. Such mutations are found in less than 5% of all cases, which is known as **"maturity-onset diabetes of the young" (MODY).** The most common cause of MODY is the mutation of the hepatic nuclear factor 1 alpha (HNF-1α).
- **Autoimmune factors.** Immune destruction of the islets of Langerhans is a typical feature of type 1 DM. These patients typically have antibodies to islet cells. The onset of clinical symptoms in type 1 DM is sudden, suggesting that the immune reaction could be initiated by a viral infection. It has been hypothesized that the destruction of islets occurs due to the action of **cytotoxic T lymphocytes,** attacking virus-infected islet cells. No definitive proof of a viral infection of islets could be found in most patients with type 1 DM. **Autoantibodies to islet cells** probably do not play a role in the islet destruction but are an important sign of islet cell injury. Such antibodies are not found in type 2 DM patients. The association of type 1 DM with certain **haplotypes** (HLA-DR3, HLA-DR4, and HLA-DQ) is yet another piece of evidence suggesting a role of autoimmunity in the pathogenesis of type 1 DM.
- **Obesity.** Accumulation of fatty acids in fat cells leads to altered fat cell response to insulin, reduction of insulin receptors, and finally to insulin resistance. This resistance is the basic change leading to all other changes in type 2 DM. Obesity does not play a significant role in the pathogenesis of type 1 DM.

Clinical and pathologic features of diabetes mellitus result from deficient action of insulin on the liver and peripheral tissues.

Insulin deficiency leads to major disturbances of intermediate metabolism of carbohydrates, lipids, and amino acids (Fig. 10-9). Insulin is an anabolic hormone stimulating accumulation of glycogen in the liver, TG synthesis in the liver and fat cells, and amino acid incorporation into proteins in muscle cells. Lack of insulin or defective action of insulin on its receptor leads to hyperglycemia, increased formation of ketone bodies (ketonemia), and protein catabolism (Fig. 10-10).

Hyperglycemia. Even though hyperglycemia is a constant finding in all forms of DM, it is often asymptomatic and discovered accidentally during routine laboratory testing. The diagnosis of DM is made if one of the following criteria set by the World Health Organization (WHO) is met and confirmed on subsequent testing:

- Random blood glucose concentration over 200 mg/dL (11.1 mmol/L) in a patient who has polyuria, polydipsia, or unexplained weight loss
- Fasting plasma glucose over 126 mg/dL (7.0 mmol/L)
- Two-hour plasma glucose over 200 mg/dL (11.1 mmol/L) during a 75-g oral glucose tolerance test

Table 10-8 Comparison of Types 1 and 2 Diabetes Mellitus (DM)

FEATURES	TYPE 1 DM	TYPE 2 DM
Prevalence	0.5%, women = men	4–5%, women > men
Concordance in identical twins	30–70%	80–90%
Autoimmunity	Yes (anti-islet antibodies)	No
Age at onset	>20 yr	>30 yr
Onset of symptoms	Sudden	Gradual
Body build	Lean	Obese
Insulin in blood	Low then absent	Increased (early) or decreased (late)
Insulin resistance	No	Yes
Ketosis	Common	Uncommon

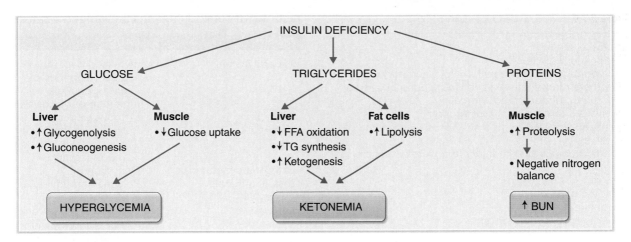

Figure 10-9 Metabolic changes in diabetes. Insulin deficiency affects the metabolism of glucose, triglycerides, and proteins. BUN, blood urea nitrogen; FFA, free fatty acid; TG, triglyceride.

Pearl

> Glucose concentration in whole blood is lower than in serum/plasma. Accordingly the values obtained by various home blood glucose monitoring devices using finger prick should not be used to diagnose diabetes.

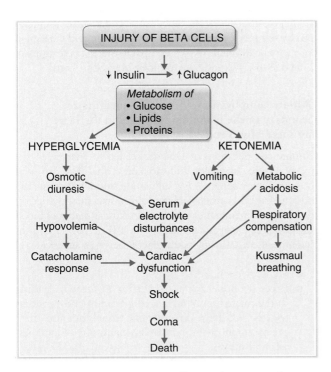

Figure 10-10 Consequences of hyperglycemia and ketonemia.

Glucose in the blood is mostly in free form, but a small fraction is linked to hemoglobin. **Glycosylated hemoglobin (HbA$_{1c}$)** accounts for 3.8% to 6.3% of total hemoglobin, and its concentration rises directly in proportion with the glucose concentration of the blood. Since red blood cells live 120 days, the level of HbA$_{1c}$ provides an insight into the level of hyperglycemia over a 3-month period. In treated diabetics the goal is the keep the HbA$_{1c}$ under 6.5% to 7%. Excessive treatment of hyperglycemia may induce **hypoglycemia,** and accordingly all diabetic patients must be taught to recognize this complication of treatment.

Glycosuria. Glucose in the urine becomes detectable whenever the capacity of the renal tubules to absorb it from primary filtrate is exceeded. In practical terms glycosuria becomes detectable when the blood glucose exceeds the concentration of 180 to 200 mg/dL. Glucosuria is typically associated with polyuria and reactive polydipsia.

Glucose measurement in the urine is a simple and inexpensive test. Urinary glucose concentration generally reflects the blood glucose level. However, in chronic diabetes, the renal threshold for glucose may be altered and thus urinary glucose measurements are not recommended for monitoring DM. Other possible causes of glycosuria are listed in Table 10-9.

Diabetic ketoacidosis (DKA). This life-threatening complication develops typically in insulin-dependent diabetic patients who are not given enough insulin to maintain normal metabolism of carbohydrates. It is defined by a triad that includes

- Hyperglycemia over 250 mg/dL
- Acidosis (serum pH < 7.3, and bicarbonate < 18 mEq/L)
- Ketonemia or ketonuria

Table 10-9 Causes of Glycosuria

Diabetes mellitus
Endocrine disorders
   Hyperfunction of adrenal, thyroid, pituitary
   Tumors of endocrine glands (e.g., adrenal cortical
     tumor, pheochromocytoma)
   Islet cell tumors (e.g., glucagonoma)
Pancreatic disease (e.g., cystic fibrosis, carcinoma of
  pancreas)
Central nervous system injury (e.g., stroke, tumors)
Burns
Sepsis
Feeding after starvation
Pregnancy
Inborn errors of metabolism
Drugs

Table 10-10 Clinical Findings in Diabetic Acidosis

FINDING	CAUSE
Hyperglycemia	Increased hepatic gluconeogenesis, glycogenolysis
	Inhibition of glycolysis
Polyuria	Osmotic diuresis
Dehydration	Polyuria and inadequate water intake (dry skin and mucosae)
Orthostatic hypotension	Dehydration
Loss of minerals (low Na$^+$, K$^+$)	Polyuria and urinary loss of minerals
Ketonemia	Increased lipolysis due to lack of insulin and excess of catecholamines and glucagon
Acetone odor	Ketonemia
Ketonuria	Ketonemia
Acidosis with anion gap	Ketonemia
Low bicarbonate	Buffering of ketone bodies in blood
Kussmaul breathing	Acidosis and excess blood CO_2
Coma	Multifactorial

Diabetic ketoacidosis is most often precipitated by factors that increase the demand for insulin or change the intermediary metabolism. In clinical practice, DKA is most often precipitated by **infection,** which is found in 30% of all cases. It can occur after the patient has forgotten or refused to take insulin (20%) or following emotional stress, alcohol abuse, and a number of intercurrent diseases, such as stroke or myocardial infarction. Surgery or trauma also may induce DKA. In about 25% of cases DKA is the first manifestation of diabetes of recent onset.

The pathogenesis of DKA is directly related to inadequate utilization of glucose and increased gluconeogenesis resulting in **hyperglycemia.** Hyperglycemia leads to **osmotic diuresis** and a loss of water and **serum electrolytes** (Na$^+$, K$^+$, Mg^{2+}, Ca^{2+}, PO$_4^{2-}$, Cl$^-$). **Hypovolemia** stimulates a release of catecholamines, which counteracts the effects of insulin and also promotes **lipolysis.** The fatty acids that are not re-esterified into TGs are metabolized into **ketone bodies** (acetoacetate and hydroxybutyrate), which are released into the circulation (see Fig. 10-10). Utilization of ketone bodies is reduced. Ketone bodies are acidic and contribute to lowering the pH of the blood. At the same time they bind bicarbonate, resulting in **metabolic acidosis with an increased anion gap.** In an attempt to compensate for the metabolic acidosis, patients breathe faster and deeper (**Kussmaul respiration**). Metabolic changes and **electrolyte disturbances** may cause **shock** progressing to **coma,** which is found in approximately 10% of all patients. If not treated properly many of these comatose patients will die. Typical findings in diabetic acidosis are listed in Table 10-10.

Hyperosmolar nonketotic coma. This complication of DM is precipitated by the same factors that cause DKA. It is much less common than DKA but has a higher mortality rate.

The precipitating factors, such a sepsis or lack of insulin intake, typically cause hyperglycemia, which may reach into several hundred milligram levels per deciliter. Ketonemia is not present, presumably because no metabolic shift has occurred

into the production of ketone bodies. Hyperglycemia is accompanied by profuse diuresis and dehydration. Osmolality of the blood is high (on average, 350 mOsm/kg). Hypovolemia and hyperosmolality of the blood cause coma, often accompanied by seizures. Lactic acidosis may be present and is a sign of poor prognosis. Table 10-11 compares the main features of coma due to DKA and hyperosmolar nonketotic coma.

Chronic complications of diabetes mellitus are secondary to the pathologic changes in the large and small blood vessels.

Chronic complications of DM are related to changes in the wall of arteries, arterioles, and capillaries. The basic nature of the pathologic changes is not fully understood, but most data indicate that DM causes biochemical and structural changes in the basement membranes and the extracellular matrix of blood vessels. These changes are multifactorial (Fig. 10-11) and include the effects of many pathogenetic factors, such as:

- Hyperglycemia
- Excessive nonenzymatic glycation of proteins leading to the formation of advanced glycation end-products (AGEs). AGEs are directly toxic to cells but also affect the basement membrane of large and small blood vessels and nerves.
- Accumulation of sorbitol due to the activation of the polyol pathway. Sorbitol stimulates the production of oxygen radicals that may damage or kill cells.

Table 10-11 Comparison of Coma Due to Diabetic Ketoacidosis and Hyperosmolar Nonketotic Diabetes Mellitus (DM)

	CAUSE OF COMA	
FEATURE	**DIABETIC KETOACIDOSIS**	**HYPEROSMOLAR NONKETOTIC DM**
Age	Young (<30 yr)	Older (>60 yr)
Onset	Sudden (<2 days)	Insidious (>1 wk)
First sign of DM	Yes (25%)	Yes (35%)
Plasma/serum findings		
Glucose in plasma	<600 mg/dL	>600 mg/dL
pH	<7.30	>7.30
Ketone bodies	+	−
Bicarbonate	<15 mEq/L	>15 mEq/L
Osmolality	<320 mOsm/kg	>320 mOsm/kg
Na^+	130–140 mEq/L	145–155 mEq/L
K^+	5–6 mEq/L	4–5 mEq/L
Insulin requirement	Yes, almost always	Yes or no
Mortality	5–10%	10–20%

- Increased production of diacylglycerol (DAG), which is a source of arachidonic acid and its derivatives (prostaglandins, leukotrienes, etc.). Arachidonic acid derivatives cause cell injury and also change the function of growth factors and cytokines.
- Dyslipidemia
- Reactive oxygen radicals and lipid peroxidation
- Hyperinsulinemia
- Hypertension
- Hypo/hyperperfusion of certain organs (e.g., glomeruli)
- Hypercoagulability of blood and platelet dysfunction

Diabetic complications can be classified as macrovascular, microvascular, or neuropathic (Fig. 10-12). In most instances these changes occur simultaneously and cannot be readily assigned to a particular defect.

Macrovascular complications. These complications are mostly related to accelerated atherosclerosis and hypertension. Included in this group are

- Coronary artery disease
- Atherosclerosis of the aorta and its major branches, such as the carotid and iliac arteries, and abdominal arteries (e.g., renal and mesenteric arteries)

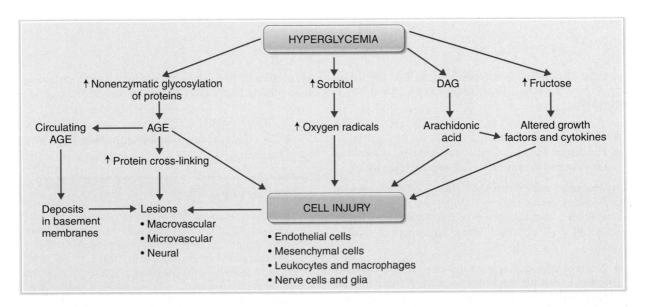

Figure 10-11 Complications of prolonged hyperglycemia. AGE, advanced glycation end-products; DAG, diacylglycerol.

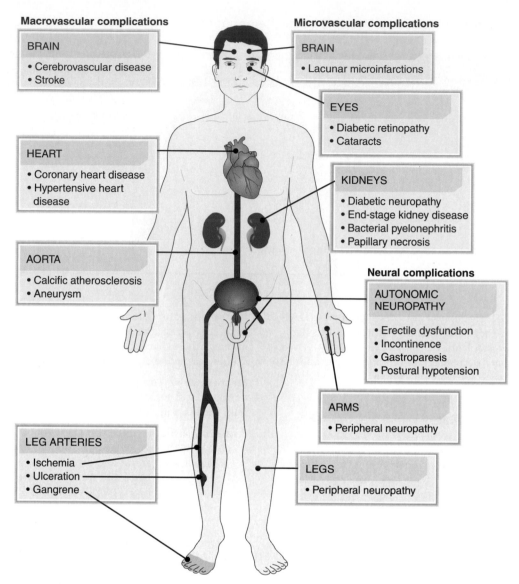

Macrovascular complications

BRAIN
- Cerebrovascular disease
- Stroke

HEART
- Coronary heart disease
- Hypertensive heart disease

AORTA
- Calcific atherosclerosis
- Aneurysm

LEG ARTERIES
- Ischemia
- Ulceration
- Gangrene

Microvascular complications

BRAIN
- Lacunar microinfarctions

EYES
- Diabetic retinopathy
- Cataracts

KIDNEYS
- Diabetic neuropathy
- End-stage kidney disease
- Bacterial pyelonephritis
- Papillary necrosis

Neural complications

AUTONOMIC NEUROPATHY
- Erectile dysfunction
- Incontinence
- Gastroparesis
- Postural hypotension

ARMS
- Peripheral neuropathy

LEGS
- Peripheral neuropathy

Figure 10-12 Clinically important complications of diabetes mellitus. Clinical findings may result from pathologic changes in large blood vessels (macrovascular complications), small blood vessels (microvascular complications), and nerves (neural complications).

■ Cerebrovascular disease
■ Peripheral vascular disease, resulting in ischemia of the extremities and diabetic gangrene (Fig. 10-13)

Microvascular complications. These complications are related to changes in the extracellular matrix of arterioles and capillaries, and the effects of hypertension or hyperperfusion of various tissues. The most important changes include

■ Nephropathy (e.g., glomerulosclerosis and arteriolosclerosis causing nephrotic syndrome, renal insufficiency, and predisposing kidneys to bacterial pyelonephritis and papillary necrosis)

■ Eye changes (e.g., retinopathy, maculopathy, and cataracts)

Pearl

> Diabetic nephropathy is the most common cause of end-stage kidney disease in the United States. It presents first with hyperfiltration and increased glomerular filtration rate, progressing to microalbuminemia (albumin in urine > 300 mg/day), overt proteinuria, hypertension, and finally resulting in renal failure.

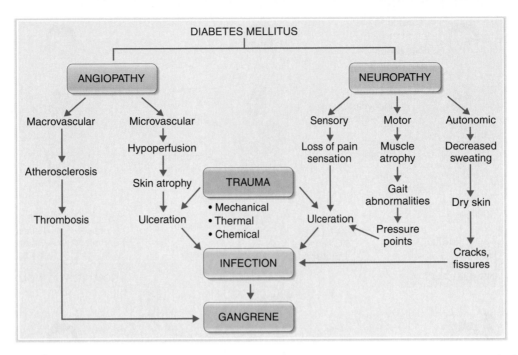

Figure 10-13 Pathogenesis of leg gangrene. Gangrene is a consequence of vascular and neural changes, which may be aggravated by infection and traumatic injury of the leg.

Neuropathic changes. These changes result from metabolic disturbances in neurons, Schwann cells, and the extracellular matrix enveloping the peripheral nerve axons. Ischemia due to macrovascular and microvascular changes also plays an important role. The most important neuropathic changes are:

- **Peripheral neuropathy,** including peripheral sensory-motor polyneuropathy, acute mononeuropathy, radiculopathy, and diabetic amyotrophy
- **Autonomic neuropathy,** including gastroparesis, chronic constipation or diarrhea, orthostatic hypotension, erectile dysfunction, bladder dysfunction, and cardiac arrhythmia

Peripheral polyneuropathy. This is the most common clinical finding. Even though it is a mixed motor-sensory neuropathy, **sensory symptoms** predominate. Paresthesia and pain in the extremities are typical. A loss of sensation of pain and vibration and decreased reflexes may be found during neurologic examination. **Postural hypotension** is the most common feature of autonomic neuropathy.

ISLET CELL TUMORS

Islet cell tumors are relatively rare neoplasms with an incidence of 1 per 1000. They account for 1% to 3% of all pancreatic tumors. The most important facts about this group of tumors are as follows:

- Histologically the tumors share the same features with other neuroendocrine tumors of the GI and respiratory tract and thus appear indistinguishable from carcinoids.
- Most (75%) are low-grade malignant tumors, except for insulinomas, which are benign in 90% of cases.
- Most tumors are hormonally active and produce typical clinical syndromes (Fig. 10-14).
- Hormonally active tumors are classified as:

  - Insulinomas (beta cell tumors)
  - Glucagonomas (alpha cell tumors)
  - Gastrinomas
  - Somatostatinomas
  - Vasoactive intestinal polypeptide-secreting tumors (VIPomas)
  - Pancreatic polypeptide-secreting tumors (PPomas)

Insulinomas cause hypoglycemia.

Insulinomas are tumors composed of beta cells. As such they secrete insulin and cause hypoglycemia. Insulinomas are the most common endocrine pancreatic tumors. In most instances they are discovered in a stage when the tumor is small (<3 cm in diameter) and clinically benign.

The typical symptoms include the classical **neuroglycopenic symptoms** such as headache, confusion, slurred speech, seizures, and fainting. These symptoms are usually associated

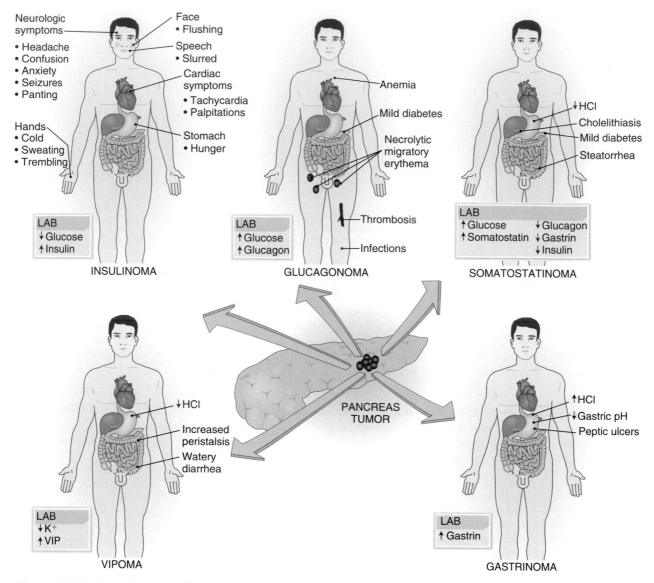

Figure 10-14 Clinical features of endocrine tumors of the pancreas. K⁺, potassium; VIP, vasoactive intestinal polypeptide.

with **adrenergic** symptoms, such as sweating, flushing of the face, and tremor. The blood glucose level is usually below 50 mg/dL, and insulin concentration is elevated.

Glucagonomas cause hyperglycemia, necrotizing migratory erythema, and hematologic changes.

Glucagonomas are tumors composed of alpha cells. These tumors secrete glucagon, which leads to hyperglycemia and mild DM. For unknown reasons the tumors also cause necrotizing, migratory erythema, venous thromboses, and anemia and predispose these patients to recurrent bacterial

infections. Typical laboratory findings include dramatically increased glucagon levels in the blood, mild hyperglycemia, and low fasting plasma amino acid levels.

Somatostatinomas inhibit the function of many endocrine cells and cause mild diabetes with gastrointestinal dysfunction.

Somatostatinomas are composed of delta cells that secrete somatostatin.

Somatostatin inhibits other endocrine cells of the pancreas and intestines, causing mild DM. Inhibition of gastrin secretion leads to hypochlorhydria (hyposecretion of HCl in the stomach) and steatorrhea and predisposes to gallstone formation. Typical laboratory findings include mild hyperglycemia; elevated somatostatin; and low insulin, glucagon, and gastrin.

Gastrinomas produce multiple peptic ulcers.

Gastrinomas are tumors composed of cells that secrete gastrin. Since the normal islets of Langerhans do not contain gastrin-secreting cells, it is presumed that the tumors originate from aberrant differentiation of undifferentiated precursor cells, which are also found in the duodenum. Indeed, 15% of all gastrinomas originate in the duodenum.

Gastrinomas manifest with signs and symptoms of Zollinger-Ellison syndrome, which includes peptic ulcers, hypersecretion of hydrochloric acid, and hypergastrinemia. Peptic ulcers are typically resistant to medical treatment and may be multiple or are found in unusual locations. Some

gastrinomas are part of the multiple endocrine neoplasia syndrome type 1 (MEN 1), which includes pituitary tumors, parathyroid tumors, or hyperplasia. Typical laboratory findings include elevated levels of gastrin in the blood and very high acidity of the gastric contents.

Vasoactive intestinal polypeptide-secreting tumors cause watery diarrhea, hypokalemia, and achlorhydria (WDHA).

Vasoactive intestinal polypeptide-secreting tumors (VIPomas) are tumors composed of cells that secrete vasoactive intestinal polypeptide (VIP). This polypeptide inhibits the secretion of hydrochloric acid in the stomach and stimulates pancreatic and intestinal secretion and intestinal motility, leading to diarrhea and hypokalemia. These clinical findings are known as WDHA syndrome or Verner-Morrison syndrome. Vasoactive intestinal polypeptide levels in the blood are elevated.

CASE STUDIES

Case 1 A 20-YEAR-OLD MAN COMPLAINING OF FREQUENT URINATION AND INCESSANT THIRST

Clinical history A 20-year-old man complained of frequent urination, excessive thirst, and easy fatigability.[1] Even though he has normal appetite and eats regularly he has lost 10 pounds over the last 2 months.[2]

Physical findings The patient is very thin. His skin and lips are dry. He is breathing fast and deeply and his breath has a fruity odor.[3]

Laboratory findings Fasting plasma sugar was 320 mg/dL.[4] Glucose and ketone bodies were detectable by dipstick in urine.[5] Blood Ace test for ketone bodies was positive.[6] Blood pH was 7.20, bicarbonate concentration was 15 mmol/L. There was an anion gap.[7]

Diagnostic procedures Blood insulin was barely detectable. Glucagon concentration was increased. Antibodies to islet cells were present in high titer.[8]

Follow-up The patient was treated and his condition improved dramatically. He was instructed how to inject himself with insulin and how to monitor his own blood sugar.[9] He was also taught how to recognize symptoms of hypoglycemia and ketoacidosis.[10]

Questions and topics for discussion

1. What are the possible causes of polyuria? Why is this patient thirsty?
2. What are the possible causes of involuntary weight loss? How is weight loss related to polyuria in this case?
3. What do these clinical findings suggest? Why are the skin and mucosae dry? Why is the patient's breathing fast and deep? What is the significance of its fruity odor? Is there evidence of Kussmaul breathing?
4. What are the possible causes of hyperglycemia?
5. Does the urine contain glucose and ketone bodies under normal circumstances? How are urinary glucose and ketone bodies measured?
6. What is the Ace test? Does it measure all ketone bodies in the blood?
7. Interpret these laboratory findings and determine whether this is acidosis or alkalosis, metabolic or respiratory.
8. What is the significance of antibodies to islet cells or insulin?
9. How long will this patient need insulin?
10. Why is it important to teach patients how to recognize the signs of hypoglycemia and ketoacidosis?

Case 2 A 58-YEAR-OLD MAN WITH LEG GANGRENE

Clinical history A 58-year-old obese man was admitted because of excruciating pain in his left leg.[1]

He was diagnosed with DM 15 years ago and he was taking antidiabetes pills more or less regularly. Every so often he would see his doctor, who would test his urine and blood and adjust the medication.[2]

He complained of frequently being short of breath. He also had tingling in his fingers and toes and occasionally felt pain in his legs, especially when walking.[3]

Physical findings The patient is obese. His pulse rate is 80/min, and his blood pressure is 150/100 mm Hg. He has bilateral pitting pedal edema. The left leg is bluish and cold below the ankle. No pulse can be palpated in this leg.[4] Funduscopic examination revealed retinal streak hemorrhages, exudates, and microaneurysms.[5] Neurologic examination revealed slower reflexes on all extremities and reduced pain sensation.[6]

Laboratory findings Fasting blood sugar was 180 mm/dL, and there was trace sugar in the urine.[7] No ketone bodies were detected in the blood or urine. Urine contained 300 mg of albumin per 24 hours.[8] Hemoglobin A_{1c} was 9%.[9]

Diagnostic procedures Arteriography revealed complete occlusion of the left tibial artery and a few other major branches of the femoral artery.[10]

Follow-up A below-the-knee amputation of the left leg was performed. He was encouraged to lose weight, and a more rigorous control of diabetes was ordered.

Questions and topics for discussion
1. What are the possible causes of leg pain?
2. How should patients with DM be monitored?
3. Explain the possible causes of shortness of breath and tingling in the fingers and toes.
4. What is the significance of this finding?
5. Explain the funduscopic findings. Are these findings caused by DM or hypertension?
6. Are these neurologic findings indicative of sensory or motor neuropathy?
7. How can the patient have hyperglycemia but only a trace of glucose in the urine?
8. Doe this patient have albuminuria? What is the predictive value of this finding?
9. What is the significance of increased HbA_{1c}?
10. What caused the occlusion of the leg arteries?

Case 3 A 50-YEAR-OLD MAN COMPLAINS OF RECENT FAINTING SPELLS ASSOCIATED WITH EXCESSIVE SWEATING

Clinical history A 50-year-old man fainted several times during the last 3 days. The fainting spells occurred in the late afternoon hours just before dinner. Each time he recovered after drinking two glasses of soda pop and eating some sugar.[1]

He also noticed that the fainting spells were associated with profuse sweating.[2]

Physical findings The patient appears well nourished and has no obvious major external signs of disease. He seems to not be in any distress, but is a bit nervous because of the fainting episodes.

Laboratory findings The only abnormality was low blood glucose (50 mg/dL).[3]

Subsequent hormonal studies revealed elevated blood insulin.[4] C polypeptide was also elevated in the blood.[5]

Diagnostic procedures Computed tomography revealed a well-circumscribed 3-cm mass in the tail of the pancreas.[6]

Follow-up A partial pancreatectomy was performed, and the tumor from the pancreas was removed. The pathology report indicated that the tumor was composed of neuroendocrine cells and was most likely benign.[7]

The final diagnosis was based on immunohistochemical data.[8]

Questions and topics for discussion
1. What are the possible causes of fainting? Does the fact that recovery occurred after drinking and eating sugar help you narrow the differential diagnosis?
2. What is the pathogenesis of sweating in this case?
3. What are the possible causes of hypoglycemia?
4. What could cause increased insulin concentration in the blood?
5. Why was the blood concentration of C polypeptide measured? Interpret these laboratory findings.
6. Is this tumor most likely benign or malignant? Which findings favor one and which favor the other possibility?
7. What are the pathologic features of neuroendocrine tumors? Are these tumors benign or malignant? How would you decide?
8. Why was an immunohistochemical study performed? Which reagents were used?

Chapter 11

THE ENDOCRINE SYSTEM

Introduction

The endocrine system is essential for the maintenance of most body functions. Endocrine disturbances may therefore manifest in many forms, as minor or major functional defects, and if not properly diagnosed may cause death. It is important to remember that:

■ Endocrine diseases affect the *overall intermediary metabolism.* Lack of thyroid hormones leads to a slowing down of the body's metabolism, whereas hyperthyroidism leads to hypermetabolism.

■ Endocrine gland dysfunction affects *body growth and maturation of many organs, mental development, and reproductive functions.*

■ Endocrine diseases may affect the *function of major organs.* For example, both hyperthyroidism and hypothyroidism cause cardiac problems and may contribute to heart failure.

■ Endocrine diseases accelerate the *progression of other chronic diseases.* For example, diabetes mellitus accelerates the development of atherosclerosis.

■ Endocrine diseases may change the *immune system and resistance to infections.* For example, an excess of corticosteroids win Cushing's syndrome may reduce resistance to infections.

In this chapter we discuss only the diseases affecting the major endocrine organs: pituitary, thyroid, parathyroids, and adrenal glands. The cells forming the dispersed endocrine system of the gastrointestinal and respiratory tract are not discussed. Diabetes mellitus, the most common and clinically the most important endocrine disease, was discussed in the Chapter 10. The relative clinical significance of various endocrine diseases is presented graphically in Figure 11-1.

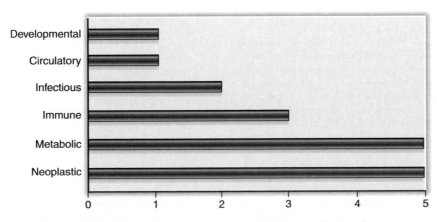

Figure 11-1 Relative clinical significance of various endocrine diseases.

Anatomy and Physiology

Adenohypophysis Anterior portion of the pituitary gland comprising the pars tuberalis, pars distalis, and pars intermedia. In standard histologic sections it is composed of three types of cells: acidophilic, basophilic, and chromophobic cells. These cells secrete polypeptide hormones and can be classified functionally or immunohistochemically into six groups: somatotrophs (growth hormone-secreting), lactotrophs (prolactin-secreting), thyrotrophs (thyroid-stimulating hormone-secreting), corticotrophs (adrenocorticotrop hormone-secreting), gonadotrophs (follicle-stimulating hormone and luteinizing hormone-secreting), and hormonally inactive cells ("null" cells, or stem cells).

Adrenal cortex Outer part of the adrenal glands. It comprises three layers: zona glomerulosa composed of mineralocorticosteroid-secreting cells, zona fasciculata composed of glucocorticoid-secreting cells, and zona reticularis composed of androgen-secreting cells.

Adrenal glands Paired endocrine glands located retroperitoneally just above the kidneys. They consist of two parts: the outer, known as the cortex, and the inner, known as the medulla.

Adrenal medulla Inner part of the adrenal glands. It is composed of catecholamine-secreting chromaffin cells. These cells develop from the neural crest cells, which have migrated to the retroperitoneal area during fetal development. The same neural crest cells give rise to paraganglia and autonomic ganglia, and thus tumors like the pheochromocytoma and neuroblastoma may originate either from adrenal or extra-adrenal sites.

Aldosterone Mineralocorticosteroid produced by the zona glomerulosa of the adrenal cortex. Its secretion from the cells of the zona glomerulosa is controlled mainly by the renin–angiotensin system. In the kidneys aldosterone promotes reabsorption of sodium and bicarbonate and the excretion of potassium and hydrogen ions. Secondary retention of water may lead to arterial hypertension.

Androgens Male sexual hormones produced by the Leydig cells of the testis and adrenal cortical cells in the zona reticularis. The most important androgens are testosterone, androstenedione, dehydroepiandrosterone (DHEA), and dehydroepiandrosterone sulfate (DHEAS).

Antidiuretic hormone (ADH, vasopressin) Octapeptide hormone synthesized by neuronal cells in the hypothalamic nuclei and stored in the posterior lobe of the pituitary. Its synthesis is regulated by the osmolality of the plasma. Antidiuretic hormone stimulates the contraction of smooth muscles. Its effects on arterioles raise the blood pressure, and its effects on the intestines promote peristalsis. The antidiuretic effect results from its action on the distal tubules of the kidney, where it promotes the resorption of water.

Catecholamines Group of biogenic amines, the most important of which are dopamine, epinephrine, and norepinephrine. Catecholamines found in the blood are derived from the adrenal medulla. Epinephrine and norepinephrine are also found in the central nervous system and peripheral nerves. Catechol-amines have many sympathomimetic effects ("fight-or-flight" reaction in stress), and raise the blood pressure.

Corticosteroids Group of 21-carbon steroids produced from progesterone by adrenal cortical cells. According to their function they are classified as mineralocorticoids or glucocorticoids.

Corticotropin (adrenocorticotropic hormone, ACTH) Glycopeptide produced in the anterior lobe of the pituitary under the control of the hypothalamic corticotropin-releasing hormone (CRH). It stimulates the adrenal cortical cells and is also excreted in large amounts during stress.

Follicle-stimulating hormone (FSH) Gonadotropic glycopeptide produced in the anterior lobe of the pituitary under the control of the hypothalamic FSH-releasing hormone. It stimulates the growth of ovarian follicles and secretion of estrogen. In males it stimulates spermatogenesis.

Glucocorticoids Steroid hormones produced by the zona fasciculata of the adrenal cortex. The most important glucocorticoids are cortisol (hydrocortisone), cortisone, and corticosterone. Their secretion is under the control of ACTH and is increased in stress. They affect the metabolism of carbohydrates, lipids, and proteins.

Growth hormone (GH) Polypeptide hormone secreted by cells of the anterior pituitary. It stimulates the liver to produce somatomedins, which promote skeletal growth. Growth hormone also acts on the intermediary metabolism of carbohydrates, lipids, and proteins.

Luteinizing hormone (LH) Gonadotropic glycoprotein produced by the anterior lobe of the pituitary under the control of the hypothalamic LH-releasing hormone. It promotes ovulation and stimulates the secretion of progesterone from the corpus luteum in women. In men it acts on Leydig cells, stimulating the production of androgen.

Neurohypophysis Posterior part of the pituitary composed of cytoplasmic extensions of neural cells in several hypothalamic nuclei. These cells secrete antidiuretic hormone (ADH, vasopressin) and oxytocin.

Oxytocin Nonapeptide synthesized by the cells of the paraventricular nucleus of the hypothalamus and stored in the posterior lobe of the pituitary. It is released on stimulation of cholinergic fibers in the areolar area of the nipple during suckling. It causes uterine contractions during delivery and milk release during lactation.

Parathormone (parathyroid hormone, PTH) Polypeptide hormone produced by the parathyroid glands. It stimulates hypercalcemia by promoting calcium release from the bone, calcium absorption in the intestine, and renal calcium reabsorption.

Parathyroid glands Four small endocrine glands located on the posterior side of the thyroid. They secrete parathyroid hormone, a polypeptide hormone essential for the metabolism of calcium and phosphorus.

Pituitary Endocrine gland located in the sella turcica and attached by a stalk to the hypothalamus. It consists of an anterior and intermediate part forming the adenohypophysis and a posterior part forming the neurohypophysis.

Prolactin Polypeptide hormone secreted by the anterior lobe of the pituitary. It plays an important role in the development of the mammary glands during pregnancy and the production of milk during lactation. It also suppresses LH secretion causing anovulation and amenorrhea.

Thyroglobulin   High-molecular-weight iodinated glycoprotein produced by thyroid follicular cells and stored in the colloid. It is taken up by follicular cells and transformed into thyroxine and triiodothyronine.

Thyroid   Bilobed endocrine gland located on the neck anterior to the trachea. It is composed of thyroid hormone-secreting cells arranged into follicles, and scattered C cells secreting calcitonin.

Thyroxine (tetraiodothyronine, T_4)   Principal hormone produced by the thyroid. It is partially diodinated into a more active form, triiodothyronine (T_3). Both T_4 and T_3 stimulate metabolism and act on most major organs in the body.

Clinical Signs and Symptoms

Amenorrhea   Lack of menstrual bleeding, usually resulting from hormonal disturbances involving the pituitary gland or the ovary. If the menstrual bleeding never occurs at the time of puberty it is called primary amenorrhea. Cessation of menstruation in a woman who was previously menstruating normally is called secondary amenorrhea.

Dwarfism (nanosomia)   Condition in which the body is considerably smaller than normal. It may have many causes, including pituitary or thyroid insufficiency in infancy and childhood.

Exophthalmos (proptosis)   Abnormal bulging of the eyes, typically seen in Graves' disease.

Galactorrhea   Abnormal production of milk unrelated to pregnancy and lactation, or an uncontrolled flow of milk during lactation.

Goiter   Diffuse, usually nodular enlargement of the thyroid caused by a variety of conditions, such as thyroiditis, iodine deficiency, or hormonal disturbances including thyroid enlargement.

Hirsutism   Condition characterized by excessive hairiness. In women it is characterized by hair growth in a male pattern (e.g., face and chest).

Myxedema   Form of nonpitting chronic edema predominantly involving the face and causing swelling of the lips and nose and deepening of facial furrows.

Osteomalacia   Form of osteopenia (reduced bone mass) characterized by inadequate mineralization of the osteoid matrix.

Osteoporosis   Form of osteopenia (reduced bone mass) characterized by a loss of mineralized bone and a tendency to fractures.

Endocrine Diseases

Acromegaly and gigantism   Syndrome caused by an excess of growth hormone (GH), usually produced by a pituitary adenoma. In children and adolescents excess GH leads to tall stature (gigantism). Acromegaly (i.e., an enlargement of the acral parts—feet, hands, nose, and jaw) is found in adults. Additional findings include hypertension, cardiomegaly, insulin resistance, and metabolic disturbances such as hyperglycemia.

Addison's disease   Adrenal cortical insufficiency due to the destruction of the adrenals by autoimmune diseases, infections (e.g., tuberculosis), or metastatic tumors. It is characterized by weight loss, weakness, hypoglycemia, hypotension and hyperpigmentation, and laboratory findings indicative of a mineralocorticoid and glucocorticoid deficiency.

Amenorrhea–galactorrhea syndrome   Syndrome related to an excess of prolactin, usually secreted by a pituitary adenoma. Clinically it manifests with spontaneous milk secretion and cessation of the menstrual cycle.

Conn's syndrome (primary hyperaldosteronism)   Syndrome caused by an excess of aldosterone, usually produced by a cortical adenoma. It is characterized by hypertension, metabolic alkalosis, polyuria, and potassium wasting. Laboratory findings include hyperaldosteronism, low renin, and low serum potassium. Secondary hyperaldosteronism is a consequence of renal diseases leading to hypersecretion of renin.

Cushing's syndrome   Syndrome caused by an excess of glucocorticoids, produced by the pathologically altered or overstimulated adrenal cortical cells, or due to an iatrogenic intake of steroids. It is clinically characterized by truncal obesity, moon facies, buffalo hump, contrasted with thin extremities affected by muscle wasting. Osteoporosis, hypertension, skin atrophy, and reduced resistance to infections are also present. Laboratory findings include excess glucocorticoids in the blood and urine and corresponding changes involving minerals and glucose. Adrenocorticotropic hormone is usually suppressed, except in patients who have Cushing's disease due to corticotropic adenoma of the pituitary.

Diabetes insipidus   Syndrome related to ADH deficiency (central diabetes insipidus) or an inability of the kidneys to respond to proper ADH stimulation (renal diabetes insipidus). In either case the kidneys cannot retain water, resulting in polyuria and dehydration. Despite polydipsia, serum osmolality is increased, as is the specific gravity of the urine. Hypernatremia and decreased osmolality are also features.

Graves' disease   Autoimmune disease characterized by overstimulation of the thyroid with antibodies to thyroid-stimulating hormone (TSH) receptors. It is clinically characterized by symmetric enlargement of the thyroid, hyperthyroidism, and exophthalmos.

Hyperparathyroidism   Syndrome caused by an excess of parathyroid hormones. It may be primary (most often due to parathyroid adenoma) or secondary (due to parathyroid hyperplasia in renal insufficiency). Clinically it manifests with hypercalcemia, loss of bone substance (osteitis fibrosa cystica), renal stones, gastrointestinal disturbances, and neurologic symptoms.

Hyperthyroidism   Syndrome caused by an excess of thyroid hormone, most often related to autoimmune disorders (Graves' disease), or functionally active thyroid tumors. Clinically it manifests with signs of hypermetabolism, such as tachycardia, sweating, and nervousness.

Hypoparathyroidism   Syndrome caused by inadequate parathyroid hormone production, most often due to surgical removal of all four parathyroid glands. The lack of PTH leads to hypocalcemia producing signs of neuromuscular irritability (e.g., tetanic spasms, Chvostek's sign, Trousseau's sign), electrocardiographic (ECG) changes.

Hypothyroidism   Syndrome caused by a lack of thyroid hormones. In infants it is most often caused by congenital thyroid aplasia and is associated with growth retardation and mental retardation (cretinism). In adults it is usually due to Hashimoto's thyroiditis or surgical resection of the thyroid. Laboratory findings include low T_4 and T_3 and high thyroid-stimulating hormone (TSH). Clinical findings include myxedema and slowed down metabolism and major vital function (e.g., bradycardia, constipation, drowsiness).

Infertility   Inability to conceive a child or become pregnant.

Pheochromocytoma   Catecholamine-secreting tumor of the adrenal medulla. Catecholamines released from the tumor cause paroxysmal hypertension and other signs of adrenergic overstimulation, such as excessive sweating, palpitations, and headaches. Excessive epinephrine and norepinephrine can be detected in the blood. Metabolized catecholamines are excreted as vanillylmandelic acid (VMA) in the urine.

Pituitary cachexia   Syndrome related to a lack of pituitary hormones, typically caused by tumors of the hypothalamic area or as a result of surgical resection or trauma. Clinically it presents with wasting and weakness and signs of hypothyroidism, adrenal cortical insufficiency, and gonadal insufficiency. Laboratory findings include hypoglycemia, hyponatremia, and reduced levels of thyroid and steroid hormones. Sheehan's syndrome is a form of panhypopituitarism found in the postpartum period. It is related to hemorrhagic infarction of the pituitary.

Normal Structure and Function

ANATOMY AND HISTOLOGY

Endocrine cells specialize in producing hormones and secreting them into the internal milieu of the blood or interstitial fluids. Some endocrine cells form organs, such as the thyroid, parathyroids, or adrenals. Others are scattered as cell groups in other exocrine glands such as the islets of Langerhans in the pancreas, the Leydig cells in the testis, and the follicular and lutein cells in the ovary. Single endocrine cells are scattered throughout the gastrointestinal and respiratory tracts. Some endocrine cells secrete biogenic amines and neurotransmitters, and some hormones are secreted by nerve cells. Such cells are thus called neuroendocrine cells. Finally note that some hormones are secreted by somatic cells that have other functions (e.g., fat cells secreting leptin), and that many biologically active proteins circulating in plasma or found at the site of inflammation may have hormone-like effects.

Based on the mode of hormone secretion (Fig. 11-2), endocrine and neuroendocrine cells can be classified into four categories:

- **Endocrine cells.** These cells secrete hormones into the blood, which carries them to a distant target organ. Typical endocrine cells are thyroid, parathyroid, and adrenal cortical cells.
- **Paracrine cells.** These cells secrete hormones into the interstitial fluid surrounding them and act on adjacent cells. Typical paracrine cells are found in the gastrointestinal tract and the islets of the pancreas. For example in the islets of Langerhans somatostatin secreted by delta cells inhibits glucagon-secreting alpha cells and insulin-secreting beta cells.
- **Autocrine cells.** These cells secrete hormones into the interstitial fluid, but the hormone binds to the cell surface of the cell that has secreted it, thus stimulating the cell itself. Many of the growth factors have autocrine properties and are especially important in promoting tumor growth.

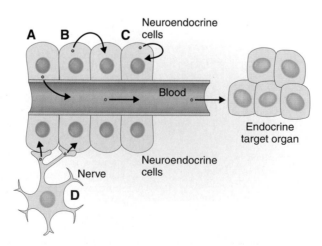

Figure 11-2 Various secretory forms of endocrine cells. **A,** Endocrine secretion. **B,** Paracrine secretion. **C,** Autocrine secretion. **D,** Neuroendocrine secretion.

■ **Neurocrine cells.** These cells have all the major features of nerve cells, but secrete hormones that act on other non-neural cells. For example, neural cells in the hypothalamus secrete releasing factors that stimulate the hormone production of pituitary cells.

PHYSIOLOGY

Biochemically hormones can be classified as steroids, polypeptides, and modified amino acids (biogenic amines). The main features of these hormones are briefly reviewed here and summarized in Table 11-1.

Steroid hormones. These hormones are continuously synthesized in the hormone-producing cells of the gonads, adrenal cortex, and placenta. The synthesis of these hormones takes place on the smooth endoplasmic reticulum, and the hormones are secreted rather than stored.

The multistep synthesis of the polycyclic backbone begins with the conversion of cholesterol into pregnenolone. This basic structure is then modified by isomerization or oxidation, leading to the formation of estrogens, progestogens, androgens, mineralocorticoids, and glucocorticoids. Steroid hormones are not water-soluble and must therefore be transported in the blood bound to transport proteins. They can enter target cells and bind to intracellular receptors, which transport them into the nucleus (Fig. 11-3). In the nucleus they bind to the hormone-response elements of the gene, stimulating protein synthesis.

Polypeptide and protein hormones. These hormones are synthesized in a stepwise manner like all other proteins in the rough endoplasmic reticulum and Golgi apparatus, where they may be glycosylated into glycoproteins. The hormones are stored in the cytoplasm in the form of membrane-bounded secretory granules. The content of these granules is released by exocytosis, which is triggered by exogenous stimuli. For example glucose triggers the release of insulin from the beta cells of the islets of Langerhans. Polypeptide and protein hormones are synthesized by cells of the pituitary, the islets of Langerhans, the parathyroids, C cells of the thyroid, gastrointestinal neuroendocrine cells, and the endocrine cells of the placenta. Polypeptide hormones are water-soluble and may be found in the plasma in a free form or bound to a transport protein. They bind to the surface plasma proteins but cannot otherwise enter into the cell cytoplasm.

Modified amino acids. These low-molecular-weight hormones are formed from amino acids, mostly tyrosine and tryptophan, in a manner similar to the production of polypeptide hormones. Typical hormones of this group are the thyroid hormones T_4 and T_3, catecholamines (epinephrine and norepinephrine), and dopamine. Most hormones in this group are stored in the cytoplasm in the form of membrane-bounded granules, except for thyroid hormones, which are secreted into the colloid and stored in the lumen of the follicles. In the plasma they circulate in a free form, but the thyroid hormones also bind to a transport protein. Catecholamines and dopamine act on cell surface receptors, whereas the thyroid hormones bind to intracytoplasmic receptors.

Clinical and Laboratory Evaluation of Endocrine Diseases

FAMILY AND PERSONAL HISTORY

In the work-up of suspected cases of endocrine disease, begin by taking a family and personal history. Some of the risk factors that can be identified in this interview are listed in Table 11-2.

PHYSICAL EXAMINATION

Symptoms and signs of endocrine disorders are often nonspecific and not readily recognizable. In some patients the endocrine disorders, such as gigantism, predominate the clinical picture, but obvious and telltale symptomatology of this sort

Table 11-1 Comparison of Steroids, Polypeptides, and Modified Amino Acid Hormones

FEATURE	STEROIDS	POLYPEPTIDES	MODIFIED AMINO ACIDS
Basic structure	Polycyclic carbon ring	Polypeptides	Amino acids
Synthesis	SER	RER, Golgi apparatus	RER, Golgi apparatus
Storage in cytoplasm	No	Yes (granules)	Yes (granules, except thyroid, which is in follicles)
Mode of release	Continuous	Triggered	Triggered
Form in blood	Bound to proteins	Free	Free (except thyroid, which is partly protein-bound)
Receptor type	Intracellular	Plasma membrane	Plasma membrane or intracellular

RER, rough endoplasmic reticulum; SER, smooth endoplasmic reticulum.
Data from Meszaros G. Endocrine and Reproductive Systems. Philadelphia, Elsevier Mosby, 2006.

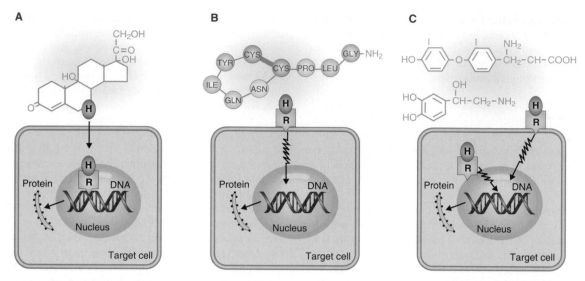

Figure 11-3 Various forms of hormones. **A,** Steroid hormones have a polycyclic structure. They bind to cytoplasmic receptors (R), which transfer them to the nucleus. In the nucleus the hormones (H) bind the hormone-responsive element of the gene and stimulate gene activity, which ultimately results in the synthesis of the proteins in the endoplasmic reticulum. **B,** Polypeptide and protein hormones are chains of amino acids, which may be glycosylated (glycoproteins). They bind to surface receptors on the cell membrane. The signal from the activated receptor is transmitted through several systems of cytoplasmic messengers to the genes in the nucleus. **C,** Modified amines can bind to the cytoplasmic receptors, as is the case with the thyroid hormone, or they bind to the cell surface receptor, as is the case with catecholamines. The receptor-generated signals are transmitted to the genetic material in the nucleus, resulting in the synthesis of the proteins.

is uncommon. Some diseases affect endocrine organs but cause few if any endocrine disturbances. For example goiter is readily detected by inspection or palpation of the neck, but it is often not associated with any disturbances in thyroid function. Many endocrine diseases are asymptomatic and are discovered only with laboratory testing.

The following is a list of some signs and symptoms of possible endocrine disease:

■ **Easy fatigability.** Fatigue is a common symptom of many endocrine disorders, most notably *hypothyroidism, hyperthyroidism,* and *adrenal insufficiency.*

Table 11-2 Risk Factors for Some Endocrine Disorders

TYPE OF RISK FACTOR	SPECIFIC DISEASES—RISK FACTOR ASSOCIATIONS
Hereditary factors	Multiple endocrine neoplasia syndromes: Medullary carcinoma of thyroid and pheochromocytoma (hypertension)
Nutritional factors	Iodine deficiency: Endemic goiter in some parts of the world
	Goitrogens in diet: Goiter
	Eating disorders: Anorexia nervosa
Diseases involving other organs	End-stage kidney disease: Secondary hyperparathyroidism
Other endocrine diseases	ACTH-secreting pituitary adenoma: Cushing's disease
Infection	Meningococcal sepsis: Acute adrenal insufficiency of Waterhouse-Friderichsen syndrome
Autoimmunity	Multiorgan autoimmune diseases: Hashimoto's thyroiditis-related hypothyroidism
Medical and surgical procedures	Neck surgery: Hypoparathyroidism
Drugs	Long-term corticosteroid therapy for rheumatoid arthritis: Hypercorticoidism and adrenal atrophy
	Lithium: Goiter
External mechanical factors	Brain trauma: Hypopituitarism

ACTH, adrenocorticotropic hormone.

- **Weight loss.** Weight loss may be associated with a loss of appetite in *bulimia* and *anorexia nervosa*. *Pituitary* and *adrenal insufficiency* cause marked wasting and cachexia.
- **Obesity.** Obesity is usually caused by overeating; pure endocrine obesity is rare. It is a feature of pituitary hypogonadism. In hypothyroidism it is typically associated with myxedema of the face, lethargy, cold intolerance, and other signs of hypometabolism. In Cushing's syndrome fat selectively accumulates on the face (moon face), back ("buffalo hump"), and in the retroperitoneum ("truncal obesity"). In polycystic ovary syndrome (PCOS) it is associated with acne, hirsutism, and amenorrhea.
- **Low stature.** Retarded growth in infancy is a typical feature of congenital hypothyroidism. Dwarfism may be caused by growth hormone deficiency in pituitary or hypothalamic diseases or a resistance to growth hormone (GH receptor mutation in Laron dwarfism).
- **Tall stature.** Excessive growth may be a sign of a GH-secreting pituitary adenoma (gigantism), but in most instances the reasons for excessive height are not found.
- **Visual problems.** *Pituitary tumors* may cause endocrine symptoms and also compress the optic chiasm, causing *bitemporal hemianopsia*. Such tumors also may cause headache due to increased intracranial pressure. *Exophthalmos* seen in *Graves' disease* may also cause visual problems.
- **Disturbances of cardiac function.** *Hyperthyroidism* causes tachycardia, and *hypothyroidism* causes bradycardia. Disturbances in the metabolism of calcium, sodium, and potassium in *parathyroid* or *adrenal* disorders may cause changes in the heart function and obvious electrocardiographic (ECG) changes.
- **Amenorrhea.** Both primary and secondary amenorrhea (lack of menstrual bleeding) may be caused by a variety of endocrine disturbances. These may involve any part of the hypothalamic–pituitary–ovarian–adrenal axis. Excessive menstrual bleeding (**menorrhagia**) may also be a sign of endocrine disturbances.
- **Hirsutism.** It is defined as an excessive growth of body hair in a male pattern on a woman. If associated with other signs of virilism, such as deep voice or male pattern baldness, hirsutism is usually related to an excess of androgens. Hirsutism associated with acne is a feature of PCOS.
- **Galactorrhea.** Spontaneous discharge of milk in a nonlactating woman is most often caused by an excess of prolactin, produced by a pituitary lactotrophic adenoma.
- **Gynecomastia.** Enlargement of the breasts in males may have many causes, and hyperestrogenism is one of them.
- **Erectile dysfunction (impotence).** This has many causes and may be classified as predominantly psychogenic, endocrine, circulatory, neurologic, or iatrogenic. Diabetes mellitus is the most common hormonal cause of impotence.

- **Polyuria.** Urgency to urinate and a large quantity of urine may be a sign of diabetes mellitus, diabetes insipidus, hypercalcemia, and several other endocrine disorders. Typically it is associated with polydipsia, but if the loss of water is not adequately replaced, dehydration may occur.
- **Hyperpigmentation of the skin.** An excess of adrenocorticotropic hormone (ACTH) may cause hyperpigmentation because in humans ACTH acts also as a melanocyte-stimulating hormone. Typically it is found in Addison's disease and bilateral adrenal gland resection for Cushing's disease *(Nelson's syndrome).* Pregnancy and use of oral contraceptives may cause hyperpigmentation on the face, known as **chloasma,** or **melasma.**
- **Osteopenia and bone fractures.** Loss of bone mass is a feature of many endocrine diseases, and it may manifest as either osteoporosis or osteomalacia. Osteopenia may be caused by a variety of conditions, such as hyperparathyroidism, Cushing's syndrome, or hyperthyroidism. Reduction of estrogens after menopause is the most common cause of osteoporosis. Both osteoporosis and osteomalacia are accompanied by an increased fragility of bones and a high frequency of spontaneous fractures.

LABORATORY STUDIES

Endocrine diseases result from either a hyperfunction or a hypofunction of endocrine organs that results in a deficiency or an excess of hormones, respectively. To diagnose an endocrine disease several of the following approaches can be taken:

- **Measure hormones in blood.** For example, the concentration of thyroxine (T_4) can be measured in the blood. To improve the precision of this test it is customary to also measure the concentration of T_3 (the more active form of T_4) and thyroid-stimulating hormone (TSH). Analyzing these three hormones in most instances determines whether hypothyroidism or hyperthyroidism is present. Furthermore, these tests can indicate whether the disease is due to a pituitary or a thyroid disorder.
- **Measure a hormone or its degradation products in the urine.** Epinephrine and norepinephrine can be measured in the blood in possible cases of pheochromocytoma. Such patients excrete a catecholamine degradation product, such as vanillylmandelic acid (VMA), which can be detected and quantitated in the urine.
- **Measure the metabolites resulting from the action of the hormone.** The best example of such a test is the plasma glucose test, which is elevated in the plasma of persons with diabetes mellitus.
- **Use of stimulation tests.** These tests are used when hormonal insufficiency is suggested, usually after initial studies have shown that the levels of a specific

Table 11-3 Endocrine Stimulation Tests

HORMONE DEFICIENCY	TEST	EXPLANATION
Growth hormone	L-Dopa, arginin, or insulin stimulation test	A lack of response → hypothalamic or pituitary disorder
Gonadotropins (FSH and LH)	GnRH stimulation	GnRH increases FSH and LH; lack of response → hypothalamic or pituitary injury or disease
Cortisol	ACTH stimulation	A lack of response to prolonged ACTH infusion → adrenal insufficiency; response to ACTH → hypothalamic or pituitary diseases

ACTH, adrenocorticotropic hormone; FSH, follicle-stimulating hormone; GnRH, gonadotropin-releasing hormone; LH, luteinizing hormone.

hormone are low. Typical stimulation tests are listed in Table 11-3.

■ **Use of suppression tests.** These tests are used when a hyperfunction of an endocrine organ is suspected. Typical suppression tests are listed in Table 11-4.

RADIOGRAPHIC IMAGING STUDIES

Enlarged endocrine glands may be readily visualized with modern radiologic techniques such as **computed tomography (CT)** or **magnetic resonance imaging (MRI)**; the latter, combined with gadolinium enhancement, is the test of choice for detecting pituitary adenomas of the pituitary region. Ectopic ACTH-secreting lung tumors can be detected using **standard chest radiographic examination.**

Functionally active endocrine cells concentrate certain radiologic markers and can be even better demonstrated with radioscanning techniques:

■ **Radioactive iodine uptake.** High uptake in thyroid lesions is seen in hyperthyroidism due to Graves' disease, toxic nodular goiter, or functioning solitary ade-

noma. Low uptake is seen in Hashimoto's thyroiditis, tumors replacing normal thyroid tissue, and in patients who are taking exogenous thyroid hormones.

■ **Radioactive I-131 iodonorcholesterol uptake.** This test may be used for detecting adrenal cortical tumors.
■ **Metaiodobenzylguanidine (MIBG) uptake.** Scintigraphy with MIBG is a sensitive technique for detecting small pheochromocytomas.
■ **Sestamibi scan.** This method is used for localizing the parathyroid glands and tumors within them. The sestamibi scan has a reported sensitivity of 85% to 90% and a specificity varying from 55% to 85%.

Clinicopathologic Correlations

PITUITARY DISEASES

The pituitary gland is in central position to the hypothalamic–pituitary–peripheral endocrine organ system (Fig. 11-4). Accordingly, pituitary diseases resulting from the hyperproduction

Table 11-4 Endocrine Suppression Tests

HORMONE OVER-PRODUCTION	TEST	EXPLANATION
Growth hormone	Oral glucose tolerance	Lack of suppression → pituitary adenoma
Cortisol	Dexamethasone suppression test	Low dose (lack of suppression) → Cushing's syndrome any type (may be false positive in obesity and stress)
		High dose suppression → pituitary ACTH tumor (no suppression in adrenal or ectopic Cushing's syndrome)
Aldosterone	Isotonic saline infusion	Lack of suppression → aldosterone tumor

ACTH, adrenocorticotropic hormone.

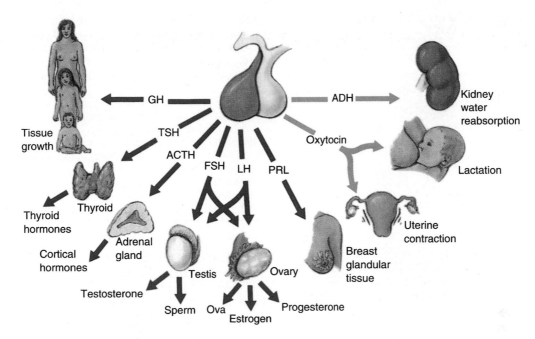

Figure 11-4 Pituitary hormones and their target tissues. Anterior pituitary is orange and posterior pituitary is yellow. ACTH, adrenocorticotropic hormone; ADH, antidiuretic hormone; FSH, follicle-stimulating hormone; GH, growth hormone; LH, luteinizing hormone; PRL, prolactin; TSH, thyroid-stimulating hormone. (From Applegate EJ: The Anatomy and Physiology Learning System. WB Saunders, Philadelphia, 1995.)

or hypoproduction of pituitary trophic hormones manifest with a hyperfunction or insufficiency of target organs or multiorgan endocrine failure.

Pituitary diseases may be caused by lesions in the pituitary gland itself, which involve the anterior or posterior lobe, or by lesions in the hypothalamus, with which the pituitary is closely linked into a single functional unit.

Anterior pituitary hyperfunction is most often caused by tumors.

Tumors are the most important lesions of the pituitary. Even so, they are quite rare. These tumors may produce hormones and cause one of the typical pituitary hormonal syndromes.

The most common pituitary tumor, the **prolactinoma,** is typically associated with **galactorrhea–amenorrhea** syndrome in women and loss of libido and impotence in men. Other syndromes related to pituitary hyperfunction are uncommon. This group of diseases includes **acromegaly/gigantism, Cushing's disease** due to corticotropic adenoma, pituitary **hyperthyroidism,** and **disturbances of reproductive function** due to gonadotropic tumors.

Prolactinoma. These tumors composed of lactotrophic cells account for approximately one third of all hormonally active pituitary adenomas. They occur eight times more

frequently in women than in men. Hyperprolactinemia stimulates the production of milk, causing galactorrhea. It also interferes with the normally pulsatile secretion of luteinizing hormone (LH) and follicle-stimulating hormone (FSH), causing amenorrhea, anovulation, infertility, and loss of libido. In men it causes erectile dysfunction, loss of libido, infertility, and gynecomastia (Fig. 11-5).

Tumors secreting prolactin may be classified as microadenomas or macroadenomas. Microadenomas do not affect the function of the surrounding normal pituitary, but the large macroadenomas may compress other cells and impede their function. The diagnosis is made by measuring prolactin in the blood and by demonstrating the tumor radiologically in the anterior lobe of the pituitary. Note, however, that hyperprolactinemia may be caused by a number of other conditions besides tumors (Table 11-5). In these conditions prolactin levels in the blood are usually less than 100 µg/L. A concentration of prolactin greater than 300 µg/L is virtually diagnostic of prolactinoma.

Normal secretion of prolactin is inhibited by dopamine. Dopamine agonists such as bromocriptine inhibit prolactin secretion even in patients who have adenomas. This type of treatment may suffice for treating microadenomas, but macroadenomas must be treated surgically.

Somatotropic adenoma. These tumors secrete growth hormone. Childhood tumors found before the closure of

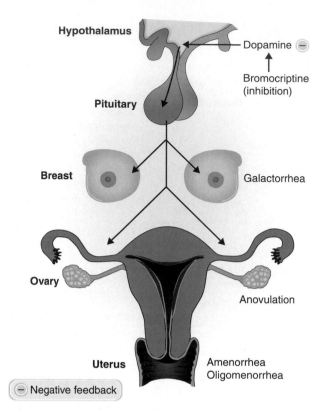

Figure 11-5 Prolactinoma. The tumor in the anterior pituitary leads to galactorrhea, anovulation, and amenorrhea. Inhibition of dopamine with bromocriptine reduces the prolactinemia.

epiphysis cause **gigantism,** and tumors of adulthood cause **acromegaly.** Gigantism is extremely rare, and acromegaly is somewhat more common. About 15% of all somatotropic adenomas also secrete prolactin and gonadotropic hormones.

Acromegaly. Acromegaly presents with acral enlargement due to thickening of the skin, excessive growth of subcutaneous tissue and bone, generalized organomegaly, and metabolic changes (Fig. 11-6). The most common findings include the following:

- Enlargement of hands and thickening of fingers, with palmar skin thickening. The patient typically complains that rings no longer fit or that gloves are tight. The patient also experiences excessive sweating.
- Enlargement of feet and toes and heel pad. The patient typically complains that shoes are too small.
- Facial changes ("acromegalic facies"). These include prominent supraorbital ridges, enlarged nose, protruding jaw, and enlarged tongue.
- Enlargement of the head. The patient complains that hats are tight. It may be associated with headaches.

Table 11-5 Causes of Hyperprolactinemia

Prolactinoma
Physiologic states
  Pregnancy, nursing, nipple stimulation
Stress
Drugs
  Dopamine receptor antagonists
  Dopamine-depleting agents
Hypothalamic and pituitary stalk lesions
  Craniopharyngioma, surgery, head injury, irradiation
Hypothyroidism
Renal failure
Cirrhosis
Neurologic diseases: seizure, spinal cord injury

- Cardiomegaly. It is part of the generalized organomegaly and in part it is caused by hypertension, which is found in most patients. Congestive heart failure develops over time.
- Musculoskeletal symptoms. Bone overgrowth and weakening of muscle is complicated by degenerative joint disease and widespread pain.
- Neuropathy. Carpal tunnel syndrome and other peripheral nerve compression-related problems are common.

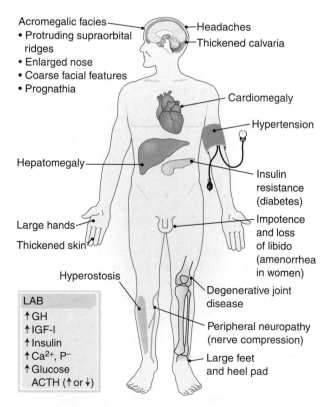

Figure 11-6 Acromegaly. ACTH, adrenocorticotropic hormone; GH, growth hormone; IGF-I, insulin-like growth factor I.

■ Genital and reproductive problems. Loss of libido and erectile dysfunction are common in males, as is oligomenorrhea in women.

■ Metabolic changes. Typically, glucose tolerance is abnormal or mild diabetes occurs. Hyperlipidemia is usually present. Hyperphosphatemia and hypercalciuria develop because of the mobilization of minerals from the bones.

The diagnosis is confirmed by measuring **GH in the blood.** Secretion of GH is pulsatile, and thus single measurements are not informative. Instead, it is recommended to give glucose by mouth and measure GH 1 hour thereafter. In normal persons glucose suppresses GH to 2 μg/L or less, but in patients with somatotropic adenomas GH levels are not suppressed and actually may paradoxically rise. Instead of GH **somatomedin C** (IGF-1) can be measured. Note that somatomedin C is a very good test for somatotropic hormones, but it must be adjusted for the age and sex of the patient. It may be abnormally low in patients who have chronic liver or kidney disease.

Tumors also may compress local structures. Compression of the optic chiasms results in **bitemporal hemianopsia.**

Hypopituitarism may be caused by many diseases affecting the anterior lobe of the pituitary, the pituitary stalk, or the hypothalamus.

Pituitary insufficiency is an uncommon condition that may manifest as panhypopituitarism or a deficiency of a single pituitary hormone or hypothalamic-releasing hormone. The latter group includes mostly genetic disorders.

A mnemonic for memorizing the causes of pituitary insufficiency is that all begin with a letter I (Table 11-6).

Clinical signs and symptoms of pituitary insufficiency do not become apparent until at least 75% of the pituitary is destroyed. The most common causes are tumors, such as

Table 11-6 Causes of Hypopituitarism

Invasive tumor (e.g., brain tumor of hypothalamus, craniopharyngioma, pituitary adenoma, meningioma, chordomas, metastases)
Iatrogenic (e.g., surgery, radiation therapy, hormonal therapy)
Infarction (e.g., Sheehan's postpartum syndrome, sickle cell anemia)
Injury (e.g., head trauma)
Infection (e.g., tuberculosis)
Immune disease (e.g., lymphocytic hypophysitis, sarcoidosis)
Inherited (e.g., isolated genetic pituitary hormone deficiencies, hormone receptor deficiencies)
Idiopathic

Data from Meszaros G: Endocrine and Reproductive Systems, Elsevier, 2006.

craniopharyngioma (in children), brain or meningeal tumors at the base of the brain, and nonfunctioning pituitary tumors. Pituitary ischemia and injury of the hypothalamus during surgery or head trauma are another important group of pituitary lesions. Sheehan's syndrome caused by hemorrhagic infarction of an enlarged pituitary is an important cause of pituitary insufficiency in underdeveloped countries.

Panhypopituitarism presents with signs of deficiency of all pituitary hormones. Growth hormone **(GH)** deficiency predisposes to hypoglycemia. Thyroid-stimulating hormone **(TSH)** deficiency causes hypothyroidism. Adrenocorticotropic hormone **(ACTH)** deficiency leads to adrenocortical insufficiency and a tendency to hypoglycemia. **Gonadotropin** deficiency leads to a loss of libido, amenorrhea, and infertility. **Prolactin** deficiency leads to cessation of lactation and typical features of Sheehan's syndrome.

Pituitary deficiency in childhood and adolescence leads to **pituitary dwarfism.** A deficiency of gonadotropins causes **delayed puberty.**

Panhypopituitarism presents with decreased secretion of pituitary, thyroid, adrenocortical, and sex hormones. The diagnosis of panhypopituitarism thus requires extensive testing for pituitary hormones as well as hormones from other endocrine glands. These findings must be subsequently confirmed by *stimulatory tests.* For example, GH secretion can be monitored after stimulation with insulin, or levodopa or L-arginine. Growth hormone and cortisol secretion can be assessed by glucagon injection.

Diabetes insipidus is caused by a deficiency of antidiuretic hormone released from the posterior lobe of the pituitary.

The posterior pituitary consists of nerve endings (i.e., axons of nerve cells) located in the hypothalamic nuclei–supraoptic nucleus and paraventricular nucleus. As such, the posterior pituitary serves as a storage site for hormones produced in the hypothalamic nuclei, most notably antidiuretic hormone (ADH) and oxytocin.

Antidiuretic hormone, also known as arginine vasopressin (AVP), is a nonapeptide synthesized by nerve cells and stored in the posterior lobe of the pituitary. It promotes the reabsorption of water in the collecting ducts of the kidneys (antidiuretic effect) and is a potent vasoconstrictor (vasopressin effect). It is released normally in response to increased osmolality of the plasma, which stimulates the osmoreceptors in the anterior hypothalamus (Fig. 11-7). Blood volume loss is yet another mechanism that leads to a release of ADH. This mechanism is initiated by low-pressure baroreceptors in the heart. Arterial hypotension, hypercapnia, hypoxia, pain, and nausea may all increase ADH release, causing vasoconstriction and antidiuresis.

Diabetes insipidus is a condition characterized by polyuria—excessive water loss through the kidneys. Two forms of diabetes insipidus are recognized (Fig. 11-8):

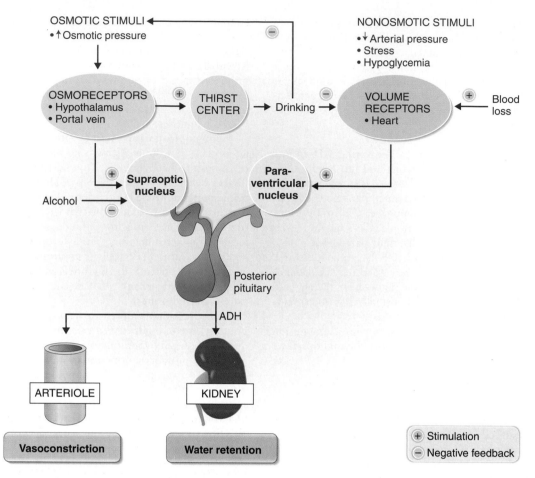

Figure 11-7 Two major antidiuretic hormone/vasopressin control loops. ADH, antidiuretic hormone.

- **Central diabetes insipidus.** The inability to concentrate urine is related to a deficiency of ADH. It is a rare disease usually caused by destruction of hypothalamic nuclei, pituitary stalk, or neurohypophysis by tumors, trauma, or surgery (e.g., hypophysectomy for anterior pituitary tumors, brain tumors).
- **Nephrogenic diabetes insipidus.** The inability to concentrate urine lies with the kidneys and can be caused by chronic renal disease, genetic inability of the kidneys to respond to ADH (e.g., ADH receptor deficiency), or drugs such as lithium.

Diabetes insipidus is characterized by **polyuria,** which may be in the range of 5 to 15 L/day. The urine is hypo-osmotic: typically the osmolality of urine is less than that of serum (<290 mOsm/kg; specific gravity < 1.010). A loss of water results in mild hypernatremia and increased serum osmolality, usually in the range of 290 to 295 mOsm/kg. Loss of water causes **polydipsia,** and thus the osmolality of the plasma returns to the normal range. If access to water is restricted, hypernatremia and increased plasma osmolality may develop. Increased sodium concentration in the serum may cause muscle weakness, prostration, fever, and coma.

Diabetes insipidus is a relatively rare condition, which must be distinguished from polyuria in diabetes mellitus and psychogenic polydipsia/polyuria.

- **Diabetic polyuria** is characterized by hyperosmotic urine (>300 mOsm/kg). Hyperglycemia and glucosuria are readily demonstrable.
- **Psychogenic polydipsia/polyuria,** a psychiatric compulsive disorder characterized by excessive water intake, resembles diabetes insipidus in that the urine is excreted in large quantities and is hypotonic. Serum osmolality is, however, normal to low, and the concentration of ADH in serum is normal.

The diagnosis of diabetes insipidus may be confirmed by the **water deprivation test** and/or injection of an analogue of ADH **(desmopressin test).** In patients with

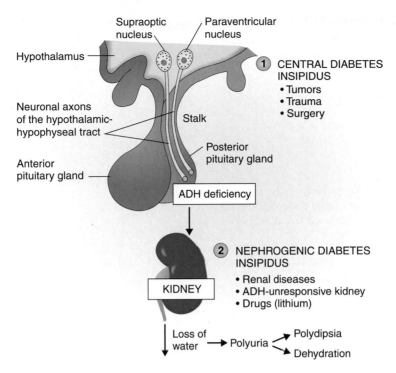

Figure 11-8 Diabetes insipidus. It may be central (1) or nephrogenic (2). ADH, antidiuretic hormone.

central diabetes insipidus water deprivation increases serum osmolality and raises the concentration of sodium, but does not increase the osmolality of the urine. Desmopressin injection increases urine osmolality over 50% from the baseline. In psychogenic polydipsia, water deprivation does not change serum osmolality and does not raise the serum sodium concentration, but the frequency of urination and the volume of urine increase, indicating that the kidney can concentrate urine. Desmopressin injection has no effect or only mildly increases serum osmolality (20–40% over the baseline).

Syndrome of inappropriate antidiuretic hormone secretion is characterized by water retention.

The syndrome of inappropriate ADH secretion (SIADH) is characterized by an excess of ADH in spite of low plasma osmolality. The syndrome of inappropriate ADH secretion may result from:

- Aberrant synthesis of ADH in malignant tumors (paraneoplastic syndrome)
- Synthesis of ADH by non-neoplastic lung tissue in chronic lung disorders
- Excessive release of ADH from the hypothalamus in brain disorders

The main causes of SIADH are listed in Table 11-7.

An excess of ADH results in retention of water and expansion of plasma volume. Serum osmolality is low (<270 mOsm/kg), sodium concentration is low (<130 mmol/L), and the urine is hypertonic (>300 mOsm/kg) compared with serum. Urine contains increased amounts of sodium in excess of 20 mmol/L.

Most patients with SIADH have no clinical symptoms, and typically there is no peripheral edema or any evidence of dehydration. In severe hyponatremia weakness, mental confusion, and lethargy begin to appear, and convulsions and coma may be encountered when the serum sodium concentration drops below 110 mmol/L.

Table 11-7 Important Causes of Syndrome of Inappropriate ADH Secretion (SIADH)

Tumors
  Carcinoma of the lung, pancreas; lymphoma; Ewing's sarcoma
Lung disease
  Chronic obstructive pulmonary disease, pneumonia, tuberculosis
Brain diseases
  Encephalitis, meningitis, brain abscess, brain tumors, subdural or subarachnoid hemorrhage, Guillain-Barré syndrome
Drugs
  Antidepressants, diuretics, cytotoxic drugs, narcotics

ADH, antidiuretic hormone.

> **Pearl**
>
> > The syndrome of inappropriate ADH secretion should be suspected in patients who have hypo-natremia and hyperosmolal urine even if they do not have any clinical symptoms.

THYROID DISEASES

The thyroid is an endocrine gland located on the anterior side of neck. It is composed of two lobes connected by an isthmus. The thyroid is mostly composed of hormone-se-creting cells, which are of two kinds:

- Follicular epithelial cells secreting tyrosine-derived thyroid hormones and thyroglobulin
- C cells secreting calcitonin, a polypeptide hormone involved in the metabolism of calcium

The secretion of thyroid hormones is under the control of the pituitary thyroid-stimulating hormone (TSH, or thyrotropin), which in turn is controlled by the hypothalamus secreting the thyrotropin-releasing hormone (TRH) (Fig. 11-9). Thyroid hormones provide a negative feedback inhibition to the hypothalamus and pituitary, inhibiting the secretion of TRH and TSH.

Follicular cells of the thyroid take up iodine and synthesize thyroid hormones from tyrosine.

Follicular epithelial cells synthesize thyroglobulin and se-crete it into the lumen of the follicles as colloid (Fig. 11-10). The synthesis of thyroid hormones requires iodine, which is taken up by the follicular cells from the interstitial fluid ("iodine trapping"). Iodine is transported to the colloidal surface by a transport protein and "organified," or attached to thyrosine to form monoiodotyrosine and diiodotyrosine. Coupling of these iodinated tyrosine derivatives leads to the formation of triiodotyronine (T_3) and tetraiodothyronine (thyroxine, T_4). Thyroglobulin is then endocytosed into the cytoplasm of follicular cells and cleaved by proteolysis, ulti-mately resulting in the formation of free T_4. This process also leads to removal of iodine from monoiodothyronene and diiodothyronine molecules. T_4 is converted in part to T_3 by 5′-monodeiodinase, and both T_3 and T_4 are secreted into the circulation. Thyroxine predominates and accounts for the bulk of thyroid hormone secretion. Thus, only 15% of the total T_3 is secreted in that form from the thyroid, whereas 85% of T_3 is produced from circulating T_4 in the periphery. Thyroxine can also be converted into a metaboli-cally inactive form, reverse T_3 (rT_3). Serum levels of rT_3 are typically elevated in acute nonthyroidal disease, reflecting a decreased concentration of T_3.

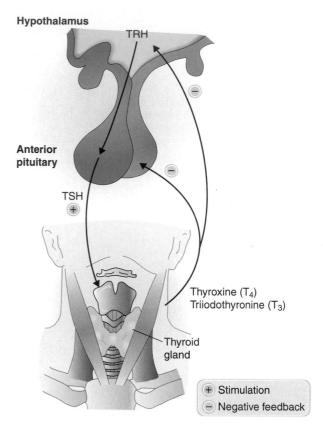

Figure 11-9 Thyroid gland. It is located on the neck and composed of two lobes interconnected with an isthmus. The thyroid hormone secretion is under the control of the hypothalamus and pituitary. A feedback mechanism pro-vided by thyroid hormones T_3 and T_4 inhibits thyrotropin-releasing hormone (TRH) and thyroid-stimulating hormone (TSH) secretion and prevents overstimulation.

Thyroid hormones circulate in the blood bound to carriers or in a free form.

The half-life of T_4 in the circulation is 1 week and that for T_3 is 18 hours. In the circulation thyroid hormones circu-late predominantly (99%) bound to carrier proteins. Ap-proximately 70% of T_4 and T_3 is bound to **thyroxin-binding globulin (TBG),** 10% to 15% is bound to **transthyretin,** 15% to 20% is bound to **albumin,** and 2% to lipoproteins.

Thyroxin-binding globulin serves as the primary reser-voir of thyroid hormones, ensuring a constant supply of hormones even if the thyroid is damaged. For example, even if the thyroid is removed surgically the TBG reservoir provides enough T_4 and T_3 to maintain the metabolic needs for at least a week. At the same time TBG prevents the loss of low-molecular-weight thyroid hormones in the urine. Transthyretin and albumin are more efficient in delivering thyroid hormones to the cells; transthyretin is especially

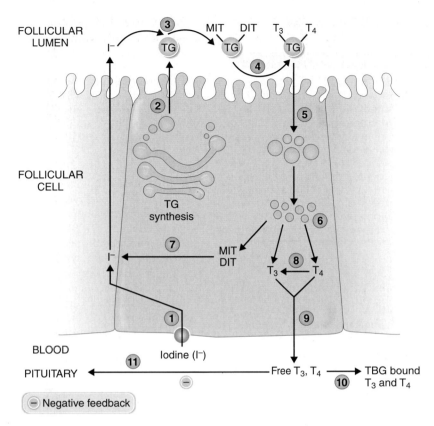

Figure 11-10 Structure and function of the thyroid follicular cell. 1, Follicular epithelial cells synthesize thyroglobulin (TG) and secrete it into the lumen of the follicles as colloid. 2, The synthesis of thyroid hormones requires iodine, which is taken up by the follicular cells from the interstitial fluid ("iodine trapping"). 3, Iodine is transported to the colloidal surface by a transport protein and "organified," that is, attached to thyrosine to form monoiodothyrosine (MIT) and diiodothyrosine (DIT). 4, Coupling of these iodinated thyrosine derivatives leads to the formation of triiodothyronine (T_3) and tetraiodothyronine (thyroxine, T_4). 5–6, Thyroglobulin is then endocytosed into the cytoplasm of follicular cells and cleaved by proteolysis, ultimately resulting in the formation of free T_4. This process also leads to removal of iodine from monoiodothyronine and diiodothyronine molecules. 7, Iodine is recirculated. 8 and 9, Thyroxine is converted in part to T_3 by 5'-monodeiodinase, and both T_3 and T_4 are secreted into the circulation 10, In the circulation thyroid hormones circulate in a free form or bound to a transport protein, thyroid-binding globulin (TBG). 11, Free T_4 and T_3 provide a negative feedback to the pituitary and hypothalamus. T_4 can be converted into a metabolically inactive form, reverse T_3. (Modified from Boon NA, Colledge NR, Walker BR, Hunter JAA [eds]: Davidson's Principles and Practice of Medicine, 20th ed. Edinburgh, Churchill Livingstone, 2006, p. 745.)

important for the delivery of T_4 and T_3 to the nervous system during development.

Free T_4 and T_3 account for only 1% of the total amount of thyroid hormone in the blood. Nevertheless, this is a very important fraction, since it represents the active form of both T_4 and T_3. Free T_4 and T_3 also provide a negative feedback to the pituitary and hypothalamus.

Thyroid hormones act on many peripheral tissues.

These hormones enter the cell cytoplasm by diffusion, whereupon all T_4 is transformed into T_3, a more active form of the hormone. T_3 binds to a cytoplasmic receptor and is transferred to the nucleus where it interacts with

the hormone reactive part of the gene. Thyroid hormones stimulate many metabolic functions of the body, increasing the metabolic rate. The most important effects on various organs are listed in Table 11-8.

Thyroid diseases may manifest clinically as thyroid enlargement, hyperthyroidism, or hypothyroidism.

Thyroid diseases belong to the most common endocrine disorders, affecting an estimated 5% to 7% of the population. Thyroid enlargement is found in 5% of all adults, hypothyroidism is found in women at a rate of 1:100 adults. Congenital hypothyroidism is found in 1 of 4000 infants. Approximately 2% to 3% of all adults have benign thyroid tumors.

Table 11-8 The Physiologic Effects of Thyroid Hormones

TISSUE	EFFECT
Heart	Tachycardia
Fat tissue	Lipolysis
Muscle	Proteolysis
Bone	Promote growth from infancy to adolescence
	Accelerated bone turnover
Nervous system	Essential for brain development and maturation in infancy and childhood
Intestine	Increased carbohydrate absorption
	Increased intestinal peristalsis

Thyroid diseases may manifest in three forms:

- **Thyroid enlargement.** In most instances this is caused by bilateral or unilateral nodular hyperplasia (goiter), but it may be also be due to diffuse hyperplasia of Graves' disease. Benign and malignant thyroid tumors may cause local or diffuse enlargement.
- **Hyperthyroidism.** Most often hyperfunction of the thyroid is caused by Graves' disease (75%), nodular goiter (15%), or solitary hyperfunctioning adenoma (5%). Other causes, such as thyroiditis and iodine-induced or TSH-induced hyperfunction of the thyroid, are less common.
- **Hypothyroidism.** Autoimmune thyroiditis (Hashimoto's disease) and surgical resection or medical thyroid ablation with radioactive iodine account for 90% of all cases of thyroid insufficiency. Uncommon causes of hypothyroidism include congenital agenesis of the thyroid, secondary pituitary hypothyroidism, iodine deficiency, and various infiltrative processes, such as tumors, sarcoidosis, and amyloidosis.

Thyroid function can best be assessed by clinical laboratory testing.

Routine clinical examination of thyroid function is based on the measurement of T_4, T_3, and TSH. In patients who have hypothyroidism, TSH is elevated and T_3 and T_4 are low. In hyperthyroidism, TSH is low and T_3 and T_4 levels are high.

Pearl

> Testing TSH is the single best method for diagnosing thyroid hyperfunction or hypofunction. This test is almost always combined with the measurement of serum T_4 and T_3.

A more complete work-up for the assessment of thyroid function includes the same basic tests and additional measurements of various fractions of thyroid hormones in blood, as follows:

- **Thyroid-stimulating hormone in serum (TSH).** This test identifies most cases of hypothyroidism or hyperthyroidism, except in the presence of hypothalamic and pituitary injury, or peripheral thyroid hormone resistance (e.g., mutation of thyroid hormone receptor). Certain drugs, such as opioids and glucocorticoids, suppress TSH secretion.
- **Total serum T_4.** These measurements include both free and bound thyroid hormones. Since most T_4 is predominantly bound to TBG, increased or decreased concentration of TBG changes the total T_4. However, the concentration of free T_4 is not altered. Thyroxin-binding globulin synthesis in the liver is increased under the influence of estrogen, and thus TBG levels in the blood are high during pregnancy. Anabolic steroids decrease TBG synthesis.
- **Total serum T_3.** This test is used to confirm T_4 results in hyperthyroidism or hypothyroidism. In over 90% of cases there is concordance between T_4 and T_3, but in 1% to 4% of all patients with hyperthyroidism T_4 is normal, but T_3 is elevated. This condition, called **T_3 thyrotoxicosis,** is especially common in areas with endemic iodine deficiency (e.g., high mountains such as Andes or Himalayas).
- **Free T_4.** This test measures the active form of the thyroid hormones. Free T_4 and T_3 must be measured when the clinical and the initial laboratory findings do not match. For example, in a condition called **euthyroid hyperthyroxemia** the patient is euthyroid but has elevated total T_4 and normal TSH. It is encountered in many chronic diseases (e.g., cirrhosis of the liver) and may be caused by drugs. In this condition free T_4 is normal, better reflecting the clinical status of the patient than total T_4. Total T_3 drops precipitously in many severe **acute nonthyroidal diseases.** Total T_4 drops also, but the free T_4 is within normal limits or even slightly elevated. Thyroid-stimulating hormone levels drop but rise later on (Fig. 11-11).
- **Thyroxin-binding globulin (TBG).** This test is performed when the clinical data are not fully accounted for by the measurements of TSH, T_4, and T_3. Since TBG serves as the main serum-binding protein for T_4 its concentration influences the total T_4 measurements but does not affect the free T_4. The concentration of T_3 is altered less, because T_3 is less protein-bound. Thyroxin-binding globulin concentration may be reduced in liver failure or as a result of malnutrition or nephrotic syndrome. Androgens also reduce TBG concentration in serum. Estrogens have the opposite effect, and TBG levels in serum rise during pregnancy. Acute liver disease is also associated with elevation of TBG. Drugs may increase or decrease TBG concentration in the blood.

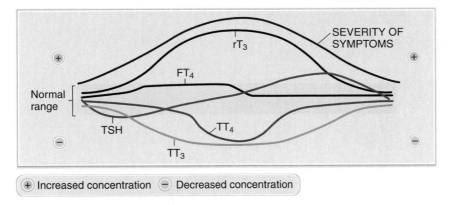

Figure 11-11 Changes in the concentration of thyroid hormones in serum during severe acute nonthyroidal disease. FT_4, free thyroxine; rT_3, reverse T_3; TSH, thyroid-stimulating hormone; TT_3, total triiodothyronine; TT_4, total thyroxine. (Modified from McPherson RA., Pincus MR: Henry's Clinical Diagnosis and Management by Laboratory Methods, 21st ed. Philadelphia, Elsevier, 2006, p. 338.)

- **Thyroglobulin.** This product of thyroid follicular cells is normally stored in the follicles, and only small amounts reach the blood. Thyroglobulin is elevated in many forms of thyroid injury, but the value of this information is limited, and this test is not routinely performed. Its main value lies in the detection of residual tumors, which secrete thyroglobulin into the blood.
- **Urine iodine.** Iodine is excreted from the body in the urine, and the urinary concentration reflects iodine stores. Remember that more than 2 billion people worldwide have iodine-deficient diets, and that iodine deficiency is an important cause of goiter.
- **Thyroid autoantibodies.** Several thyroid autoantibodies are used in clinical practice, but the most important are the **antibodies to thyroperoxidase (TPO).** Anti-TPO antibodies are found in more than 90% of patients with Hashimoto's thyroiditis and hypothyroidism and are useful for diagnosing this autoimmune disease. However, anti-TPO antibodies are also present in up to 40% of patients with nodular goiter, and up to 25% of normal adults have anti-TPO antibodies, limiting the diagnostic value of this test. **Antibodies to the TSH receptor** are found in 90% of patients with Graves' disease and are highly specific for that disease.
- **Radioactive iodine uptake.** Scintigraphy with iodine-131 is useful for demonstrating thyroid hyperfunction. In Graves' disease uptake is diffuse, whereas in toxic adenoma the uptake is localized to "hot nodules." Nonfunctioning thyroid tumors manifest as "cold nodules."

Pearl

> The thyroglobulin test may be useful for detecting drug-induced hyperthryroidism ("hyperthyroidismus medicamentosa"). In these patients the serum thyroglobulin is within normal limits, in contrast to high levels of T_4 and T_3.

Hyperthyroidism is characterized by an increased metabolic rate and acceleration of many physiologic functions.

Hyperthyroidism is a common disease occurring in adults at a rate of 1:50 in women and 1:250 in men. In 75% of all cases, hyperthyroidism is caused by Graves' disease, which manifests with the following clinical features (Fig. 11-12):

- **Signs of hypermetabolism.** Increased metabolic rate results in fatigue, heat intolerance, and excessive sweating. Weight loss occurs despite increased appetite. Palmar erythema is common.
- **Cardiovascular changes.** These include tachycardia, palpitations, systolic hypertension, angina, and atrial fibrillation. Cardiac failure develops at an increased rate.
- **Digestive system changes.** Symptoms include occasional vomiting and changes in bowel habits.
- **Neuromuscular system changes.** The patients show signs of anxiety, increased irritability, and emotional instability. Muscle weakness, tremor, hyper-reflexia, and occasionally even paralysis occur.
- **Reproductive system changes.** Women may experience changes of the menstrual cycle, which may include oligomenorrhea or amenorrhea. Infertility spontaneous abortions are encountered at an increased rate. Men experience a loss of libido and impotence.
- **Eye changes.** Exophthalmos with retraction of the lid and a lid lag are demonstrable during eye movement. Lacrimation is excessive, and the incidence of corneal ulceration is increased. These external changes may be associated with visual problems and even papilledema.
- **Skin changes.** The skin is moist, and profound itching may occur. Loss of hair (alopecia), focal skin depigmentation (vitiligo), and pretibial myxedema are probably related to autoimmune disturbances and are useful signs of Graves' disease.

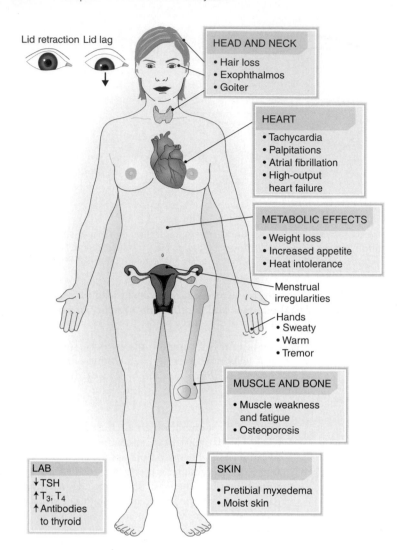

Lid retraction Lid lag

HEAD AND NECK
• Hair loss
• Exophthalmos
• Goiter

HEART
• Tachycardia
• Palpitations
• Atrial fibrillation
• High-output
  heart failure

METABOLIC EFFECTS
• Weight loss
• Increased appetite
• Heat intolerance

Menstrual
irregularities

Hands
• Sweaty
• Warm
• Tremor

MUSCLE AND BONE
• Muscle weakness
  and fatigue
• Osteoporosis

LAB
↓TSH
↑T_3, T_4
↑Antibodies
  to thyroid

SKIN
• Pretibial myxedema
• Moist skin

Figure 11-12 Hyperthyroidism due to Graves' disease. T_3, triiodothyronine; T_4, tetraiodothyronine (thyroxine); TSH, thyroid-stimulating hormone.

Pearl

> Thyroid storm is a life-threatening complication of hyperthyroidism, most often precipitated by infection. It manifests with fever, agitation, confusion, and irregular heartbeats (tachycardia, atrial fibrillation) leading to heart failure (especially in older patients).

Clinical features of hypothyroidism vary and depend on the duration and severity of the hormone deficiency.

Hypothyroidism is a common disease affecting 1:100 adults, but occurring six times more often in females than males. It is most often caused by autoimmune lymphocytic thyroiditis (Hashimoto's disease) or iatrogenic interventions (e.g., surgery or radioactive iodine treatment).

Deficiency of thyroid hormones in general slows down the metabolism, but the clinical presentation depends on the duration and severity of hormone deficiency. An accumulation of mucopolysaccharides, such as hyaluronic acid and chondroitin sulfate, in tissue causes many findings. Most typical is the myxedema of the hands, feet, and face, which is often accompanied by a typical periorbital puffiness. The speech is slurred due to enlargement of the tongue and swollen lips. Changes in the vocal cords lead to hoarseness, whereas changes in the ear cause poor hearing. The most common findings in hypothyroidism listed by organ systems are illustrated in Figure 11-13, and are as follows:

■ **Signs of hypometabolism.** Reduced metabolic rate results in weight gain, somnolence, cold intolerance, and fatigue.
■ **Cardiovascular changes.** These include bradycardia, pericardial and pleural effusion, and hypertension.

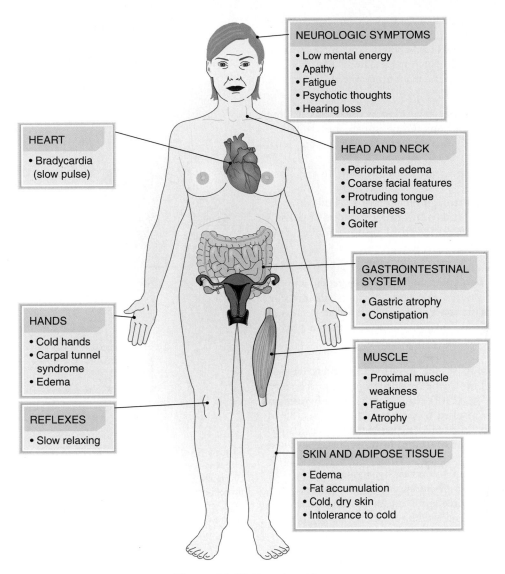

NEUROLOGIC SYMPTOMS
- Low mental energy
- Apathy
- Fatigue
- Psychotic thoughts
- Hearing loss

HEART
- Bradycardia (slow pulse)

HEAD AND NECK
- Periorbital edema
- Coarse facial features
- Protruding tongue
- Hoarseness
- Goiter

GASTROINTESTINAL SYSTEM
- Gastric atrophy
- Constipation

HANDS
- Cold hands
- Carpal tunnel syndrome
- Edema

MUSCLE
- Proximal muscle weakness
- Fatigue
- Atrophy

REFLEXES
- Slow relaxing

SKIN AND ADIPOSE TISSUE
- Edema
- Fat accumulation
- Cold, dry skin
- Intolerance to cold

Figure 11-13 Hypothyroidism.

- **Digestive system changes.** Symptoms include constipation and increased incidence of ileus due to sluggish peristalsis.
- **Neuromuscular system changes.** The patients show signs of depression and may even develop major mental disturbances ("myxedema madness"). Deafness is another common problem. Aches and pains due to muscle stiffness or peripheral nerve compression syndromes (e.g., carpal tunnel syndrome) are common features. There is delayed relaxation of tendon reflexes.
- **Reproductive system changes.** Women may experience menorrhagia and infertility. In men the symptoms are less prominent and mostly include a loss of libido.

- **Skin changes.** The skin looks puffy, especially on the face, hands, and feet (myxedema). Yellow discoloration of the skin is due to hypercarotenemia. Loss of lateral eyebrows it characteristic.

PARATHYROID DISEASES

The parathyroid glands are located on the posterior side of the thyroid. Most people have four parathyroids, which are all of approximately the same size, measuring 2 to 3 mm in the longer diameter.

Parathyroid chief cells secrete parathyroid hormone (PTH), a single-chain polypeptide that is important for the regulation of calcium homeostasis. A rise in serum calcium concentration inhibits the synthesis of PTH, but the synthesis is reactivated as soon as the concentration of serum calcium drops.

Parathyroid hormone is closely linked with the metabolism of vitamin D with which it regulates the metabolism of calcium (Fig. 11-14). The main functions of PTH can be summarized as follows:

- Stimulation of bone resorption by osteoclasts, leading to a release of calcium and phosphate into the blood
- Stimulation of calcium reabsorption in the renal tubules
- Inhibition of phosphate reabsorption in the renal tubules
- Stimulation of renal production of 1,25 dihydroxyvitamin D_3 (1,25$(OH)_2D_3$), the active form of vitamin D, which promotes intestinal absorption of calcium and phosphorus

As a result of these direct and indirect effects of PTH on calcium absorption, metabolism, and excretion, and the excretion of phosphorus, the blood calcium concentration increases, whereas the concentration of phosphate decreases.

Parathyroid diseases may manifest as hyperfunction or hypofunction of the parathyroid glands.

- **Hyperfunction of the parathyroid glands.** Hyperparathyroidism may be classified as primary, secondary, or tertiary (Fig. 11-15). **Primary hyperparathyroidism** is most often caused by parathyroid adenomas (85%) and less often by primary hyperplasia of all four glands. **Secondary hyperparathyroidism** is most often caused by chronic renal disease. **Tertiary hyperparathyroidism** evolves from secondary hyperparathyroidism. In this complication of chronic renal failure the parathyroid glands become autonomous and unresponsive to normal physiologic stimuli.

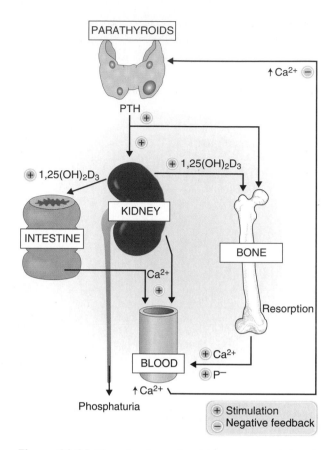

Figure 11-14 The role of parathyroid hormone and vitamin D in the metabolism of calcium. 1,25$(OH)_2D_3$, 1,25 dihydroxyvitamin D_3; P^-, phosphate; PTH, parathyroid hormone. (Modified from Boon NA, Colledge NR, Walker BR, Hunter JAA [eds]: Davidson's Principles & Practice of Medicine, 20th ed. Edinburgh, Churchill Livingstone, 2006, p. 772.)

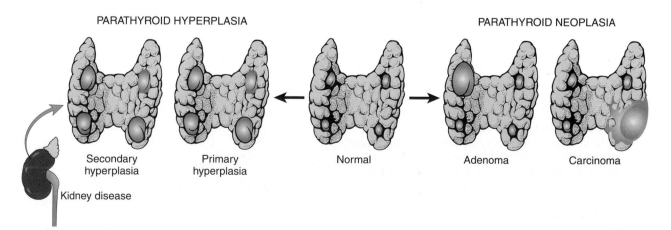

Figure 11-15 Hyperparathyroidism. Hyperfunction of parathyroids can be classified as primary due to tumors (adenoma, carcinoma) or hyperplasia of the parathyroid glands, or secondary, usually due to renal disease. Hypofunction is a consequence of destruction or removal of the parathyroid glands. (From Damjanov I: Pathology for Health Professions, 3rd ed. WB Saunders, St. Louis, 2005, p. 404.)

- **Hypofunction of the parathyroid glands.** Hypoparathyroidism results mostly from destruction or surgical removal of the parathyroid glands.

Laboratory tests are essential for diagnosing parathyroid diseases.

The function of the parathyroid glands can be assessed in most cases by measuring serum calcium and phosphate and PTH concentration. In a complete work-up and in complex cases it is necessary to also measure vitamin D concentration and include markers of bone proliferation, such as alkaline phosphatase. In some patients with tumor-related hypercalcemia it is useful to include in the laboratory panel the measurement of parathyroid-related polypeptide (PTHrP).

The following is a list of the laboratory tests included in a complete parathyroid panel:

- **Calcium.** Serum calcium varies physiologically in a narrow range. Hyperparathyroidism leads to a rise in serum calcium; hyperparathyroidism causes hypocalcemia. Other causes of hypercalcemia and hypocalcemia are discussed in greater detail in Chapter 1.
- **Phosphorus.** Serum levels of phosphorus are primarily regulated by the extent of phosphate reabsorption in the kidneys. Hypoparathyroidism is associated with high serum phosphorus due to increased renal reabsorption. Hyperparathyroidism leads to a decline of serum phosphorus due to an increased renal loss. Other causes of hypophosphatemia and hyperphosphatemia are discussed in greater detail in Chapter 1.
- **Parathyroid hormone.** This hormone is measured in serum primarily for evaluating hypercalcemia and in cases of suspected hyperparathyroidism or hypoparathyroidism. The interpretation of serum PTH levels should be correlated with serum calcium levels as illustrated in Figure 11-16.
- **Alkaline phosphatase.** Serum alkaline phosphatase stems mostly from the liver, but a significant amount of this enzyme may come from growing bones. It is expressed on osteoblasts; hence it is elevated in the serum of children and adolescents during active bone growth. In adults it may be elevated during healing of bone fractures, in Paget's disease, and with osteomalacia due to vitamin D deficiency.
- **Vitamin D.** Precursors of vitamin D derived from food or formed in the skin are hydroxylated in the liver and then again in the kidneys to produce the biologically active form of vitamin D. Both of these vitamin forms (i.e., the one formed in the liver, 25(OH)D [calcidiol], and the one formed in the kidney, 1,25(OH)$_2$D$_3$ [calcitriol]), may be measured in the serum. Parathyroid hormone and phosphate depletion act independently on the kidney to form more calcitriol. Low serum calcium stimulates the production of PTH, which stimulates the hydroxyl-

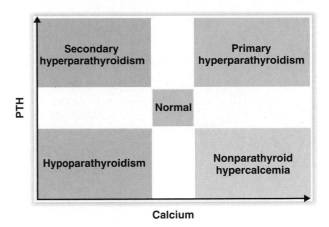

Figure 11-16 Interpretation of serum calcium and parathyroid hormone levels. (Modified from McPherson RA, Pincus MR: Henry's Clinical Diagnosis and Management by Laboratory Methods, 21st ed., Philadelphia, Saunders Elsevier, 2007, p. 179.)

ation of vitamin D in the kidney. Hypercalcemia suppresses PTH, thus reducing the renal hydroxylation of vitamin D. Calcitriol stimulates absorption of calcium and phosphorus in the intestines, reabsorption of calcium in the kidney, and deposition of these minerals in the bones (Fig. 11-17).

- **Parathyroid-related polypeptide (PTHrP).** Although biochemically distinct from PTH this polypeptide hormone binds to the same receptor as PTH. Hence, it has the same effects on calcium and phosphorus homeostasis. Parathyroid-related polypeptide is secreted by many tumors and is found in 50% to 90% of cases of tumor-related hypercalcemia.
- **Calcitonin.** This polypeptide hormone produced by C cells of the thyroid lowers serum calcium and phosphorus levels. Calcitonin counteracts the effects of PTH. It inhibits osteoclasts and stimulates loss of calcium and phosphate in urine. Nevertheless, calcitonin is not measured routinely in the work-up of parathyroid disorders. Currently it is used mostly as a marker of medullary carcinoma of the thyroid, a tumor derived from C cells. Medullary carcinoma is a hallmark of multiple endocrine neoplasia syndrome type 2 (MEN-2), and calcitonin could be used for early diagnosis of these familial cases.

Primary hyperparathyroidism is characterized by hypercalcemia.

Hyperparathyroidism is a relatively common disease affecting up to 1% of the adult population. Its peak incidence is in the third and fourth decade, but it may be found in younger and older patients as well. Some parathyroid adenomas are familial and are found in patients who have MEN-1.

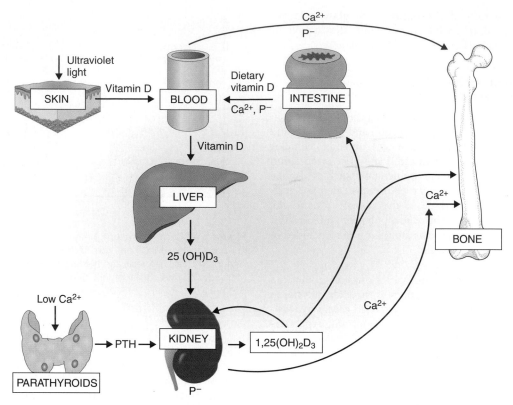

Figure 11-17 The interaction between vitamin D, parathyroid hormone (PTH), and calcium (Ca^{2+}) and phosphorus (P^-). $1,25(OH)_2D_3$, 1,25 dihydroxyvitamin D_3.

Clinical presentation of hyperparathyroidism is highly variable. Up to 80% patients may be asymptomatic or have nonspecific generalized symptoms and are diagnosed accidentally. Symptomatic patients typically demonstrate symptoms pertaining to the kidneys and bones.

The most important clinical features of hyperparathyroidism (Fig. 11-18) are as follows:

- **Bone changes.** Parathyroid hormone has both short-term and long-term effects on the bones. Short term, PTH activates osteoclasts, which degrade bone, and leads to a release of calcium and phosphate into the blood. Long term, PTH promotes proliferation of many bone cells, including osteoclasts, osteoblasts, and fibroblasts, which leads to the typical pathologic changes known under the name of *osteitis fibrosa cystica.* Clinically the bones are painful and are prone to fractures. Typical changes are seen on radiographic examination. Brown tumors of hyperparathyroidism are rare today. These lytic lesions are histologically composed of osteoclasts and resemble giant-cell bone tumors.
- **Renal changes.** Hypercalcemia is associated with polyuria and nocturia. Loss of water leads to polydipsia.

Calciuria also occurs, predisposing to nephrocalcinosis and renal stone formation. The incidence of renal failure is increased.
- **Gastrointestinal changes.** These include nausea, vomiting, and constipation. Peptic ulcers and pancreatitis occur at an increased rate.
- **Neurologic symptoms.** Typically, patients are tired and lethargic and experience muscle weakness. Memory loss, confusion, and coma may be found in advanced cases.
- **Cardiovascular changes.** Electrocardiographic changes and arrhythmia are related to the effects of calcium on the contracting cardiac myocytes. The incidence of arterial hypertension is increased.

Pearl

> The most popular mnemonic for the symptoms of hypercalcemia of hyperparathyroidism states that it manifests with "painful bones, renal stones, abdominal groans, and mental moans."

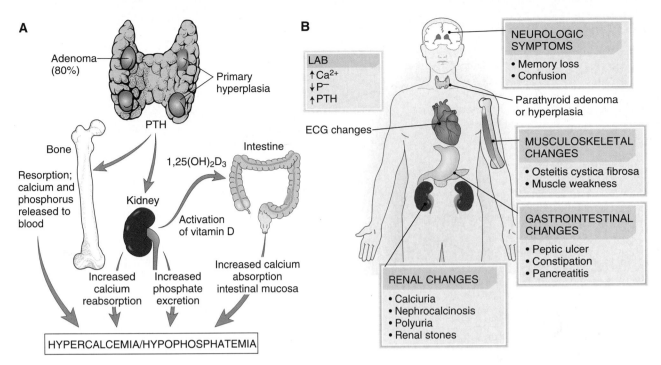

Figure 11-18 Pathogenesis of hypercalcemia (**A**) and the principal clinical signs and symptoms of hyperparathyroidism (**B**). Ca^{2+}, calcium; ECG, electrocardiogram; $1,25(OH)_2D_3$, 1,25 dihydroxyvitamin D_3; P^-, phosphorus; PTH, parathyroid hormone.

Secondary hyperparathyroidism is a consequence of chronic renal failure.

Secondary hyperplasia of the parathyroid glands occurs most often as a complication of **chronic end-stage kidney disease.** The parathyroid glands enlarge in response to **hypocalcemia.** that develops in these patients for several reasons, as illustrated in Figure 11-19. Several factors play a role in the pathogenesis of hyperplasia of parathyroid glands, but the three most salient ones are listed here.

- **Hyperphosphatemia.** Reduced excretion of phosphorus in the urine is caused by a loss of glomeruli and reduced glomerular filtration of phosphorus into the primary filtrate. Since the concentration of phosphorus is inversely related to calcium, a reactive hypocalcemia results.
- **Reduced hydroxylation of vitamin D in the kidneys.** Damaged kidneys cannot properly activate vitamin D to form $1,25(OH)_2D_3$, leading to a virtual vitamin D deficiency. Vitamin D deficiency results in a **decreased intestinal absorption of calcium.** It also leads to **osteomalacia** and inadequate calcification of the organic matrix of bones. Without $1,25(OH)_2D_3$, PTH cannot properly act on the bones either.
- **Renal leak of calcium.** The loss of tubular function prevents reabsorption of calcium, and it is lost in urine.

In the first phase of secondary hyperparathyroidism serum phosphorus is typically very high, whereas calcium is low. Subsequently, when the parathyroid glands enlarge due to hyperplasia, the additional PTH corrects the calcium levels, and thus in later stages of the disease both phosphorus and calcium are elevated. Most of the calcium and phosphorus is derived from the bones, which become demineralized and show the typical pathologic features of **renal osteodystrophy.**

Other less common causes of secondary hyperparathyroidism are listed in Table 11-9. In such cases hypocalcemia is usually less severe, because PTH usually enhances bone resorption in an effort to compensate for the calcium deficiency.

Hypoparathyroidism is a rare condition characterized by hypocalcemia.

Hypothyroidism is much less common than hyperparathyroidism. Most often it results from **accidental surgical removal** of all four glands during neck surgery for thyroid tumors or some other condition. **Autoimmune hypoparathyroidism** is a rare condition, but overall it is still the second most common cause of hypoparathyroidism. It usually occurs as a part of **polyendocrine deficiency syndrome** manifesting as adrenal insufficiency, hypogonadism, atrophic gastritis and pernicious anemia, and autoimmune hepatitis. Such patients also develop mucocutaneous candidiasis.

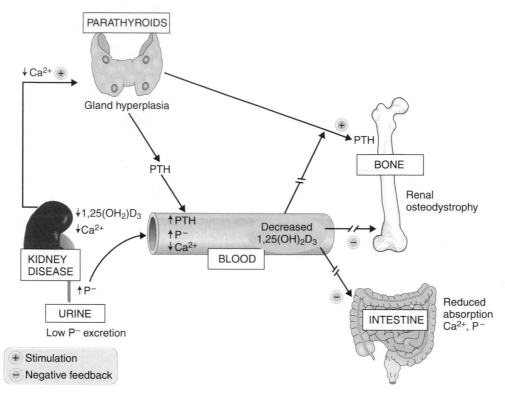

Figure 11-19 Secondary hyperparathyroidism. In the first phase of hyperparathyroidism, renal failure leads to hyperphosphatemia and hypocalcemia, which stimulates parathyroid hormone (PTH) synthesis. Reduced hydroxylation of 25-hydroxyvitamin D leads to a deficiency of active vitamin D [1,25(OH)$_2$D$_3$], which in turn results in osteomalacia and reduces intestinal absorption of calcium and phosphorus. In later stages of the disease hypercalcemia and hyperphosphatemia (not shown) occur, and the bones show typical signs of renal osteodystrophy. P$^-$, phosphate.

The signs of hypoparathyroidism include

- Hypocalcemia
- Hyperphosphatemia
- Reduced PTH in serum
- Neurologic signs of hypocalcemia—paresthesia and tingling of fingers and toes, Chvostek's sign, muscle cramps, and generalized tetany

Table 11-9 Causes of Secondary Hyperparathyroidism

Chronic renal failure
Vitamin D deficiency
    Lack of sun exposure (e.g., rickets in children)
    Dietary deficiency (e.g., elderly and poor, malnourished persons)
    Drug-induced increased metabolism of vitamin D (e.g., rifampicin, anticonvulsants)
Reduced calcium intake or absorption
    Dietary calcium deficiency
    Postgastrectomy states
    Small-bowel resection
    Crohn's disease

- Cardiovascular effects of hypocalcemia—ECG changes such as prolonged QT interval and arrhythmias

DISEASES OF THE ADRENAL CORTEX

The adrenal cortex forms the outer part of adrenal glands, which are located above the kidneys in the retroperitoneal spaces (Fig. 11-20). The cortex consists of three layers:

- **Zona glomerulosa.** The outer layer of the cortex produces mineralocorticoids.
- **Zona fasciculata.** The middle zone produces glucocorticoids.
- **Zona reticularis.** The inner zone produces androgens and a very small amount of estrogens.

The zona fasciculata and zona reticularis are under the control of the pituitary ACTH, which has only a minor effect on the zona glomerulosa. The secretion of mineralocorticoids in the zona glomerulosa is mostly regulated by the renin–angiotensinogen–angiotensin system.

Steroid hormones produced by the adrenal cortex have several important functions, as follows:

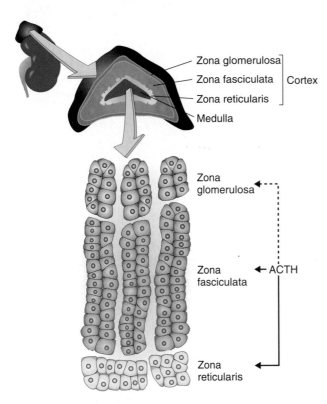

Figure 11-20 Adrenal glands. Each gland consists of cortex and medulla. The cortex has three layers: zona glomerulosa, zona fasciculata, and zona reticularis.

- **Aldosterone.** This mineralocorticoid acts on distal tubules and collecting ducts to promote uptake of Na^+ in exchange for K^+ or H^+.
- **Cortisol.** This glucocorticoid has anti-insulin activity, decreasing glucose uptake in muscle and adipose tissue. It enhances the effects of glucagons and epinephrine, favoring glycogenolysis and lipolysis. It also has anti-inflammatory effects and inhibits ADH.
- **Androgens.** The adrenal zona reticularis secretes androstenedione, dehydroepiandrostenedione (DHEA), and dehydroepiandrostenedione sulfate (DHEAS). They are much weaker androgens than testosterone. In peripheral tissues 17-ketosteroid reductase can convert androstenedione to testosterone and thus increase its androgenic effects.

The synthesis of steroid hormones is a multistep process involving several hydroxylases (Fig. 11-21). Once the hormones are synthesized they are secreted into the blood bound to transport proteins. Cortisol is transported bound to **corticoid-binding protein (CBG,** or **transcortin),** a plasma protein produced by the liver. Most of cortisol is bound to CBG, and only 10% is found in the free form. The synthesis of CBG is increased by estrogen and thus its concentration in plasma is high during pregnancy. Approximately 25% of

aldosterone is also bound to CBG, but 40% of it is bound to albumin, and 35% is in a free form in plasma. Androgens released from the zona reticularis circulate mostly bound to albumin.

Degradation products of steroid hormones are excreted in the urine. Cortisol is excreted as **17-hydroxycorticoids.** Androgens are excreted in the urine as **17-ketosteroids.** These steroid metabolites can be measured in the urine and are important for the evaluation of adrenal diseases.

Adrenal cortical diseases manifest as hyperfunction or hypofunction of cortical cells.

Hypersecretion of corticosteroids may result from

- Hyperplasia of adrenal cortical cells
- Benign tumors (adenomas)
- Malignant tumors (carcinomas)

Hyperplasia may involve all three zones of the cortex, but quite often it manifests with hypersecretion of hormones characteristic for a particular zone of the normal adrenal cortex. Hyperplasia may be primary and of unknown origin, or secondary due to stimulation by ACTH.

Benign adrenal cortical tumors are typically monoclonal and are thus composed of cells corresponding to those found in one of the three zone of the normal adrenal cortex. As such, these tumors secrete hormones that are typical for the zone from which they have arisen.

Malignant tumors synthesize hormones in a more unpredictable manner. Hormones found in the blood of such patients often do not allow one to conclude from which zone of the cortex the tumor arose. Some tumors secrete mineralocorticoids, glucocorticoids, and androgens at the same time.

Adrenal cortical hyperfunction may manifest clinically in the form of three distinct syndromes:

- **Hyperaldosteronism.** This disease is characterized by an excess of aldosterone, a mineralocorticoid that leads to hypertension and hypokalemia.
- **Cushing's syndrome** (hypercortisolism). This syndrome is characterized by an excess of glucocorticoids leading to disturbances of the intermediary metabolism of carbohydrates, lipids, and proteins.
- **Adrenogenital syndrome.** It is characterized by an excess of androgenic hormones.

Adrenal cortical hypofunction results from the destruction of the adrenal cortex. It manifests as **Addison's disease,** a chronic wasting disease characterized by a deficiency of all steroid hormones produced by the adrenal cortex.

Hyperaldosteronism is characterized by hypertension and hypokalemia.

Hyperaldosteronism is characterized by hypersecretion of the mineralocorticoid aldosterone. Two forms of hyperaldosteronism are recognized:

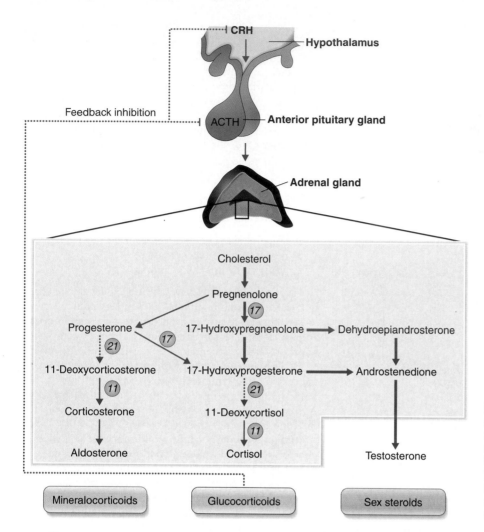

Figure 11-21 Steroidogenesis. ACTH, adrenocorticotropic hormone; CRH, corticotropin-releasing hormone. (Modified from Kumar V, Abbas AK, Fausto N [eds]: Robbins and Cotran Pathologic Basis of Disease, 7th ed. Philadelphia, Elsevier Saunders, 2005, p. 1213.)

■ **Primary hyperaldosteronism (Conn's syndrome).** This form of hyperaldosteronism is most often caused by cortical adenomas (75%). It most often affects women between the ages of 30 and 50 years. **Idiopathic hyperaldosteronism** is used for the form of the disease in which no adrenal tumors are found. This disease of unknown origin is associated with micronodular hyperplasia of the cortex, but in some cases the glands may even be of normal size.

■ **Secondary hyperaldosteronism.** This complication of chronic renal disease is caused by overstimulation of the zona glomerulosa by angiotensin II formed from angiotensinogen under the influence of renin (Fig. 11-22).

In both primary and secondary forms of hyperaldosteronism aldosterone occurs in excess. In primary hyperaldosteronism excess of aldosterone suppresses the secretion of renin (**hyporeninemic hyperaldosteronism**). In secondary hyperaldosteronism both the renin and aldosterone levels are high (**hyper-reninemic hyperaldosteronism**).

An excess of aldosterone leads to increased renal reabsorption of sodium, increased sodium concentration in the blood, and an expansion of extracellular fluid causing arterial hypertension (Fig. 11-23). Aldosterone itself acts on smooth muscle cells or arterioles causing vasoconstriction, which contributes to hypertension. In secondary hyperaldosteronism angiotensin II acts on arterioles causing their constriction, which also promotes hypertension.

The **clinical features** of primary hyperaldosteronism result from the effects of aldosterone on homeostasis of sodium and potassium as follows:

■ **Hypertension.** Arterial hypertension is the most important clinical finding. It is associated with hypernatremia and hypokalemia. Headaches are common, and hypertensive retinopathy is seen in long-standing disease. In approximately 50% of patients hypertension persists even after the removal of the aldosteronoma, suggesting that the vascular changes persist and might be irreversible.

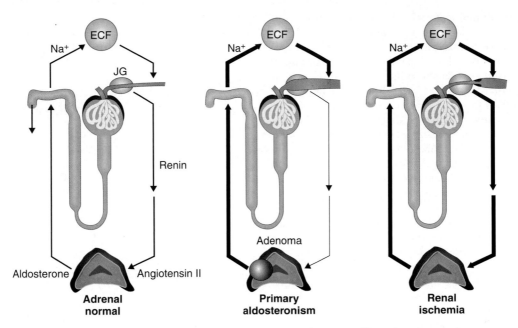

Figure 11-22 Hyperaldosteronism. Primary hyperaldosteronism is most often caused by adrenal cortical tumors, and secondary hyperaldosteronism is a consequence of excessive renin–angiotensin stimulation of the zona glomerulosa of the adrenal cortex. ECF, extracellular fluid; JG, juxtaglomerular apparatus. (Modified from Sodeman WA, Sodeman TH: Sodeman's Pathologic Physiology Mechanism of Disease. WB Saunders, Philadelphia, 1985, p. 1018.)

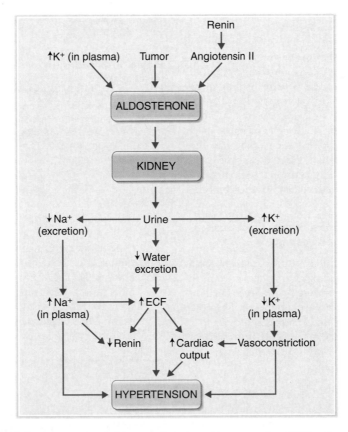

Figure 11-23 Pathogenesis of aldosterone-induced hypertension. ECF, extracellular fluid.

- **Hypernatremia.** Aldosterone leads to a retention of sodium (Na^+), leading to initial hypernatremia. Elevation of Na^+ in serum leads to a reactive release of **atrial natriuretic hormone** (ANH), which promotes excretion of Na^+ in the urine (natriuria). Hence, in most patients serum Na^+ is within normal limits, and they usually do not have generalized edema.
- **Hypokalemia.** Aldosterone promotes excretion of potassium (K^+) in urine. Urine contains increased amounts of K^+, whereas the concentration of K^+ in the blood is reduced. Hypokalemia may cause muscle weakness and fatigue. The ECG shows changes such as flattening of T waves and the appearance of U waves.
- **Nocturnal polyuria.** Long-standing hypokalemia may damage the kidneys **(hypokalemic nephropathy),** rendering them resistant to ADH. Since the kidneys cannot retain the water, polyuria results accompanied by polydipsia. Polyuria typically occurs during the night, a period of the day when normal kidneys conserve water. Loss of K^+ is associated with retention of bicarbonate (HCO_3^-), which contributes to metabolic alkalosis.
- **Metabolic alkalosis.** In response to K^+ loss in the urine and resultant hypokalemia, the body releases the intracellular K^+ into the blood. The loss of intracellular K^+ is accompanied by an intracellular influx of H^+ and Na^+. The loss of H^+ reduces the pH of the blood and causes metabolic alkalosis.

Tumor-derived hyperaldosteronism must be distinguished from essential hypertension, which is best done with a **saline loading test.** This test is performed by intravenously infusing isotonic NaCl over a period of 2 hours and by measuring aldosterone and cortisol in the blood during the loading. Expansion of the extracellular space reduces serum aldosterone levels in patients who have essential hypertension but does not affect those who have primary hyperaldosteronism. Furthermore, such patients have much more aldosterone than cortisol in their blood.

Hypercortisolism causes complex metabolic changes clinically known as Cushing's syndrome.

Cushing's syndrome is a clinical condition caused by an excess of glucocorticoids. In clinical practice it is most often caused by exogenous hormones (i.e., medicinal or self-motivated intake of synthetic corticosteroids). The nonmedicinal (endogenous) form of hypercortisolism can be classified as **ACTH-dependent** or **ACTH-independent** (Fig. 11-24). The most important causes of endogenous forms of hypercortisolism are

- **Pituitary** corticotropic adenoma (70%). These ACTH-secreting tumors were first described by the famous neurosurgeon Harvey Cushing, hence the name of the syndrome and related disease.

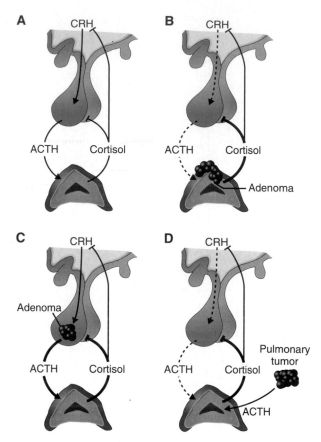

Figure 11-24 Adrenocorticotropic hormone (ACTH)-dependent and ACTH-independent Cushing's syndrome. CRH, corticotropin-releasing hormone. **A,** Normal. **B,** Adrenal cortical adenoma. **C,** Pituitary adenoma. **D,** Pulmonary ACTH-secreting tumor. (Modified from Sodeman WA, Sodeman TM: Sodeman's Pathologic Physiology. Mechanisms of Disease, Philadelphia, WB Saunders, 1985, p. 1016.)

- **Adrenal** cortical adenoma, carcinoma, or hyperplasia (20%). Adenomas account for approximately one half of all cases, carcinomas are less common, and primary hyperplasia accounts for only 15% of all hyperfunctioning adrenal lesions.
- **Ectopic** ACTH overproduction by nonpituitary tumors (10%). Most often this paraneoplastic syndrome is caused by small-cell lung cancer, but it may be related to bronchial or gastrointestinal carcinoid tumors, islet cell tumors, and many other neoplasms.

Pearl

> The mnemonic for the causes of hypercortisolism is **ACTH: a**drenal lesions, **C**ushing's disease, **t**umoral ACTH, and **h**ormonal therapy.

The clinical features of hypercortisolism result from the effects of cortisol on the intermediary metabolism of carbohydrates, lipids, and proteins. The most important clinical findings are as follows (Fig. 11-25):

■ **Weight gain, moon face, truncal obesity, and accumulation of fat on the back ("buffalo hump").** These changes are related to cortisol-induced hyperglycemia and reactive hyperinsulinemia, which stimulates **fat accumulation.** Cushing's syndrome is also associated with **sodium and water retention** due to the weak mineralocorticoid effects of cortisol and its precursors (e.g., deoxycorticosterone, DOC). Most patients are constantly hungry and engage in **hyperphagia.**

■ **Muscle wasting on the extremities and anterior abdominal wall.** Patients with Cushing's syndrome typically have thin arms and legs and weak abdominal muscles, resulting in a protruding belly. These changes are related to **atrophy of the skeletal muscles** caused by increased **proteolysis.** Amino acids released from the muscles are transported to the liver and used for **gluconeogenesis.** These metabolic processes are stimulated by cortisol and insulin.

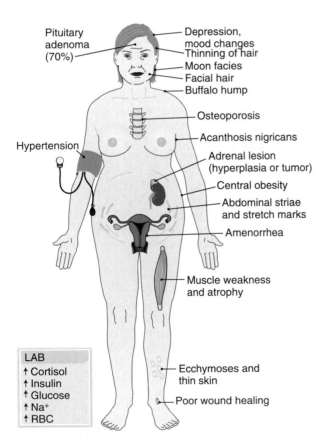

Figure 11-25 Clinical features of Cushing's syndrome. RBC, red blood cell count.

Pituitary adenoma (70%)
Depression, mood changes
Thinning of hair
Moon facies
Facial hair
Buffalo hump
Osteoporosis
Hypertension
Acanthosis nigricans
Adrenal lesion (hyperplasia or tumor)
Central obesity
Abdominal striae and stretch marks
Amenorrhea
Muscle weakness and atrophy
LAB
↑ Cortisol
↑ Insulin
↑ Glucose
↑ Na⁺
↑ RBC
Ecchymoses and thin skin
Poor wound healing

■ **Hypertension.** It is characterized by increased **diastolic pressure,** which is caused by **retention of sodium and water** in the kidneys.

■ **Glucose intolerance.** Cortisol has **anti-insulin** activity and stimulates **gluconeogenesis and glycogenolysis** in the liver. Hyperglycemia is typically associated with hyperlipidemia. In 20% of cases overt **diabetes mellitus** is present.

■ **Skin changes.** Typical changes include **violaceous striae, stretch marks,** and **ecchymoses.** These changes reflect weakness of the **connective tissue** and **vascular fragility** induced by the direct effects of cortisol on **collagen synthesis** and other extracellular matrix components in fibroblasts. **Delayed wound healing** is related to the same inhibitory effects of cortisol. Hyperpigmentation in intertriginous areas (**acanthosis nigricans**) results from changes in glycosaminoglycans of the extracellular matrix and dermal blood vessels.

■ **Osteoporosis.** Cortisol inhibits collagen synthesis and thus has a profound effect on the formation of osteoid. It also accelerates bone breakdown. **Healing** of **fractures** is delayed.

■ **Polycythemia.** Cushing's syndrome patients typically have a plethoric ruddy face, which is related to an increased red blood cell count. Cortisone stimulates **erythropoietin,** which in turn promotes erythropoiesis in the bone marrow.

■ **Reproductive changes and virilization.** Cushing's syndrome in women is associated with menstrual irregularities, such as oligomenorrhea or amenorrhea, and infertility. They also may have signs of virilization, such as hirsutism, and an increased incidence of acne on the face and the back. These changes are related to the **androgenic effects** of 17-ketosteroids. Males suffer from impotence and a loss of libido.

■ **Depression, sleep disturbances, and memory loss.** Many patients are initially euphoric but then become depressed. Sleep disturbances like insomnia or lethargy are common. Short-term memory may be impaired. These mental changes are related to the complex effects of cortisol on the central nerovous ystem (CNS).

Pearl

> A mnemonic to help you recall the most important features of Cushing's syndrome is **adipose** (just think that there is truncal adiposity, buffalo hump, and moon face): **a**diposity, **d**iabetes, **i**nfertility, **p**sychologic problems, **o**steoporosis and muscle wasting, **s**kin changes (striae, hirsutism, bruises), **e**levated blood pressure/**e**rythrocytosis.

The laboratory tests that may be useful for the diagnosis of Cushing's syndrome include

- **Blood cell counts.** Hemoglobin, hematocrit, and red blood cell count are high. Total white blood cell count is normal, but there might be fewer than normal eosinophils and lymphocytes.
- **Serum electrolytes.** Most often minerals are within normal limits, but in some patients who have adrenal carcinomas hypokalemic alkalosis might be present.
- **Cortisol in serum.** Total cortisol and free cortisol (5% of total) can be measured. A random blood cortisol test does not provide useful information because the secretion of cortisol is cyclical during the day. Blood concentration is at its highest in the morning and its lowest at midnight. Cortisol blood concentration also may rise significantly during stress and in the course of various diseases. Accordingly, several blood samples collected during day and night must be analyzed. Alternatively a **midnight free cortisol** could be measured, and if elevated it is suggestive of Cushing's syndrome. To avoid blood collection at midnight, one may measure **cortisol in the saliva.**
- **Free cortisol in urine** collected over 24 hours. Urinary free cortisol correlates well with total blood cortisol and free blood cortisol calculated over the same period. For practical purposes this test is the best screening test and usually the first test used for distinguishing Cushing's syndrome from simple obesity.
- **Low-dose dexamethasone suppression test.** Dexamethasone, a cortisol analogue injected intravenously in a *low dose* at bedtime, suppresses the normal morning rise of cortisol in the blood. In patients who have Cushing's syndrome such suppression does not occur. Some drugs and renal failure may cause false positive results, and thus the positive dexamethasone test must be confirmed by additional testing such as dexamethasone suppression followed by a **corticotropin-releasing hormone (CRH) stimulation test** or a **high-dose dexamethasone suppression test.**
- **ACTH in serum.** Serum corticotropin (ACTH) is *high* in patients who have Cushing's disease due to pituitary adenoma or in patients with nonpituitary tumors that secrete ACTH. Cushing's syndrome caused by adrenal tumors or primary hyperplasia or that occurring in patients treated with steroids is characterized by a *low* serum ACTH. Overall, the concentration of ACTH in the blood is higher in patients with tumors than in those with small pituitary adenomas. However, finding the source of ACTH might not be simple, because the ACTH values vary over a broad range. If one suspects that the pituitary is the source of ACTH, the pituitary must be proved to contain a tumor, or a sample of venous blood draining from the sella turcica must be measured for ACTH (**inferior petrosal sinus sampling**).
- **High-dose dexamethasone suppression test.** Dexamethasone injected in a *high* dose suppresses below 50% increased levels of ACTH in patients with pituitary adenoma (Cushing's disease), but does not suppress ACTH produced by malignant nonpituitary tumors.

Adrenal androgen excess causes reproductive problems and virilization in women but is of no major consequence in men.

Adrenal androgenic steroids include **androstenedione, dehydroepiandrostenedione (DHEA),** and **dehydroepiandrostenedione sulfate (DHEAS).** Excessive production of these weak androgens occurs to some extent in many adrenal cortical tumors and cortical hyperplasia. Since the production of these hormones is also under the control of ACTH, they are overproduced in Cushing's disease as well. In men these androgens produce no obvious changes, but in women they may cause menstrual irregularities, infertility, hirsutism, or virilization.

Hirsutism. It is defined as abnormal and excessive hair growth (**hypertrichosis**) in a male pattern. It affects approximately 10% of adult white women. It is more common in some ethnic groups, such as women of Mediterranean extraction, who have more androgen-sensitive areas on their bodies than other women. Hirsutism is rare in women of East Asian origin.

The extent of hairiness varies and may be graded on a scale from 1 (mild) to 4 (severe) according to the scale proposed by Ferriman and Gallwey (Fig. 11-26). Over 95% of white women in the United States and Europe have a hirsutism score below 8 points on that scale.

Most often the causes of hirsutism are unknown, so it is labeled idiopathic. In some cases hirsutism is hereditary. Identifiable causes of hirsutism include hyperandrogenism of ovarian or adrenal origin, uncommon pituitary tumors, and drugs (Table 11-10). Irregular menstrual periods since puberty suggest ovarian origins. Galactorrhea or acromegaly suggests pituitary disorders. Adrenal androgen production can be usually suppressed with low-dose dexamethasone, which is useful in distinguishing adrenal from ovarian causes of hirsutism. Certain drugs (e.g., minoxidil and cyclosporine) stimulate hair growth in an androgen-independent manner.

Congenital adrenal hyperplasia (CAH). This form of female pseudohermaphroditism may manifest as *neonatal virilization* of female babies, with or without salt wasting, or in a *late-onset form*, which becomes apparent only at the time of puberty. The incidence of the disease is approximately 1:12,000, but it is more common in some ethnic groups (e.g., Hispanics and Jews). The mutation may involve the genes encoding one of the hydroxylases involved in the synthesis of steroids: 21-hydroxylase, 11-hydroxylase, or 17-hydroxylase (Fig. 11-27).

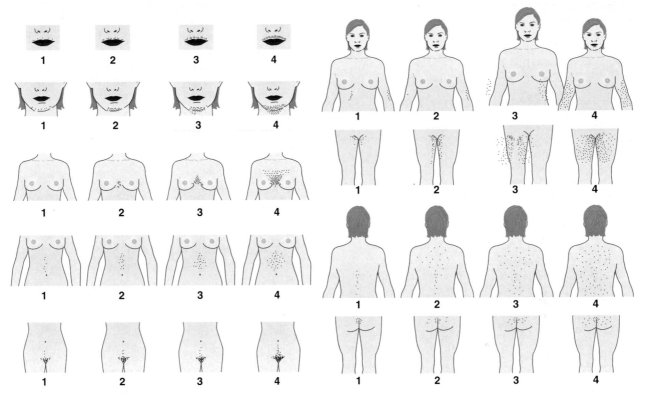

Figure 11-26 Hirsutism scoring scale. The nine body areas known to respond to androgens are scored according to Ferriman and Gallwey from 0 (no terminal hair) to 4 (frankly virile). For healthy women a normal hirsutism score is less than 8. (Redrawn from DeGroot LI, Jameson JL [eds]: Endocrinology, 4th ed. Philadelphia, WB Saunders, 2000, p. 2125, and the original drawings in Ehrman D, Rosenfeld R, J Clin Endocrinol Metab 71:1, 1990.)

The inactivation of the gene encoding steroid 21-hydoxylase (cytochrome P_{450c21}), an enzyme that is essential for the production of cortisol, accounts for 95% of cases of CAH. Typically there is a point mutation of the corresponding gene *P450c21B*, transforming it into a gene that resembles the inactive pseudogene $P_{450c21A}$, a change called "microgene conversion." Without this enzyme no cortisol could be synthesized, and all the cortisol precursors are shunted into the production of androgens. In some cases the synthesis of aldosterone is also affected. The deficiency of 11-hydroxylase or 17-hydroxylase may produce similar effects.

Due to a lack of cortisol, which normally provides the negative feedback inhibition of ACTH, the production of pituitary ACTH becomes unchecked. The serum concentration of ACTH is high, which in turn further stimulates the production of adrenal androgens. Treatment with cortisol reduces ACTH secretion and improves the clinical picture.

Clinically CAH has several forms:

■ **Deficiency of 21-hydroxylase with virilization and salt wasting.** This is the most common form of 21-hydroxylase deficiency recognized in infants. It is typically associated with a block in the production of cortisol and the shunting of intermediary steroids into androgen production. Virilization of female external genitalia begins in utero during pregnancy, and by the time of birth the baby has ambiguous external genitalia with clitoromegaly and fusion of labioscrotal folds. The synthesis of aldosterone is also affected, resulting in a renal loss of sodium and water. Typically, the patient has signs of hyponatremia, hyperkalemia, dehydration, and metabolic acidosis, leading to hypovolemic shock.

■ **Deficiency of 21-hydroxylase with virilization.** In this form of CAH the only symptom is virilization of the external genitalia. An excess of androgen synthesis in the adrenal cortex is associated with no cortisol synthesis and reactive overproduction of ACTH.

■ **Late-onset form of 21-hydroxylase deficiency.** This mildest form of 21-hydroxylase deficiency does not produce virilization of the external genitalia. Many patients are asymptomatic or have only mild signs of virilization. Clinically, no genital abnormalities are present at the time of birth, but at the time of puberty the affected girls show menstrual irregularities and some signs of virilization, such as hirsutism. The diagnosis is made by means of laboratory testing.

Table 11-10 Causes of Hirsutism

Idiopathic*
  Familial
Ovarian hyperandrogenism
  Polycystic ovary syndrome
  Idiopathic hyperthecosis of the ovary
  Sex cord stromal ovarian tumors (e.g., Sertoli-Leydig cell tumor)
  Pregnancy-related hyperandrogenism (e.g., hyper-reactio luteinalis)
Adrenal hyperandrogenism
  Congenital adrenal hyperplasia
  Cushing's syndrome
  Adrenal cortical neoplasia (adenoma, carcinoma)
Pituitary tumors
  Prolactinoma
  Somatotropic adenoma
Obesity with peripheral testosterone production
Exogenous hormones
  Anabolic androgens (e.g., athletes, body builders)
  Oral contraceptives
Drugs
  Monoxidil
  Phenytoin
  Cyclosporine
True hermaphroditism

*The most common form of hirsutism.

■ **Deficiency of 11-hydroxylase.** This form of CAH is rare in most parts of the world, but in some Arab countries and Israel it is the most common form of the disease. The synthesis of cortisol and aldosterone is inhibited, leading to increased synthesis of androgens and virilization of the genitalia. The accumulation of 11-deoxycorticosterone, which acts as a mineralocorticoid, prevents salt wasting and dehydration, and in most patients causes hypertension. Loss of potassium in the urine may evolve into hypokalemic alkalosis.

Adrenal insufficiency (Addison's disease) is characterized by a deficiency of mineralocorticoids and glucocorticoids.

Addison's disease is a rare chronic adrenal cortical insufficiency that may result from destruction or surgical removal of the adrenal glands, pituitary destruction, or atrophy of adrenals caused by long-term therapy with corticosteroids. Destruction of the adrenal glands is most often caused by **autoimmune adrenalitis.** The adrenals may be destroyed by the deposition of amyloid in systemic amyloidosis or hemosiderin in hemochromatosis or by metastatic malignant tumors. Human immunodeficiency virus (HIV) and cytomegalovirus (CMV) infection may also cause adrenal insufficiency. Tuberculosis, histoplasmosis, and similar chronic infections are less common today in the United States. Acute meningococcal sepsis may cause Waterhouse-Friderichsen syndrome, which leads to massive bleeding into the adrenals and sudden onset of adrenal insufficiency.

Signs and symptoms of Addison's disease result from the deficiency of glucocorticoids and mineralocorticoids. Adrenal androgens are also missing, but this deficiency is less obvious clinically. Clinical signs and symptoms, most of which are rather nonspecific, are presented in Figure 11-28 and listed here as follows:

■ Weakness and easy fatigability
■ Weight loss and anorexia
■ Hyperpigmentation of the skin and mucous membranes
■ Nausea and vomiting
■ Abdominal pain
■ Diarrhea or constipation
■ Electrocardiographic changes of hyperkalemia, such as high-peaked T waves and a prolonged PR interval
■ Cardiac arrhythmia, including cardiac block
■ Salt craving
■ Orthostatic hypotension and syncope

Laboratory testing of serum typically shows the following findings:

■ Low Na^+, Cl^-, and HCO_3^-
■ High K^+
■ Dehydration
■ Hypoglycemia
■ Low serum aldosterone and cortisol
■ High ACTH

Stimulation of adrenals with ACTH, which under normal circumstances raises the concentration of cortisol in the blood, gives negative results. Primary adrenal insufficiency can be distinguished from pituitary insufficiency by measuring aldosterone in the same blood sample: if the patient has pituitary insufficiency, aldosterone rises, but if the disease is caused by adrenal destruction, aldosterone does not rise.

DISEASES OF THE ADRENAL MEDULLA

The adrenal medulla consists of cells that synthesize the catecholamines epinephrine and norepinephrine. Epinephrine and norepinephrine are stored in cytoplasmic granules of the adrenal medullary cells and are released in response to numerous stimuli. Typically they are released into the circulation during exercise, in response to stress, following massive hemorrhage, following trauma, or during surgery.

Epinephrine and norepinephrine circulate bound to albumin. When released they bind to α-adrenergic and β-adrenergic receptors in various organs, thus causing many physiologic reactions. The most important organs and the reactions provoked by catecholamine are listed here:

■ Heart—tachycardia and stronger myocyte contraction
■ Blood vessels—vasoconstriction, but also vasodilation in some vessels

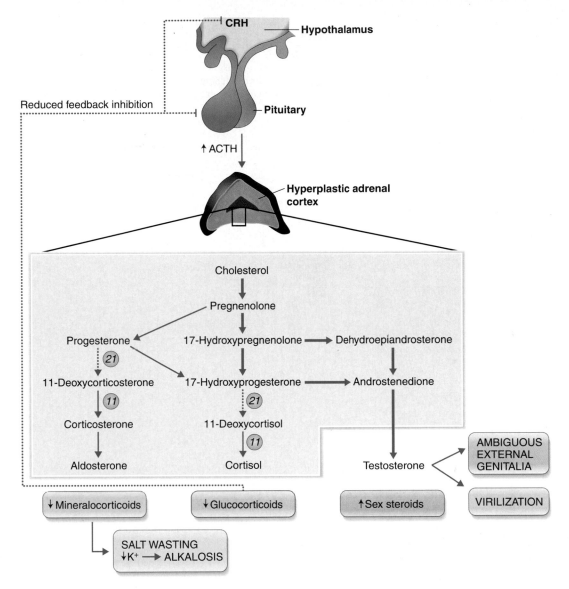

Figure 11-27 Congenital adrenal hyperplasia (CAH). The most common form of CAH characterized by ambiguous external genitalia and salt wasting is related to the deficiency of 21-hydroxylase and a block in the synthesis of cortisol and aldosterone. Deficiency of 11-hydroxylase inhibits the synthesis of cortisol and aldosterone, but the accumulation of 11-deoxycorticosterone, which acts as a mineralocorticoid, prevents salt wasting. ACTH, adrenocorticotropic hormone; CRH, corticotropin-releasing hormone. (Modified from Kumar V, Fausto N, Abbas A [eds]: Robbins and Cotran Pathologic Basis of Disease, 7th ed. Philadelphia, Elsevier Saunders, 2005, p. 1213, with permission.)

- Kidney—renin release
- Liver—glycogenolysis leading to hyperglycemia
- Fat tissue—lipolysis
- Intestine—smooth muscle cell relaxation and loss of peristalsis
- Skin—sweating with cold and pale extremities due to constriction of peripheral arterioles

Epinephrine and norepinephrine are metabolized into **metanephrine** or **normetanephrine,** respectively, and then converted to **vanillylmandelic acid (VMA).** These degradation products are excreted in the urine, where they may be measured biochemically (Fig. 11-29).

The most important diseases of the adrenal medulla are tumors. In childhood most tumors are composed of primitive neuroblastic precursors of adrenal medullary cells and are classified as neuroblastomas. In adults, the tumors are composed of well-differentiated cells secreting epinephrine or norepinephrine and are called pheochromocytomas.

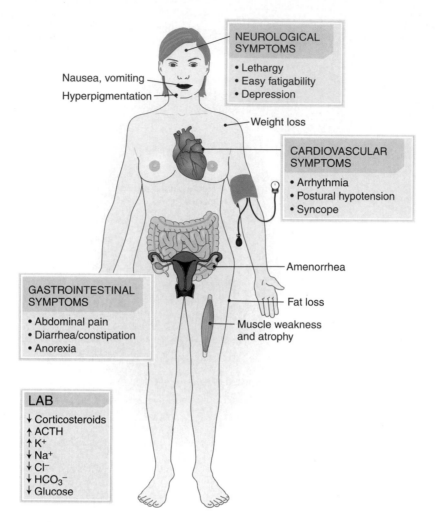

Nausea, vomiting

Hyperpigmentation

NEUROLOGICAL SYMPTOMS
• Lethargy
• Easy fatigability
• Depression

Weight loss

CARDIOVASCULAR SYMPTOMS
• Arrhythmia
• Postural hypotension
• Syncope

Amenorrhea

Fat loss

Muscle weakness and atrophy

GASTROINTESTINAL SYMPTOMS
• Abdominal pain
• Diarrhea/constipation
• Anorexia

LAB
↓ Corticosteroids
↑ ACTH
↑ K^+
↓ Na^+
↓ Cl^-
↓ HCO_3^-
↓ Glucose

Figure 11-28 Clinical features of Addison's disease. ACTH, adrenocorticotropic hormone.

Pheochromocytomas are tumors that secrete catecholamines and thus cause paroxysmal hypertension.

Pheochromocytomas are rare tumors, typically associated with hypertension. Although not more than 1 in 1000 hypertensive patients have a pheochromocytoma, it is important to recognize the tumor because surgical removal of the tumor may cure an otherwise recalcitrant hypertension. The most important clinical findings in patients who have a pheochromocytoma are as follows:

■ **Hypertension.** It is typically paroxysmal because catecholamines are stored in tumor cells and are released in bouts. The hypertension results from vasoconstriction of arterioles and increased cardiac output due to better venous return and the positive inotropic effect of catecholamines on the myocardium. In about 50% of cases the hypertension may be sustained and show only minor fluctuations from one measurement to another. It usually does not respond to standard antihypertensive treatment.

■ **Paroxysmal sympathetic effects.** The release of epinephrine and norepinephrine causes numerous sympathomimetic effects, such as sudden onset of headache,

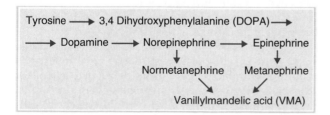

Tyrosine ⟶ 3,4 Dihydroxyphenylalanine (DOPA) ⟶
⟶ Dopamine ⟶ Norepinephrine ⟶ Epinephrine
                              ↓   ↓
                    Normetanephrine   Metanephrine
                              ↘   ↙
                        Vanillylmandelic acid (VMA)

Figure 11-29 Synthesis and degradation of catecholamines.

sweating, palpitations, tachycardia, facial flushing, nausea, vomiting, and blurry vision. Typically these attacks last not more than an hour.

- **Postural hypotensive episodes and syncope.** These episodes follow hypertensive episodes, or, in patients who have sustained hypertension, they occur at random and are caused by exhaustion of the adrenergic effect and inadequate perfusion of vital organs.
- **Increased metabolic rate.** It may manifest as fever with sweating, tachycardia, easy fatigability, and, in prolonged disease, as weight loss.
- **Hyperglycemia.** Catecholamines have an anti-insulin effect and promote glycogenolysis in the liver, leading to a rise of serum glucose. Hyperglycemia is accompanied by hyperlipidemia due to the lipolytic effect of catecholamines on peripheral fat stores.

Pearl

> A pheochromocytoma should be suspected if the hypertension is diagnosed in a young person, it does not respond to standard antihypertensive treatment, and is episodic. Paroxysms of hypertension can be precipitated by exercise, anesthesia, or even palpation of the abdomen.

The diagnosis of pheochromocytoma is based on laboratory findings, functional suppression tests, and radiologic demonstration of the tumor.

- **Laboratory testing.** Typically, catecholamines or their derivatives are increased in the blood and urine. Because catecholamines are released from the tumors episodically, it is best to collect urine over a 24-hour period and then test it. The measurement of urinary **metanephrine** is the best screening test, but urinary free **epinephrine** or **norepinephrine** or **vanillylmandelic acid (VMA)** can also be measured. The increased amounts of metanephrine and VMA stem from the catecholamines degraded in the tumor itself and to a lesser extent from such degradation in the peripheral tissue.
- **Clonidine suppression test.** The test is based on the fact that clonidine, an α_2-agonist and antihypertensive agent, blocks the centrally regulated sympathomimetic nerves. Thus, if one were to measure catecholamines in the blood and the blood pressure 3 hours after clonidine administration in normal people and those who have essential (primary) hypertension a suppressive effect would be evident. However, in patients with pheochromocytoma clonidine does not lower the arterial pressure, and the blood catecholamines remain high.
- **Radiologic localization of the tumor.** Larger tumors may be seen on a CT scan or MRI of the abdomen, but for smaller tumors adrenal scanning with ^{131}I-metaiodobenzylguanidine (MIBG) is best. Approximately 90% of pheochromocytomas are solitary, localized in the adrenals, and benign, but in 10% of cases they may be either extra-adrenal, or multiple or malignant.

HORMONAL DISEASES OF THE OVARY

The ovaries have a dual function: to produce germ cells (oocytes) and to produce hormones. Both functions must be coordinated to initiate normal pregnancy and thus fulfill the reproductive role in a woman.

Hormonal activity of the ovaries is regulated by pituitary gonadotropins, **follicle-stimulating hormone (FSH)** and **luteinizing hormone (LH),** which in turn are under the control of hypothalamic **gonadotropin-releasing hormone** (Fig. 11-30). These central regulators are released in a pulsatile manner. Inhibition of FSH with synthetic estrogens/progesterones is the basis of oral contraceptive medications.

During the first part of the menstrual cycle FSH stimulates the follicular granulosa cells to produce **estrogens.** Luteinizing hormone stimulates the theca cells at the periphery of the follicles to produce androgens, which diffuse through the basement membrane into the follicle and are then converted to estrogen. Granulosa cells also secrete the polypeptide hormones **inhibin** and **activin,** which regulate the local estrogen-to-androgen ratio. Inhibin promotes androgen synthesis but inhibits its conversion to estrogen. Activin has the opposite effect: it inhibits androgen synthesis and promotes androgen conversion to estrogens. Inhibin also provides negative feedback to the pituitary, whereas activin activates it.

Estrogens are the predominant hormones produced during the first part of the menstrual cycle (Fig. 11-31). The principal target organs for estrogens are the primary and secondary female reproductive organs. Many other organs are affected as well, as follows:

- **Uterus.** The development and growth of the uterus during puberty and pregnancy depends on estrogen. Endometrium proliferates in response to estrogen.
- **Vagina.** Estrogen is essential for the normal development of the vagina. In adult women it promotes the proliferation and maturation of the vaginal epithelium and accumulation of glycogen.
- **Fallopian tubes.** Estrogen regulates the function of ciliated cells, mucus production, and smooth muscle contraction in the Fallopian tube.
- **Breast.** Breast development and enlargement at the time of puberty depend on estrogen.
- **Fat tissue.** Estrogen stimulates accumulation of fat on the hips and the breasts.
- **Hair growth.** Estrogen stimulates the growth of axillary and pubic hair.
- **Bone growth.** Estrogen stimulates bone growth and is important for the maintenance of normal bone structure.

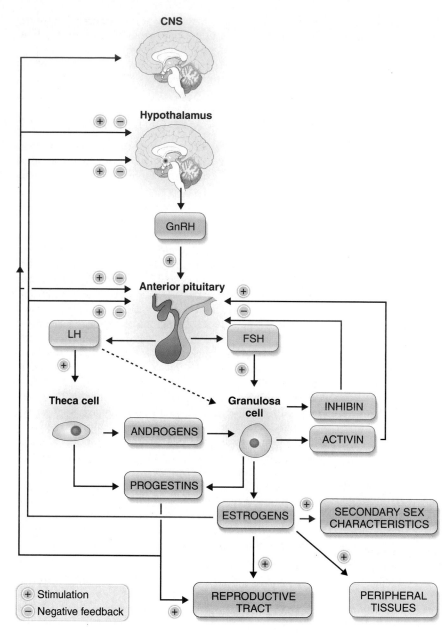

Figure 11-30 Hypothalamic–pituitary–ovarian axis. Gonadotropin-releasing hormone (GnRH) stimulates the pituitary, which secretes the follicle-stimulating hormone (FSH) and luteinizing hormone (LH). FSH and LH stimulate granulosa and theca cells to produce estrogens, progestins, androgens, inhibins, and activins, which provide negative or positive feedback to the hypothalamus or the pituitary. Inhibin inhibits the pituitary, whereas activins activate it. CNS, central nervous system. (Modified from Boron WF, Boulpaep EL [eds]: Medical Physiology, Philadelphia, WB Saunders, 2003, p. 1148.)

Estrogens provide both a negative and a positive feedback on the hypothalamus and the pituitary. The feedback effect depends on the concentration of hormones and the conditioning of the hypothalamic nuclei and pituitary. During most of the cycle, estrogens and progestins have a negative effect and inhibit the secretion of gonadotropin-releasing hormone (GnRH), FSH, and LH. However, the rise of the estrogens during the last few days of the proliferative phase has a reverse effect, and the feedback becomes positive. A smaller rise of progestins has the same effect. This leads to a preovulatory midcycle rise of LH, which triggers the ovulation and the

transformation of the follicle into a corpus luteum. The corpus luteum secretes estrogens and progesterone.

Progestins, the most important of which is progesterone, act predominantly on the reproductive organs, but they also provide negative feedback to the hypothalamus and the pituitary.

■ **Uterus.** Progesterone maintains the integrity of the endometrium during the second phase of the menstrual cycle. It also stimulates the endometrial glands to secrete and helps prepare the endometrium for

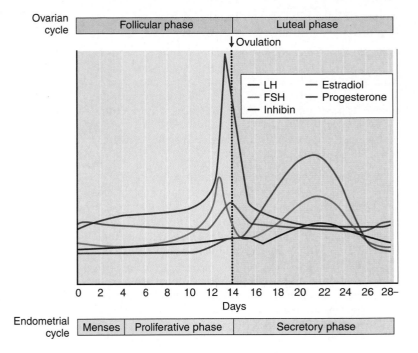

| Ovarian cycle | Follicular phase | Luteal phase |

↓Ovulation

— LH   — Estradiol
— FSH   — Progesterone
— Inhibin

0 2 4 6 8 10 12 14 16 18 20 22 24 26 28–
Days

| Endometrial cycle | Menses | Proliferative phase | Secretory phase |

Figure 11-31 Hormonal changes during the menstrual cycle. The surge of luteinizing hormone (LH) on day 13 leads to ovulation, a point that divides the proliferative from the secretory phase. Estrogen is the prevalent ovarian hormone during the proliferative (follicular) phase. Progesterone predominates in the secretory phase. FSH, follicle stimulating hormone.

implantation of the fertilized oocyte. Progesterone also changes the viscosity of the cervical mucus and the composition of the fallopian tube secretions.

■ **Breast.** Progesterone supports the cyclic changes of the ducts, lobules, and the stroma contributing to the enlargement of breast during the secretory phase of the menstrual cycle.

The first menstrual bleeding (menarche) begins usually after the age of 9 years.

The hormonal changes the precede puberty include activation of the hypothalamic pituitary–ovarian axis. Menarche, the first menstrual bleeding, usually begins after a girl reaches the age of 9 years. It is typically preceded by budding of the breasts. Breast budding before the age of 8 years or the menarche before the age of 9 years constitutes precocious puberty.

Precocious puberty may occur due to a variety of reasons, but in more than 90% of all cases the cause is never identified **(constitutional precocious puberty).** Other causes such as organic brain diseases or tumors of the brain, ovary, or adrenals are less common.

Puberty is characterized by an increased production of estrogens, which accounts for the development of most female secondary sex characteristics. Genital organs develop and the breasts grow to full size. Estradiol and the ovarian and adrenal androgens are responsible for the growth of pubic and axillary hair. Estrogens stimulate bone growth and account for the pubertal growth spurt. This is accomplished by the direct action of estrogens on the cells of the epiphyseal growth plate. Estrogens contribute to the strength of bone, but not as efficiently as testosterone.

Ovarian involution at menopause results in cessation of menstruation.

The ovaries contain a limited number of oocytes and follicles, and, with age, fewer and fewer of them are available to sustain regular ovulation and the menstrual cycle. After all the oocytes have been spent normal menstrual cycles do not occur, and the woman enters menopause. In most women menopause begins between the age of 45 and 55 years, but in some it may occur much earlier. If it begins before the age of 40 years, as seen in approximately 1% of all women, it is called **premature menopause.**

Menopause is characterized by a cessation of menstrual cycles and a reduced production of estrogens. Ovaries produce less and **less estrogen,** the synthesis of which shifts to peripheral fat tissue, which becomes the major source of estrogen in these women. Low serum estrogen levels are associated with high FSH and LH in the blood. The synthesis of androstenedione, which before menopause is produced in equal amounts in the adrenals and the ovaries, is also reduced, but the synthesis of testosterone in the ovaries remains at the premenopausal level.

The hormonal changes that occur during menopause lead to episodes of **hot flushes,** or **hot flashes.** They are caused by an unregulated discharge of central sympathetic activity that occurs in parallel with pituitary discharge of FSH and LH. These two changes are, however, unrelated.

Decreased ovarian production of estrogens results in trophic changes affecting many organs. The uterus involutes, and the endometrial mucosa becomes atrophic. Vaginal mucosa is also atrophic.

Amenorrhea results from an interruption of the hypothalamic–pituitary ovarian function.

Amenorrhea is a condition in which the menstrual cycle does not take place, and menstrual bleeding never occurs. It may be preceded by menstrual irregularities, characterized by weak bleeding (*oligomenorrhea*), painful and irregular menses (*dysmenorrhea*), or massive menstrual bleeding (*menorrhagia*).

On the basis of etiology, amenorrhea may be classified as primary or secondary.

- **Primary amenorrhea.** For clinical purposes primary amenorrhea is a condition in which menarche did not occur by the age of 16 years. It is related to abnormal development of the female genital organs or of the pituitary or results from genetic metabolic disorders involving the pituitary, ovarian, or adrenal hormones.
- **Secondary amenorrhea.** These women have menstrual periods at the time of puberty but later on they stop ovulating and do not have menses. For clinical purposed amenorrhea is diagnosed if a women does not have menstrual bleeding over the period of her three normal cycles. Amenorrhea of this type occurs typically during pregnancy and it can be induced by oral contraceptives. The most common causes of secondary amenorrhea are hormonal changes, including pituitary, thyroid, adrenal cortical, and ovarian hormones. Hypothalamic–pituitary dysfunction caused by anorexia nervosa or bulimia is an important cause of amenorrhea. Stress itself may cause amenorrhea. Polycystic ovary syndrome is yet another very common cause of chronic amenorrhea. The most important causes of amenorrhea are listed in Table 11-11.

Table 11-11 Causes of Amenorrhea

Developmental disorders
   Chromosomal disorders (e.g., Turner's syndrome)
   Agenesis of the uterus
   Gonadal dysgenesis
   Inborn errors of hormone synthesis (e.g., CAH)
Hypothalamic causes
   Anorexia nervosa
   Depression
   Tumors of the base of the brain
Pituitary causes
   Prolactinoma
   Panhypopituitarism (e.g., Sheehan's syndrome)
Ovarian causes
   Polycystic ovary syndrome
   Chemotherapeutic injury of the ovary
   Premature menopause
Uterine/vaginal abnormalities

CAH, congenital adrenal hyperplasia.

Pearl

> Amenorrhea occurs in 2% of all women who have used oral contraceptives and then have stopped taking them to become pregnant. However, such amenorrhea is not more common than in nonusers and is thus not a consequence of contraception.

Polycystic ovary syndrome is a syndrome related to a dysfunction of the hypothalamic–pituitary–ovarian–adrenal axis.

Polycystic ovary syndrome (PCOS) derives its name from the typical pathologic findings—enlargement of the ovaries, which contain numerous follicular cysts. Initially it was thought that these women could not ovulate because of an anatomic barrier in the ovary, but later it became obvious that the causes for anovulation are hormonal.

This rather common disease of unknown origin most likely represents the common outcome of several interlinked hormonal and metabolic disturbances. The ovaries apparently do not respond to pituitary gonadotropins and cannot ovulate, but the exact mechanism of anovulation is unknown. It seems that the granulosa cells do not respond to LH and thus cannot mature to the point where the follicle ruptures and releases the oocyte. The oocytes die and the unruptured follicles transform into fluid-filled cysts lined by granulosa cells. The theca cells of these follicular cysts produce increased amounts of androgens.

Although the pathogenesis of PCOS is not entirely clear, the overall consensus is that the changes in various organs are caused by a dysfunction of the hypothalamic–pituitary–ovarian–adrenal axis. Hormonal abnormalities are complex, but in most cases include increased serum levels of the following hormones:

- Luteinizing hormone (LH). The LH:FSH ratio is in excess of 2.5:1.
- Adrenal androgens
- Estrogens
- Insulin

Clinical signs and symptoms that characterize PCOS are as follows:

- **Menstrual irregularities.** These vary from oligomenorrhea to prolonged anovulatory cycles and amenorrhea. Polycystic ovary syndrome accounts for approximately 30% of all cases of secondary amenorrhea in young women. Infertility is common.
- **Hirsutism.** Excess hair on the face and the chest are associated with increased incidence of acne.
- **Obesity.** Excess of fat tissue contributes to hyperestrogenism due to peripheral conversion of adrenal androgens to estrogens.

- **Spotting and vaginal bleeding.** Bleeding is related to endometrial hyperplasia caused by hyperestrogenism.
- **Insulin resistance.** It may result in hyperglycemia or overt diabetes mellitus.
- **Dyslipidemia.** It results from obesity and insulin resistance.
- **Hypertension.** Together with hyperlipidemia it accelerates atherosclerosis.

Clomiphene citrate is effective in inducing ovulation in women who desire to become pregnant.

HORMONAL DISEASES OF THE TESTIS

The testis, the male gonad, has two functions: to produce, sperm and to secrete androgens.

Spermatogenesis takes place inside the somniferous tubules, which contain germ cells in various stages of maturation and **Sertoli cells.** The intertubular interstitial spaces contain **Leydig cells,** which secrete androgens.

Like the ovaries, the testes are under the control of the hypothalamic GnRH and pituitary gonadotropic hormones FSH and LH (Fig. 11-32). Gonadotropic hormones stimulate

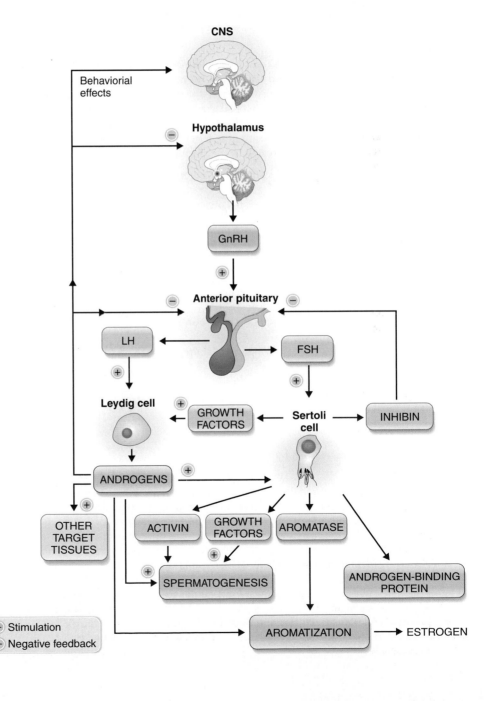

Figure 11-32 The hypothalamic–pituitary–testicular axis. (Modified from Boron WF, Boulpaep EL [eds]: Medical Physiology, Philadelphia, WB Saunders, 2003, p. 1125.)

the Sertoli and Leydig cells, which in turn cooperate in supporting spermatogenesis.

■ **Sertoli cells.** Their primary function is to support spermatogenesis. These cells also produce a polypeptide called inhibin, which inhibits the release of pituitary gonadotropins by negative feedback. Sertoli cells also produce growth factors that promote the growth of Leydig cells, an androgen-binding protein, and estrogens.

■ **Leydig cells.** These interstitial cells are the primary source of testosterone and other androgens in the male body. Androgens act locally on Sertoli cells and spermatogenic cells and are also released into the circulation.

Testosterone acts by transforming into dehydrotestosterone (DHT), which is transported into the nucleus so that it can interact with the hormone-responsive part of the gene and stimulate protein synthesis. Over 95% of all testosterone is derived from the testis, and more than 80% of circulating DHT is derived from peripheral conversion of testosterone.

The most important effects of testosterone are as follow:

■ Development of internal and external male genital organs during fetal life
■ Growth and development of male sexual organs at the time of puberty
■ Initiation and maintenance of spermatogenesis
■ Formation of the secondary male sexual characteristics at puberty
  ■ Deepening of the voice
  ■ Growth of pubic, axillary, and chest hair
  ■ Sebaceous and sweat gland development
■ Pubertal growth spurt and bone growth in coordination with growth hormone
■ Closure of the growth plates of long bones at the end of puberty
■ Maintenance of sexual function, libido
■ Development of skeletal muscle
■ Effects on the brain to promote certain male traits

Hypogonadism is characterized by low production of testosterone.

Hypogonadism is characterized by a hypofunctioning of the testes. The consequences of testicular hypofunction depend very much on the patient's age at diagnosis and the pathogenesis of the disease. It may be classified as

■ **Primary testicular hypogonadism.** In this condition the cause of the disease lies in the abnormal development of the testes. The serum testosterone is low, and the gonadotropins are high.
■ **Hypothalamic–pituitary hypogonadism.** In this condition the serum testosterone and gonadotropin levels are low.

■ **Secondary testicular hypogonadism.** In this condition the normally functioning testes are injured at a certain point of adult life and testicular failure develops. Hormonal functions of the testes may be preserved, but spermatogenesis is usually reduced.

Primary testicular hypogonadism. This condition is a consequence of abnormal testicular development. The best example of primary hypogonadism is **Klinefelter's syndrome,** a disease caused by chromosomal abnormalities. These patients are genetically male, meaning that they have a Y chromosome, but in addition to it, they have two or more X chromosomes (47,XXY or 48,XXXY). The testes are atrophic and produce inadequate amounts of testosterone. Puberty never occurs, and spermatogenesis is never established.

The diagnosis of Klinefelter's syndrome is made on the basis of clinical, laboratory, and cytogenetic data. Clinically, the patients are tall and have eunuchoid features and gynecomastia. The penis is small, and the testes atrophic. At the time of adolescence, puberty does not occur, and the secondary male characteristics never develop. Laboratory data supporting the diagnosis are low serum testosterone and high serum FSH levels. If the FSH levels in serum are three times higher than normal, and aspermatogenesis is confirmed, there is no need to perform a testicular biopsy, especially if the clinical findings are consistent with the diagnosis of Klinefelter's syndrome. Cytogenetic studies demonstrating additional X chromosomes confirm the diagnosis.

Hypothalamic–pituitary hypogonadism. This group of diseases, also known as hypogonadotropic hypogonadism, is characterized by low serum testosterone and low FSH and LH. The basic defect lies with the release of GnRH from the hypothalamus or pituitary gonadotropins. For example in Kallmanns syndrome the hypothalamic defect results in defective release of GnRH and a loss of olfactory neurons, leading to anosmia. Brain tumors, trauma with hemorrhage, and surgical interventions may all cause injury to the hypothalamus. The destruction of the pituitary stalk or the pituitary itself by tumors, trauma, or surgery also may reduce or completely abolish the pulsatile secretion of FSH and LH.

Secondary testicular hypogonadism. Testicular failure may be induced by infections (e.g., mumps orchitis), cytotoxic drugs, irradiation, trauma, surgery, and other similar extraneous influences. Systemic diseases, starvation, chronic liver disease, and many multiorgan hormonal disturbances affect the testes, but in some cases they also may disrupt the normal hypothalamic–pituitary–testicular axis. Probably the most common cause of testicular injury is **cryptorchidism,** found in 0.5% of all male children. It is usually unilateral, and the unaffected testis may compensate adequately for the loss or injury of the contralateral one.

Depending on the cause of testicular injury the testis may undergo visible atrophy or remain of normal size and show only histologic signs of seminiferous tubule hyalinization and a loss of spermatogenesis. Serum testosterone is usually in the normal range. Ejaculate may contain a reduced number of spermatozoa *(oligospermia),* but infertility occurs only when the injury is very severe and bilateral.

Male infertility is characterized by a reduced number or spermatozoa in the ejaculate.

Male infertility is characterized by a lack of spermatozoa or severely reduced number of spermatozoa in the ejaculated sperm. Normally 1 mL of ejaculated sperm contains approximately 60 million spermatozoa. If the number is reduced below 20 million, the condition is called **oligospermia**. If no viable spermatozoa or no spermatozoa at all are seen during microscopic examination, the condition is called **azoospermia.**

The statistics of infertility show that 80% of all women who are trying to become pregnant with a steady male partner are able to during a year of unprotected sexual intercourses. Of the remaining 20% percent of women, some become pregnant during the next year, but approximately 15% of couples are unable to have a baby and are thus considered to be infertile. In about 60% of these infertile couples the cause lies with the woman, in 30% with the man, and in about 10% the cause is never found. Hence, in the work-up for infertility, both the female and male partner must be considered. The problem may be classified as primarily pertaining to one of the following aspects of the reproductive process:

- **Hormones.** The hormonal defect may involve the hypothalamic–pituitary–gonadal axis. Disruption of the menstrual cycle or the suppression of hypothalamic–pituitary hormones may occur due to overproduction of other hormones (e.g., prolactin) or intake of androgens (e.g., body building). Oral contraceptives act by suppressing the release of FSH from the pituitary. Severe disease, starvation, or anorexia nervosa all disrupt normal hormone production.
- **Spermatogenesis.** In congenital testicular developmental conditions like **Klinefelter's syndrome,** the testes do not produce sperm because of a lack of testosterone and a lack of spermatogenic cells. In the condition called **Sertoli-only syndrome** (del Castillo's syndrome), the man has a genetic defect characterized by a lack of germ cells in the seminiferous tubules. **Spermatogenic maturation arrest** is a condition in which spermatogenesis cannot be completed but is arrested at a specific stage of maturation. **Hypospermatogenesis** includes a spectrum of congenital and acquired diseases characterized by reduced spermatogenesis.
- **Obstructions.** Anatomic defects or acquired lesions secondary to infection or trauma or surgery may interrupt the normal pathway between the ovaries and the uterus (most often in the Fallopian tube) and thus prevent fertilization or implantation of the oocytes. In males obstruction of the epididymis or the vas deferens may prevent the entry of spermatozoa into the terminal parts of the genital system, and thus an **obstructive azoospermia** is present. Vasectomy is a contraceptive procedure that has the same effect.

CASE STUDIES

Case 1 A 30-YEAR-OLD MAN WITH HEADACHES, INDISTINCT SPEECH, AND BLURRY VISION

Clinical history A 30-year-old man complained that he has constant headaches, which of late have been associated with blurry vision.[1] Furthermore he noticed problems in talking, and his voice has become deeper.[2]

Physical findings The most striking finding was a protruding lower jaw and a large protruding nose. The teeth appeared separated from one another by wide interdental spaces, and the tongue appeared enlarged. His speech was slurry. In comparison with the picture on his drivers' license (taken 3 years previously), his facial features were coarse. The hands and feet were enlarged, and the fingers and toes appeared thicker than normal. The liver was enlarged.[3] He had hypertension and systolic cardiac murmurs. The heart appeared enlarged on the anteroposterior radiograph.[4]

Laboratory findings The fasting plasma sugar was slightly elevated above normal, but there was no glucosuria.[5] Other routine tests gave normal results.

Diagnostic procedures Detailed radiologic studies, including CT and MRI, were performed. The bones of the head appeared thicker than normal, and the sella turcica was enlarged. The bones of hands and feet showed cortical thickening, with widening of distal phalanges.[6] The visual field showed bitemporal hemianopsia.[7] Special testing included the measurement of growth hormone following glucose administration and the measurement of somatomedin C (IGF-I). These tests confirmed the suspected diagnosis.[8]

Follow-up The patient underwent transphenoidal hypophysectomy and improved markedly.

Questions and topics for discussion
1. What could cause headache and blurry vision? Is headache a sign of endocrine diseases? Which endocrine diseases are associated with headache? What is the pathogenesis of headache in each of the diseases that you listed?
2. What could be the cause of slurred speech? Why has his voice become deeper?
3. What are the possible common denominators for all those clinical findings? You just made a "driver's license-assisted diagnosis." Explain.
4. Explain the cardiovascular findings.
5. Does this patient have diabetes mellitus or glucose intolerance? How would you prove it? Explain the pathogenesis of hyperglycemia. Why is it not associated with glycosuria?
6. Interpret these radiologic findings. Which one is most directly linked to the basic pathologic change that caused all other changes?
7. What caused the bitemporal hemianopsia?
8. Why is it necessary to give glucose before measuring serum growth hormone concentration? Is somatomedin produced by the pituitary? How do GH and somatomedin C test results correlate with one another?

Case 2 A 40-YEAR-OLD WOMAN COMPLAINING OF FREQUENT PALPITATIONS AND SWEATING

Clinical history A 40-year-old woman noticed that her heart beats fast and "pounds in the chest."[1] She also said her face feels warm and she feels comfortable only in a cold air-conditioned room. She has constantly sweaty palms and feet.[2] She has lost weight, 10 pounds over the last 3 months.[3]

Physical findings The patient appears nervous and anxious.[4] She has protruding eyes with a prominent lid lag.[5] She has a mild fever and warm and sweaty palms. She is tachycardic and her systolic pressure is elevated, whereas the diastolic pressure is normal.[6]

The thyroid is enlarged and warm, and a bruit is evident.[7]

Laboratory findings The routine laboratory tests gave normal results. TSH was low, T_4 and T_3 were elevated.[8] Antibodies to TSH receptor and thyroglobulin were positive in a high titer.[9]

Diagnostic procedures Scintigraphy of the thyroid with radioactive iodine revealed diffuse uptake in the entire thyroid gland.[10]

Follow-up Treatment with antithyroid drugs gave good results, and the patient improved.

Questions and topics for discussion
1. Does this patient have palpitations? Explain.
2. What are the possible causes of these symptoms?
3. What are the possible causes of involuntary weight loss in a 40-year-old woman?
4. Why is she nervous and anxious?
5. Does she have exophthalmos? What is the pathogenesis of this finding?
6. Why does this patient have an elevated systolic pressure? If the disease is not treated could she develop heart failure? Would this be a high-output or low-output heart failure?
7. What could cause thyroid enlargement? What is the most common cause of thyroid enlargement? Does she have a goiter?
8. Explain this thyroid panel of tests. What is the significance of elevated TSH?
9. Which antibodies are useful for diagnosing thyroid diseases?
10. How is thyroid scintigraphy performed?

Case 3 A 35-YEAR-OLD WOMAN WITH HYPERTENSION

Clinical history A 35-year-old woman was found to have arterial hypertension during a routine pre-employment medical examination. She was given diuretics and a beta-blocker, but the blood pressure could not be controlled and actually became worse.[1]

Physical findings The patient had systolic and diastolic hypertension. There was no edema or any other sign of heart failure.

Laboratory findings Serum sodium was high and potassium was low, whereas the concentration of potassium in urine was high and the concentration of sodium was low.[2]

Serum aldosterone was high and serum renin was low.[3]

Diagnostic procedures A salt-loading test was performed and showed that the aldosterone secretion could not be repressed.[4] A radioscan was performed, and a tumor was found in the left adrenal gland.[5]

Follow-up The pathologist reported that the adrenal gland contained a yellow tumor, which histologically had the typical features of a benign adrenal cortical tumor (adenoma).[6] The patient was treated surgically and the tumor was removed. She improved dramatically.

Questions and topics for discussion

1. What are the possible causes of hypertension in a young person? Which forms of hypertension do not respond to standard antihypertensive treatment?
2. What is the pathogenesis of hypernatremia and hypokalemia? Why does this patient not have edema?
3. What is the significance of high aldosterone and low renin, especially when compared with the cases that have high renin and high aldosterone?
4. What is a salt-loading test and how is it performed? Please interpret these results.
5. How are adrenal lesions visualized radiologically? Do you expect to find a small or a large tumor in this case?
6. How did the pathologist make the diagnosis of adenoma? Why was the tumor yellow?

Case 4 A 25-YEAR-OLD OBESE WOMAN WITH IRREGULAR MENSTRUAL PERIODS AND INFERTILITY

Clinical history A 25-year-old woman complained that her menstrual bleeding is irregular and that each time the blood flow is less abundant than before. Occasionally she has no menstrual bleeding for 3 to 4 months.[1] She also complains of a frequent urge to urinate. She produces copious amounts of urine and drinks a lot because she is constantly thirsty.[2] She is married but has been unable to become pregnant during the last 2 years.[3]

Physical findings The patient is overweight and moves around with difficulty. She has thick facial hair on her upper lip and on the chin and has acne.[4]

Laboratory findings Fasting plasma sugar was markedly elevated, but all other routine tests gave normal results. Serum insulin was high.[5] Luteinizing hormone was high and the ratio of LH:FSH was high.[6] Serum androstenedione and testosterone were slightly elevated above normal.[7]

Diagnostic procedures Gynecologic examination revealed enlarged ovaries with smooth external surfaces.[8]

Follow-up The patient was treated with clomiphene and became pregnant.[9]

Questions and topics for discussion

1. Does this woman have oligomenorrhea, amenorrhea, or dysmenorrhea?
2. Interpret these findings. Why would an obese woman have polyuria?
3. Define *infertility* and discuss its causes. Does this woman meet your definition of infertility?
4. What is the significance of hair growth on the face of this woman?
5. Why is the serum insulin level high? Does this woman have diabetes? If so, what kind?
6. What is the significance of increased levels of LH and the LH:FSH ratio?
7. What is the source of androgens in this case?
8. Do these gynecologic palpatory findings suggest a neoplastic or reactive functional ovarian lesion?
9. How does clomiphene act and how did it make it possible for this woman to become pregnant?

Chapter 12

THE KIDNEYS

Introduction

The kidneys are part of the urinary system (tract). The clinical significance of urinary tract diseases may be best illustrated by the fact that urinary tract infections (UTIs) are among the most common infections encountered in general medical practice. Between 1% and 2% of all visits to doctors' offices are prompted by UTIs. One in 5 women between the ages of 20 and 45 years has periodic problems with urination, and 5% of all women in that age group experience a UTI. The rate of infection rises to 15% by the age of 65 years. Urinary tract tumors account for 10% of all malignant tumors in men and 4% in women. The relative clinical significance of various renal diseases is presented graphically in Figure 12-1.

The kidneys are vital organs essential for maintaining the normal internal milieu and for the excretion of waste products in the urine. In this chapter, rather than spending time on common infections and tumors of the urinary tract or developmental abnormalities, since these diseases are covered in greater detail in pathology and microbiology textbooks, we concentrate on diseases that affect basic renal function. The importance of these diseases is best highlighted by considering the following facts:

- Acute tubular necrosis with significant retention of metabolic by-product and waste material occurs in most patients who have undergone prolonged major surgery, and in many patients who have been in shock or have suffered major trauma.
- Renal dysfunction is encountered in the course of many systemic diseases, such as diabetes mellitus, arterial hypertension, or systemic lupus erythematosus (SLE).
- Renal failure may develop due to a failure of another organ, such a prerenal failure due to congestive heart disease or hepatorenal syndrome as a complication of cirrhosis.

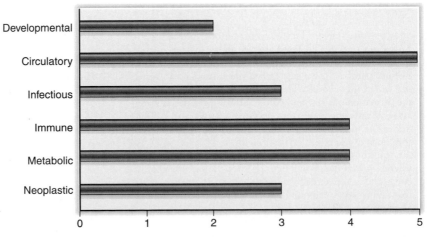

Figure 12-1 The relative clinical significance of various renal diseases.

KEY WORDS

Normal Anatomy and Physiology

Afferent arteriole Small branch of the interlobular renal artery that enters the glomerulus on its vascular pole. It brings arterial blood into the glomerulus. The afferent arteriole branches into glomerular capillaries, which by confluence form the efferent arteriole. Blood leaves the glomerulus through the efferent arteriole, which branches into peritubular capillaries or vasa recta. At its entry into the glomerulus the afferent arteriole wall contains juxtaglomerular cells.

Blood supply The kidneys receive 20% to 25% of the cardiac output. Approximately 90% of the arterial blood remains in the cortex, 9% enters the outer medulla, and only 1% reaches the inner medulla. Kidneys maintain a constant blood flow by autoregulation that functions when the perfusion pressure is in the range from 60 to 180 mm Hg.

Glomerular basement membrane (GBM) Selectively permeable specialized vascular basement membrane outlining the glomerular capillaries. It regulates the ultrafiltration of plasma and the formation of the primary urinary filtrate. Together with the fenestrated endothelial cells and the foot processes forming epithelial cells (podocytes), the GBM forms the glomerular capillary wall (GCW).

Glomerular filtration rate (GFR) Rate at which the plasma is filtered in the glomeruli to form the glomerular urinary filtrate. The GFR can be expressed as milliliters of fluid per minute or liters per day. Since the renal plasma flow is 600 mL/min and the ratio of renal plasma flow to GFR is constant at 5:1, the GFR is approximately 120 mL/min.

Glomerular tuft Convolution of fenestrated capillaries that have a highly specialized membrane designed for selective ultrafiltration of plasma. The glomerular tuft contains three cell types: the endothelial, epithelial, and mesangial cells.

Glomerulus Initial portion of the nephron interposed between the afferent and efferent arterioles on one side and the proximal convoluted tubule on the other. It is composed of a tuft of fenestrated capillaries enclosed by Bowman's capsule.

Juxtaglomerular (JG) apparatus Structure composed of specialized renin-secreting cells localized in the wall of the afferent arteriole at the vascular pole of the glomerulus, along with the cells of macula densa a specialized part of the distal convoluted tubule.

Kidneys Paired organs located in the retroperitoneum, connected on one side to renal arteries and veins and on the other to the ureter. On cross section, the kidney has two distinct parts: an outer part called the cortex and an inner one called the medulla. The main function of the kidney is the formation of urine and elimination of superfluous water and minerals, metabolic waste products, drugs, and xenobiotics. The kidneys secrete some hormones and growth factors, such as renin and erythropoietin.

Mesangium Connective tissue framework of the glomerulus extending into the glomerular tuft from the vascular pole. It consists of mesangial cells and nonfibrillar extracellular matrix that fills the space delimited by the confluence of three to four glomerular capillaries.

Nephron Basic functional unit of the kidney comprising the glomerulus, the proximal convoluted tubule, the loop of Henle, the distal tubule, and the collecting ducts. On one side the nephron is linked to the arterial blood supply and on the other with the excretory urinary ducts. There are two types of nephrons: cortical nephrons (which have short loops of Henle) and juxtamedullary nephrons (which have long loops of Henle extending into the medulla). The former are surrounded by capillary networks and the latter by vasa recta, the only blood supply for the deep medulla and the papillae.

Renal arteries There are two renal arteries both of which originate from the abdominal aorta. In the kidneys they branch, forming large interlobar arteries, which in turn give rise to arcuate arteries running along the corticomedullary junction. The arcuate arteries give rise to the cortical interlobar arteries, which give rise to the afferent arterioles. The efferent arteriole exiting the glomerulus gives rise to peritubular capillaries and vasa recta, which drain into the small renal veins.

Renin Enzyme secreted by the juxtaglomerular cells in response to reduced blood supply to the kidneys. It acts on angiotensinogen, transforming it into angiotensin, which stimulates aldosterone production in the adrenal cortex. Through this mechanism renin raises the blood pressure.

Ureter Tubular organ serving as the conduit for urine from the renal pelvis to the urinary bladder.

Urethra Tubular organ serving as the final conduit for the fluid exiting the urinary bladder during micturition. In males it also serves as a passageway for semen.

Urinary bladder Hollow organ whose primary function is to store urine prior to micturition.

Urine Fluid formed in the kidney from ultrafiltered plasma, containing, in addition to water, minerals, organic waste material, and possibly some xenobiotics. Urine is formed in the nephron through a stepwise process that includes ultrafiltration of the plasma, selective and site-specific reabsorption of some minerals and water, and secretion of others.

Urothelium (transitional epithelium) Specialized epithelium lining the renal calices, pelvis, ureters, urinary bladder, and the posterior part of the urethra.

Vitamin D Lipid-soluble vitamin hydroxylated in the liver and thereafter in the kidney, where the active form of the vitamin, $1,25(OH)_2D_3$, is formed. With parathyroid hormone it regulates the absorption and metabolism of calcium.

Pathophysiology

Anuria Absence of urine, or in practical terms less than 100 mL of urine per day. Anuria is a sign of renal failure and may be classified as prerenal (e.g., due to reduced renal perfusion in heart failure), intrarenal (e.g., due to glomerulonephritis or toxic tubular necrosis), or postrenal (e.g., due to the obstruction of the ureters or bladder outflow tract).

Azotemia Increased blood concentration of nitrogen-containing compounds, such as urea or creatinine. The blood concentration of urea is conventionally expressed as blood urea nitrogen (BUN). Azotemia is usually a sign of renal failure, which may be prerenal, intrarenal, or postrenal.

Glycosuria Appearance of glucose in the urine in excess of the minimal amounts normally found in the urine (<200 mg/24 hours). It is a consequence of hyperglycemia, most often owing to diabetes mellitus.

Hematuria Appearance of blood in the urine. It may be macroscopic and visible to the naked eye or microscopic and detectable only by microscopic examination of the renal sediment.

Lipiduria Appearance of lipid droplets or lipid casts in the urine. Typically found in nephrotic syndrome and hyperlipemic states.

Oliguria Production of urine in small amounts. Typically it is a sign of renal failure, which may be prerenal, intrarenal, or postrenal. In adults oliguria is generally diagnosed when the total urinary output is below 400 mL/day.

Polyuria Production of large quantities of urine, reflected in both an increased frequency of urination (pollakisuria) and an abnormally large volume of fluid excreted over a 24-hour period. Empirically it is diagnosed in adults when the urine production exceeds 3 to 5 L/day.

Proteinuria Excretion of proteins in the urine in excess of the normal amount for the age of the patient. In healthy adults urine contains less than 500 mg of protein in 24 hours, but in children the urine contains less protein. Proteinuria is usually a sign of glomerular injury and occurs in nephritic and nephrotic syndromes. Bence Jones proteinuria is a feature of multiple myeloma and is characterized by urinary excretion of immunoglobulin light chains.

Pyuria Excretion of pus in the urine. Typically it is caused by bacterial infection.

Urinary casts Cylindrical structures found in the urine, typically formed from protein-rich contents of the renal tubules. Hyaline casts are normal components of urine and are formed predominantly from Tamm-Horsfall protein, which is secreted into the lumen of the distal tubules. Red blood cell casts contain deformed or fragmented red blood cells and are a sign of glomerular hematuria. Granular casts are composed of granules formed from disintegrated cells in tubular necrosis. White blood cell casts contain fragmented neutrophils and are found in inflammatory conditions.

Renal Diseases

Acute glomerulonephritis Inflammatory glomerular disease mediated by immune complexes. Immune complexes may be formed in situ in the glomeruli or may be deposited in the glomeruli from the circulation. Immune complexes can be formed between immunoglobulins and bacterial antigens, autoantigens, or glomerular antigens. The disease is characterized by an infiltrate of neutrophils or macrophages and proliferation of mesangial cells. Clinically it presents in the form of a nephritic syndrome.

Acute tubular necrosis Acute renal failure caused by necrosis of the renal tubular cells. It may result from ischemia (prerenal renal failure) or the action of toxins. Clinically it manifests with a loss of renal function. Typically the tubules cannot form urine or concentrate the primary filtrate. It manifests first with oliguria, followed by polyuria. In most instances tubular cells regenerate, and renal function is reestablished.

Acute tubulointerstitial nephritis Allergic reaction, most often precipitated by drugs. It is characterized by interstitial infiltrates of lymphocytes, eosinophils, and plasma cells and destruction of tubular cells. Clinically it manifests with acute renal failure.

Amyloidosis Systemic disease characterized by deposition of amyloid in many organs. It may be most often associated with the deposition of AA type amyloid, encountered in chronic inflammatory diseases, or AL amyloid, seen in multiple myeloma. Clinically it usually manifests with a nephrotic syndrome.

Crescentic glomerulonephritis Severe form of acute glomerulonephritis characterized by exudation of inflammatory cells into the pericapillary urinary space of the glomeruli, leading to the formation of crescents. It usually occurs after a focal necrotizing glomerulonephritis, typically caused by Goodpasture's syndrome or Wegener's granulomatosis, or less often after a severe form of acute postinfectious glomerulonephritis. Clinically it manifests as rapidly progressive glomerulonephritis (RPGN). Renal failure develops within 1 to 3 months of the onset of the disease.

Diabetic glomerulosclerosis Glomerular lesion induced by long-standing diabetes mellitus. Pathologically it has two forms: nodular glomerulosclerosis (Kimmelstiel-Wilson disease) with mesangial hyaline nodule formation, and diffuse glomerulosclerosis with diffuse thickening of the glomerular basement membranes. Both forms of glomerulosclerosis lead to proteinuria that may ultimately result in nephrotic syndrome, progressing to renal failure.

Focal glomerulosclerosis (FGS) Glomerular disease that may be idiopathic (primary) or secondary to so-called hyperperfusion injury of the glomeruli or another renal or systemic disease (e.g., AIDS). It is found in a subset of children who have nephrotic syndrome and are initially found to have minimal-change nephropathy (lipoid nephrosis). Morphologically it is recognized by partial obliteration of glomerular capillary tufts with hyaline material. Such changes are found only in some glomeruli, hence the name: focal, meaning some glomeruli, and segmental, meaning parts of the glomerular capillary tufts. Clinically it manifests as nephrotic syndrome unresponsive to treatment. Focal glomerulosclerosis is the most common cause of nephrotic syndrome in adults.

Glomerulonephritis Inflammation of the glomerulus, most often caused by immune mechanisms. It may be acute or chronic. Several morphologic variants of glomerulonephritis are found, such as necrotizing, proliferative, mesangial, crescentic, focal, and diffuse.

Goodpasture's syndrome Renal–pulmonary syndrome mediated by cytotoxic antibodies to type IV collagen in glomerular and pulmonary capillary basement membranes. These antibodies cause focal and segmental necrotizing glomerulonephritis, which progresses to crescentic glomerulonephritis over a period of a month or two. Clinically it manifests as a RPGN with pulmonary hemorrhage.

Hydronephrosis Dilatation of the renal pelvis and calices with flattening of the renal papillae. If chronic hydronephrosis leads to an atrophy of the entire kidney parenchyma.

It is typically caused by obstruction of the ureters with urinary stones, tumors, or extraureteral pathologic lesions (e.g., retroperitoneal fibrosis). The urine inside the hydronephrotic kidneys may become infected, leading to pyelonephritis or pyonephrosis (pus-filled hydronephrotic kidney).

Lupus nephritis   Chronic glomerulonephritis, which occurs in approximately 75% of patients with systemic lupus erythematosus (SLE). It results from the deposition of circulating immune complexes in the glomeruli.

Membranous nephropathy   Immune complex-mediated glomerular disease manifesting clinically as a nephrotic syndrome. Immune complexes are deposited on the epithelial side of the basement membranes and do not evoke inflammation.

Minimal-change disease   Also know as "nil disease" or lipoid nephrosis, it is a disease of unknown origin. It manifests as nephrotic syndrome that usually responds well to treatment with steroids. Typically it occurs in children, but it may be found in adults as well. By light and immunofluorescence microscopy the glomeruli appear normal, and the only visible abnormality is the fusion of foot processes of the epithelial cells seen by electron microscopy.

Nephritic syndrome   Clinical syndrome related to glomerulonephritis and characterized by oliguria, hematuria, proteinuria, hypoalbuminemia, and edema. Patients are typically hypertensive and have acute azotemia related to a reduced GFR. The urine is reduced in amount and dark brown. The urinary sediment contains red blood cell casts and dysmorphic and fragmented red blood cells. Most often it is a manifestation of postinfectious glomerulolonephritis and thus it heals in more than 90% of cases. In a minority of cases it follows a rapid downhill course, and in some cases it persists or progresses to chronic glomerulonephritis and end-stage renal failure.

Nephrosclerosis   Term used to describe renal pathologic changes related to hyaline sclerosis of the arterioles and fibrosis of the intrarenal arteries. Benign nephrosclerosis is associated with hypertension and gradual loss of renal function leading to uremia. Accelerated nephrosclerosis, which shows fibrinoid necrosis of the arterioles and proliferative arteriolitis, is typically associated with malignant hypertension in African American men.

Nephrotic syndrome   Clinical syndrome characterized by proteinuria, lipiduria, hypoalbuminemia, hyperlipidemia, and generalized edema. In children it is most often caused by minimal-change disease. In adults it is most often caused by focal glomerulosclerosis, but it may be due to membranous nephropathy, diabetic glomerulosclerosis, amyloidosis, or systemic lupus erythematosus (membranous type, class IV).

Pyelonephritis   Bacterial inflammation of the kidney, which may be acute or chronic. Infection may reach the kidney upstream through urine backflow from the urinary bladder (ascending infection) or hematogenously (descending infection). Most often it is caused by uropathogens (i.e., *E. coli, Proteus, Klebsiella, Enterococcus, Seratia* sp.). The complications of acute pyelonephritis include papillary necrosis, pyonephrosis and perinephric abscess, or systemic sepsis ("urosepsis"). The most important complications of chronic pyelonephritis are arterial hypertension and, in bilateral cases, renal failure (uremia).

Rapidly progressive glomerulonephritis (RPGN)   Term used for any form of renal failure of sudden onset associated with severe glomerular injury. Pathologically it manifests with crescentic glomerulonephritis. It is typical of anti-GBM cytotoxic antibody-mediated glomerulonephritis (Goodpasture's syndrome) and pauci-immune glomerulonephritis (e.g., Wegener's granulomatosis). It is lethal if not treated, but if immunosuppressive treatment is given in time, the patient may recover.

Renal cell carcinoma   The most common malignant tumor of the kidneys. It originates from cells of the proximal tubules. Most often the tumor manifests with hematuria (50%) or nonspecific symptoms. It is thus called "internist's tumor" because it is usually diagnosed by internists rather than urologists. It metastasizes through the renal veins to the lungs or locally to the lymph nodes.

Renal failure   Loss of renal function, which may be classified as prerenal, intrarenal, or postrenal; acute or chronic. The most common cause of acute renal failure is prerenal renal failure, related to hypoperfusion of the kidneys due to low blood pressure. It occurs in heart failure, shock, hypotension after surgery, or trauma. Intrarenal renal failure is caused by primary glomerular or tubulointerstitial diseases. Postrenal renal failure is caused by urinary tract obstruction. Acute renal failure is usually reversible. Chronic renal failure is irreversible. It may be mild or severe (uremia).

Transitional cell carcinoma   Malignant tumor originating from the renal calices and pelves. Histologically it is identical to urothelial carcinoma of the urinary bladder. It is usually papillary but may also be flat or invasive. Grade I tumors have an excellent prognosis but tend to recur. Grade III tumors have poor prognosis.

Tubulointerstitial nephritis   Group of renal diseases affecting tubules and interstitium and clinically manifesting as reduced renal function. It may be related to an adverse reaction to drugs, abuse of analgesics, urate deposition, hypercalcemia, or multiple myeloma. Bacterial infections of the kidney are by convention not included under this heading but are called pyelonephritis.

Uremia   Synonym for end-stage kidney failure. In this state the body cannot excrete the urinary waste products. Retention of these waste products results in azotemia (elevation of BUN and creatinine), metabolic acidosis, and dysfunction of many vital organs. Without renal dialysis or renal transplantation it is invariably lethal.

Urolithiasis   Synonym for urinary stone disease. Urinary stones (uroliths) are chemically classified as (1) calcium oxalate/phosphate, (2) uric acid, (3) ammonium magnesium calcium phosphate ("struvite"), or (4) cysteine stones. Stones may form in the renal pelvis, ureters, or urinary bladder. Clinically most often they manifest with renal colic related to the impaction of stones in the ureters. Chronic obstruction leads to hydronephrosis and loss of renal function. Urinary stones also predispose to urinary infection.

■ The overall incidence of chronic renal disease is approximately 150 per million persons, and most of these patients require long-term dialysis or renal transplantation.

Urinalysis is performed during the routine yearly medical check-up, for health employment, for insurance purposes, and essentially for all hospitalized patients. It provides a rough insight into the function of the kidneys and the urinary tract, but it also may give some indication about a person's general health status. A more complex assessment of renal function requires additional testing and a higher degree of expertise, and therefore a consultation with a nephrologist is one of the most often required consultations in most hospitals.

Normal Structure and Function

NORMAL ANATOMY AND HISTOLOGY

The kidneys are paired organs located in the retroperitoneal space of the abdomen. Each kidney receives arterial blood from the abdominal aorta through a renal artery, whereas a renal vein links each of them to the inferior vena cava. The renal calices and pelves form the conduit for the urine formed in the kidneys, linking the kidneys with the ureters and the urinary bladder. The urine is voided through the urethra, which passes through the penis in men but is embedded in fibromuscular stroma and is relatively short in women.

The nephron is the basic functional unit of each kidney.

Each kidney is composed of approximately 1 million nephrons. **Nephrons** form the basic functional units and are composed of several components: the glomerulus, proximal convoluted tubule, loop of Henle, distal convoluted tubule, and collecting ducts (Fig. 12-2). The main function of the nephrons is the formation of urine, which begins by the filtration of the plasma in the glomeruli, followed by reabsorption of some components of the filtrate, secretion of additional substances, and final concentration of the filtrate into urine.

The filtration of the blood occurs in the glomeruli and involves the passage of filtered plasma ("glomerular ultrafiltrate") into the lumen of the proximal tubule. The barrier between the blood and the urinary space is formed by the **glomerular capillary wall** (GCW), which has three components:

■ **Endothelial cells,** the fenestrated capillaries lining the inside of the capillaries.
■ **Glomerular basement membrane (GBM),** the semipermeable membrane composed of collagen type IV, laminin, and some other extracellular matrix components. It has an inner layer called the *lamina rara interna,* an external layer called the *lamina rara externa,* and a

central portion called the *lamina densa.* It is electrically charged and has a specific structure and permeability that allows the passage of molecules that have a molecular weight less than albumin (68,000 daltons). Larger molecules do not pass through the GBM ("selective permeability of the GBM").
■ **Visceral epithelial cells** (podocytes), which form the foot processes that are tightly linked to the external basement membrane. These cells are in continuity with parietal epithelial cells lining the inside of Bowman's capsule, thus delimiting them from the glomerular urinary space. The glomerular urinary space freely communicates with the lumen of the proximal tubules.

Within each kidney are two types of nephrons: the more numerous cortical nephrons, which account for 75% of all nephrons, and the less numerous juxtamedullary nephrons. **Cortical nephrons** have short loops of Henle, which are located mostly in the cortex and penetrate only at a short distance into the outer medulla. **Juxtamedullary nephrons** have long loops of Henle, which extend deep into the medulla and sometimes even to the tip of the renal papillae.

Renal vessels have several functionally distinct segments.

The blood vessels of the kidney form a complex meshwork that comprises several functionally distinct segments.

■ **Renal arteries.** These arteries originate from the abdominal aorta. On entry into the kidneys they branch and give rise to interlobal arteries, which give rise to arcuate arteries running along the corticomedullary junction. Interlobular arteries enter the cortex in the direction of the renal capsule, in their course giving rise to lateral branches called afferent arterioles.
■ **Glomerular arterioles. Afferent arterioles** enter the glomeruli, branching into the glomerular capillaries, which become confluent on the other end so that the blood that remains following filtration leaves the glomeruli through the efferent arterioles. **Efferent arterioles** leaving the cortical glomeruli form specialized capillaries.
■ **Peritubular capillary network.** This network of capillaries forms from efferent arterioles exiting from high cortical glomeruli. They drain into small renal veins. The arterioles exiting the juxtamedullary glomeruli form the **vasa recta,** fenestrated capillaries which loop through the medulla before draining into the renal veins.
■ **Renal veins.** Renal veins do not differ significantly from veins in other organs. They drain into the vena cava. Obstruction of the renal veins (e.g., renal vein thrombosis) may adversely affect the function of nephrons.

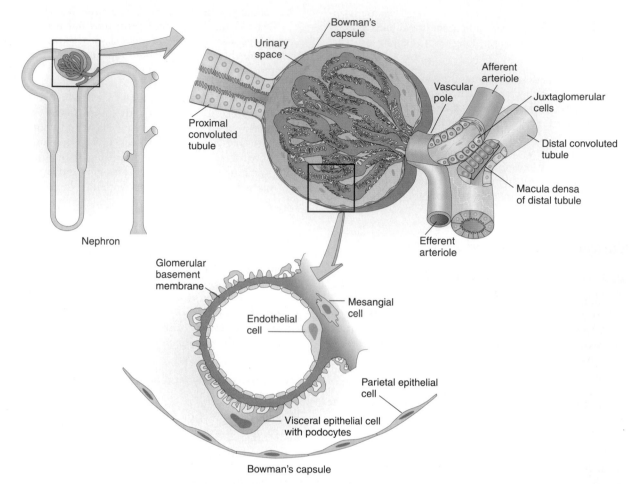

Figure 12-2 The nephron and its vasculature. Nephrons form the basic functional units of each kidney. Arterial blood from the interlobular artery passes through the glomerulus, where it is filtered into the lumen of the proximal convoluted tubules, enters into the peritubular capillaries, and then exits by the way of veins. (Modified from Boron WF, Boulpaep EL: Medical Physiology, Philadelphia, WB Saunders, 2003, p. 740.)

Note that the kidneys have two distinct capillary networks arranged in sequence: a *high-pressure* one, forming glomerular capillaries and favoring filtration of blood into the urine, and a *low-pressure* one, composed of the peritubular network and vasa recta, favoring the reabsorption of fluids back into the circulation.

The kidneys contain hormone-secreting cells and cells that activate vitamins.

In addition to the nephron and the vasculature, which are involved in the formation of urine, the kidneys contain metabolically active regulatory and secretory (endocrine) cells. The most important among these cells are

- **Cells of the juxtaglomerular (JG) apparatus.** These include the specialized sensor cells of the distal tubule

(called the **macula densa**) and granular renin-secreting JG cells in the outer wall of the afferent arteriole.
- **Erythropoietin-secreting cells.** These cortical interstitial cells respond to hypoxia by secreting erythropoietin, which stimulates the production and maturation of red blood cells in the bone marrow.
- **Vitamin D-activating cells.** Vitamin D, which is first hydroxylated in the liver into $25(OH)D_3$ and released into the blood, is filtered in the glomeruli and reabsorbed by the proximal renal tubules, which hydroxylate it into the active form of vitamin, $1,25(OH)_2D_3$, and release it back into the blood.
- **Angiotensin II-forming cells.** Circulating angiotensin I, formed from hepatic angiotensinogen through the action of renin, is taken up by the endothelial cells in renal vessels and transformed into angiotensin II. Angiotensin II is a very potent vasoconstrictor and is

important for the autoregulation of renal blood flow. Prostaglandins produced in the kidneys cause vasodilatation and counteract the action of angiotensin II.

NORMAL PHYSIOLOGY

The principal functions of the kidneys are as follows:

- Formation and excretion of urine
- Excretion of waste products, drugs, and toxins
- Regulation of body water and mineral content of the body
- Maintenance of the acid–base balance
- Regulation of blood pressure through the secretion of renin
- Regulation of hematopoiesis through the secretion of erythropoietin
- Synthesis of the active form of vitamin D

Most of these functions were discussed in other chapters, so we limit our discussion here to the formation of urine.

The formation of urine depends on proper blood flow and the coordinated function of all parts of the nephron.

The kidneys receive 20% to 30% of the total cardiac output. In practical terms that means that in the average adult male **renal plasma flow** (RPF) is 600 mL/min. Renal blood flow is **autoregulated** by the humoral factors, such as angiotensin II, which leads to vasoconstriction, and by prostaglandins, which cause dilatation. At a constant plasma inflow into the glomeruli, the **glomerular filtration rate (GFR)** also remains constant. Normally, the ratio of RPF to GFR is 5:1, and the GFR is thus 120 mL/min, or approximately 170 L/day. The factors that could reduce the GFR are listed in Table 12-1.

Table 12-1 Causes of Reduced Glomerular Filtration Rate

PATHOGENETIC MECHANISM	DISEASE
Decreased renal blood flow	Heart failure
Hypotension–hypoperfusion of kidneys	Massive blood loss
Constriction of afferent arterioles	Hypertension (angiotensin II ↑)
	Trauma, brain injury, and other states with ↑ sympathetic activity (norepinephrine ↑)
Glomerular inflammation	Acute glomerulonephritis
Endothelial cell swelling	Eclampsia
Glomerular thrombi	DIC, TTP, ITP
Increased urinary back pressure	Urinary obstruction, hydronephrosis
Decreased glomerular capillary bed	Chronic glomerulonephritis

↑, increase; DIC, disseminated intravascular coagulation; ITP, idiopathic thrombocytopenic purpura; TTP, thrombotic thrombocytopenic purpura.

The **excretion of urine** is a stepwise process that includes several site-specific physiologic events aimed at preserving the essential balance of minerals and organic compounds and eliminating the waste products (Fig. 12-3):

Filtration. The plasma filtered in the glomeruli forms the glomerular filtrate, which enters into the lumen of the proximal tubules. The red blood cells (RBCs) and the white blood

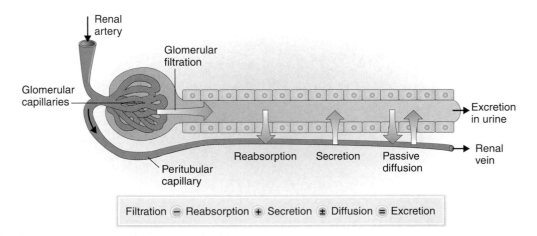

Filtration ⊖ Reabsorption ⊕ Secretion ± Diffusion ⊜ Excretion

Figure 12-3 Excretion of urine. It depends on the filtration, reabsorption, and secretion of water and solutes, and in some instances their passive diffusion in and out of the tubules.

cells (WBCs) cannot pass the endothelial cell barrier and are thus not found in the glomerular filtrate. The semipermeable GBM allows only the passage of proteins that have molecular weights lower than albumin (68,000 daltons). Almost all proteins reaching the proximal tubule are reabsorbed, and the final urine contains thus less than 150 mg of protein per 24 hours.

Reabsorption. Different minerals and metabolites are handled by different parts of the nephrons (Fig. 12-4). The proximal tubule is the most active site and thus reabsorbs almost all the amino acids, glucose, and bicarbonate and 70% of the sodium, potassium, calcium, and phosphate. Additional reabsorption of calcium in the distal tubule is regulated by **parathyroid hormone** (PTH) and the reabsorption of sodium by aldosterone. Reabsorption of sodium phosphate in the proximal tubule may be inhibited by PTH. The reabsorption of water in the collecting duct occurs under the control of **antidiuretic hormone (ADH),** also known as **vasopressin.**

Secretion. The renal tubules can acidify urine by actively secreting *hydrogen ions* (H^+). Active secretion of *potassium* (K^+) takes place under the control of aldosterone in the distal tubules. **Aldosterone** also stimulates secretion of H^+ in the distal tubules and collecting ducts. Several *organic acids* and *organic bases* are also secreted into the lumen or the renal tubules.

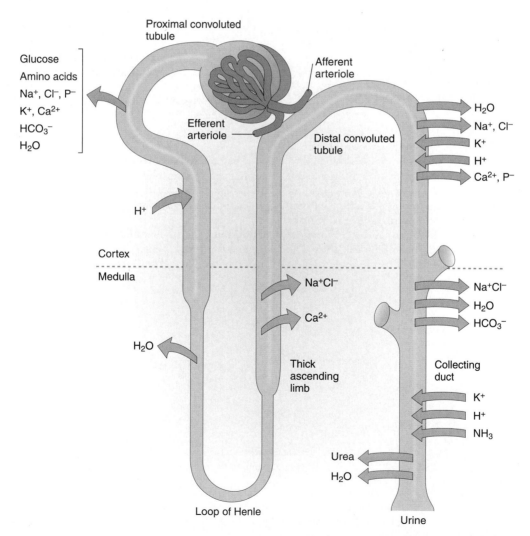

Figure 12-4 Renal handling of major minerals. The net flow of water and solutes (*arrows*) varies from one portion of the nephron to another. Aldosterone and parathyroid hormone (PTH) act on the distal tubule, and antidiuretic hormone (ADH) acts on the collecting ducts.

Passive diffusion. Water passively follows the movement of sodium and chloride in most parts of the nephron or moves toward areas of high osmolality. Diffusion of water out of the tubules can occur anywhere except in the ascending loop of Henle, which is impermeable to water. **Urea,** the concentration of which increases progressively as the filtrate passes along the collecting duct, also diffuses from the distal parts of the collecting duct into the interstitial fluid of the medulla, which has a lower concentration of urea than the lumen of the collecting ducts.

The kidneys conserve or excrete water according to the needs of the body.

Although the kidneys can concentrate urine, they are limited in how much they can concentrate it. Normal kidney cannot concentrate urine beyond 1200 mOsm/kg. Hence, to excrete the daily waste load, the kidneys must excrete 500 to 700 mL of water per day. Beyond this **obligatory minimal urine volume,** the kidneys reabsorb most of the fluid filtered in the glomeruli and thus conserve it for other purposes. On the other hand, if the body is overhydrated, the kidneys excrete several liters of water. This is primarily a result of increased extracellular fluid (ECF) content,

which stimulates osmoreceptors in the hypothalamus to release antidiuretic hormone (ADH).

Urine produced in the presence of high ADH concentration in the blood is **hyperosmotic** (Fig. 12-5). Remember that the primary glomerular filtrate is **isosmotic** with plasma (285–295 mOsm/kg). The water in the glomerular filtrate moves out of the proximal tubule in parallel with the minerals that are reabsorbed, so that the osmolality of the intratubular fluid does not change until the fluid enters the thick ascending limb of the loop of Henle and the early distal tubules. These parts of the nephron are impermeable to water, and thus the reabsorption of Na^+Cl^- is not followed by water. Accordingly the tubular fluid entering the late distal tubule is diluted. This hyposmolar tubular fluid diffuses through the wall of the late distal tubule, because it is made water-permeable by ADH. Antidiuretic hormone-mediated water diffusion continues to occur in the collecting duct as well, leading to a concentration of the tubular contents all the way to 1200 mOsm/kg.

Hypo-osmotic urine is produced in the presence of low ADH levels in blood. Antidiuretic hormone diminishes somewhat the tubular fluid in the thick ascending limb of the loop of Henle and the early distal tubule, but the most prominent effects of ADH deficiency are seen in the late distal

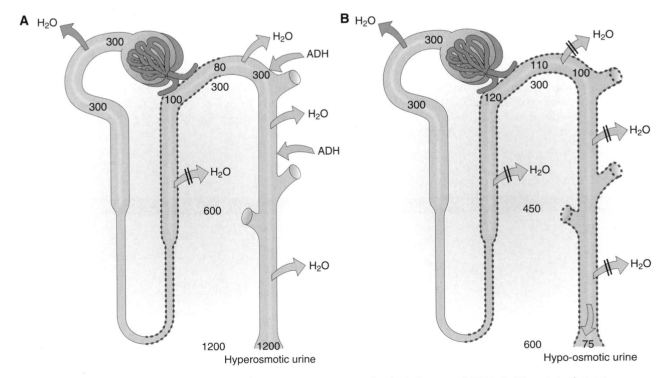

Figure 12-5 Production of hyperosmotic and hypo-osmotic urine under the influence of ADH. **A,** Diuresis in the presence of high serum antidiuretic hormone (ADH). **B,** Diuresis in the presence of no ADH. The thicker, dotted line indicates impermeability to water. P⁻, phosphate. (Modified from Constanzo LS: Physiology, Philadelphia, WB Saunders, 1998, pp. 258–259.)

tubule and the collecting duct. Without ADH these parts of the nephron become impermeable to water, and water is excreted in large amounts, thereby diluting the urine.

Serum ADH concentration may be increased or decreased. Antidiuretic hormone is increased in serum during **water deprivation,** and it is reduced following water intake. The **syndrome of inappropriate ADH secretion (SIADH),** a paraneoplastic condition, is characterized by high serum ADH, whereas in **central diabetes insipidus** due to hypothalamic or pituitary lesions, ADH is low. In **nephrogenic diabetes insipidus** serum ADH is high, since it is released from the hypothalamus in high quantities in response to high plasma osmolality.

The salient features of the main clinical conditions related to ADH water conservation or loss are listed in Table 12-2.

The kidneys can modify the excretion of sodium to maintain a constant serum concentration of sodium.

Sodium is filtered in the glomeruli in large amounts, but more than 99% of that Na^+ is reabsorbed in the nephron (Fig. 12-6). Actually, even the small amount of Na^+ that is excreted in the urine can be conserved to a great extent if need be, as is the case when extrarenal Na^+ loss increases in the gastrointestinal tract or through sweating.

Most of the reabsorption of Na^+ occurs in the **proximal tubules,** which reabsorb approximately 70% of the filtered Na^+. The rate of reabsorption can increase when Na^+ is lost through the GI tract due to vomiting or diarrhea and the ECF volume contracts. Expansion of the ECF, as occurs during infusion of isotonic saline solution, decreases tubular reabsorption and increases the urinary loss of sodium.

Sodium is also reabsorbed in the **ascending loop of Henle and the early part of the distal tubule.** The reabsorption is directly proportional to the amount of Na^+ reaching this part of the nephron. In contrast to the

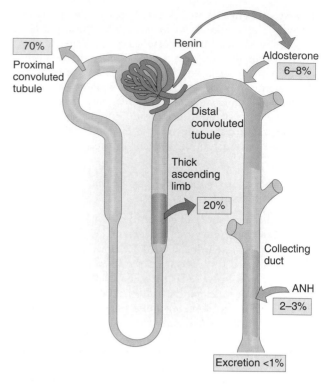

Figure 12-6 Sodium handling by the kidneys. Most of the sodium filtered in the glomeruli is reabsorbed, and less than 1% is excreted in the urine. ANH, atrial natriuretic hormone. (Modified from Constanzo LS: Physiology, Philadelphia, WB Saunders, 1998, p. 236.)

proximal tubule, this part of the nephron is not permeable to water, and the tubular fluid thus becomes diluted. Reabsorption of sodium can be inhibited by so-called loop diuretics, which are widely used in the treatment of hypertension.

Table 12-2 Antidiuretic Hormone-Related Water Loss or Conservation Syndromes

CONDITION	SERUM ADH	PLASMA OSMOLALITY	URINE OSMOLALITY	URINE OUTPUT
Water deprivation	↑	↑ or N	↑	↓
SIADH	↑	↓	↑	↓ (water "intoxication")
Polydipsia	↓	↓ to N	↓	↑ (hypo-osmotic polyuria)
Central diabetes insipidus	↓	↑	↓	↑ (hypo-osmotic polyuria)
Nephrogenic diabetes insipidus	↑	↑	↓	↑ (hypo-osmotic polyuria)

ADH, antidiuretic hormone; SIADH, syndrome of inappropriate antidiuretic hormone secretion; N, normal; ↑, high; ↓, low.

The later part of the distal tubule and the collecting ducts reabsorb 6% to 8% of filtered Na^+. Nevertheless, this part of the nephron is very important in regulating Na^+ excretion, because these cells function under the control of aldosterone. **Aldosterone** increases Na^+ reabsorption and increases K^+ secretion. **Atrial natriuretic hormone (ANH)** promotes renal Na^+ excretion by inhibiting Na^+ reabsorption in the inner medullary collecting duct. Atrial natriuretic hormone acts on other parts of the kidney, such as by dilating the afferent arterioles increasing the GFR, by increasing the medullary blood flow, and by decreasing the release of renin. Atrial natriuretic hormone also inhibits the secretion of aldosterone and the release of ADH.

Potassium excretion in the urine is predominantly regulated by aldosterone, the requirements for sodium excretion, and acid–base status.

The kidneys excrete 90% to 95% of daily K^+ intake, whereas the rest is excreted in the feces. The excretion of K^+ depends on filtration, reabsorption, and secretion, which take place in different parts of the nephron.

The serum concentration of K^+ depends on food intake and the distribution of K^+ in tissues. In alkalosis, cells release H^+ in an attempt to reduce the blood pH, and K^+ enters the cells, leading to hypokalemia. In acidosis, the opposite happens and the cells release K^+, the principal intracellular cation, and the blood is hyperkalemic. In either case the concentration of K^+ is still much lower than that of Na^+.

Both K^+ and Na^+ are filtered in the glomeruli, and the glomerular filtrate contains the same concentration of these electrolytes as the plasma. As in plasma the concentration of K^+ is much lower. Nevertheless, like sodium, the K^+ is mostly (approximately 70%) reabsorbed in the proximal tubules (Fig. 12-7). Like Na^+ it is also reabsorbed in the ascending loop of Henle and in the distal nephron. Aldosterone stimulates the distal tubule and the collecting ducts to secrete K^+, which is diametrically opposite from the effects of aldosterone on Na^+. This typically occurs when the blood concentration of potassium is increased due to high dietary intake of K^+ or in acidosis. Under normal conditions urine contains only 2% of the K^+ that was initially filtered in the glomeruli, but in hyperkalemia its concentration in urine may increase 50 times.

Calcium and phosphorus concentrations in the serum critically depend on renal excretion of these minerals.

Calcium circulates in the blood in a free form and bound to albumin. Free calcium (Ca^{2+}) is filtered in the glomeruli and most of it is reabsorbed in the proximal tubule (Fig. 12-8). The remaining Ca^{2+} reaches the distal parts of the nephron, which reabsorb most of it, allowing only 1% of the filtered Ca^{2+} to be excreted. The excretion of Ca^{2+} is under the influence of PTH, which promotes Ca^{2+} reabsorption in the distal tubule (**"hypocalciuric effect of PTH"**). Calciuria may occur in hypercalcemia, when more Ca^{2+} is filtered in the glomeruli. Natriuresis and acidosis also increase Ca^{2+} excretion in the urine.

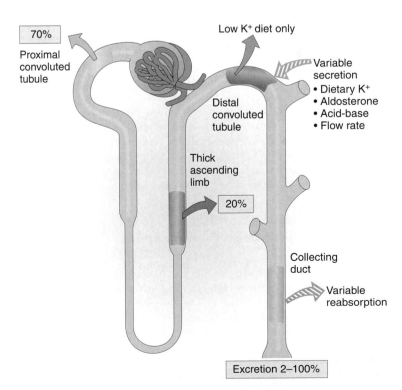

Figure 12-7 Potassium handling by the kidneys. (Modified from Constanzo LS: Physiology, Philadelphia, WB Saunders, 1998, p. 245.)

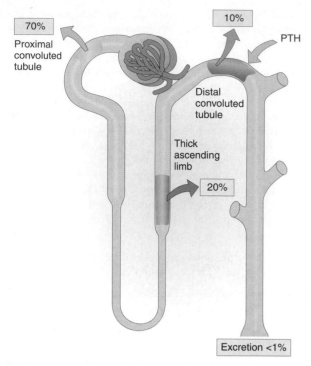

Figure 12-8 Calcium handling by the kidneys. Most of the filtered calcium is reabsorbed in the proximal tubule. The reabsorption of calcium in the distal tubules is under the influence of parathyroid hormone (PTH). Less than 1% of filtered calcium is excreted in the urine. (Modified from Constanzo LS: Physiology, Philadelphia, WB Saunders, 1998, p. 250.)

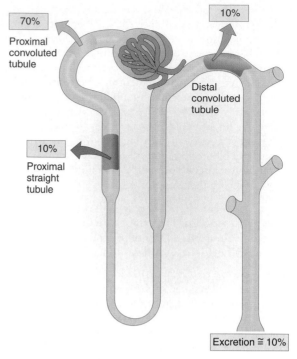

Figure 12-9 Phosphorus handling by the kidneys. Most of the filtered phosphorus is reabsorbed. Reabsorption in the distal tubule is under the influence of parathyroid hormone (PTH). Approximately 10% of phosphorus is excreted in the urine. (Modified from Constanzo LS: Physiology, Philadelphia, WB Saunders, 1998, p. 250.)

Phosphorus circulates in the blood as phosphate or bound to proteins. Phosphorus, mostly in form of phosphates, is filtered in the glomeruli, and up to 90% of it is reabsorbed in the nephron (Fig. 12-9). Most of the reabsorption (up to 70%) occurs linked to Na^+ (**"sodium–phosphate cotransport"**) in the proximal convoluted tubule and to a lesser extent (up to 10%) in the proximal straight tubule. Approximately 10% of phosphorus is absorbed in the distal tubule. Parathyroid hormone inhibits the cotransport of sodium and phosphate, promoting the excretion of phosphorus (**"phosphaturic effect of PTH"**).

The kidneys are important for the maintenance of acid–base balance.

The kidneys play an important role in the maintenance of the acid–base balance through the following mechanisms:

- **Excretion of fixed acids.** These acids are produced from incomplete oxidation of proteins, lipids, and carbohydrates.
- **Reabsorption of bicarbonate and excretion of hydrogen.** Eighty percent to 90% of bicarbonate

(HCO_3^-) filtered in the glomeruli is reclaimed in the proximal tubules. Active secretion of H^+ in the distal tubules serves to exchange H^+ for HCO_3^- and thus save the remaining 10% to 20% of filtered HCO_3^- (Fig. 12-10). Sodium is used in this interchange and is linked to the transport of K^+. Hydrogen reacts in the tubular fluid with HCO_3^-, thus forming H_2CO_3, which dissociates into CO_2 and H_2O. Free CO_2 diffuses back into the cytoplasm of the tubular cells and under the action of carbonic anhydrase again forms HCO_3^-, which is returned into the blood.

- **Excretion of ammonia and phosphate.** Hydrogen ions excreted into the tubular fluid must be buffered, which is achieved by the secretion of ammonia and filtered phosphates (Fig. 12-11).

The kidneys excrete metabolic waste products, drugs, and toxins.

The kidneys excrete many metabolic waste products, drugs, and toxins. Among these the most important are urea and creatinine, two major end products of intermediary metabolism.

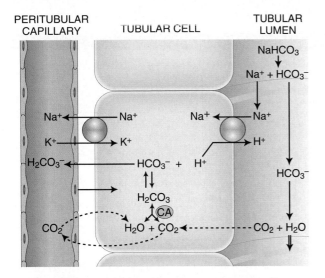

Figure 12-10 Bicarbonate recovery by the kidneys. Bicarbonate cannot be reabsorbed directly, but it is reclaimed from the glomerular filtrate in exchange for hydrogen ions (H^+). Carbonic anhydrase (CA) forms bicarbonate (HCO_3^-) from the CO_2, which has diffused into the cytoplasm of tubular cells. Bicarbonate then returns into the blood to serve as a buffer. This interchange is linked to the flux of sodium (Na^+) and potassium (K^+) mediated by an Na^+/K^+ ATPase.

Urea. It is filtered in the glomeruli, and approximately one half of it is reabsorbed in the proximal tubule. The ascending loops of Henle secrete urea into the lumen, the distal tubules resorb 30%, and then finally the inner medullary collecting duct resorbs large amounts of the remaining urea. Hence only 15% of the filtered urea is excreted. In conditions that increase urine production urea excretion may increase up to 60% of the filtered urea concentration.

Creatinine (Cr). Most of Cr is thus derived from creatine phosphate in skeletal muscles; a small fraction is from the heart. Ingestion of meat may increase the concentration of creatinine. It is filtered in the glomeruli and excreted without further processing in the distal tubules. A small amount of Cr is secreted in the tubules, but this amount is negligible, and thus Cr is used for measuring the GFR.

The kidneys have endocrine functions.

Kidney cells respond to hormones, but at the same time the kidneys are also a source of major hormones. Previously we mentioned that the kidneys respond to aldosterone, PTH, ADH, and angiotensin II. The kidneys produce several hormones, the most important of which are

- **Renin.** This blood-regulating hormone is produced by the JG apparatus cells. It acts on angiotensinogen, transforming it into angiotensin I. Angiotensin I is transformed into angiotensin II through the action of angiotensin-converting enzyme. Angiotensin II acts on the adrenal cortex to produce aldosterone. At the same time angiotensin II is a potent vasoconstrictor and has several other effects on the kidneys.
- **Erythropoietin.** This hormone acts a growth factor for erythroid precursors of the bone marrow and also promotes differentiation and maturation of these cells.
- **1,25(OH)$_2$D$_3$ vitamin.** This active form of vitamin D is produced in the kidneys and released into the circulation, where, in tandem with PTH, it regulates the homeostasis, absorption, and deposition of calcium.

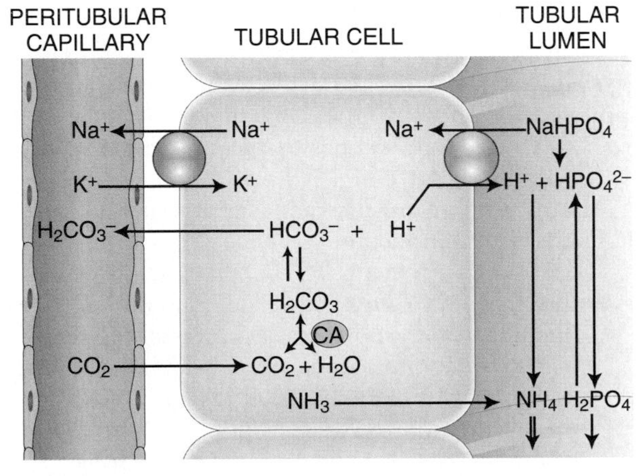

Clinical and Laboratory Evaluation of Renal Disease

FAMILY AND PERSONAL HISTORY

Family and personal history can point to some important risk factors that play a role in the pathogenesis of renal diseases. A few examples of such links and associations are given in Table 12-3.

PHYSICAL EXAMINATION AND HISTORY OF PRESENT DISEASE

Symptoms and signs of renal diseases depend on the type of disease and on the location of the lesions. The most important signs and symptoms are as follows:

- Pain
- Frequent urination
- Polyuria

Figure 12-11 Buffering of excreted hydrogen ions (H^+). Hydrogen excreted into the fluid in the lumen of the tubules must be buffered so that the pH of urine does not become too acidic. This is accomplished by formation of phosphate and ammonia buffers. CA, carbonic anhydrase.

Table 12-3 Risk Factors for Renal Diseases

TYPE OF RISK FACTOR	SPECIFIC DISEASES—RISK FACTOR ASSOCIATIONS
Hereditary factors	Autosomal dominant polycystic kidney disease Autosomal recessive polycystic kidney disease Sickle cell anemia: Papillary necrosis Familial form of Wilms' tumor
Social factors/infections	Drug addiction: Focal glomerulosclerosis HIV: HIV nephropathy Bacterial endocarditis: Glomerulonephritis in IV drug users
Other systemic diseases or diseases of other organ systems	Diabetes mellitus: Diabetic nephropathy Multiple myeloma: Myeloma kidney disease or renal/systemic amyloidosis Chronic suppuration: Amyloidosis
Environment	Hot climate: Higher incidence of renal stones in the "stone belt" states in the southern United States
Surgical procedures	Surgery: Prerenal renal failure Renal transplantation: Transplant rejection Urinary tract surgery/instrumentation: Ascending urinary tract infections
Drugs	Analgesic abuse: Analgesic nephropathy Antibiotics: Acute tubulointerstitial nephritis as a hypersensitivity reaction
Pregnancy	Acute ascending pyelonephritis Eclampsia: Proteinuria and renal hypertension

HIV, human immunodeficiency virus; IV, intravenous.

- Oliguria/anuria
- Dysuria and urinary retention
- Incontinence
- Edema
- Hypertension

Pain may originate from any part of the urinary system.

Pain caused by urinary tract diseases may originate from the kidneys, ureters, or the urinary bladder and urethra.

Renal pain. It is dull and visceral and is felt in the flank and lower back. It may be caused by mass lesions such as renal tumors or cysts, or acute enlargement of the kidneys due to acute pyelonephritis, glomerulonephritis (GN), or tubulointerstitial nephritis. Circulatory disturbances such as infarct of the kidney due to emboli or renal vein thrombosis also cause pain. Hemorrhage from trauma is associated with acute pain.

Ureteric colic. Colic is caused by spastic contraction of the ureter due to an obstruction. Such obstructions may be related to an impacted stone, intraluminal blood clot, sloughed-off renal papillae in papillary necrosis, or tumors. The pain may be felt in the flank, upper or lower abdomen, and pelvis, or it may radiate into the groin and scrotum. Ureteric obstruction initiates the so-called ureteric–renal reflex, which results in a constriction of renal arteries and reduced production of urine.

Bladder pain. Pain is typically caused by an obstruction of the bladder outlet and is felt inside the pelvis. It is often associated with disturbances of urination, such as increased frequency, hematuria, or inability to urinate. Bladder pain may be caused by stones, tumors, or acute or chronic cystitis.

Frequency of urination and the volume of urine produced vary under normal conditions and if increased may be a sign of disease.

Normal kidneys produce about 1500 mL of urine per day. Since the urinary bladder has the capacity to hold approximately 500 mL and is somewhat smaller in women, a normal person has the need to urinate four to six times a day.

The frequency of urination and total urine output depend on several factors, including

- **Fluid intake.** Fluid intake depends on individual drinking habits and may be increased considerably under stress or in psychogenic polydipsia, a condition characterized by compulsive drinking. Bear in mind that alcoholic beverages contain not only alcohol but also water, and that a typical heavy beer drinker may consume huge amounts of extra water a day.
- **Extrarenal fluid loss.** Fluid may be lost due to insensible evaporation (e.g., in airplanes), increased sweating (e.g., hot weather), and gastrointestinal loss (e.g., diarrhea or vomiting).

- **Renal function.** Loss of renal function may reduce or increase the volume of urine. Polyuria is associated with increased frequency of urination.
- **Capacity of the urinary bladder.** The bladder is somewhat smaller in women than in men, but even so its capacity varies from one person to another. Chronic infections and hypertrophy due to obstruction of the bladder neck reduce the capacity of the bladder.
- **Drugs.** Diuretics and many other drugs affect the renal handling of salts and water and thus influence urine production.
- **Local conditions modifying the micturition reflex.** The micturition reflex is initiated by stimuli acting on sensory nerves in the posterior urethra and bladder neck. Irritation of these nerve endings by inflammation, urinary stones, or prostatic hyperplasia is associated with increased frequency.
- **Frequent urination (pollakisuria)** can be divided clinically into two major groups: urination with polyuria and urination without polyuria. The causes of polyuria are listed in Table 12-4.

Urgency is a need to urinate even when the urinary bladder is not full.

The need to urinate even when the urinary bladder is not completely full is usually a sign of disease, although it may be psychogenic and a sign of nervousness. Urgency typically results from the increased sensitivity of the stretch sensors in the posterior bladder neck and posterior urethra. It is most often caused by inflammation or prostatic hyperplasia.

One should recall that the emptying of the bladder is physiologically regulated by a **micturition reflex,** which is initiated by the intravesical pressure acting on the stretch receptors in the bladder neck and posterior urethra. The sensory impulses cause contraction of the detrusor muscle, followed by "self-regeneratively" increased sensitivity of the sensors. Thus a new cycle is initiated and followed by yet another cycle. The reflex can be overcome voluntarily, but as the filling of the urinary bladder continues and the pressure rises, each reflex cycle becomes shorter and more intense, until the point is reached when the micturition cannot be prevented voluntarily. At that point, another reflex is activated, leading to the relaxation of the external sphincter and the beginning of the urination. In pathologic conditions this reflex is hyperactive and cannot be controlled voluntarily as easily as under normal conditions.

Polyuria results from increased water intake or the inability of the body to hold water.

Urine production exceeding 3000 mL/day is considered polyuria. It may be caused by increased water intake, abnormal regulation of water maintenance, or abnormal water excretion (see Table 12-3). Pathogenetically polyuria may be related to the following mechanisms:

Table 12-4 Causes of Frequent Urination

FREQUENT URINATION WITHOUT POLYURIA	FREQUENT URINATION WITH POLYURIA

Congenital disorders
  Congenitally small bladder
  Ureterovesical reflux in girls
  Congenital stricture of meatus or urethra
Aging related changes
  Atrophic vaginitis
  Pelvic floor relaxation
  Cystocele
  Prostatic hyperplasia
Inflammation
  Cystitis
  Prostatitis
  Vulvitis–vaginitis
Mechanical irritation
  Urinary stones
  External compression (e.g., pregnancy)
Neoplasms
  Bladder cancer
  Prostatic neoplasia
  Gynecologic cancer
Neurologic diseases
  Multiple sclerosis
  Spinal cord injury
  Autonomic neuropathy (e.g., diabetes)
	Congenital renal tubular diseases
	Psychogenic or intentional polydipsia
	Central diabetes insipidus
	  Hypothalamic lesions (e.g., tumors, meningitis, trauma, surgery)
	  Stalk lesions (e.g., trauma, surgery)
	  Pituitary lesions (e.g., tumors of the anterior pituitary, surgery, trauma)
	Renal diabetes insipidus (e.g., chronic renal diseases)
	  Glycosuria (e.g., diabetes)
	  Metabolic disorders (e.g., hypercalcemia, hypokalemia)
	  Drugs (e.g., lithium, diuretics)
	  Alcohol, caffeine

- **Excessive water intake.** Some people drink habitually large quantities of water, tea and coffee, or beer and other alcoholic beverages. Psychogenic polydipsia is characterized by compulsive drinking of water in large quantities.
- **Osmotic diuresis.** The most common cause of osmotic diuresis is hyperglycemia of diabetes mellitus. Some diuretic acts the same way.
- **Abnormal water excretion.** The most common cause of this form of polyuria is chronic renal failure, which leads to nephrogenic diabetes insipidus. The kidneys lose the capacity to conserve water. Metabolic diseases such as hypokalemia or hypercalcemia also may cause polyuria. Central diabetes insipidus due to ADH deficiency is an important but fortunately rare cause of polyuria.

Nocturia is a form of polyuria characterized by an urge to urinate during the night. Normal persons produce less urine while asleep, so that they do not usually need to get up to urinate during the night. The common causes of nocturia are as follows:

- **Polyuria of any type.** Excessive production of urine usually disrupts the normal wake/sleep cycle of urine production and causes polyuria.
- **Drugs.** Many diuretics increase nocturnal urine production. Drugs that improve cardiac functions could have the same effects.
- **Excessive drinking of water or alcohol.** These are the most common causes of nocturia.
- **Edematous states.** Edema accumulation in several chronic conditions, such as congestive heart failure, cirrhosis, or chronic renal failure, predisposes to nocturia. The fluid accumulating in the lower extremities and the abdomen is mobilized by lying down, returns into the venous circulation, and is excreted in the kidneys.
- **Urinary/pelvic problems.** Reduced capacity of the urinary bladder due to chronic inflammation or muscular hypertrophy of the bladder wall may cause an urge to urinate during the night. This is most common in elderly persons with prostatic hyperplasia or chronic cystitis. Pelvic floor relaxation on reclining is a cause of frequency in sleeping women who have had previous pelvic surgery or complications of pregnancy.

Urination may be painful, incomplete, or associated with obvious changes in the appearance of urine.

The most important disturbances of urination are dysuria, urinary retention, and incontinence.

Dysuria. It refers to pain, which may occur during, before, or immediately after micturition. The patients describe the feeling as "burning" or urgency to urinate. It may be associated with increased frequency of urination, hesitancy, or incomplete evacuation of urine. Most often it is caused by cystitis.

Retention of urine. Incomplete evacuation of urine may be noticed by the patient, but it may be also demonstrated as residual urine by ultrasound or by catheterization after the patient has voluntarily emptied the bladder. It usually results from obstruction of the bladder neck, as occurs in prostatic hyperplasia, or a loss of strength of the detrusor muscle, as happens in chronic cystitis. **Acute urinary retention** due to bladder obstruction may be painful. **Chronic retention** develops gradually and is either asymptomatic or associated with incontinence or a frequent urge to urinate. It is more common in men than women. If the volume of residual urine exceeds 100 mL, the risk of infection is increased.

Changes in the color of urine. Urine is normally clear and yellow due to its content of urea. Concentrated urine appears darker yellow, but the real changes in the color of urine are related to substances found in it. **Deep yellow** urine may be a consequence of tetracycline ingestion. **Cloudy white** urine is usually related to increased amounts of phosphates, and it clears on the addition of acid. It may be also due to bacteria, pus, or desquamation of epithelial cells from the bladder. **Orange urine** may reflect high concentration of bilirubin, rhubarb, cathartics like senna, or anthracycline. **Red urine** may be caused by beets, blackberries, food colors in candies, cathartics like phenolphthalein and cascara, and drugs such as rifampin. Freshly voided urine may be red due to hemoglobinuria or myoglobinuria. **Blue-green** urine may be due to bilirubin/biliverdin, methylene blue, or infection with *Pseudomonas aeruginosa*. **Brown or black** urine after standing is caused by porphyrin, melanin, or homogentisic acid.

Incontinence is involuntary passage of urine that may occur due to many reasons.

Normally, during the filling of the bladder the sympathetic impulses predominate, leading to a relaxation of the detrusor muscle and contraction of the internal sphincter (Fig. 12-12). The external sphincter is under voluntary control. During urination the cholinergic impulses predominate, stimulating the contraction of the detrusor muscle and the relaxation of the internal sphincter. The reduced sympathetic impulses contribute to bladder emptying. This control of urination may be lost under many conditions and lead to incontinence ("inability to retain urine").

The pathogenesis of incontinence varies from one person to another and includes among others

- **Inadequate sphincter control.** This is seen physiologically in small children but may occur occasionally in adults as well ("stress incontinence").
- **Overflow incontinence.** This typically occurs in urinary retention due to prostatic hyperplasia or uterine prolapse with compression of the urinary bladder in females.
- **Urge incontinence.** An inability to delay urination is found in patients with urinary bladder diseases, prostatic hyperplasia, or neurologic diseases.

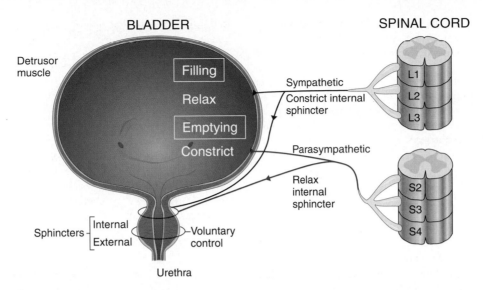

Figure 12-12 Control of bladder function. During the filling of the bladder sympathetic impulses cause relaxation of the detrusor muscle and constriction of the internal sphincter. Cholinergic impulses predominate during urination, causing constriction of the detrusor and relaxation of the internal sphincter. The external sphincter is under voluntary control.

■ **Neurologic disturbances.** A loss of urinary sensation and autonomic innervation is seen in autonomic neuropathy of diabetes, and many chronic neurologic diseases, such as multiple sclerosis or Parkinson's disease, or dementia.

■ **Loss of consciousness.** Comatose patients have no voluntary control of the external sphincter.

■ **Drugs.** Deep anesthesia and many psychotropic drugs are typically associated with loss of bladder control. The mechanisms include loss of voluntary control and the effects on the sympathetic or parasympathetic part of the bladder control.

■ **Stress incontinence.** Urine leaks when abdominal pressure is increased. The underlying cause is usually urethral sphincter weakness or pelvic floor weakness in multiparous women.

■ **Old age.** In the elderly, incontinence is usually multifactorial, but even with the most intensive examinations sometimes it is not possible to find its true cause and it must be labeled as **idiopathic.** Loss of mental function and the inability to reach the toilet in time because of restricted mobility are common causes of incontinence in the elderly. Congestive heart failure or fecal impaction in the rectum may be the cause or incontinence in some cases.

The most common causes of incontinence are listed in Table 12-5.

In the work-up for a patient who has incontinence it is important to determine whether it is related to an urge to urinate, and to identify the conditions under which it occurs. The patients are usually asked to keep a detailed "bladder journal" for at least 2 weeks to help identify the

Table 12-5 Clinically Important Causes of Incontinence

Infants and small children (normal to a certain age)
Infections
  Cystitis
  Urethritis
  Prostatitis
Tumors and related conditions
  Benign prostatic hyperplasia
  Tumors of the prostate, bladder
  Rectal tumors invading sacral plexus
  Gynecologic cancer
  Spinal cord tumors ("cauda equina syndrome")
  Epidural cord compression
Mechanical/traumatic events
  Childbirth injury of pelvic floor
  Sphincter injury
  Cystocele
Neurologic diseases
  Stroke
  Spinal cord injury
  Dementia
  Multiple sclerosis
Autonomic and peripheral neuropathies (e.g., diabetes)
Muscular paralysis
Drugs
Idiopathic/multifactorial
  Stress incontinence
  Old age incontinence

possible causes. A detailed medical history, including the review of medications, and a complete physical examination are required to identify possibly treatable causes of incontinence.

Enuresis is a special form of incontinence that occurs during sleep. **Primary enuresis** in childhood is a failure to attain full bladder control. **Secondary enuresis** develops in persons who had full control, but have lost it due to some known or unknown reasons.

Edema resulting from renal disease is caused by hypoalbuminemia and reduced osmotic pressure of the plasma or water retention.

Edema, an accumulation of fluids in extracellular spaces, is a common feature of renal diseases. It is especially prominent in nephrotic and acute nephritic syndrome.

In nephritic syndrome it tends to appear rapidly, whereas in nephrotic syndrome it usually develops insidiously.

The edema of nephrotic syndrome is a consequence of glomerular injury, which leads to increased filtration of albumin into the urinary space and the lumen of the proximal tubules (Fig. 12-13). Large quantities of albumin in the glomerular filtrate cannot be absorbed by the proximal tubules, resulting in proteinuria. Depletion of albumin from the circulation results in hypoalbuminemia and consequent reduction of the colloid osmotic pressure of the plasma. The fluid cannot be retained in the circulation, and thus water leaks into the interstitial spaces. Reduced plasma volume elicits a hormonal adaptive response, including excretion of ADH, atrial natriuretic hormone, and renin. The net effect is retention of Na^+ and water, which still cannot be retained in the circulation, thus aggravating the edema.

Hypertension in renal disease is initiated by a release of renin.

Arterial hypertension is a common complication of renal diseases. Renal diseases are the most common cause of secondary hypertension. Hypertension of sudden onset is a constant feature of acute glomerulonephritis, but it is also found in end-stage kidney disease. Problems with renal perfusion in polycystic kidney disease, or in the scarred kidneys characteristic of chronic pyelonephritis, have the same consequences. Narrowing of the orifices of the renal arteries in atherosclerosis is a cause of chronic renal failure and hypertension.

Renal hypertension may be mediated through the renin–angiotensin–aldosterone system or it may be multifactorial, as in chronic renal disease.

Renin-mediated hypertension may occur in several diseases known to be associated with an increased production of renin. The most important of these conditions are as follows:

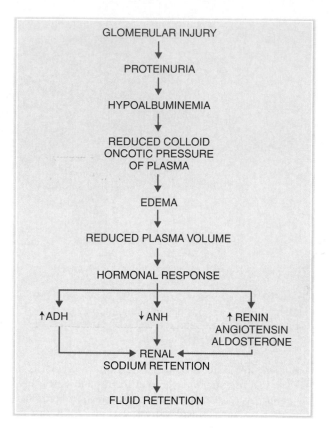

Figure 12-13 Pathogenesis of edema in nephrotic syndrome. Edema is predominantly caused by a loss of serum albumin, the primary oncotic protein preventing the escape of water from blood vessels. Reduced plasma volume elicits a hormonal reaction, which further contributes to sodium and water retention in the kidneys. ADH, antidiuretic hormone; ANH, atrial natriuretic hormone.

- **Renal artery stenosis.** This form of hypertension, often called **renovascular hypertension,** may be related to congenital changes in the renal arteries (e.g., fibromuscular dysplasia of the renal arteries) or acquired, as in atherosclerosis involving the orifices of the renal arteries as they exit the aorta. External compression of the renal arteries is a rare cause of hyper-reninemia.
- **Reduced arterial pressure.** Hypotension caused by congestive heart failure acts as a stimulus on mechanoreceptors in the afferent arterioles of the glomeruli, stimulating the synthesis of renin in the juxtaglomerular apparatus. Such conditions are also associated with a reduced delivery of sodium to the macula densa portion of the distal tubule, which also stimulates renin release.
- **Reduce glomerular blood flow.** These changes are typically seen in acute glomerulonephritis, an inflammatory disease characterized by increased

glomerular cellularity. Inflammatory reaction leads to a narrowing of glomerular capillaries. The glomerular filtration surfaces are covered by inflammatory cells and immune complexes, and thus the glomerular filtration rate is reduced. Accordingly, less Na^+ reaches the sensors in the macula densa, which stimulates the renin-producing cells to release renin.

Hypertension of chronic renal failure is usually multifactorial. It occurs in chronic glomerulonephritis, chronic pyelonephritis, chronic diabetic renal disease, polycystic kidney disease, and any other kidney disease associated with a reduced renal mass. The causes of hypertension are not fully understood but include

- **Reduced glomerular filtration rate.** Loss of glomeruli leads to a retention of salt and water, resulting in an expansion of the plasma volume. **Salt and water retention** are the most important reasons for hypertension in these patients.
- **Increased peripheral vascular resistance.** Even though increased peripheral vascular resistance involving arterioles and capillaries is one of the most common abnormalities in renal hypertension, its pathogenesis is not fully understood. It has been proposed that it results from inhibition of Na^+/K^+ **ATPase** due to increased extracellular fluid, but the real cause of vascular changes is unknown. **Endothelin**, a potent vasoconstrictor, is increased in chronic renal failure, probably because its inhibitors have been inactivated.
- **Vasoconstriction.** This is in part related to **"nephroangiosclerosis"** (i.e., arteriolosclerosis and fibrosis of the renal artery branches), which increases the intrarenal resistance to blood flow. A loss of **renal vasodilatory substances** produced in the renal medulla, such as medullipin, prostaglandins, and kinins, probably also contributes to vasoconstriction.
- **Sympathetic nervous system. Sympathetic overreactivity** may in part be due to the overstimulation of the sympathetic nervous system in renal failure or be due to **reduced clearance** of epinephrine and norepinephrine in the urine.
- **Activation of the renin–angiotensin–aldosterone system.** In many patients with chronic renal disease, renin production is normal. However, some patients overproduce renin, which is most likely secondary to the disturbances in the handling of Na^+ and water.

Renal hypertension should be suspected in the presence of chronic renal insufficiency or other signs of uremia. It should be also considered in elderly patients who have hypertension of sudden onset or hypertension that has become resistant to conventional medical treatment.

URINALYSIS

The diagnosis of renal disease is to great extent based on laboratory findings. Thus it is important to examine not only the blood but also the urine and carefully search for signs of kidney or urinary tract disease.

Routine urinalysis includes gross examination of the urine, biochemical analysis, and microscopic examination of the urinary sediment. In some instances the volume of the total daily urinary output must be measured. Bacteriologic studies may be indicated if infection is suspected. Special biochemical tests are indicted in cases of suspected metabolic diseases (e.g., porphyria) or paraneoplastic kidney diseases (e.g., detection of immunoglobulin light chains in multiple myeloma or vanillylmandelic acid [VMA] in pheochromocytoma). Cytopathologic examination is indicated in patients who might have tumors of the urinary system.

The most important abnormalities detected by urinalysis are as follows:

- Changes in the urine volume and composition
- Proteinuria
- Glycosuria
- Hematuria
- Abnormal urinary sediment
- Abnormal bacteriologic findings

Routine urinalysis includes physical and chemical analysis of the urine and microscopic examination of the urinary sediment.

Routine examination of the urine is one of the most common laboratory tests performed in the doctor's office or the hospital. It includes inspection of the urine, dipstick analysis for pH and some common analytes, and microscopic examination of the urinary sediment. Normal urine has the following properties:

- **Color.** The urine is normally clear and straw-colored. The most common cause of color changes is drugs, but the color may also change due to various metabolites such as bilirubin, hemoglobin, and porphyrins, and among others.
- **Clarity.** The normal urine is clear. Turbidity most often results from precipitation of solutes, and less commonly from the presence of leukocytes, erythrocytes, and bacteria. Urates precipitate in acid urine, whereas phosphates tend to precipitate in alkaline urine. Turbid urine must be examined microscopically to determine the cause of this change.
- **pH.** Normal urine is slightly acidic and has a pH 4.5 to 7.5. The pH of urine varies, and thus the first urine collected in the morning it is usually more acidic due to retention of CO_2 during sleep. Postprandial urine is alkaline because of the excretion of hydrochloric acid into the stomach. The most common cause of

alkaline urine is bacteria, which are found in the presence of infection. Proteinuria may render urine acidic. Increased excretion of ammonia in acidosis lowers the pH of urine, whereas decreased excretion of ammonia in metabolic alkalosis makes the urine alkalotic. Increased excretion of HCO_3^- in respiratory alkalosis makes the urine alkaline.

■ **Specific gravity.** Normal urine contains minerals and low-molecular-weight compounds such as urea and thus has a low specific gravity in the range from 1.016 to 1.022. Urea accounts for 20%, chloride for 25%, and phosphate and sulfate for 15% of the specific gravity. A low specific gravity of urine below 1.007 (**hyposthenuria**) results from excess water excretion or renal inability to concentrate urine in various tubular diseases. Increased specific gravity (**hypersthenuria**) results from high-molecular-weight molecules such as proteins, glucose, or radiographic contrast material. **Isosthenuria** is characterized by a fixed urine specific gravity of 1.010 and is typically a sign of severe renal injury and loss of the ability to concentrate urine.

■ **Protein.** Normal urine contains less than 100 mg/L of protein. The dipstick method, which is inexpensive but not too sensitive, can detect protein in excess of 150 to 300 mg/L. Note that concentrated urine may give positive results even in the absence of proteinuria. On the other hand, a large volume of urine may dilute the protein concentration, thus giving a negative result. Bence Jones protein does not react with the dipstick and thus may be missed with this approach.

■ **Glucose.** Normal urine does not contain glucose, because it is reabsorbed from the glomerular filtrate in the proximal tubules. Glucose is detected in urine as a reducing substance in a copper reduction or enzymatic tests. The **copper reduction test** may become positive even in the presence of other reducing substances, such as other sugars (e.g., lactose, fructose), ascorbic acid, uric acid, creatinine, and various drug metabolites. **Glucose oxidase strips** do not give these false positive results and are specific for glucose. Ascorbic acid and ketones may inhibit the test, however, resulting in false negative results.

■ **Blood.** The urine does not contain blood, but the urinary sediment may contain up to two erythrocytes and up to two white blood cells per high-power field. The presence of RBCs is a sign of hematuria, whereas WBCs are a good indication of bacterial infection. A WBC count in excess of 50 per high-power field is a reliable sign of acute bacterial infection, whereas lower counts are usually found in chronic or localized infection. Bacteria form nitrites from nitrates, and thus a **nitrite test** is positive in infected urine.

Pearl

> Normal urine is negative for acetone ("Ace test"), ketone bodies, bilirubin ("Ictotest"), hemoglobin, and nitrite, but contains urobilinogen.

Proteinuria is a sign of renal or lower urinary tract disease.

Normal persons excrete less than 150 mg of proteins in urine. As indicated earlier the glomeruli do not allow the passage of plasma proteins exceeding the molecular weight of albumin, which has a molecular weight of 68,000 daltons. Furthermore most of the low-molecular-weight proteins and amino acids that are filtered in the urinary space are absorbed in the proximal tubules. Proteins found in urine collected over 24 hours include albumin (20–30 mg), low-molecular-weight proteins filtered in the glomeruli (10–20 mg), and proteins secreted by the distal tubule such as Tamm-Horsfall protein and IgA (40–60 mg). Proteins released from the cytoplasm of epithelial cells desquamated from the lining of the urinary system also contribute to the total protein content of urine.

Proteinuria may result from increased permeability of the glomerular capillary wall or defective reabsorption of proteins in the proximal tubules. Such proteinuria may be clinically classified as mild (<500 mg/24 hours), moderate (<3 g/24 hours), or severe (>3 g/24 hours) (Table 12-6).

Table 12-6 Clinically Important Causes of Proteinuria

MILD PROTEINURIA (<500 mg/24 hr)	MODERATE PROTEINURIA (<3 g/24 hr)	SEVERE PROTEINURIA (>3 g/24 hr)
Fever	Urinary tract infection	Preeclampsia
Hypertension	Chronic pyelonephritis	Nephrotic syndrome
Obstructive uropathy	Acute glomerulonephritis	Diabetic nephropathy
Diabetic kidney disease	Chronic glomerulonephritis	Multiple myeloma
Chronic pyelonephritis	Acute tubular necrosis	Amyloidosis

Hematuria, or blood in the urine, may be macroscopic and diagnosed by naked eye examination or it may be visible only microscopically.

Hematuria is the appearance of blood in the urine. If grossly visible during urination or on naked eye examination of the urine, it is called macroscopic. Macroscopic hematuria originates mostly from the urethra and the bladder: initial hematuria is of urethral origin, terminal hematuria is from the bladder neck and trigonum, and total hematuria is of either bladder or renal origin. Microscopic hematuria is defined as a finding of more than four red blood cells per high-power field during the examination of the urinary sediment. It is typically diagnosed by examining fresh urine after centrifugation—the sediment is found in the final drop of urine that remains after is centrifuged urine has been decanted. Microscopic hematuria is an important sign of renal disease, but it may be caused by minor bleeding due to cystitis or irritation of the bladder. Hematuria of glomerular origin is associated with changes in the morphology of RBCs ("dysmorphic RBC") and their fragmentation, as well as the formation of RBC casts. Bleeding from the lower urinary tract does not affect the morphology of RBCs.

The most important causes of hematuria are urinary stones (20%), malignant tumors (15%), bacterial infections of the urinary bladder (10%), and prostatic hyperplasia (10% of hematuria in men). Clinically important causes of hematuria are listed in Table 12-7.

Glycosuria is, in most instances, a consequence of hyperglycemia.

Glucose is a low-molecular-weight molecule that is filtered in the glomeruli, so that its concentration in the glomerular filtrate is the same as in the plasma. All the glucose filtered in the glomeruli is absorbed in the proximal tubules. Glycosuria appears when the concentration of glucose in the blood exceeds approximately 200 mg/dL, at which point its concentration in the glomerular filtrate exceeds the absorptive capacity of the proximal tubules. Hence, glycosuria is in most instances a consequence of hyperglycemia, and it is most often caused by **diabetes mellitus.** Inborn defects of tubular function are a rare cause of **renal tubular glycosuria.** These relatively rare childhood diseases may be associated with other abnormalities, such as amino aciduria and phosphaturia.

Bacteriologic studies should be performed only on fresh and properly collected urine.

The urinary tract is in contact with the external environment, and thus the distal portion of the urethra normally contains bacteria. Small numbers of bacteria may gain access to the bladder as well, more commonly in women than in men, because the female urethra is relatively short.

Bacteriologic studies must be performed on freshly collected urine, which should be placed on bacteriologic plates as soon as possible. Infection is confirmed if the urine contains more than 100,000 bacterial colonies per milliliter of urine. In symptomatic patients even lower numbers of bacteria may be taken as evidence of infection.

Urine that has not been refrigerated after collection but was sitting at room temperature for more than 2 hours almost invariably shows an increased number of

Table 12-7 Clinically Important Causes of Hematuria

Renal and ureteric diseases
    Glomerulonephritis
    Polycystic kidney disease
    Suppurative inflammation (e.g., pyelonephritis)
    Papillary necrosis
    Renal infarcts
    Renal or ureteric stones
    Tumors
Urinary bladder and urethral diseases
    Cystitis, prostatitis, urethritis
    Urinary stones
    Instrumentation (e.g., cystoscopy, catheterization)
    Therapy related—surgery, radiation therapy, cytotoxic drugs
    Tumors
Hematologic bleeding disorders
    Hemophilia
    Thrombocytopenia (e.g., leukemia, TTP, DIC)
    Sickle cell anemia
Trauma

DIC, disseminated intravascular coagulation; TTP, thrombotic thrombocytopenic purpura.

bacteria. Fresh urine may also be examined microscopically, and if more than 20 bacteria are seen in the urinary sediment per high-power field, one may conclude that an infection is present, especially if the sediment also contains WBCs.

Urine must be collected in conditions that are as aseptic as possible. To this end the external orifice of the urethra must be cleaned, and a "midstream" urine sample collected. Fractionated urine collection, which may be combined with prostatic massage, is performed in some cases. Finally, in some cases it is necessary to use catheters to collect urine, which reduces the chances of contaminating urine. Collection of urine in small children is an especially complicated procedure.

Pearl

> Catheterization is not an absolutely risk-free procedure. It is associated with subsequent infection in 1% to 3% of patients. Indwelling catheters account for a huge number of hospital-acquired infections.

RENAL FUNCTION TESTS

The function of the renal glomeruli and tubules can be assessed by measuring the efficiency at which the kidneys clear the blood of waste products such as creatinine and urea and by estimating the ability of the kidneys to concentrate urine.

Creatinine clearance is proportionate to the glomerular filtration rate and thus is the most widely used test for assessing renal function.

Creatinine, a cyclic anhydride of creatine, is a low-molecular-weight normal by-product of muscle metabolism. It is formed from creatine and creatine phosphate in the muscles at a constant rate of 20 mg/kg of body weight. Creatinine released from the muscles into the blood is excreted almost exclusively by the kidneys, and thus it can serve as a marker of renal function. Intestinal excretion accounts for 2% of creatinine excretion and can be ignored in most instances. The measurement of creatinine in urine collected over 24 hours is the most widely used test for checking whether the 24-hour urine collection was properly performed.

Creatinine production is constant for each individual, but it depends on the muscle mass of the body. Thus it is normally higher in men than in women, and in muscular than asthenic or undernourished persons. Creatinine production decreases with age, since muscle mass has a tendency to decrease with age. However, since the creatinine clearance also decreases with age, the plasma concentration of creatinine remains in the normal range of 0.6 to 1.2 mg/dL (53–106 μmol/L) throughout adult life.

Glomerular filtration accounts for 85% of renal excretion of creatinine, and thus creatinine clearance provides a reliable measure of glomerular filtration rate (GFR). Tubular secretion accounts for a small fraction (15%) of total urinary creatinine content. This aspect of creatinine excretion becomes important only in advanced chronic renal failure when it may account for 50% of total creatinine excretion.

Creatinine clearance (C_{Cr}) is the most widely used test of glomerular filtration rate. C_{Cr} is expressed in milliliters per minute (mL/min), and it is normally in the range of 95 to 105 mL/min/1.75 m². It is calculated by measuring creatinine concentration in the plasma (P_{Cr}) and urine (U_{Cr}) and the amount of urine produced during one minute (V_U). Since the production of urine varies during the day, the V_U is calculated from the total 24-hour urine divided by 1440 (24 hours × 60 minutes = 1440 minutes).

If one assumes that the GFR is the total volume of blood cleared of creatinine, then the amount of creatinine in plasma should equal the amount of creatinine in urine:

$$C_{Cr} \times P_C = V_U \times U_C$$

or stated otherwise

$$C_{Cr} = \frac{U_{Cr} \times V_U}{P_{Cr}}$$

where,

C_{Cr} = creatinine clearance in mL/min
U_{Cr} = concentration of creatinine in urine in mg/dL
V_U = volume of urine in mL/min, calculated from the total urine volume collected over 24 hours divided by 1440 minutes
P_{Cr} = concentration of creatinine in plasma in mg/dL

Since creatinine production is proportionate to total muscle mass, creatinine clearance can be estimated from serum creatinine concentration (S_{Cr}) even without total 24-hour urine collection, using empirical formulas. The most popular is the **Cockroft-Gault formula** for measuring the GFR, as follows:

$$C_{Cr} = \frac{(140 - age) \times IBW}{72 \times S_{Cr}} (\times\, 0.85\ for\ females)$$

Ideal body weight (IBW) is calculated in men by starting with 50 kg and adding 2.3 kg for each inch over 5 feet. In women IBW is calculated by starting with 45.5 kg and adding 2.3 kg for each inch over 5 feet. Because women have a smaller muscle mass, the correction factor of 0.85 must be introduced.

Creatinine clearance is inversely proportional with the extent of renal functional impairment, and thus serum creatinine concentration rises as the creatinine clearance decreases (Fig. 12-14). As seen in Figure 12-14, serum creatinine concentration remains within normal limits and starts to rise only after more than two thirds of the total functional kidney reserve is destroyed. In renal insufficiency creatinine clearance is in the range of 20 to 50 mL/dL, and in end-stage kidney disease requiring dialysis it is typically 5 to 20 mL/dL.

Blood urea concentration rises in renal failure.

Urea is the end product of amino acid metabolism, and in blood it is usually measured as blood urea nitrogen (BUN). Its concentration in the blood depends on the rate of production in the liver and the rate of excretion in the urine. Increased BUN is an early sign of renal failure, but in many instances renal dysfunction is secondary to extrarenal causes ("prerenal renal failure"). The most common causes of elevated BUN are listed in Table 12-8.

Urea is filtered in the glomeruli, but 50% of it is passively absorbed in the tubules. Thus the clearance of urea is approximately 50% of the GFR. Reabsorption of urea is increased in dehydration and when urine flow rate is decreased.

Table 12-8 Causes of Elevated Blood Urea Nitrogen

Renal diseases
Prerenal renal failure
Congestive heart failure
Massive blood loss
Dehydration
Prolonged surgery
Trauma
Burns
Intrarenal renal failure
Postrenal renal failure
Increased protein intake
Gastrointestinal bleeding
High-protein diet
Increased protein catabolism
Sepsis
Steroid therapy
Drugs

BUN is a much less reliable sign of renal failure than creatinine, and therefore it is best to interpret it as a BUN/creatinine ratio. Normally the BUN/creatinine ratio is 10:1. In intrarenal renal failure BUN and creatinine in the blood rise in parallel, and thus the ratio remains normal. In dehydration and prerenal failure the BUN/creatinine ratio increases to 15:1 or 20:1. Postrenal failure caused by obstruction also increases the BUN/creatinine ratio. Nonrenal causes for an increased BUN/creatinine ratio include high-protein diet, increased absorption of proteins from the intestine after massive gastrointestinal bleeding, and hypercatabolic states such as sepsis or thyrotoxicosis.

URINARY SEDIMENT EXAMINATION

Urinary sediment is best examined while fresh, that is, immediately after the urine has been centrifuged in the office laboratory. Thus the sediment is decanted from the test tube onto a slide and examined microscopically without any additional staining. Occasionally it will, however, be necessary to apply some stains or perform more complicated examinations, such as examination under polarized light.

Native urinary sediment should be examined for the presence of cells, casts, crystals, and bacteria.

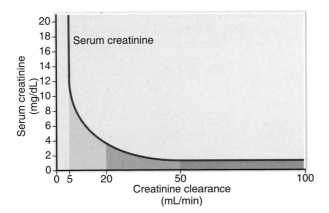

Figure 12-14 Relationship between serum creatinine concentration and creatinine clearance. Note that the glomerular filtration rate must drop well below 50% of normal before creatinine in serum becomes elevated. In renal insufficiency creatinine clearance is in the range of 20 to 50 mL/dL, but if it drops to 5 to 20 mL/dL, dialysis must be started.

Cells found in urinary sediment include desquamated epithelial cells, occasional RBCs, and WBCs. More than four **RBCs** per high-power field is a sign of microscopic hematuria. **Dysmorphic RBCs,** that is, cells that have an abnormal shape and vary in size, are usually a sign of glomerulonephritis. **WBCs** in excess of 3 per high-power field in men and 10 per high-power field in women is usually a sign of infection; it may be accompanied by bacteriuria. **Eosinophiluria** is found in tubulointerstitial hypersensitivity nephritis.

Urinary casts are composed of protein that has changed from the sol state into the gel state and thus reflects the inside shape of the tubule in which it has condensed (Fig. 12-15). Several casts may be found in urine, and some of them have diagnostic value as follows:

- **Hyaline casts.** These clear translucent cylinders composed of protein only are normally found in the urine.
- **Fatty casts.** These casts consist of a proteinaceous matrix and lipid droplets or cholesterol crystals. They are found in nephrotic syndrome.
- **RBC casts.** These casts consist of a proteinaceous matrix studded with red fragmented RBCs. They are typical of acute glomerulonephritis, in which they are usually admixed with dysmorphic RBCs.
- **WBC casts.** These casts consist of a proteinaceous matrix intermixed with nucleated and fragmented neutrophils. These casts are typically found in pyelonephritis and tubulointerstitial nephritis.
- **Renal tubular casts.** These casts consist of fragmented cytoplasm of tubular cells and are usually dark brown.
- **Granular casts.** These casts are composed of cellular debris. Typically they are derived from small granules.
- **Waxy casts.** These refractile casts have sharp outlines, and although there are no cellular fragments in their matrix they are still readily visible. Waxy casts are a sign of chronic renal failure.

- **Broad casts.** These bland or finely granular casts are wider than normal tubules and are typically found in end-stage kidney disease.

Crystals form in both acid and alkaline urine. Acid urine contains uric acid, sodium urate, or calcium oxalate crystals. Alkaline urine contains mostly triple phosphate ("coffin lid-like") crystals. Cystine crystals are hexagonal and found in cystinuria.

SEROLOGIC BLOOD TESTS

Many renal diseases are immune-mediated, and thus it is often necessary to perform serologic tests and search for antibodies that may play an important pathogenetic role or antibodies that might provide some clues about the nature of the renal disease. The most commonly performed tests are as follows:

- **Antinuclear antibodies (ANAs).** This relatively sensitive test is positive in many autoimmune diseases, such as SLE, scleroderma, and rheumatoid arthritis. The test is useful for screening purposes but has a low specificity. If SLE is suspected antisingle-strand DNA, antidouble-strand DNA, and anti-Sm antibody tests should be performed.
- **Anti-GBM antibodies.** These antibodies are present in the serum of patients who have Goodpasture's syndrome.
- **Antineutrophil cytoplasmic antibodies (ANCAs).** These antibodies, most particularly c-ANCA, are positive in Wegener's granulomatosis and are useful for the diagnosis of this disease. In the kidneys, Wegener's granulomatosis it typically manifests as rapidly progressive glomerulonephritis. Kidney biopsy shows crescentic glomerulonephritis, similar to that seen in Goodpasture's syndrome. In contrast, Wegener's granulomatosis does not manifest with deposits of immunoglobulins in the glomeruli ("pauci-immune glomerulonephritis").

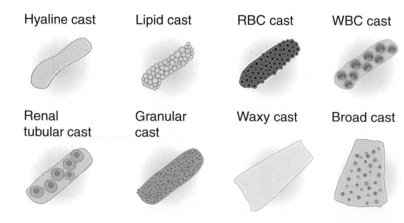

Hyaline cast   Lipid cast   RBC cast   WBC cast

Renal tubular cast   Granular cast   Waxy cast   Broad cast

Figure 12-15 Urinary casts. RBC, red blood cell; WBC, white blood cell. (Modified from Goljan EF: Pathology, Philadelphia, WB Saunders, 1998, p. 370.)

- **Complement.** Immune complexes activate complement, and accordingly its concentration decreases in immunologically mediated renal disease. Total serum complement concentration is thus a sensitive marker of the activity of immune-mediated glomerulonephritis, and it is typically used for assessing the activity of lupus nephritis.

Clinicopathologic Correlations

Renal disease can be classified as acute or chronic. According to the pathogenesis of these diseases they can be classified as related to a **multisystemic disease,** such as septic shock or diabetes mellitus; **primary renal diseases** involving the glomeruli, tubules and interstitium, or renal blood vessels; or **lower urinary tract diseases,** causing obstruction of urinary outflow or allowing an ascending infection (Fig. 12-16).

On the basis of the underlying pathology kidney disease may be classified with regard to the primary lesions, which may be found in the glomeruli, tubulointerstitial compartment of the kidney, or the vascular compartment. In many instances more than one renal compartment is involved.

Glomerular diseases. The glomerular diseases may be classified by their pathogenesis as follows:

- **Immune-mediated glomerulonephritis.** This group includes postinfectious glomerulonephritis, lupus nephritis, membranoproliferative glomerulonephritis, and membranous nephropathy.
- **Multisystemic disease-associated glomerulopathies.** The most important diseases of this group are diabetes mellitus, hypertension, and amyloidosis.
- **Glomerular diseases of unknown pathogenesis.** This group comprises entities such as minimal-change disease (lipoid nephrosis), IgA nephropathy, and focal glomerulosclerosis.
- **Congenital glomerulopathies.** The best known examples are Alport's syndrome and "thin-membrane disease."

Tubulointerstitial diseases. This group of diseases includes the following:

- **Infectious diseases.** The most important diseases in this group are acute pyelonephritis and chronic pyelonephritis.
- **Toxic kidney injury.** The most important lesions of this type include tubular necrosis due to the effect of toxins, drugs, and heavy metals.
- **Immune-mediated disease.** The best example is drug-induced tubulointerstitial nephritis.
- **Metabolic diseases.** The tubules may be damaged by hypercalcemia, uric acid in hyperuricemia, multiple myeloma, and many other metabolic diseases. Diabetes mellitus predisposes to infections and papillary necrosis.
- **Congenital nephropathies.** These are rare diseases but are still important causes of morbidity in children. Polycystic kidney disease is a genetic disease that begins in childhood but becomes clinically evident only in adulthood.

Vascular diseases. This group of diseases is usually associated with systemic diseases that affect blood vessels in other organs as well, such as hypertension, atherosclerosis, or systemic sclerosis. Some immune diseases that affect the glomeruli, such as SLE, may affect the renal vessels as well. Systemic metabolic diseases such as diabetes cause arteriolar changes in the glomeruli, and amyloidosis affects both the glomeruli and the blood vessels.

For clinical purposes it is more convenient to classify renal diseases according to their manifestation. Thus, several **renal syndromes** are recognized including the following:

- Acute renal failure
- Nephritic syndrome
- Rapidly progressive renal failure
- Nephrotic syndrome
- Asymptomatic urinary abnormalities
- Renal infections
- Renal and urinary tract stones
- Tubulointerstitial diseases
- Chronic renal failure
- Renal tumors

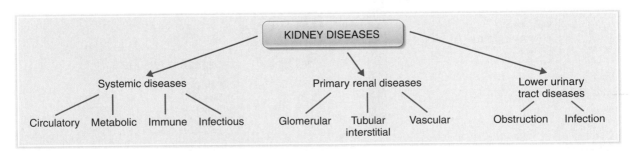

Figure 12-16 Classification of kidney diseases.

ACUTE RENAL FAILURE

Acute renal failure is a term used to describe a sudden loss of renal function characterized by

- Reduced production of urine, clinically recognized as oliguria or anuria
- Retention of water, H^+, and minerals, resulting in metabolic acidosis; retention of metabolic waste products in the blood, most notably BUN and creatinine

Acute renal failure may be caused by numerous renal or systemic diseases, but it also may result from trauma, burns, dehydration, or surgery. For clinical purposes it may be classified as prerenal, intrarenal, or postrenal (Fig. 12-17). In most instances the kidneys show signs of tubular necrosis, which is caused by ischemia in about 50% of all cases.

Toxic tubular necrosis, primary renal diseases, and urinary tract obstructions are less common causes of acute renal failure. In most hospital-based patients acute renal failure is multifactorial.

Pearl

> Prerenal renal failure due to blood or fluid loss may present with low jugular vein pressure and reduced skin turgor, whereas renal failure due to congestive heart failure is characterized by increased venous pressure and high jugular vein pressure. Renal and postrenal failure are characterized by fluid overload and high venous pressure.

Acute prerenal renal failure is caused by reduced renal perfusion.

Acute prerenal renal failure is in most instances related to reduced effective extracellular fluid (ECF) volume, that is, intravascular fluid volume that determines the renal perfusion. In an adult man weighing 70 kg the effective ECF volume is approximately 700 mL. Reduced intra-arterial volume (e.g., due to massive blood loss) activates the baroreceptors in the carotid sinus and the aortic arch and is sensed by the afferent arterioles in the kidneys, evoking the typical release of sympathomimetic substances, vasopressin (ADH), and activation of the renin–angiotensin–aldosterone system (Fig. 12-18). The combined effect of all these interconnected reactions is hypoperfusion of the kidneys, resulting in a reduced GFR and retention of water and Na^+ in the kidneys.

The most common causes of prerenal renal failure are as follows:

- **Blood loss.** Massive blood loss due to trauma or surgery reduces the total ECF, resulting in reduced cardiac output and peripheral vasoconstriction.
- **Fluid loss.** Loss of fluid may occur in patients with extensive burns, watery diarrhea, or vomiting. All these conditions reduce the effective ECF and cause renal hypoperfusion.
- **Cardiac failure.** Cardiac output is reduced due to "pump failure" and results in hypoperfusion of the kidneys and many other organs. Reactive vasoconstriction, aimed at retaining the blood pressure and the normal ratio between the cardiac output and the vascular lumen that needs to be filled, contributes to ischemia. In addition venous stasis is present, which contributes to generalized edema and altered fluid distribution in the body.

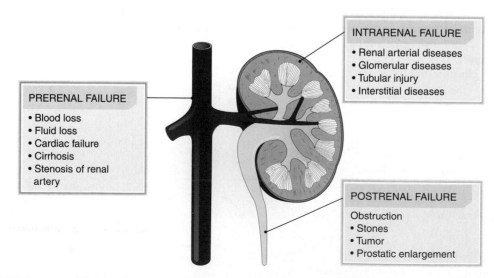

PRERENAL FAILURE
- Blood loss
- Fluid loss
- Cardiac failure
- Cirrhosis
- Stenosis of renal artery

INTRARENAL FAILURE
- Renal arterial diseases
- Glomerular diseases
- Tubular injury
- Interstitial diseases

POSTRENAL FAILURE
Obstruction
- Stones
- Tumor
- Prostatic enlargement

Figure 12-17 Acute renal failure. Three major forms of acute renal failure are recognized clinically: prerenal, intrarenal, and postrenal.

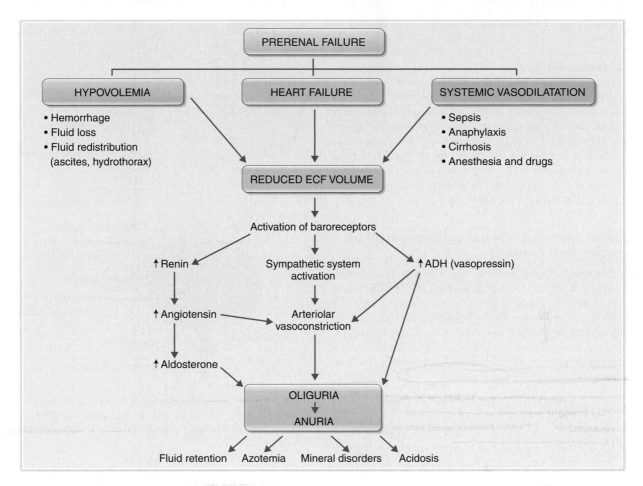

Figure 12-18 Prerenal renal failure. Reduction of the effective extracellular fluid (ECF) volume may develop due to hypovolemia, heart failure, or systemic vasodilatation. Reduced ECF volume activates baroreceptors, leading to renin and antidiuretic hormone (ADH) secretion and ultimately resulting in oliguria, fluid retention, azotemia, mineral disorders, and acidosis.

■ **Cirrhosis.** Peripheral vasodilatation and formation of ascites lead to redistribution of body fluids, thereby reducing the effective ECF. This leads to an activation of the renin–angiotensin–aldosterone system and vasoconstriction of renal arterioles and reactive oliguria typical of hepatorenal syndrome.

■ **Sepsis.** Endotoxins produced by bacteria cause peripheral vasodilatation, and the heart output, although increased, cannot maintain normal perfusion of the major organs. Reactive intrarenal vasoconstriction typically reduces the glomerular perfusion even more.

Intrarenal acute renal failure may be caused by an injury to the blood vessels, glomeruli, or tubules.

Intrarenal failure may develop due to a variety of causes, including vascular occlusion; immunologic injury of the vessels, glomeruli, or tubules; toxic injury of the tubules; and destruction of all three renal compartments by bacterial

infection. The typical examples of these pathologic processes are given here as follows:

■ **Vascular occlusion.** Major renal arteries can be occluded by thromboemboli originating from cardiac valves in endocarditis. Cholesterol emboli originating in ruptured aortic atheromas may completely occlude the renal arterial system and cause acute renal failure.

■ **Glomerular diseases.** The most important glomerular cause of acute renal failure is crescentic glomerulonephritis, clinically presenting as rapidly progressive renal failure. Most often renal failure is part of Wegener's granulomatosis and is typically associated with pulmonary hemorrhage and upper respiratory tract lesions. The glomeruli contain cellular crescents, obliterating the urinary space and compressing the glomerular capillary tufts.

■ **Tubular injury.** Tubular injury may be caused by exogenous toxins (e.g., mercury poisoning), drugs, or endogenous metabolites (e.g., uric acid crystals in gout, or immunoglobulin light chains in multiple myeloma).

- **Interstitial disease.** Acute bacterial infection may begin in the interstitial spaces or inside the tubules. The same is true for immune reactions caused by drugs or in renal transplants. Hence it is customary to classify these diseases as **tubulointerstitial.** In view of the fact that the vessels are often involved as well, it is probably best not to try to establish the site of the primary injury but to label these diseases with a noncommittal term, **nephritis** or **nephropathy** (e.g., "transplant nephropathy").

Postrenal acute renal failure results from obstruction of outflow for the urine.

Urinary tract obstruction can occur at the level of the ureters, bladder neck, or urethra (Fig. 12-19). Unilateral obstruction of one ureter can be readily compensated for by the unobstructed kidney. Major obstruction of the bladder neck or urethra, however, can cause renal failure, which must be treated immediately. Ureteric obstruction in a single kidney or a renal transplant obviously produces the same life-threatening emergency.

> **Pearl**
>
> > Urinary bladder obstruction due to prostatic disease is the most common cause of acute postrenal obstruction in nonhospitalized patients.

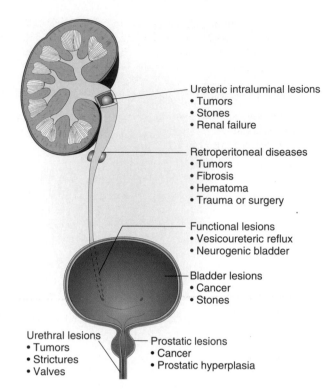

Figure 12-19 Causes of urinary tract obstruction. The obstruction can occur at the level of the ureter, bladder, or urethra. It may be related to structural or functional changes.

Ureteric intraluminal lesions
- Tumors
- Stones
- Renal failure

Retroperitoneal diseases
- Tumors
- Fibrosis
- Hematoma
- Trauma or surgery

Functional lesions
- Vesicoureteric reflux
- Neurogenic bladder

Bladder lesions
- Cancer
- Stones

Urethral lesions
- Tumors
- Strictures
- Valves

Prostatic lesions
- Cancer
- Prostatic hyperplasia

Acute renal failure results in the retention of water, minerals, and metabolites that are normally excreted in the urine and in acidosis.

Acute renal failure typically manifests with reduced urine output (oliguria), which may progress to anuria. The symptoms of the condition that caused the renal failure dominate the clinical presentation. Biochemical changes in the blood and urine provide the most important clues suggesting renal failure. Typical findings include

- **Azotemia** (i.e., increased serum levels of organic waste products)
  - BUN
  - Creatinine
  - Uric acid
- Water retention
  - Intravascular volume overload
- Electrolyte imbalance
  - Hyperkalemia
  - Hyponatremia
  - Hyperphosphatemia
  - Hypocalcemia
- Acidosis
  - Decreased serum HCO_3^-

Water and waste products are not excreted because of the reduced GFR. Water retention leads to dilutional hyponatremia. It may manifest as generalized edema or edema involving particular internal organs such as the lungs, causing dyspnea, or the brain, causing somnolence. Retention of urea and ammonia affects the central nervous system, causing drowsiness, loss of appetite, nausea, and vomiting. In severe cases it may even cause coma.

Retention of K^+ and phosphate reflects both a reduced GFR and tubular injury. Hyperkalemia may be aggravated by an increased influx of K^+ into the circulation from damaged tissues, as in cases of major trauma, rhabdomyolysis, or hemolysis. Hypocalcemia, which is reactive and secondary to hyperphosphatemia, is seen in the early stages of acute renal failure, but it usually corrects itself spontaneously. Nevertheless, the changes in the serum concentration of K^+ and Ca^{2+} may have profound effects on the heart, causing arrhythmia and electrocardiographic changes. Disturbances of mineral homeostasis may even cause death from cardiac arrest.

Acidosis results from the retention of organic acids that are normally excreted in the urine and the inability of the kidneys to remove excess H^+. Bicarbonate is consumed, and its concentration in the blood is typically reduced. Lactic acid released from other ischemic tissues in hypotensive shock contributes to acidosis.

Pearl

> Some patients with acute renal failure and azotemia may have polyuria, that is, urinary output over 3 L/24 hours. This is typical of tubular necrosis in which the GFR is preserved. Partial urinary tract obstruction may also manifest with polyuric renal failure.

Acute renal failure affects the function of vital organs.

Acute renal failure causes metabolic changes that affect all major organs in the body, as follows:

- **Cardiopulmonary complications.** Heart failure results from fluid overload, which may be complicated by irregularities of cardiac contractions due to hyperkalemia and hypocalcemia. Pump failure leads to cardiac ischemia, which further reduces the cardiac output. Renin-mediated acute hypertension reduces the cardiac output even more. Left heart failure leads to pulmonary congestion and edema, which in severe cases does not respond to diuretics.
- **Neurologic complications.** Urea and other toxic waste products combined with electrolyte disturbances and acidosis cause CNS depression, seizures, and even coma or death.
- **Disturbances of coagulation.** Bleeding from mucosal surfaces often occurs, resulting most likely from the effects of metabolic changes on platelets and blood vessels. Most profound bleeding occurs in the gastrointestinal tract, especially in patients who are in shock.
- **Predisposition to infection.** Metabolic changes adversely affect the body's natural defenses. Thus it is not uncommon to encounter recurrent infections in these patients. Reduced food intake due to a loss of appetite and nausea further weakens the body's resistance to infections.

Acute renal failure is a serious condition that requires prompt treatment. In mild cases correction of the fluid and metabolic balance prevents major complications, but in most patients peritoneal dialysis or extracorporeal hemodialysis must be used. The usual **indications for dialysis** are severe pulmonary edema not responding to diuretics, hyperkalemia over 6.5 mmol/L, a pH of 7.2 or less, pericarditis, encephalopathy, and worsening renal failure as evidenced by progressive oliguria and rising azotemia.

The clinical course of acute tubular necrosis includes three phases: **azotemic, diuretic,** and **recovery phase.** The outcome of acute renal failure due to acute tubular necrosis depends on the severity of the renal injury and the causes and duration of the injury. Patients with severe oliguria and anuria have a worse prognosis than those with mild oliguria or polyuria. The cause of prerenal renal injury is also important: the worst outcome is after trauma and surgery, but is much better after medical diseases, and is best if renal failure occurs as a complication of pregnancy and delivery.

The cause of renal failure may be diagnosed clinically and by means of laboratory studies.

The causes of acute renal failure can be diagnosed by taking into account the clinical and laboratory data. The **patient's history** may provide important clues, and the clinician must inquire about recent accidents, trauma, surgery, drugs, and radiologic procedures. **Urinalysis** should include measurement of urinary volume to diagnose oliguria and an estimate of the amount of Na^+ or creatinine excretion, protein, or blood. Red blood cells, RBC casts, leukocytes, or tumor cells may be seen in urinary sediment. Eosinophiluria is a typical finding in allergic tubulointerstitial nephritis. Renal tubular necrosis is characterized by the presence of pigmented cellular casts formed from tubular cells ("muddy urinary sediment"). Microbiologic studies should be performed on the urine of all patients with acute renal failure.

As mentioned earlier prerenal renal failure is characterized by a **BUN/creatinine ratio** of over 20:1. **Renal failure index** (RFI) can be calculated by measuring the ratio of urinary Na^+ and creatinine to serum creatinine, expressed in percentages as follows:

$$RFI = \frac{(U_{Na}/U_{Cr})}{P_{Cr}} \times 100$$

RFI is typically below 1% in prerenal failure, and if above 1% it suggests renal tubular necrosis.

Fractional excretion of sodium (FE_{Na}) is calculated by taking into account urine and plasma Na^+ and creatinine concentration as follows:

$$FE_{Na} = \frac{U_{Na}/P_{Na}}{U_{Cr}/P_{Cr}} \times 100$$

Values below 1% are typically found in prerenal failure.

Other tests that must be performed in patients with acute renal failure include studies aimed at identifying possible causes of postrenal urinary tract obstruction. The most useful in this respect is **ultrasound,** which may detect dilatation of the ureters and renal pelvis (hydronephrosis), possible masses obstructing the urinary tract, urinary calculi, tumors, clots, renal vein thrombosis, and many other pathologic changes. **Computed tomography (CT)** may also be useful. **Cystoscopy** is indicated if a urinary bladder lesion is suspected. **Renal biopsy** may be indicated if a rapidly progressive glomerulonephritis or acute allergic tubulointerstitial nephritis is suspected.

NEPHRITIC SYNDROME

Nephritic syndrome is a set of clinical signs and symptoms that accompany immune-mediated glomerulonephritis. The syndrome is defined by the following clinical findings:

- Proteinuria
- Hematuria of glomerular origin
- Oliguria
- Hypertension
- Edema

Nephritic syndrome may be related to a primary renal disease or it may be a secondary complication of an infection in some other site. It may also occur in the context of a systemic immune disease, such as SLE, which also affects the kidneys, producing a secondary glomerulonephritis. The most important causes of acute nephritic syndrome are listed in Table 12-9.

Clinical signs and symptoms of nephritic syndrome are a consequence of the immune-mediated inflammation of the glomeruli.

Clinical signs and symptoms of nephritic syndrome are best illustrated by analyzing the glomerular changes that occur in acute poststreptococcal glomerulonephritis (PS-GN). This

Table 12-9 Most Common Causes of Acute Nephritic Syndrome

Primary glomerulonephritis
    IgA nephritis*
    Membranoproliferative glomerulonephritis type I
    Membranoproliferative glomerulonephritis type II
Postinfectious glomerulonephritis
    Poststreptococcal glomerulonephritis*
    Nonpoststreptococcal glomerulonephritis (e.g.,
        meningococcal sepsis, pneumonia, "shunt
        nephritis")
    Bacterial endocarditis associated glomerulonephritis
    Syphilis
    Viral infections (e.g., viral hepatitis B or C, infectious
        mononucleosis, measles)
    Protozoal infections (e.g., malaria, toxoplasmosis)
Secondary glomerulonephritis of systemic diseases
    Lupus nephritis (systemic lupus erythematosus)*
    Pulmonary renal syndromes
        Wegener's granulomatosis
        Goodpasture's syndrome
    Henoch-Schönlein purpura
    Microscopic polyarteritis
    Serum sickness and postvaccination glomerulonephritis

---

*Most important disease in each of the three groups.

acute disease typically develops within 2 weeks after an acute streptococcal throat infection. A similar reaction can occur due to infection of other tissues, and less often even in bacterial infections caused by other bacteria. It is not known why some infections cause PS-GN and others do not.

Bacterial infection with certain "nephritic" strains of group A beta-hemolytic streptococci is typically associated with production of antibodies reacting with bacterial antigens. Immune complexes formed between bacterial antigens and antibodies in circulation may deposit in the glomeruli, activate the complement system, and thus induce glomerulonephritis (Fig. 12-20). Bacterial antigens also may be "implanted" during filtration in the glomeruli, and the immune complexes may be formed locally along the glomerular basement membrane and the mesangial areas. Activation of complement generates chemotactic fragments and intermediate complexes, which attract inflammatory cells and stimulate the proliferation of mesangial cells. These cells produce various mediators of inflammation such as interleukins, interferon, tumor necrosis factors, prostaglandins, and others, which damage the basement membrane and make it more permeable.

Glomerular inflammation has the following consequences:

- **Increased permeability of the basement membrane.** This allows albumin and even larger proteins to pass into the glomerular filtrate and ultimately results in **proteinuria.**
- **Microscopic defects in the glomerular basement membrane.** This allows RBCs to pass through the glomerular barrier and thus enter into the lumen of the proximal tubules. **Hematuria** accounts for the brownish red discoloration of the urine, which is typically described as "bouillon-like." The RBCs passing thought the GBM are deformed or fragmented (**"dysmorphic red blood cells"**). Some of the RBCs are incorporated into the casts forming in the lumen of the proximal tubules from protein-hypersaturated fluid. These **RBC casts,** typical of glomerular hematuria, are passed into the urine where they can be detected by examining the urinary sediment microscopically (see Fig. 12-15).
- **Reduced glomerular filtration rate.** Inflammatory cells attach to the endothelial surface of the glomeruli, narrow the capillary lumen, and thus physically impede blood flow through those glomeruli. Proliferation of mesangial cells contributes further to the narrowing of the capillary lumina. The reduced GFR results in **oliguria.**
- **Reduced sodium filtration.** Due to reduced glomerular filtration less fluid and even more importantly less Na^+ reach the tubular sensors in the macula densa. These events stimulate the production of **renin** and the activation of the renin–angiotensin–aldosterone system. Together with the tubular–glomerular autoregulation, aldosterone causes constriction of the afferent

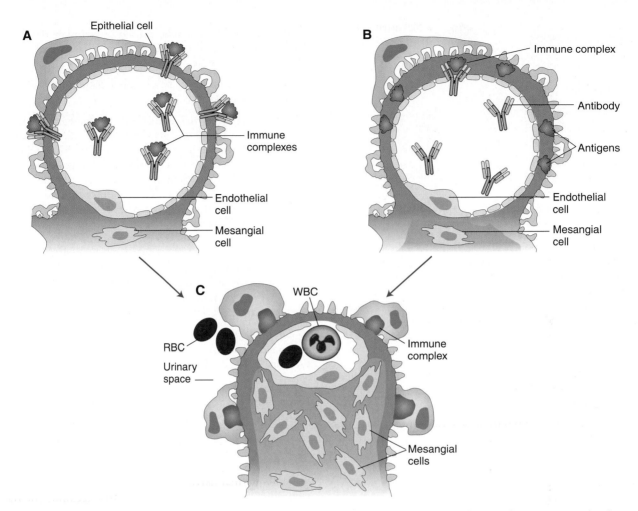

Figure 12-20 Acute poststreptococcal glomerulonephritis. The diagram shows the two pathways of immune complex formation as seen by electron microscopy. **A,** Deposition of preformed circulating immune complexes that reach the glomerular capillaries through the bloodstream. **B,** Formation of immune complexes in situ between implanted bacterial antigens and circulating antibodies. **C,** The outcome of immune complex deposition in the glomeruli, evidenced as subepithelial "humps," is identical in both instances. The immune complexes are chemotactic and attract neutrophils, which attach to the glomerular capillaries. Proliferation of mesangial cells is present, leading to a narrowing of the capillary lumen. Red blood cells pass through the damaged capillary wall into the urinary space and are seen on the epithelial side of the basement membrane. RBC, red blood cell; WBC, white blood cell.

arterioles, further reducing glomerular blood flow. In addition this leads to arterial **hypertension.**

■ **Edema.** Retention of Na⁺ and water in the kidneys, combined with hypoalbuminemia due to proteinuria, causes edema of the soft tissues. Typically this is best seen on the face, which appears "puffy." The hands and feet are swollen, and there might be fluid accumulation in the thoracic and abdominal cavity. Edema of the brain makes the affected children sleepy and in severe cases it may even cause coma. Pulmonary edema causes shortness of breath and easy fatigability.

The typical clinical features of acute glomerulonephritis are illustrated in Figure 12-21. The disease most often

occurs in children, but it may follow various infections in adults. In children it has an excellent prognosis, and over 90% of children recover completely. In the remaining 9% the disease may have a somewhat protracted course and last several months. In 1% of all childhood cases acute PS-GN leads to end-stage kidney disease. In adults the recovery is often not as complete as in children and a significant number of cases.

NEPHROTIC SYNDROME

Nephrotic syndrome is a set of clinical signs and symptoms encountered in diseases that cause increased permeability of

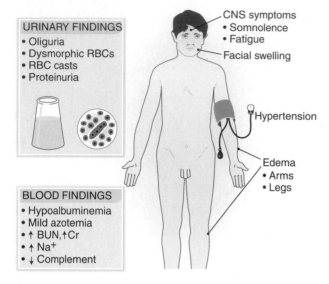

URINARY FINDINGS
• Oliguria
• Dysmorphic RBCs
• RBC casts
• Proteinuria

CNS symptoms
• Somnolence
• Fatigue

Facial swelling

Hypertension

Edema
• Arms
• Legs

BLOOD FINDINGS
• Hypoalbuminemia
• Mild azotemia
• ↑ BUN, ↑ Cr
• ↑ Na⁺
• ↓ Complement

Figure 12-21 Clinical features of acute poststreptococcal glomerulonephritis. BUN, blood urea nitrogen; CNS, central nervous system; Cr, creatinine; RBC, red blood cell.

the glomerular capillaries. The syndrome is defined by the following clinical findings:

■ Proteinuria
■ Hypoalbuminemia
■ Hyperlipidemia
■ Edema

Nephrotic syndrome can be caused by primary renal disease, or it may occur as a renal complication of multisystemic disease.

Nephrotic syndrome can be classified pathogenetically as primary or secondary.

■ **Primary nephrotic syndrome** results from primary renal diseases, most of which are of unknown origin. The most important diseases in this category are lipoid nephrosis ("minimal-change disease"), idiopathic membranous nephropathy, and focal glomerulosclersosis, or membranoproliferative glomerulonephritis type I or type II.
■ **Secondary nephrotic syndrome** occurs in the course of multisystemic diseases, which may be immune-mediated (e.g., SLE), metabolic (e.g., diabetes mellitus), neoplastic (e.g., amyloidosis of multiple myeloma), or infectious (e.g., membranous nephropathy due to chronic viral hepatitis, or focal glomerulosclerosis due to HIV infection).

The most common causes of nephrotic syndrome and associated clinical findings that may suggest its cause are listed in Table 12-10.

Renal biopsy is essential for the diagnosis of nephrotic syndrome.

As shown in Table 12-10, nephrotic syndrome may be associated with some clinical findings that could point to the cause of the disease. Further data that could suggest the diagnosis are the age of the patient, because some forms of nephrotic syndrome are more common in children and some are more common in adults (Table 12-11).

Table 12-10 Common Causes of Nephrotic Syndrome

DISEASE	PATHOGENESIS	ASSOCIATED CONDITIONS AND FINDINGS
Lipoid nephrosis (minimal-change disease)	Unknown	Usually none Atopic dermatitis, Hodgkin's disease
Focal segmental glomerulosclerosis	Unknown	Usually none Heroin abuse, HIV infection
Membranous nephropathy	Immune	Usually none Drugs (e.g., gold, penicillinamine) Malignancy Viral hepatitis B or C
Membranoproliferative GN	Immune	Usually none
Lupus nephritis	Immune	SLE (skin rash, arthritis, ANA, etc.)
Amyloidosis	Unknown	Multiple myeloma Chronic infection
Diabetic glomerulosclerosis	Metabolic	Diabetes mellitus (hyperglycemia, etc.)

ANA, antinuclear antibodies; GN, glomerulonephritis; HIV, human immunodeficiency virus; SLE, systemic lupus erythematosus.

Table 12-11 Age-related Incidence of Various Forms of Nephritic Syndrome

DISEASE	PREVALENCE	
	CHILDREN (<15 yr, as % of total)	ADULTS (as % of total)
Lipoid nephrosis	75	10
Focal segmental glomerulosclerosis	8	35
Membranous nephropathy	2	20
Membranoproliferative GN	5	<1
Diabetes mellitus	<1	20
Amyloidosis	0	5
SLE and other GN	10	10

The data are estimates and rounded up so that the total sum is not exactly 100 in either column.
GN, glomerulonephritis; SLE, systemic lupus erythematosus.

Renal biopsy is indicated in most instances, and it is essential for establishing the cause of nephrotic syndrome. The only exception is lipoid nephrosis (minimal-change disease), the most common cause of nephrotic syndrome in children. Lipoid nephrosis responds in most instances to steroid treatment, and thus it is customary to treat such children rather than perform a biopsy on them. If the nephrotic syndrome does not respond or recurs shortly after the completion of therapy, a renal biopsy might be necessary to establish the diagnosis and exclude the possibility that proteinuria is actually caused by some other glomerular disease, such a focal glomerulosclerosis.

The histopathologic findings seen in renal biopsy are usually typical, but must be interpreted in the context of immunofluorescence (IF) and electron microscopy (EM) findings.

Some of these typical changes seen in the most common forms of nephrotic syndrome are shown in Figure 12-22 and summarized here as follows:

- **Lipoid nephrosis.** This disease of unknown origin is also known as minimal-change disease ("nil disease") because the glomeruli show no microscopic changes and no IF findings. Electron microscopy shows fusion of the foot processes of epithelial cells. This change is not specific and most likely represents a reaction to increased leakage of proteins through the hyperpermeable GBM.
- **Focal glomerulosclerosis.** Light microscopy shows focal and segmental hyalinization of the capillary loops. Such sclerotic capillary loops may trap immunoglobulins, which are visible by IF, but otherwise no immunoglobulin deposits are evident. Electron microscopy shows fusion of the foot processes of the epithelial cells like in lipoid nephrosis.
- **Membranous nephropathy.** By light microscopy one may see thickening of the GBM. Granular deposits of immunoglobulin and complement ("immune complexes") on the epithelial side of the GBM are evident by IF. These immune complexes are visible by EM. Similar changes are seen in the membranous type of lupus nephritis (class V), which, however, also contains mesangial deposits of immune complexes.
- **Diabetic glomerulosclerosis.** Nephrotic syndrome results from metabolic changes in the GBM and mesangial matrix. By light microscopy a thickening of the GBM and widening of the mesangial areas are evident, which may become nodular ("nodular sclerosis of Kimmelstiel-Wilson"). The thickened GBM may be impregnated with albumin, globulin, and other plasma proteins, but no immune complex deposits are visible by IF or EM.

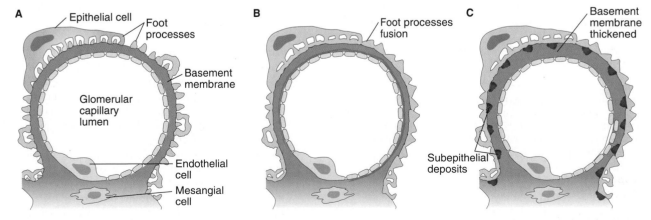

Figure 12-22 Pathologic changes in common forms of nephrotic syndrome as seen by electron microscopy. **A,** Normal glomerulus. **B,** Lipoid nephrosis (minimal-change disease) shows only fusion of the foot processes. **C,** Membranous nephropathy shows deposits of immune complexes on the epithelial side of the glomerular basement membrane.

■ **Amyloidosis.** Amyloid is fibrillar material that is deposited in the glomeruli and renal blood vessels. It may be identified by Congo red staining, which appears red but becomes green when examined under polarized light. Biochemically amyloid deposits may be derived from light-chain immunoglobulins (amyloid AL, typically encountered in multiple myeloma) or from serum amyloid A precursor protein (amyloid AA) produced by the liver in response to chronic inflammation.

The clinical features of nephrotic syndrome are a consequence of massive protein loss in the urine.

Proteinuria resulting from increased glomerular permeability is massive and typically exceeds 3.5 g of protein in urine collected over 24 hours. This "nephrotic range proteinuria" over time depletes albumin from the plasma. Prolonged **hypoalbuminemia** (≤2.5 g/dL) reduces the oncotic pressure of the plasma and allows the water to escape into the tissue, leading to generalized **edema** (anasarca) (see Fig. 12-13). Such patients may show signs of **circulating volume depletion syndrome** and experience syncope, hypovolemic shock, and even renal failure.

The liver cannot produce enough albumin to compensate for the renal loss of albumin and instead releases lipoproteins, which leads to **hyperlipidemia.** Long-term hyperplipidemia contributes to the development of atherosclerosis, which is further accelerated by **hypertension** that develops in some patients with nephrotic syndrome, especially if it is caused by focal glomerulosclerosis. The depletion of the intravascular volume stimulates the renin–angiotensin–aldosterone syndrome and the activation of the sympathetic system.

Loss of other proteins may be initially overshadowed by the loss of albumin, but note that albumin is not the only protein lost in the urine. Loss of **anticoagulation proteins,** such as antithrombin III, protein C, and protein S, accounts for the hypercoagulability of blood and increased incidence of thrombosis. Loss of **complement proteins, cytokines,** and **immunoglobulins** is associated with an increased incidence of infection. Loss of thyroid and steroid **hormone-binding proteins** may result in hypothyroidism, amenorrhea, and menstrual irregularities. Loss of **vitamin D-binding protein** may cause osteomalacia.

CHRONIC RENAL FAILURE

End-stage kidney disease represents irreversible loss of renal function usually below 20% of normal. It is the final outcome of many renal and multisystemic diseases, the most important of which are:

■ Diabetes mellitus (30%)
■ Hypertension and vascular diseases (20%)
■ Glomerular diseases (15%)
■ Pyelonephritis and other renal diseases (10%)
■ Systemic autoimmune diseases (5%)

■ Polycystic kidney disease (5%)
■ Unknown (15%)

Uremia is the term used for the clinical syndrome resulting from end-stage renal disease. It is incompatible with life, and these patients can be kept alive only by dialysis or renal transplantation.

Clinical manifestations of end-stage kidney disease reflect the loss of major renal function.

Clinical manifestations of end-stage kidney disease result from a loss of renal excretory function, inability of the kidneys to take part in the regulation of acid–base balance, and a loss of various metabolic and endocrine renal functions. The principal consequences are as follows:

■ **Fluid and electrolyte retention.** There is fluid overload and expansion of the ECF with dilutional hyponatremia. Retention of K^+ and phosphorus results in hyperkalemia, hyperphosphatemia with reactive hypocalcemia, and metabolic acidosis.
■ **Azotemia.** Retention of urea, creatinine, and ammonia affects the central nervous system, leading to nausea and vomiting, and results in pruritus due to the deposition of urate crystals on the surface of the skin and mucosae ("uremic frost"). Irritation of serosal surfaces leads to uremic pericarditis and pleuritis and effusions into the body cavities.
■ **Hypertension.** It is in part related to the hypersecretion of renin and in part to fluid retention and hypervolemia.
■ **Endocrine and metabolic disturbances.** Hyperphosphatemia and reactive hypocalcemia stimulate the parathyroid glands to produce PTH, which acts on the bone to cause renal osteodystrophy and leaking of Ca^{2+} and phosphate from the bones. Inadequate hydroxylation of vitamin D results in a deficiency of $1,25(OH)_2D_3$, which contributes to osteomalacia and reduced Ca^{2+} absorption in the intestines. Hormonal disturbances include sexual dysfunction, menstrual disturbances, and amenorrhea.
■ **Hematologic disturbances.** Reduced production of erythropoietin leads to reduced production of erythroid cells and normochromic normocytic anemia with a low reticulocyte count. Platelet dysfunction predisposing to bleeding also occurs. Bleeding time is usually prolonged. Leukopenia and T-cell dysfunction are present, predisposing to infections.
■ **Neurologic disturbances.** These changes are multifactorial and related to the retention of metabolites and various poorly defined "urotoxins," disturbances of electrolytes, and acidosis. Symptoms include fatigue, somnolence, headaches, seizure, loss of mental functions, and may even progress to coma. Peripheral sensorymotor neuropathy presents with reduced sensation, paresthesia, and reduced reflexes.

The metabolic consequences of chronic renal failure affect all major organ systems.

Chronic renal failure may remain clinically unrecognized for a long time because the human organism may adapt and tolerate for prolonged periods the metabolic changes resulting from renal malfunction. Once the symptoms and clinical signs become evident they may relate to all organs (Fig. 12-23). The clinical manifestations of chronic renal failure are listed by major organs in Table 12-12.

URINARY STONES

Urolithiasis, or the formation of renal stones, is a very common cause of urinary tract disturbances. It has been estimated that it may occur in up to 10% of all Americans and is especially common in the Southern states ("stone belt"). Urinary stones tend to recur. The rate of recurrence is 15% during the first year after diagnosis, 35% at 5 years, and 60% at 10 years.

Urinary stones form in abnormal urine.

Urinary stones may form inside the renal pelvis, ureters, or the urinary bladder. Stones form from substances that are normally excreted in the urine under the following conditions:

■ **Hypersaturation of urine with lithogenic substances.** Normal urine contains calcium phosphate and calcium oxalate, uric acid, and several other chemicals. If these chemicals are excreted in increased amounts, the urine becomes hypersaturated, and crystals of these minerals start forming, finally aggregating into stones. The most common cause of stone formation is hypercalciuria.

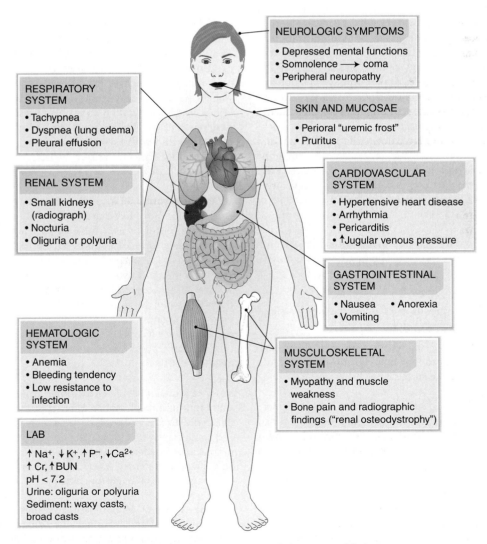

Figure 12-23 Clinical features of chronic renal failure.

Table 12-12 Clinical Manifestations of Chronic Renal Failure Listed by Organ System

ORGAN SYSTEM	CLINICAL FINDINGS
Urinary	Oliguria, less often polyuria
	Azotemia, retention of fluids and minerals
Cardiovascular	Hypertension, arrhythmias, congestive heart failure, pericarditis and pericardial effusion or tamponade
Respiratory	Tachypnea, hyperventilation, dyspnea, pulmonary edema, pleural effusion
Gastrointestinal	Nausea, vomiting, peptic ulcer, erosive gastroenteritis, diarrhea
Hematologic	Anemia (pallor, fatigue), platelet dysfunction (bleeding), leukopenia (infections), and T-cell dysfunction (infections)
Endocrine	Secondary hyperparathyroidism of deficient function, vitamin D, loss of sexual functions, amenorrhea, hyperprolactinemia, gynecomastia
Musculoskeletal	Myopathy and muscle weakness, renal osteodystrophy
Nervous	Mental fatigue and function loss and central nervous system depression
	Peripheral neuropathy

■ **Loss of natural inhibitors of lithogenesis.** Normal urine contains substances that prevent nucleation of crystals and stone formation. The best known inhibitors of lithogenesis are pyrophosphate, diphosphonate, citric acid, and Tamm-Horsfall mucoprotein, but many other substances also inhibit stone formation. Patients who lack these inhibitors in the urine have a tendency to produce urinary stones.

■ **Infection.** Bacteria may damage the urothelium, and fragments of this tissue may serve as a nidus for stone formation. In addition, urease-producing bacteria such as *Proteus mirabilis* may make the normally acidic urine alkaline and thus predispose to the precipitation of minerals.

Note that in 20% to 25% of patients with urinary stones the cause of stone formation and their pathogenesis remain unknown.

The biochemical composition of urinary stones varies, but most contain calcium salts.

Urinary stones can be classified according to their biochemical composition into four major groups: calcium, uric acid, struvite, and cystine stones.

Calcium stones (70%). Calcium complexed to phosphate or oxalate accounts for most urinary stones. More than half of these patients have **idiopathic hypercalciuria** without hypercalcemia, but in about 10% **hypercalcemia** related to hyperparathyroidism, sarcoidosis, malignant tumors, or some bone disease is found. Approximately 20% of patients have **hyperuricemia,** some have **hyperoxaluria** (due to intestinal overabsorption of oxalate) or congenital **hypocitraturia.** In a significant number of patients (20%) the cause of urinary stone formation is never established, and the condition is considered idiopathic.

Calcium stones form in slightly alkaline urine. Most patients have normal serum Ca^{2+} levels, but those who have hypercalcemia must be evaluated further for hyperparathyroidism. Note that gout and hyperuricemia may be associated with the formation of calcium stones, as well as with uric acid stones. Hyperoxalosis is found in vegetarians, whose diet contains increased amounts of oxalates, and in patients who absorb increased amounts of oxalates due to intestinal disease. Chronic diarrhea also may produce hypocitraturia, which promotes urinary stone formation.

Uric acid stones (10%). These stones are typically a complication of hyperuricemia and hyperuricosuria, which are found in over 50% of patients. Most of these patients have idiopathic gout. Other causes of hyperuricemia, such as hyperproliferative diseases like lymphoma and leukemia and psoriasis, are less common. In close to 50% of all patients neither hyperuricemia nor uricosuria is evident, and the cause of stone formation is unknown. Uric acid stones form in acidic urine. Pure uric acid stones are not visible in routine radiographs, but often they contain specks of calcium, which makes them radiopaque.

Struvite stones (20%). These stones, composed of magnesium ammonium phosphate, are typically formed in urine infected with urea-splitting bacteria such as *Proteus mirabilis* and some staphylococci, which generate ammonia and thus make the urine alkaline. These stones are often large, irregularly shaped, and may take the shape of the dilated renal pelvis and calices ("staghorn calculi").

Cystine stones (<1%). These stones are uncommon and are found in children who have hereditary cystinosis. Such children have cystinuria and form radiolucent stones in acidic urine.

Urinary stones may obstruct the ureters or damage the urothelium.

Most urinary stones are formed in the upper urinary tract, from which they enter the ureter. Impaction of stones in the ureter causes spasms, which manifests clinically as ureteric colic. The pain begins gradually, escalating in severity over a period of 20 to 60 minutes. It is usually associated with nausea and vomiting. If the stone descends lower into the ureter, the pain may radiate to the groin and testicles or labia. Urinary urgency and frequency are signs that the stone has lodged at the ureterovesical junction.

Hematuria is common, but typically it occurs after the onset of renal colic. Pyuria and fever are found in patients with superimposed infection. Many urinary bladder stones may be asymptomatic or cause only microscopic or macroscopic hematuria.

Urinary stones are visible radiographically in over 90% of cases. Ultrasound and spiral CT are also used. Most stones are small and pass spontaneously with analgesia and hydration. All stones should be submitted for chemical analysis if possible. Hydration is the mainstay to preventing recurrence, and it may be combined with dietary modifications or drugs. Lithotripsy or surgical lithotomy may be indicated for larger stones.

The work-up of a case of urinary stones that has been diagnosed for the first time should include serum electrolytes, BUN and creatinine, and complete urinalysis. Hypercalcemic patients should be examined further for hyperparathyroidism, and uric acid should be measured in suspected cases of hyperuricemia.

Complications of chronic urinary stone disease are the consequences of obstruction or infection.

Urinary stones may cause obstruction of urinary outflow and also predispose to infections. The most common complications are

- **Hydronephrosis and hydroureter.** Obstruction is most common in patients who have large struvite stones. Hypoperfusion of the hydronephrotic kidney may cause **arterial hypertension** due to oversecretion of renin. **Renal papillary necrosis** is yet another complication that occurs at an increased rate.
- **Complete loss of renal function.** Complete obstruction of urinary outflow may cause atrophy of the renal parenchyma and complete loss of renal function. Bilateral loss of renal function may cause uremia.
- **Infection.** Stagnant urine may easily be infected, and thus urolithiasis is often accompanied by bacterial **cystitis.** Ascending infections may cause **pyelonephritis.** Accumulation of pus in the obstructed renal pelves and calices is called **pyonephrosis.**

URINARY TRACT TUMORS

Most tumors of the urinary tract are malignant, and the benign tumors are considerably less common in all sites. The most common tumors are those of the kidney and the urinary bladder. Renal tumors account for approximately 2% and bladder tumors account for approximately 5% of all visceral tumors.

Renal cell carcinoma often manifests with nonspecific symptoms.

Most kidney tumors of adults originate from the renal tubular epithelium and are classified as renal cell carcinomas. Wilms' tumors are the most common tumors of children. Histologically, most renal cell carcinomas are composed of clear cells, but also papillary carcinomas and a few other less common histologic forms of cancer also occur.

Renal cell carcinomas have a peak incidence in the 55 to 65 age group. Clinical findings are often nonspecific, and the tumor is often referred to as "internist's tumor" since many of them are diagnosed while the patient is being evaluated for symptoms unrelated to the urinary system. Overall the most common findings are as follows:

- Hematuria (60%)
- Back pain (30%)
- Fever, night sweats (20%)
- Weight loss (20%)
- Anemia (20%)
- Paraneoplastic syndromes such as hypercalcemia, polycythemia, or hypertension (20%)

The diagnosis of renal carcinoma is most often made radiologically by CT or other diagnostic modalities. All tumors are treated surgically: smaller ones can be removed by partial nephrectomy; larger ones need more radical surgery including complete nephrectomy and dissection of the lymph nodes. The prognosis depends on the stage of the tumor at the time of diagnosis: small tumors limited to the kidney have a good prognosis, but large tumors and those that have metastasized have a poor prognosis. These tumors are relatively resistant to chemotherapy, and accordingly, any that have metastasized or recur have a poor prognosis.

Urinary bladder carcinoma may occur in an aggressive and a less aggressive form.

Urinary bladder carcinomas are most often classified as transitional (urothelial) carcinomas. Adenocarcinoma and squamous cell carcinomas or sarcomas are less common.

Transitional cell carcinomas most often present as low-grade papillary carcinomas; such tumors can be removed during cystoscopy, and although they tend to recur they have a good prognosis. Invasive poorly differentiated carcinomas have a poor prognosis.

Clinical findings typically include
- Hematuria (75%)
- Recurrent urinary infections (15%)
- Bladder irritability, urgency, frequent urination (15%)

The diagnosis is made by cystoscopy, cytopathologic examination of urinary sediment, and tumor biopsy. The prognosis depends on the histologic type of tumor and the stage (i.e., extent of tumor spread). The treatment is surgical, which in high-grade tumors is combined with radiation therapy and chemotherapy.

CASE STUDIES

Case 1 DARK BROWN URINE IN A PROFOUNDLY SWOLLEN 6-YEAR-OLD CHILD

Clinical history   A 6-year-old boy had a throat infection that improved on its own without treatment.[1] Two weeks after the infection the mother noticed that the child was somnolent and appeared sick, even though he did not have a fever. He refused to eat and did not want to go to school. The mother also noticed that his face was swollen.[2] The urine was dark brown and the amount of urine seemed to be less than normal.[3] Otherwise the child was healthy.

Physical findings   The child appears well developed and is mobile. His movements are sluggish, and he is a bit subdued. No localizing symptoms were recorded, and he has no pain in the throat or anywhere else. He appears to have periorbital edema and his lips seem to be swollen. His fingers and toes are also swollen. He is also slightly short of breath. His pulse rate is 90 beats/minute, and the blood pressure is 145/95 mm Hg.[4]

Laboratory findings   At the time of admission the serum WBC and RBC counts were within normal limits. Serum showed slight elevation of BUN and creatinine, with a normal BUN:Cr ratio of 10:1. Serum electrolytes were within normal limits.[5] Albumin was slightly lower than normal.[6]

Urine was positive for 3+ protein and for 3+ blood by dipstick.[7] The examination of urinary sediment revealed numerous RBCs, many of which were dismorphic. Red blood cell casts were also present.[8] Urine culture was negative.

Follow-up laboratory testing reveled oliguria, proteinuria in the range of 1.5 g protein/24 hours, persistent hematuria, and RBC casts in the urine.

Outcome   The child was treated symptomatically and recovered completely.[9]

Questions and topics for discussion
1. What is the most likely cause of a throat infection in a 6-year-old child? Does he require treatment?
2. What is the significance of facial swelling? List the possible causes of facial swelling.
3. What are the possible causes of dark urine?
4. Please interpret these physical findings. What is the cause is hypertension?
5. Please interpret these laboratory findings. Does this child have renal failure?
6. What is the cause of hypoalbuminemia? Which clinical finding could be attributed to hypoalbuminemia?
7. What is the cause of proteinuria and hematuria? How could one quantify better the dipstick data?
8. What is the significance of dismorphic RBCs and RBC casts in the urinary sediment?
9. Do all patients with this disease recover completely?

Case 2 A 40-YEAR-OLD MAN WITH GENERALIZED EDEMA

Clinical history   A 40-year-old man noticed swelling of his legs and widening of his girth. He also complained of shortness of breath while at rest as well as while walking.[1]

Physical findings   He has pitting edema of all four extremities, and fluid could be demonstrated in the thorax and abdominal cavity. His blood pressure is normal, and all his vital signs were within normal limits.

Laboratory findings   All the hematologic parameters were normal in the peripheral blood.

Serum albumin is low, and low-density lipoproteins (LDLs) are high.[2] Immunoglobulins are normal, and total complement is slightly lower than normal. The ANA test and the serologic tests for viral hepatitis B and C and syphilis and HIV are negative.[3] Urine shows 4+ protein by dipstick analysis. The urinary sediment contains lipid casts, but no RBCs or neutrophils.[4]

Follow-up Detailed examination revealed no other disease and no signs of chronic infection or neoplasia. He underwent a renal biopsy, which showed thickening of the glomerular basement membranes ((GBMs) by light microscopy. By immunofluorescence microscopy the GBMs showed numerous "lumpy-bumpy" granular deposits, which were also visualized by electron microscopy.[5]

Outcome No specific treatment was prescribed, and the patient lived 10 more years until he finally had to undergo renal dialysis.[6]

Questions and topics for discussion

1. What is another term for generalized edema? What could cause generalized edema?
2. What are the possible causes of hypoalbuminemia? How do you explain the elevation of LDLs?
3. Why is it important to perform all these tests?
4. Please interpret all these urinary findings.
5. Are these pathologic findings diagnostic or would it be necessary to perform additional tests to arrive at the final diagnosis?
6. Why was he not given any specific treatment? What is the usual prognosis of this disease?

Case 3 OLIGURIA IN A 60-YEAR-OLD MAN WITH PNEUMONIA AND SEPSIS

History and clinical findings A 60-year-old man was hospitalized for pneumonia. At the time of admission he had a high fever, was short of breath, and had tachypnea and tachycardia. He also noticed that his urine output had decreased.[1]

Laboratory findings Blood cultures were positive for *Streptococcus pneumoniae*. He had leukocytosis but RBC and platelet counts were normal. He had mild hypernatremia, prominent hyperkalemia, normal chlorides, and low bicarbonate in serum.[2] The blood pH was low. Blood urea nitrogen and creatinine were elevated, and the BUN:Cr ratio was 20:1.[3] Urinary output was low (500 mL/24 hours). Serum osmolality was slightly increased (310 mmol/kg), and urine osmolality was high (630 mmol/kg).[4]

Outcome He was treated, and on the fifth day started producing more urine.[5] The urine output increased to 5 L/day and then came back and he recovered completely. The electrolytes, BUN, and creatinine were normal at the time of his discharge from the hospital.

Questions and topics for discussion

1. What could be the possible explanations for the decreased urine output in a patient who has pneumonia?
2. Please interpret these laboratory findings.
3. What is the significance of BUN and creatinine elevation?
4. Are these findings indicative of prerenal or intrarenal renal failure? Does this patient have anuria or oliguria?
5. What is the significance of these findings?

Case 4 A 60-YEAR-OLD DEPRESSED WOMAN WITH END-STAGE KIDNEY DISEASE WHO REFUSED TO HAVE HEMODIALYSIS

Clinical history A 60-year-old woman, known to have chronic glomerulonephritis, was regularly going to hemodialysis, until one day she decided to refuse this treatment and stay home.[1] She was found unconscious and hospitalized.[2]

Clinical findings The woman was comatose. Her blood pressure was 190/120 mm Hg, and she appeared edematous. Fluid was evident in the pleural and pericardial spaces, and the pulse rate was fast. The skin had good turgor. Several ecchymoses were present on the extremities, and her gingivae were suffused with blood.[3]

Laboratory findings She had pronounced anemia, which was normocytic and normochromic.[4] The leukocytes and platelet counts were normal. Serum electrolyte disturbances included hyperkalemia, hyperphosphatemia, hypocalcemia, and low bicarbonate.[5] The pH of the blood was low.[6] Urea and creatinine were markedly elevated.[7]

Follow-up She underwent emergency hemodialysis and recovered.

Questions and topics for discussion

1. Why is dialysis performed? How could one measure the efficiency of dialysis?
2. Why did this woman lose consciousness?
3. Why does she have hypertension? Is she dehydrated or does she show signs of water retention? Why does she have a bleeding tendency?
4. Why does this woman have anemia? How could this anemia be treated?
5. Please interpret these laboratory findings. What are the possible consequences of hyperkalemia and the other electrolyte disturbances?
6. What is the cause of acidosis?
7. Does this patient have azotemia?

Index